Psychopharmacology
FOR MENTAL HEALTH PROFESSIONALS
AN INTEGRATIVE APPROACH

Psychopharmacology

FOR MENTAL HEALTH PROFESSIONALS

AN INTEGRATIVE APPROACH

2nd Edition

R. Elliott Ingersoll

Cleveland State University

Carl F. Rak

Cleveland Psychoanalytic Center

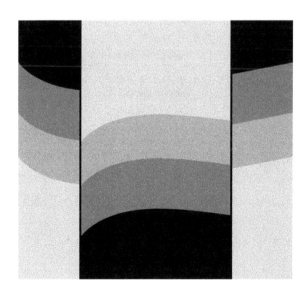

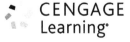
CENGAGE
Learning·

Australia • Brazil • Mexico • Singapore • United Kingdom • United States

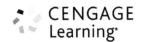
CENGAGE
Learning·

Psychopharmacology for Mental Health Professionals: An Integrative Approach, **Second Edition**
R. Elliott Ingersoll and Carl F. Rak

Product Director: Jon David Hague

Product Manager: Julie Martinez

Product Assistant: Nicole Richards

Marketing Manager: Shanna Shelton

Art and Cover Direction, Production Management, and Composition: Lumina Datamatics, Inc.

Manufacturing Planner: Judy Inouye

Cover Image: © Living Art Enterprises, LLC / Science Source

For product information and technology assistance, contact us at **Cengage Learning Customer & Sales Support, 1-800-354-9706.**

For permission to use material from this text or product, submit all requests online at **www.cengage.com/permissions.** Further permissions questions can be e-mailed to **permissionrequest@cengage.com.**

Library of Congress Control Number: 2014943048

Student Edition:
ISBN: 978-1-285-84522-7

Cengage Learning
20 Channel Center Street
Boston, MA 02210
USA

Cengage Learning is a leading provider of customized learning solutions with office locations around the globe, including Singapore, the United Kingdom, Australia, Mexico, Brazil, and Japan. Locate your local office at **www.cengage.com/global**.

Cengage Learning products are represented in Canada by Nelson Education, Ltd.

To learn more about Cengage Learning Solutions, visit **www.cengage.com**.

Purchase any of our products at your local college store or at our preferred online store **www.cengagebrain.com**.

Printed in the USA
1 2 3 4 5   29 28 27 26 25

Contents

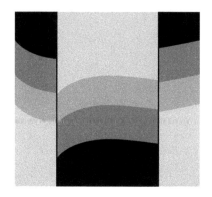

4   Psychological, Social, and Cultural Issues in Psychopharmacology   52

PART TWO

Introduction   81

5   The Antidepressant Era   82

7   Antipsychotic Medications: The Evolution of Treatment   150

Preface

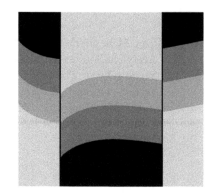

These early years of the 21st century are a time of great opportunity for nonmedical mental health professionals. For the first time since the inception of the mental health fields we have excellent research on how to treat many mental health symptoms like depression and anxiety. Perhaps more importantly, the lay public is learning what many of us in mental health fields have known for years: we don't know what causes mental disorders and when medications work; we don't fully understand why medications work. There is no support for the overused cliché that mental disorders are caused by chemical imbalances in the brain. We know this now. Just because we can intervene chemically (in some but not all cases) in no way means the chemicals affected by the intervention were "unbalanced" to begin with. The truth is we still don't know what balanced brain chemistry is, let alone unbalanced brain chemistry. So why is this a great time of opportunity for nonmedical mental health professionals? Because the public is learning that there are no psychotropic medications that act as "magic bullets" that will "cure" mental disorders. Now that that misconception is dispelled we have a chance to teach laypeople which symptoms may respond to talk therapy, which seem to require medications and which will likely respond to a combination of medications and therapy. This sort of education and advocacy is critical in all mental health professions to inform clients and their families about what we know and what we do not know. An informed client can then make informed choices. The medications discussed in this book are like any tool. They can be used wisely or mendaciously misused. We have tried to present both the benefits and risks of these medications as well as their implications for our society. We hope dear reader that you find what you are seeking in the following pages.

ACKNOWLEDGMENTS

I (Ingersoll) want to thank my research assistants over these years, Kevin Blake, Laura McIntyre and Doreen George Thomas. Thanks to Carlene Ortiz for her selfless support when I was losing faith in my ability and my sense of vocation. Finally thanks to Cleveland State University for giving me sabbatical time to finish this project. CSU has been an excellent place for me to work and I appreciate the support I have gotten there.

I (Rak) also wish to thank Drs. Patrick Enders, Zinovi Goubar, Kay McKenzie, and Luis Ramirez. They are all careful and thoughtful psychiatrists working in the Cleveland area. They always took time to answer my questions and speak with me about the dilemmas of medicating children and adults. Thank you!

Finally, we both are so grateful to Julie Martinez who believed enough in this project to give us a much needed extension when our lives were "off the rails" and we needed more time.

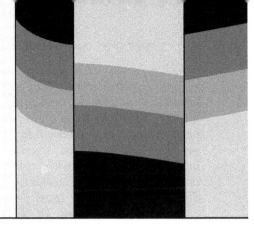

PART ONE

An Overview of the New Edition

This book is an introductory level text on psychopharmacology for students preparing for careers in psychology, counseling, and social work. Like other texts, we cover pharmacodynamics and pharmacokinetics for each class of psychotropic medications. We also discuss psychosocial treatments that are recommended concurrent with medications. In addition, we discuss the psychological, cultural, and social issues around psychopharmacology. In the United States, the pharmaceutical industry is an enormous economic force with at least two lobbyists for every Senate and Congressional representative (Petersen, 2009). The industry's power (like any other) can be used constructively or destructively but it forms much of the cultural and social discourse. Given this, it is unrealistic and irresponsible to omit discussion of the relevant issues, which include influence on diagnosis, the creation of *DSM-5* (American Psychiatric Association, 2013), and the increasing medicating of children and adolescents despite scant evidence supporting the practice.

Although this book is a revised edition of *Psychopharmacology for Helping Professionals: An Integral Exploration*, it is a different book. Our aim is that this text meets your needs. Having used the first edition for six years, our students have taught us a great deal about how we can help them organize and learn this material. We have presented the basic information (updated) in a more traditional manner and deleted much of the historical discussion. This allowed us to add sections on psychosocial treatments, expand the discussion of medication and children, and add chapters on psychotropic medications and the elderly as well as drug replacement therapy for addictions. Rather than simply listing study questions at the end of each chapter, we have added learning objectives for each main heading in the chapters and then review questions *at the end* of each section that should tell the student whether or not they met the objectives. Our students have said that because much of this information is new, this style helps them "digest material" in "small bites." This makes sense to us as we want the journey to be nourishing for all readers.

WHAT IS AN INTEGRATIVE APPROACH?

Integrative approaches have been around in psychology and psychotherapy for decades and are making their way into psychiatry and thinking about psychopharmacology. In the 21st century, with a new diagnostic manual (*DSM-5*), the truth is we still do not know definitively why people develop mental and emotional disorders and, when medications work, precisely how they work. An integrative approach is one that takes multiple perspectives on the topic being discussed. In this book, we will examine psychotropic medications from four perspectives.

The first perspective is from a biological or physiological point of view. Because this model is frequently called the *medical model*, we will use that phrase when writing about this perspective. This perspective examines what seems to be happening in the nervous system when people are suffering mental illness and what medications seem to do in the nervous system that correlates with a decrease or remission of symptoms. The second perspective is a psychological one. This is not usually part of psychopharmacology books but if you are a clinician you know it is important. What does the client think/feel about taking medication? How might medications change the subjective, phenomenological experience of the client? The psychological perspective is more concerned with the client's "mind" than their brain.

The other two perspectives are cultural and social. The cultural perspective reflects the subjective shared experience of particular groups. It reflects shared beliefs of groups whether they be groups of people identified with an ethnic label (e.g., Orthodox Jews) or the shared worldview of a client's family of origin (e.g., "we don't believe in mental illness or taking medication"). The social perspective reflects that more objective aspects of our society. Things like laws governing psychotropic medications, power to prescribe medications, and the economic power of the pharmaceutical industry would all be views from the social perspective.

These four perspectives derive from Integral Theory (Wilber, 2000) and, although the theory is far more complex than these four perspectives, it emphasizes that the more perspectives you account for, the more complete your understanding of the topic in question. For example, because this book is aimed at nonmedical mental health professionals or students training to enter those professions, it would not make sense to omit the psychological perspective that offers ideas on how to work with clients around medication issues that are more psychological than physiological. Equally, no discussion of pharmaceuticals can omit the power of the industry without becoming two-dimensional and unrealistic. Given that, as we progress we will be very clear which perspectives we are using at different points in the book. Although a majority of the material is focused on the biological perspective (that we will call the "medical model") these other points of view will give a fuller picture of psychopharmacology and help clinicians advocate for their clients across cultures.

CHAPTER ONE

Introduction

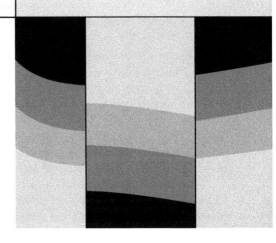

Learning Objectives

- Be able to conceptualize the "information explosion" and how it relates to the brain sciences.
- Be able to describe pharmacodynamics and pharmacokinetics.
- Be able to articulate the benefits of an integrative approach to psychopharmacology.

ENCOURAGEMENT TO THE READER

Some of you may begin this book with some anxiety because this is a new area for you. You may imagine that psychopharmacology is exclusively a "hard science," and perhaps you don't think of yourself as a "hard science" kind of person. You may even feel uncertain about your ability to master basic psychopharmacological concepts. First, let us assure you one more time that our goal is to make this topic accessible to readers who are practicing as or studying to be mental health professionals, many of whom may not have a background in the physical or organic sciences. Second, we recommend to those teaching a course in psychopharmacology that, because of the rapid nature of change in the field, teaching styles that rely on memorization are of limited use in this area. We recommend helping students master basic concepts and then applying these concepts to cases. To facilitate that process, we supply cases and objectives/review questions for main sections of the book. Finally, we invite you students to join us in an incredible journey centering on the most complex organ known to humanity—the human mind and brain. We hope you can revel in the complexity of the brain and the sheer magnitude of its power. We hope you can resist the temptation to want simple and concrete answers to many of the questions this journey will raise. We also hope you learn to appreciate the ambiguous nature of "mind" and its relationship to the brain. As authors and researchers who have traveled this path before us will attest, there are no simple or even known answers to many of the questions that arise (Grilly & Salmone, 2011; Schatzberg & Nemeroff, 1998). We encourage a mixture of trying to comprehend the information while dwelling in the mystery that is the context for the information. Before moving on, we offer a mantra to help you implement this recommendation.

A MANTRA

Even though psychopharmacology is in its embryonic stage, it is a vast and complex topic. Several years ago I (Ingersoll) engaged in some multicultural counseling training with Paul Pederson. In that training, Dr. Pederson commented, "Culture is complex, and complexity is our friend." We offer a paraphrase as a mantra for psychopharmacology students: "Reality is complex, and complexity is our friend." We remind the reader of this mantra throughout the book. You might try saying it aloud right now: "Reality is complex, and complexity is our friend." If you reach a passage in this book that is challenging for you or that arouses anxiety, stop, take a deep breath, and practice the mantra.

The primary audience for this book is mental health clinicians who may not have had much training in biology, neurology, and psychopharmacology. This includes counselors, psychologists, clinical social workers, marriage and family therapists, and substance abuse counselors. We will refer specifically to these different mental health professionals throughout the book as well as including all of them in the phrase "mental health professionals." Although there are significant differences in the training models of these different professionals, they all draw on the same knowledge base when treating clients in school or clinical settings. We also want to add that there are several labels used to describe the therapeutic relationships clients have with mental health professionals. These labels include "counseling," "therapy," "talk therapy," "psychosocial interventions," and "psychotherapy." There is great debate across the mental health professions about whether and how these labels differ, but in this book we use them synonymously for the sake of simplicity. While reading this book, you will notice technical terms highlighted with bold print the first time they appear. These terms are defined in the Glossary at the end of the book. Although not all key terms are highlighted, those that nonmedical mental health professionals are less likely to have been exposed to are defined in the Glossary. We encourage you to keep a dictionary handy for other terms that may be new to you. If you come across a word you do not understand, stop reading and check the definition in the glossary or a dictionary. Many readers skip over unfamiliar words assuming the meaning will become clear in a later sentence. Clarifying unfamiliar words when they occur adds to the enjoyment of reading the book and facilitates a better understanding of the topic.

SCIENTIFIC TRUTH AND THE ACCELERATION OF KNOWLEDGE

It is no secret that knowledge accumulation is accelerating. We are familiar with the label "information explosion" to describe this phenomenon. In the early 1970s, the French economist Georges Anderla (1973, 1974) prepared a statistical estimate of how quickly knowledge has been growing, based on a variety of indicators. According to Anderla, if you begin in the year 1 c.e. (which stands for Current or Common, Era) it took 1500 years for knowledge to double. The second doubling took only 250 years (1750). The third doubling took only 150 years (1900), the fourth 50 years (1950), and the fifth doubling only 10 years (1960). If there is any accuracy in Anderla's model, knowledge began doubling almost monthly in the late 20th century (Wilson, 1992). Increase in knowledge about the human brain is particularly pronounced.

The final decades of the 20th century unearthed more knowledge about the human brain than all prior centuries combined. One of the most exciting fields benefiting from these developments is psychopharmacology. *Pharmacology* is the science of the preparation, uses, and effects of drugs. *Psychopharmacology* is the branch of pharmacology related to the psychological effects of drugs and the use of drugs to treat symptoms of mental and emotional disorders. These drugs are called *psychotropic medications*. "Psyche" colloquially refers to "mind," and "tropic" means "acting on" or "moving toward" but many in the field would say these medications act on the brain and this affects the mind.

Developing neuroscience technologies have helped accelerate brain research and change in the field of psychopharmacology by letting scientists peer more deeply into the brain and nervous system. The latest technological advances include positron emission tomography (PET) scans, magnetic resonance imaging (MRI), Diffusion Tensor Imaging (DTI), Voxel-Based Morphometry, and magneto-encephalography. PET scans for brain functions work thus: The technician injects a radioactive form of oxygen into a person and then asks the person to perform a particular task under a PET scanner. Because the brain area most active during the task requires more oxygen, the PET scanner can trace the radioactive oxygen to those sites in the brain used in the task. The computer scanner then generates a picture that maps the brain activity. MRI scans generate images by magnetizing hemoglobin (the iron-containing colored matter in red blood corpuscles that carry oxygen to tissues) and by tracing changes in blood oxygen levels in the brain. Like the PET scan, MRI images of the brain can be used for diagnostic or research purposes. DTI is a type of MRI that can highlight microstructural changes in the white matter of the brain or glial cells (Emsell & McDonald, 2009). This is becoming more important because we discovered that, far from being only glue or insulation for neuronal axons (*glia* comes from the Greek word for *glue*), glial cells actually send neurotransmission and communicate with other cells (Fields, 2009, 2010; Sasaki, Matuski, & Ikegaya, 2011).

Magnetoencephalography measures the magnetic field associated with electrical currents in the brain to trace activity levels across brain structures when subjects are engaged in a particular task (Bloom, Nelson, & Lazerson, 2001).

There are also multiple techniques for extracting information from MRI scans. The most common quantitative techniques are "region of interest" (ROI) and computational morphometry studies. In ROI analysis, a trained rater manually traces a brain region of interest using "boundary rules" to compare sizes between different brains scanned. *Computational morphometry* is an automated method of comparing brain structures between different populations in a study. The most common variation is called voxel-based morphometry (VBM), which allows viewing of gray matter, white matter, and cerebrospinal fluid (Emsell & McDonald, 2009).[1] Voxel-based morphometry is neuroimaging analysis technique that uses a type of mapping (statistical parametric mapping) to identify regions of interest in the brain and calculate their volume. Finally, there are also deformation-based morphometry (DBM) and tensor-based morphometry (TBM). Both techniques are used to compare brain structures, but they rest upon different theoretical assumptions.

Computer technology has also enabled pharmaceutical researchers to generate three-dimensional models of brain cell receptors and the drug molecules that bind to them. Brain-scanning technologies have allowed us to see how the drugs act on the nervous system (**pharmacodynamics** covered in Chapter Two) and how the body metabolizes and eliminates drugs (**pharmacokinetics** covered more extensively in Chapter Three). These are only some of the advances that have contributed to the exponential increase in the number of drugs developed annually.

Despite the explosion of advances in psychopharmacology in the last 30 years, the field can still be thought of as in an embryonic stage (Advokat, Comaty, & Julien, 2014). Although scientists know a lot about the physiological mechanisms of many psychotropic medications, we know little about how they actually change mood. Researchers are just now beginning to explore how the effects of psychotropic medication differ depending on the age, sex, and race of the person taking them (Heinrich & Gibbons, 2001). Although Western society is emerging from a postmodern era where multiculturalism was heavily emphasized, little research has been done on differing cultural worldviews regarding psychotropic agents, let alone how such agents differentially affect people of various racial and ethnic backgrounds. In addition, people are now rethinking whether current diagnostic categories for mental and emotional disorders apply to younger children (Ingersoll & Marquis, 2014; McClure, Kubiszyn, & Kaslow, 2002a) and how medications affect the dozens of developmental variables in this age group. Although the Human Genome Project has initiated efforts to understand human DNA, in the late 20th century scientists were still unclear about the role of over 90% of human DNA (Suurkula, 1996). In 2012, teams of scientists agreed that much of the DNA previously thought to be "junk" are actually "switches" that regulate how genes work or turn "off" and "on" (Doolittle, 2013). Efforts to describe the human genetic code and mechanisms of gene expression hold great promise for drug development, but there is still a great deal to be learned.

---

[1]As with any approach, VBM has received criticism because of the assumptions on which it is based. See Ashburner and Friston (2001) and Bookstein (2001).

As recently as 30 years ago, psychopharmacology was a medical subspecialty for psychiatrists in particular. At that time, nonmedical mental health providers could ethically practice with little knowledge of psychotropic medications. As long as they had a medical professional to whom they could refer clients, their knowledge of psychotropic medications could be minimal. This is no longer the case. Most (if not all) mental health professionals work with clients taking psychotropic medications and need to be knowledgeable about the drugs their clients are taking. The integrative perspective we emphasize in this book provides a template that, when applied properly, suggests that understanding the physiological properties of psychotropic medications is merely the beginning of the journey. We use the integrative Model to address many pressing issues rarely discussed in books on psychopharmacology. For example, most psychopharmacology books simply discuss what medications are used for particular symptoms but do not address how to deal with cultural issues that may influence a client's resistance to taking a prescribed medication. Another example is the place of **direct-to-consumer advertising.** Although mental health professionals may know that changes in federal law in the 1980s allowed pharmaceutical companies to advertise directly to consumers via television ads and other media, they may not know that there is a fierce debate over whether such advertising for psychotropic medications is ethical.

Pharmacologists working in controlled conditions in laboratories may have the luxury of limiting their focus to interactions between drug molecules and neurotransmitters. But mental health professionals in the field must understand clients' perceptions and subjective experiences of taking medications, cultural views of psychotropic medications, group differences in response to the medications (according to sex, age, race, etc.), developmental considerations, socioeconomic institutions that mediate access to medications, and competing worldviews and theories on what causes mental health symptoms. The four perspectives of our integrative framework requires consideration of these topics and sets this book apart from other books on psychopharmacology. Although this consideration requires more effort, it contributes to a well-rounded knowledge of psychopharmacology that translates into better clinical practice.

Review Questions

- What is meant by "information explosion" and how is it reflected in psychopharmacology?
- Describe pharmacodynamics and pharmacokinetics.
- What are the benefits of an integrative approach to psychopharmacology?

CHAPTER ONE: SECTION TWO

Learning Objectives

- Be able to describe why therapists need more than just a physiological or medical understanding of psychotropic medications.
- Discuss the differences between what is commonly thought of as "mind" and what is thought of as "brain."

Everybody Is Right (About Something): The Many Faces of Truth

History shows that extremists, despite the strength of their convictions, are rarely correct (Radin, 1997, p. 205).

In this book, we consider multiple dimensions of and perspectives on psychopharmacology. Although it would be convenient to state that all mental and emotional symptoms derive from some malfunction of brain chemistry, there is no evidence to support this statement. Many people are surprised to hear this, so it is important to restate: There is no evidence that all mental and emotional symptoms derive from some *malfunction or imbalance* of brain chemistry. Today pharmaceutical companies advertise directly to consumers and often give the impression that psychological disorders are really "medical disorders" that can be alleviated with a particular medication, much as antibiotics can alleviate a bacterial infection. If psychological disorders were like medical disorders, then studying the brain, brain chemistry, and scientific method would suffice. Even the *International Classification of Diseases, tenth edition (ICD-10)* has a separate volume for mental and behavioral disorders (WHO, 1992). So although the medical model provides an important perspective, we also need to study the mind, the sociocultural contexts in which mind and brain function, and the consciousness underlying mind and brain.

The entire truth of psychopharmacology cannot be explored solely through scientific method. Like a diamond, truth has many facets, which are complementary (but not necessarily competing). As philosopher Ken Wilber (2003) notes, no mind is capable of 100% error, so everyone is right about something but not everyone is equally right about everything. Given that insight, exploring the different perspectives of psychopharmacology need not produce warring factions championing mutually exclusive theories of **etiology** and treatment. Taking different perspectives in exploring psychopharmacology reveals different truths about it.

Lest you think we are lapsing into some type of **radical constructivism** or **relativism** (we are not), consider these questions: What sort of blood test would you use to determine your political philosophy? How might exploring your feelings about your mother help diagnose a streptococcus infection? How can a firsthand understanding of a person's religion be used to tell you how much money he or she earns? How could data about your yearly income be used as an indicator of your sexual orientation? These questions are meaningless, because each proposes an incorrect tool for finding the answer. Because different perspectives reveal different faces of truth, they require tools matched to the task. There are different forms of truth and knowledge and different tools are employed in exploring them. We emphasize this point because many people believe that medical science (or science in general) is the only tool and that it can solve any problem.

The Medical Model Perspective

The perspective of medical science (and science in general) clearly reflects one type of truth, and we draw amply from it in this book. Whereas a relativist would say that one perspective or type of truth is just as good as another for any job, we maintain that some perspectives and tools are better than others for particular tasks. Everyone knows that no blood test can determine a person's political philosophy. Does this mean one's preference for a political philosophy does not exist? No. It simply means a blood test is not a good tool to use to explore the issue. In this case, dialogue is far better than a blood test. To find out a person's political philosophy, you talk with the person to learn what his or her political philosophy is. Regarding the diagnosis of streptococcus infection, a throat culture is a far better test than discussing feelings about one's mother.

Scientific truth is objective truth that can be verified by some observable measurement. This is the type of truth emphasized by the tools of scientific method, the medical model, and most psychopharmacology books. The perspective of scientific truth is an important cornerstone of psychopharmacology. This is what we are referring to as the **medical model perspective**. It is characterized by its focus on objective, measurable data related to individuals. Although labeled "medical model" for the purposes of this book, this perspective also includes schools of psychology that rely heavily on objective measurement (such as behaviorism). In psychopharmacology, the medical model perspective helps us understand parts of the brain that seem correlated with symptoms of mental or emotional disorders and things such as the molecular structure of drugs. But mental health professionals are concerned with more than the correlations of symptoms with brain functions or the molecular structures of drugs. As professionals, we are also concerned with *how clients feel* about taking medications, how and whether psychotropic medications alter their consciousness, relevant cultural issues that may affect their attitudes or increase their preference for alternatives to psychotropic medications, aspects of group membership (race, sex) that may predict differential responses to psychotropic medications, as well as how our clients' place in society affects their ability to get the drugs they may need.

The Psychological Perspective

Other perspectives complement the medical model and help mental health professionals build a well-rounded understanding of psychopharmacology. These other perspectives reveal other faces of truth that the medical model is not equipped to explore but that are equally important for mental health professionals. As Wilber (1997) noted, the techniques of the medical model perspective can trace the electrical currents in a subject's brain but can only give scientific verification about the electrical activity in that brain—they cannot tell whether the person is thinking about opening a homeless shelter or robbing a liquor store. Further, there is no evidence that the experience of consciousness is caused solely by electrical activity in our brains (Chalmers, 1995).

Information about what other people (including our clients) are thinking can only be obtained through truthful dialogue with them. This introduces the second perspective we use in this book, the **psychological perspective**. Psychology's name is derived from the goal of studying the mind or soul. Despite that origin, it has evolved into the scientific study of mind and behavior and has come to greatly resemble the medical model. Schwartz and Begley (2002) assert that psychologists have become overly attached to a version of the medical model that dismisses conscious experience and focuses only on what is observable or measurable. They conclude, "Surely there is something deeply wrong, both morally and scientifically, with a school of psychology whose central tenet is that people's conscious life experience … is irrelevant" (p. 6). It is that conscious experience that we are referring to when we use the phrase "psychological perspective" or what consciousness feels like from the inside. We include the psychological perspective because clients' **phenomenological** experiences of the world cannot be dismissed as irrelevant and are often a key ingredient in their growth.

Our psychological perspective deals with consciousness. Although one of the most ambitious pursuits of scientific knowledge is the Human Genome Project, there exists an equally ambitious (even if less well known) human consciousness project. The psychological perspective as revealed by the consciousness project is summarizing millennia of knowledge about the human mind, the subjective human experience, consciousness, the domain of the unconscious, and the farther reaches of human nature (be they existential or spiritual). For more on the human consciousness project go to http://www.nourfoundation.com/events/Beyond-the-Mind-Body-Problem/The-Human-Consciousness-Project.html. This knowledge is different from knowledge generated by the medical model perspective, but is no less important for mental health professionals who deal with the whole person. The subjective knowledge about oneself that counseling, psychotherapy, or meditation explore is different from the type of knowledge that science produces to tell us about how nerve cells fire in our brain. It is truly odd that although psychotropic medications are actually supposed to modify experienced consciousness, very few books on the topic actually address that and instead prefer just to discuss how drug molecules bind to neuronal receptors.

Suppose, for example, that you experience an insight about yourself that leads to more effective ways of living. For the sake of the example, assume the insight is that you fear emotionally depending on others, so you tend to push them away and isolate yourself. When you experience this insight, certainly nerve cells will fire in your brain, but no one can prove the cells are "causing" the insight—in some cases they accompany it and in others they fire slightly before your conscious knowledge of the insight. Further, others cannot learn about the insight by reading a PET scan of your brain taken when you had the insight. You must truthfully share the insight in order for others to learn about it—no physical measurement of any type (brain cells firing, heart rate, blood pressure, and so forth) will reveal the insight—you must share it. This is an important type of knowledge of the sort commonly shared and explored in counseling sessions.

The psychological perspective also includes people's unconscious life experience. The many tools we use to explore the psychological perspective include introspection, dialogue about that introspection, interpreting dialogue, and sharing our interpretation to assess its accuracy. Although we can only be aware of those things that are conscious, by definition, the tools of the psychological perspective can help clients bring to awareness things that were previously unconscious. As Wilber (2003) noted, psychotherapy is always about increasing awareness and this increase in awareness is experienced through the psychological perspective. These tools are familiar to anyone trained in the mental health professions, but it is amazing how easily we forget their importance.

The Cultural Perspective

A third perspective or type of truth concerns how people should treat one another as well as the beliefs and worldviews people may share. These shared beliefs constitute aspects of culture. Culture, ways of living that groups of humans transmit from one generation to another, includes the shared beliefs and worldviews that different groups develop to understand the world and their place in it. Because shared worldviews are so important to culture, we refer to this third perspective as the **cultural perspective**. The word *culture* may refer to a subgroup of people who share similar genetic and social histories, as in "African-American culture" or a subgroup that comes about for other reasons, such as a business or industry, as in the culture of a pharmaceutical company. Again, no number of PET or MRI scans of brains can show what worldview a person holds, which ways of relating or worldviews are better than others, or whether a person prefers to be "in time" or "on time." As Wilber (1995) puts it, scientific knowledge can never tell us why compassion is better than murder, why social service is better than genocide. Michael Polanyi (1958) also articulated this insight. Polanyi was a Nobel Prize–winning chemist who realized during the communist revolutions in Europe that the revolutionaries were trying to build a culture and a society on scientific principles (the Lenin-Trotsky five-year plan) and that

those principles were the wrong tools for the task. Polanyi understood that the tools of science could never help these revolutionaries build a culture or a society worth living in. History has validated his judgment. Although the design of the Soviet Union tried to account for and control all the measurable aspects of society, it severely underestimated the cultural/ethnic differences that, since its dissolution, have erupted between former member nations. Scientific truth can tell us which psychotropic medication has the greatest probability of easing a client's suffering. But the scientific truth and the medication cannot erase nonbiological sources of suffering nor address what this suffering means to the client. For example, if the client shares a worldview that is highly suspicious of taking psychotropic medication, the client is unlikely to comply with the prescription.

The Social Perspective

A fourth type of truth, which concerns the structure and impact of social institutions, we call the **social perspective**. Social institutions are based in shared beliefs, policies, and laws that affect people in observable, measurable ways. Whereas the medical model perspective deals with measurable, observable data about individuals, the social perspective deals with measurable, observable data about groups and particularly institutions. One good example in psychopharmacology is the ongoing debate about whether a person can and should be medicated against his or her will (Gelman, 1999). Although the legal system is ideally based on the public's shared understanding of how we need to be regulated with laws, laws prohibiting or permitting forced pharmacological treatment have profound impact on individuals. Besides the legal institutions of our society, other institutions relevant to psychopharmacology include the government (e.g., the Food and Drug Administration, the Drug Enforcement Agency) and the pharmaceutical industry in general. Issues such as whether people in the United States should be able to import medications from Canada are the domain of the social perspective. (Again, imagine the absurdity of trying to resolve this import question through the medical model perspective.)

Most books on psychopharmacology focus on scientific or medical model perspectives of what medications seem to do, how they correlate with symptom relief, how much of the medication is needed, and so on. Although we cover these issues in detail, we also discuss the other perspectives that are pertinent to mental health professionals. For example, what does it mean to a client to take a psychotropic medication (psychological perspective)? What does it mean that a significant number of children in this society are referred for medication instead of for counseling (social perspective)? How should we interpret and interact with a family that believes psychotropic medication is spiritually damaging (cultural perspective)? It is time for humanity to integrate the various types of knowledge people have access to, and a study of psychopharmacology can benefit by such integration.

We have mentioned the power of the pharmaceutical industry particularly in the United States. Like all power it can be used well or misused. One of the most striking things since the publication of the first edition of this book is the increase in lawsuits prosecuting pharmaceutical companies for illegal practices related to psychotropic medication. Some examples:

- In 2011, Massachusetts filed a lawsuit against Janssen for "deceptive" marketing of the antipsychotic resperidone (Mental Health Weekly, 2011) and settled for $158 million.
- Since 2004, the United States has collected nearly $8 billion from fraud enforcement actions against pharmaceutical companies for illegally promoting drugs for off-label uses (Avorn & Kesselheim, 2011).
- In 2009, Eli Lilly Company pled guilty to illegal marketing of the antipsychotic olanzapine and paid a $1.42 billion fine (Associated Press, 2009).
- In 2010, AstraZeneca was fined $520 million for illegal marketing of the antipsychotic quetiapine (Wilson, 2010).

What seems to be happening is that the culture of the pharmaceutical industry is being more closely monitored by government agencies due to a history of ethically questionable actions. This definitely

affects clinicians and clients. For example, what if one of your clients was taking a drug that is not FDA approved for a serious disorder like Bipolar I Disorder and that has no documented efficacy? Certainly the client's welfare is at stake and this is where clinicians advocating for clients and maintaining healthy relationships with prescribing professionals is important.

PSYCHOPHARMACOLOGY AND MAGICAL THINKING

R. Stivers, in his book *Technology as Magic* (2001) suggests that as different technologies "disenchant" our sense of the world, people may respond with magical thinking by endowing those technologies with magical attributes. "Today our expectations for technology are magical" (p. 7). You can see this change particularly in psychopharmacology. We have had clients who thought that if they took antidepressant medication prescribed for their symptoms it would (almost magically) erase all suffering from their lives. We agree with Stivers that this society has almost magical expectations of pharmaceutical companies, their products, and the medical professionals who prescribe those products. One practice tied to this expectation is what we call "word magic."

"Word magic" is the use of words in such a way so as to create the illusion of certainty where certainty does not exist. Word magic is used to increase one's control over the world (and other people), to artificially reduce the complexity of reality, and to help one deal with the insecurity experienced in the face of complexity. Particularly in the service of control, word magic can be used to trigger strong emotions in a reader or listener for the purpose of increasing the speaker's own power. Former U.S. Attorney General A. Mitchell Palmer and Senator Joseph McCarthy engaged in word magic, wielding the key term "communist" to increase their political power during "red scares" in the early- and mid-20th century. The same type of word magic was used in the witch hunts, in the Inquisition, and is still being used in the current "war on drugs" (which is really a war on drug users) in the United States (revisited in Chapter Ten).

How does this relate to psychopharmacology? When various professionals, groups, or companies use words to convey pharmacological certainty where little certainty exists, they are engaging in word magic and in some cases trying to increase their own power. An example of this is the flawed idea that mental illness is caused by a chemical imbalance in the brain. As noted this "hypothesis" has been falsified multiple times. This can result in what Charles Tart (1997) refers to as scientism: "a dogmatic, psychological hardening of materialistic belief systems with emotional attachments, rather than authentic science" (p. 22). Frequently this hardening of belief systems with emotional attachments takes the form of proclaiming something to be much simpler than it is in reality. An example is when pharmaceutical companies, in ads for antidepressants, state, "Depression is a serious medical disease." The payoff for pharmaceutical companies in framing depression this way is that if the general public thinks of depression first and foremost as a medical disease, their first response if feeling depressed will be to go to a medical doctor for a prescription rather than to a mental health professional for counseling. As we will show, depression is an overdetermined set of symptoms that may be biological, psychological, or spiritual in etiology. Just because depression is described in the *ICD-10* (the diagnostic manual for physicians) does not mean it is a medical disease in the same sense that influenza is a disease. Tart goes on to explain that we are conditioned to assume people in lab coats are dealing with certainty and that sometimes people in lab coats perpetuate that misunderstanding.

MOVING ON: WHAT WE KNOW, WHAT WE DO NOT KNOW

To avoid falling into word magic, people must be willing to admit what they do not know. Studying the mind and brain moves us all to the knowledge frontier of the 21st century. Consider this: Despite considerable success in developing medications that ease the symptoms of mental and emotional disorders, scientists have little understanding of how most of these medications work. Researchers are learning more about how psychotropic agents act on the brain and body (pharmacodynamics) and how the body disposes of them (pharmacokinetics), but scientists still know very little about why certain drugs decrease certain symptoms and contribute to emotional and behavioral changes. Even more interesting (although less publicized) is that in a great number of studies (and with particular symptoms like depression), as many participants respond to placebos as respond to the actual medications being investigated (Fisher & Greenberg, 1997; Khan, Leventhal, Khan, & Brown, 2002). There are many unanswered questions about the brain, the mind, and the relationship between the two. All together now: "Reality is complex, and complexity is our friend."

An example of this complexity is the case of Louise. Throughout the book, we provide cases that illustrate good responses to medications, treatment-resistant symptoms, side effects, client psychological issues related to medications, and cultural and social considerations. The cases illustrate the complementary types of truths we have summarized as the medical model, psychological, cultural, and social. Although it would be much simpler only to use cases where clients have symptoms, take medications, then get better, this has seldom been our experience. Lawrence's case illustrates many of the perspectives we have introduced in this chapter. It does not lend itself to a single interpretation that relies solely on one perspective. Read the case, and consider the questions following it.

The Case of Lawrence

Lawrence is a 35-year-old lawyer who anguishes with a very poor self-image, terrible anxiety, depression, and lability of mood. He is the oldest of three and his mother left the family permanently when he was five. At that time, his father expected him to be the little man of the house and take care of his younger sisters. Lawrence remembers that he always complained to his father that he didn't feel right, not like the other boys. His father would always reply with the same phrase, "Just move on, son." Lawrence always believed that no one got him, not even his new stepmom. Both at home and in school he was a loner. He was very bright and got more than acceptable grades. He grew very anxious whenever he had to interact with others. His father had no patience for his isolation. Lawrence gradually developed what seemed to be a social phobia.

From an intrapsychic perspective, this client suffered a serious loss of the mothering one at a critical time in development. Just as he began to enter the latency age of child development, he loses his primary relationship with whom he can share insights and changes that he is experiencing. This aspect of his development was delayed or foreclosed while his father expected him to accelerate his development to an advanced stage of caretaker of his sisters. In both roles he became very passive. By the time he reached high school he was in a suicidal depression and had to be hospitalized for attempting suicide. Each day of his life was a burden. The attending physicians at the hospital tried to get him to take an antidepressant. He refused.

Lawrence graduated from college, served in the army, and married. Eventually, he attended law school with very little alteration of his mood or self-efficacy. He failed the law boards and his wife threatened to divorce him if he did not pass them the second time. He was distraught and angry. He felt betrayed by his wife who had almost forced him to attend law school. He sought out therapy and consultation with a psychiatrist. The therapist recommended twice-a-week psychotherapy and the psychiatrist put him on 100 mg of sertraline (brand name Zoloft). Lawrence tried the sertraline for three months and indicated that he felt no improvement. The psychiatrist added 250 mg of bupropion (brand name Wellbutrin) to be taken along with the sertraline. Lawrence expressed his concern about being over medicated, but the psychiatrist encouraged him to try both medications.

After four months, Lawrence spoke to both his therapist and psychiatrist that he believed the medications were not really helping him. After much consultation and discussion with Lawrence, the psychiatrist decided to titrate him off the buprorion and to add 2 mg of aripiprazole (brand name Abilify a newer antipsychotic used at very low doses in the treatment of depression). Within a week, Lawrence was unable to sleep, was very agitated, and could not focus on his work. The psychiatrist, although puzzled, was not totally baffled by this development in Lawrence. He expanded his clinical interview, consulted in-depth with the therapist, and concluded that Lawrence had been masking a bipolar presentation with some moderate drinking. He started Lawrence on a course of lithobid (Lithium) after discontinuing his other medications. This course of treatment served Lawrence well for several years and he periodically had his blood levels checked for lithium poisoning. The course of pharmacological treatment that Lawrence received is far more the norm for the patient of 2013.

THE MIND–BRAIN PROBLEM

If you were on a game show and the host asked you (for $1000) to clearly define mind, brain, and the difference between the two, how would you answer? How you answer is basically how you conceptualize the mind–brain problem. The mind–brain problem is an old philosophical issue that addresses whether or not the mind and brain are distinct entities and what their relationship is. Scientific knowledge of both the mind and the brain is incomplete. No one knows what the mind is, where it comes from, or how it interacts with the brain (Dossey, 2001). However, numerous scholars have noted that even if there were complete knowledge of the mind and brain, the problem might still be unsolvable (Koch, 2012). Consider being asked to define "the mind." At first glance this might seem a simple task for a mental health counselor or a student training in one of the mental health professions. In fact, it is a rather vexing question with a multitude of answers depending on your theoretical orientation. As much as many hate to admit it, to "define" what "mind" means first requires a leap of faith in the theory or theories you believe most accurately reflect the reality of what the mind is. To say you adhere to a particular theory of the mind–brain problem is fine; to claim a particular theory is ultimately true at this point in history is scientism, not science. Generally, the mind–brain problem has been explored through two hypotheses, the epiphenomenon hypothesis and the dual-substance hypothesis, discussed as follows.

The Epiphenomenon Hypothesis

The first hypothesis is called the **epiphenomenon** hypothesis (sometimes called the "side effect" hypothesis—the mind is a side effect of the brain). The theory underlying this is what might be called *radical materialism*. The basis of radical materialism is that all things, including the mind, derive from other things that can be objectively observed and measured. This hypothesis states that the mind derives from the brain. In other words, the mind is an epiphenomenon of the brain. In a sense, this theory claims that your mind, including your sense of self, is a "side effect" of having a developed brain. The 19th-century biologist Thomas Huxley (known as "Darwin's Bulldog" for his fervent support of Darwin's theory of evolution) popularized this hypothesis. More recently Damasio (2000), Dennett (1991), and Churchland (1995, 1999) have set forth varieties of the theory. Sometimes the theory is not stated outright but implied, as if this were the only acceptable theory on mind and brain. Richard Thompson (2000) gave one example when he wrote, "What is consciousness and how does it arise from the brain?" (p. 481). His implication that it does arise from the brain is a theoretical assumption, not an indisputable fact even though he presents it as such. This is another example of word magic—using words to create an illusion of certainty where there is none.

Advocates of the epiphenomenon hypothesis support it by first noting a brain structure responsible for a particular function (such as the relationship of Broca's area to speech, for example). Next they point out that, for example, if Broca's area is damaged, speech is impaired. The reasoning is that one's sense of self (one's mind) is a consequence of brain functioning and if those parts of the brain responsible for the sense of self are damaged, the sense of self is either impaired or vanishes, just as speech becomes impaired if Broca's area is damaged.

Perhaps the most time-worn example used to support the epiphenomenon hypothesis is the 19th-century case of Phineas Gage. Gage was a railroad construction worker who had a tamping iron driven through his skull as the result of an explosion. Although he miraculously survived the accident, the story used to be that his personality became so altered that those who knew him say Gage was a different person after the accident. Damasio (1995) hypothesized that from a materialist perspective Gage, the person, had changed because the areas of his brain that maintained and expressed personality had changed when damaged in the accident. Of course, as in most things, there is now a difference of opinion on Gage. Kean (2014) wrote that descriptions of Gage's personality change are greatly exaggerated. In fact, he noted that historical documents show that Gage went to South America and worked as a stage coach driver. Even if the stories about his drinking and aggression after the accident are true, how much of that may have been related to pain or depression (the psychological perspective)?

Our sense of self is somewhat more complicated than other functions that are traced to specific brain areas, so researchers do not yet know exactly which areas, and the relationships between them, result in the sense of self. Damasio (2010) and others have begun to tackle this problem, but science is far from an explanation. Thus to accept the radical materialist position is a statement of faith that neuroscientists will be able to completely map out the brain and its functions (and that they are correct in thinking such knowledge would resolve the mind–brain problem).

As you can imagine, those who adhere to the medical model of mental and emotional disorders often support the epiphenomenon hypothesis. This model is the basis of allopathic medicine. Allopathic medicine (as opposed to homeopathic or osteopathic) is the branch of medicine that adheres to the philosophy that to treat or cure a disease process, you introduce an agent (such as a drug) that acts in a manner opposite to the disease process you are trying to treat or cure. Although it is often assumed that if scientists know a disease process they also know its etiology (cause), this is far from true. Thus, there is no foundation for the allopathic assumption that identifying a disease process (depressive symptoms for example) and decreasing or stopping that process means that the process had a physical origin. Strict adherence to the medical model leads to unfounded assumptions that all mental or emotional disorders derive from faulty functioning in the brain or nervous system. Many follow this strict adherence despite strong evidence that the mind (at least the thought processes and emotions of the mind) influences the body as much as any organ like the brain and particularly disorders like depression and anxiety. Although we would agree that severe mental disorders like Schizophrenia will almost certainly turn out to be primarily physiological in their etiology, others like depression are overdetermined (meaning there are many ways one may develop depression).

The Dual-Substance Hypothesis

The dual-substance hypothesis is often dated back to the philosopher René Descartes who lived in the early 17th century, although it certainly predates Descartes, because it exists to some extent in both Hindu and Buddhist philosophy. Descartes proposed both that a divine being exists and that this divine being created thinking things (*res cogitans*) and material things (such as bodies) that extend into the material realm (*res extensa*). He thought thinking things do not actually exist in time and space and cannot be externally observed. The extended beings do exist in time and space and can be externally observed. Although Gabbard (2001) believes that substance dualism has fallen out of favor, there is still ample support for variations on the hypothesis. Most variations equate "mind" with "consciousness."

Those holding a spiritual worldview often accept the dual-substance argument (in various formulations). Such a worldview may endorse a belief in a God or Divinity of some sort and possibly some notion of an eternal soul. This is not necessary, however, because the Buddhist view, for example, refers to different types of consciousness. One such type is a nonmaterial, ever-present "subtle consciousness" that we are thought to be most in touch with in deep sleep, advanced meditation, sneezing, and orgasms (think about that next time you sneeze!). From the Tibetan Buddhist perspective, epiphenomenalism and radical materialism fall into the trap of reifying physical phenomena (Descartes's *res extensa*) and denying the existence of mental phenomena (Descartes's *res cogitans*) (Wallace, 1999). From this perspective, to say that consciousness depends on the brain for existence is akin to saying that food depends on a stomach for existence. Psychologist Dean Radin (1997) wrote, "The average neuron consists of about 80 percent water and about 100,000 molecules. The brain contains about 10 billion cells, hence about 10^{15} molecules. Each nerve cell in the brain receives an average of 10,000 connections from other brain cells, and the molecules within each cell are renewed about 10,000 times in a lifetime" (p. 259). Radin then asked why, despite this continuous change, the patterns of our sense of self remain stable even though the physical material supporting that sense of self is in constant flux. The body you have while reading this (including your brain) is not at all the same body you had three years ago, but your sense of self is.

In addition to these two perspectives on the mind–brain problem, there are also variations such as interactionism (mind and brain are different but mutually causal) and parallelism (mind and brain are totally separate and do not communicate).

The mind–brain problem is an important context for the study of psychopharmacology. If this context is ignored, it is far easier to ignore things, such as the placebo effect, that hold important truths, as yet untapped, that may contribute to our knowledge of healing the symptoms of mental/emotional disorders. Ignoring the mind–brain problem also makes it easier to commit category errors and support them with word magic (such as asserting that all depression is caused by a "chemical imbalance").

THE LAYOUT OF THIS BOOK

Part One

The first part of this book covers introductory material on the basic principles of psychopharmacology derived from the medical model as well as material representing the different truths or perspectives that complement the medical model. The information in Chapter Two focuses on pharmacokinetics: how the body acts on drugs. Chapter Three focuses on pharmacodynamics: how drugs act on the body. Chapter Four is an overview of the nervous system and tells the story of neurotransmission. The story of neurotransmission is the story of how brain cells (neurons) communicate both electrically and chemically. If you know this story, you have a general understanding of how psychotropic medications are designed and what they are supposed to do. The story of neurotransmission gives you a sense of the complexity of neurotransmission and a sense of how much people have yet to learn about it. By understanding the story of neurotransmission you will also be able to conceptualize what we currently know about mechanisms of action of psychotropic medications and about strategies pharmaceutical companies use to develop newer drugs.

Chapter Five gives an overview of relevant issues from the psychological perspective—the subjective sense of our experience of life. Psychological issues also include interpersonal issues relevant to mental health practitioners working with clients and other professionals. These issues include how to talk with clients about medication and compliance, how to approach collaboration with prescribing professionals, and how to process particular issues in supervision. In Chapter Six, the last chapter in Part One, we cover important social and cultural issues. We give an overview of cultural, racial, and gender differences regarding responses to psychotropic medication and then discuss the relevance of powerful institutions such as the pharmaceutical industry and the Food and Drug Administration.

Part Two

The second part of the book contains four chapters covering classes of commonly prescribed psychotropic drugs used to treat depression, anxiety, psychosis, mood instability, and a host of other conditions. Each chapter includes some history on the discovery and use of each category of drugs. This history provides the context that informs the four perspectives we comment on in each chapter. In addition to the history, we present medical model theories of how the drugs work and cover common drugs in each category including their side effects. Then, in each chapter, we include relevant material from the psychological, cultural, and social perspectives. Note that a medication approved by the FDA for some use has both a generic name and a brand name (or brand names). For example, Prozac is a brand name for a drug, the generic name for which is *fluoxetine*. Throughout the book when we refer to a drug in an example we try to provide the reader with both generic and brand names. The *PDR*, the *Physicians' Desk Reference*, is the standard reference book on drug names, both generic names and brands. It is available both at the reference desk of most public libraries and online.

Part Three

Part Three of the book, titled "Newer Issues," addresses psychotropic medications for children (including stimulant medications), the elderly and psychotropic medication, an update on herbaceuticals, a chapter on drug replacement therapy and the conclusion. The chapters in this part differ from those in Part Two in that these are newer areas and often have been the subject of fewer research studies. Many of the agents discussed in Part Two and used with adults are still being investigated for efficacy with children. Although scientists have done a great deal of research on the medical model of how stimulants affect children, they have only just begun to deal with which children are really good candidates for stimulant therapy and what the medicating of young children means for this society. Note that each chapter contains study questions and exercises for the reader.

STUDY QUESTIONS AND EXERCISES

1. Describe the four perspectives derived from the Integral Model introduced in this chapter.

2. Outline some of the differences between a medical disorder that can be treated allopathically, such as a bacterial infection, and a mental/emotional disorder, such as depression.

3. Discuss with your classmates the mind–brain problem and your beliefs about the role of the mind and brain. In the context of your beliefs, discuss why you chose to enter a mental health profession.

CHAPTER TWO

Introduction to the Nervous System, Neurons, and Pharmacodynamics

INTRODUCTION

This chapter has six sections. The first introduces the central and peripheral nervous systems. The second takes a closer look at the central nervous system. The third section introduces glial cells and neurons. The fourth section introduces neurotransmitters. The fifth tells the story of neurotransmission and the sixth discusses pharmacodynamics or how drugs act on the brain.

SECTION ONE: AN OVERVIEW OF PHYSIOLOGY RELEVANT TO PSYCHOPHARMACOLOGY

Learning Objectives

- Know the basic parts of the central nervous system.
- Know the divisions of the peripheral nervous system.
- Understand that side effects can impact the central and peripheral nervous systems.

In this chapter, we provide an overview of the central nervous system, the brain, the brain's individual cells (called *neurons*) and **pharmacodynamics** (how drugs act on your body). This material has been the focus of most psychopharmacology texts, but remember, it is only part of the story—an important part that discloses truth—but not the whole truth.

In studying this material, some students become anxious, thinking, "I don't really have any background in biology or physiology." Relax. If "hard science" doesn't come naturally to you, think of the brain and the nervous systems as miraculous works of art that you can experience even if you cannot fully understand them. Set aside quiet study time to read this material. If it is new to you, don't expect to grasp it reading in 20-minute intervals or in a distracting environment. Approach this chapter as a "brain appreciation" tour. Remembering our mantra and the fact that the best "hard science" minds in the world are really just starting to understand the brain, sit back with a warm drink and join us for this tour through the most complex organ known to human beings.

A FEW BASICS

We start with a sketch of the **central** and **peripheral nervous systems**. Figure 2.1 illustrates key parts in both systems. Although we focus on central nervous system effects from various medications, it is important to understand some basics of the peripheral nervous system, because many drugs have **side effects** on this system. Much of the information in this section is drawn from Advokat, Comaty and Julien (2014), Bloom, Nelson, and Lazerson (2005), Carlson (2012), and Thompson (2000). Readers interested in full expositions of the brain and central nervous system are referred to their work.

The central nervous system includes the brain and spinal cord. The peripheral nervous system (the nervous system outside the brain and spinal cord) is divided into the **somatic** and **autonomic** (or visceral) **nervous systems**. The somatic nervous

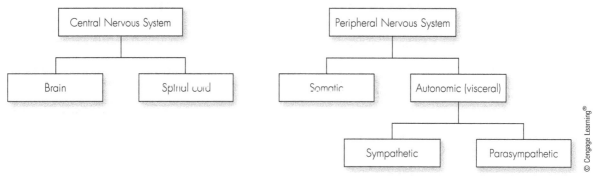

FIGURE 2.1 Basic Overview of Human Nervous Systems

system connects with sense receptors and skeletal muscles while the autonomic nervous system controls involuntary functions related to the glands, smooth muscles, heart, and viscera. This is important, because the goal for **psychotropic** drug compounds is to get them into the central nervous system. Remember that "psychotropic" means acting on or moving toward the mind, but because we lack a clear understanding of the relationship between mind and brain (as discussed in Chapter One) the medical model perspective assumes most psychotropic medications have to reach the brain. Note that there is also ample evidence that what we call "mind" may have correlates in other parts of the body, such as the bacterial signature we each carry in the gut which may also affect mental disorders (Bested, Logan, & Selhub, 2013; Forsythe, Kunze, & Bienenstock, 2012; Rodriguez, 2013; Stafford, 2012).

The nerves in your body and head that send information to and from the central nervous system are peripheral nerves. As you can see in Figure 2.1, the peripheral nervous system consists of the somatic and autonomic nervous systems. The somatic nervous system consists of peripheral nerves (nerves outside the central nervous system) that connect with sense receptors (receptors for vision, taste, and so on) and with skeletal muscles. The somatic nervous system regulates voluntary activity and relays information from the sensory organs to the central nervous system and from the central nervous system to the skeletal muscles. Thus, when you see a pint of Haagen-Dazs ice cream,

the somatic nervous system relays the visual stimulus to the central nervous system where you decide to reach for the pint (and a spoon). Next the signal for reaching for the ice cream is relayed back to the skeletal muscles, and that signal brings a creamy delight within your reach.

The autonomic (visceral) nervous system regulates activities that are primarily involuntary. For example, once you have enjoyed your ice cream, the autonomic nervous system is correlated with activities such as digesting, so you can just bask in the afterglow of a good "sugar high." The autonomic nervous system is further subdivided into the sympathetic nervous system (active during arousal such as fight, flight, or freeze responses) and the parasympathetic nervous system (active during conservation of energy). Activation of the sympathetic nervous system mobilizes your bodily resources and prepares you to expend energy. For example, if you left the Haagen-Dazs on the counter and your dog spied it just before you reached for it, your sympathetic nervous system would help you spring into action, thwarting Fido and capturing your prize. The activation of the parasympathetic nervous system deactivates organs that the sympathetic nervous system activated. Once the ice cream is safe in your grasp, your parasympathetic nervous system returns your body to **homeostasis** so you can settle down.

A ready example of how a drug affects the peripheral nervous system is the popular antidepressant fluoxetine/Prozac (when referencing drugs in a chapter we will use the generic name, a forward slash ("/") and then the brand name). Physicians often recommend that patients take fluoxetine/Prozac with food. This is because a common side effect of fluoxetine/Prozac (and most similar antidepressants) is nausea. This nausea occurs because the fluoxetine/Prozac affects serotonin receptors, and the peripheral nervous system in our digestive tracts is rich in these receptors. Because the drug must pass through these peripheral nervous system structures to get into the bloodstream and eventually the central nervous system, along the way any receptors to which the drug binds are affected. This also returns us to the interesting point about the "mind" being linked with the "gut." Could antidepressants acting on these gut receptors be causing more than just "side effects"? Even if the mind did turn out to be totally generated by the brain (the epiphenomenon hypothesis in Chapter One), what if the "brain" we are referring to includes the entire nervous system? Until researchers can secure funding to think beyond the limits of the current models, such questions remain unexplored.

Review Questions

- What are the two general parts of the central nervous system?
- What are the functions of the somatic and autonomic nervous systems?
- Why can drugs cause side effects in areas like the gut?

SECTION TWO: EXPLORING THE CENTRAL NERVOUS SYSTEM

Learning Objectives

- Be able to generally describe functions related to the brain stem, midbrain, and neocortex.
- Know what sorts of mental health symptoms may be directly related to the functioning of the limbic system.
- Understand the structural relationship between different parts of the brain.

As noted, the central nervous system consists of the brain and the spinal cord. The brain has three general "layers" that developed through evolution, commonly called the **brain stem** or **reptilian brain**, the midbrain or **mammalian brain** (which is technically part of the brain stem), and the **neocortex**. There is also the cerebellum (Latin for "little brain") that controls motor functions and posture. The brain has structures in and across these layers that we have correlated with particular functions. There are several ways to classify brain structures. We have followed the systems used by Advokat et al. (2014) and Carlson (2012), because these authors are highly respected in the field. Note that although some names of the brain structures may seem unfamiliar, they are usually Latin or Greek words for rather mundane objects and we will translate them as we go.

Exploring the Brain Stem

The brain stem includes structures that function to keep us alive. Figure 2.2 illustrates the structures of the brain stem and midbrain. When drugs interfere with the function of these structures, the results can be life threatening. For example, when a person drinks so much alcohol that it inhibits the neurons in these structures, the result can be coma and death.

The medulla oblongata is described as "the continuation of the spinal cord in the brain" (Thompson, 2000, p. 14) and controls breathing, heart rate, blood pressure, skeletal muscle tone, and digestion. This small, complex structure forms many connecting links between brain and spinal cord. Shaped like a pyramid, it is about an inch long and less than an inch across at its widest area. Its name comes from the Latin for "long marrow." The structure is so dense in neurons that the tissue looks dark, like bone marrow. Sometimes it is simply called the "medulla."

There is an important cluster of neurons in the brain stem called the **locus coeruleus** (pronounced *sa **roo** lee us*), from the Latin for "blue disc"; the cluster of neurons has a blue appearance. This structure consists of neurons that release norepinephrine and appear to help the person set priorities on

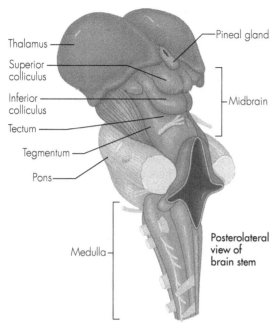

Thalamus

Superior colliculus

Inferior colliculus

Tectum

Tegmentum

Pons

Medulla

Pineal gland

Midbrain

Posterolateral view of brain stem

FIGURE 2.2 The Brain Stem and Midbrain

Source: From *Biological Psychology*, 7th ed., by J. W. Kalat.

incoming signals and decide where to place attention. Because of this link with attention, the role of the locus coeruleus is being investigated for links to the symptoms of attention deficit hyperactivity disorder (ADHD).

The pons (from the Latin for "bridge") connects the medulla oblongata and the midbrain. It also connects the two halves of the cerebellum. The pons extends into the reticular formation (part of the midbrain) and governs alertness, waking, sleeping, muscle tone, and some reflexes. The reticular formation has a netlike appearance (from the Latin *reticular*, "netlike"). The brain stem also includes the raphe nuclei (meaning "nerve cells forming a seam"). The raphe nuclei contain serotonin neurons and are thought to trigger slow-wave sleep. You can imagine the importance of understanding this if a client is going to take a drug that radically increases levels of serotonin in the brain. By increasing serotonin in this area, the drug is also going to cause sleepiness and possibly disrupt the sleep cycle, because serotonin is involved in sleep functions in the brain.

Exploring the Midbrain

The midbrain is also labeled **mesencephalon** (Greek for "midbrain") and is a continuation of the brain stem (see Figure 2.2). It merges into the thalamus and hypothalamus and encompasses what Advokat et al. (2014) call the "subthalamus." The subthalamus, combined with the basal ganglia, constitutes one of our motor systems called the **extrapyramidal motor system**. All information that passes between the brain and the spinal cord travels through the midbrain. As mentioned, the reticular formation is an interconnected network of neurons that extends from the spinal cord into the midbrain. These neurons are implicated in sleep, arousal, and a number of vital functions. The medulla, pons, and midbrain are thought to have developed early in human evolution (thus the common name "reptilian brain").

The Cerebellum

The cerebellum (from the Latin, meaning "little brain") looks like a little brain attached onto the larger cerebrum (illustrated in Figure 2.3). The cerebellum lies over the pons and is crucial to things such as balance and smooth, coordinated movement. It has connections with the vestibular system (the balance system located in the inner ear), the auditory, and the visual systems. The cerebellum, the subthalamus, and the basal ganglia make up the **extrapyramidal system**, which helps coordinate movement, including initiation, smoothness, and termination of movement. If people take a medication that interferes with the functioning of the extrapyramidal system, they will likely suffer from involuntary movements called **extrapyramidal side effects**. We discuss these in detail in our treatment of antipsychotic medications.

Exploring the Diencephalon

"**Encephalon**" is a Greek word that simply means "brain." "Di" means "between," so the diencephalon

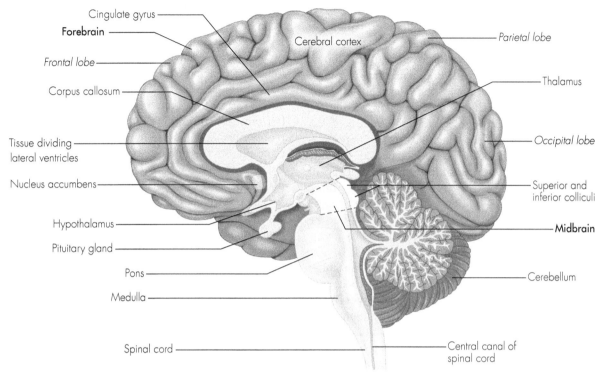

Cingulate gyrus

Forebrain

Frontal lobe

Corpus callosum

Tissue dividing
lateral ventricles

Nucleus accumbens

Hypothalamus

Pituitary gland

Pons

Medulla

Spinal cord

Cerebral cortex

Parietal lobe

Thalamus

Occipital lobe

Superior and
inferior colliculi

Midbrain

Cerebellum

Central canal of
spinal cord

FIGURE 2.3 A Sagittal Section Through the Human Brain

Source: From *Biological Psychology*, 7th ed., by J. W. Kalat.

is between the telencephalon and the brain stem. There are several important structures in this brain area. The thalamus, a large group of nerve cells, acts as the final relay area for the major sensory systems that project to the cerebral cortex: the visual, auditory, and somatic sensory systems (Thompson, 2000). Oddly enough, the translation of the Latin word *thalamus* is "bedroom" or "receptacle." Although "receptacle" means basically "final relay area," we have yet to figure out how "bedroom" fit in for the ancient translators, but feel free to use your imagination.

The hypothalamus ("below the thalamus") is a collection of cells that lie above the pituitary gland and immediately in front of the midbrain. The hypothalamus controls the autonomic nervous system and endocrine system and maintains the body's homeostasis (internal state). It also regulates temperature, fluids, metabolism, appetite

for specific nutrients, as well as what are called the "four Fs" (Fighting, Feeding, Fleeing, and Mating—again, use your imagination). Hormones secreted by the hypothalamus control the pituitary gland. Part of the wide-ranging influence of the hypothalamus is related to its control over the pituitary gland. Together, they act as a "master control system." "The hormones they release act on the other **endocrine glands** such as the thyroid, adrenal, and pituitary glands that secrete certain substances, particularly hormones, directly into the blood. The hormones released by the endocrine glands then act back on the pituitary gland and hypothalamus to regulate their activity, an example of feedback control" (Thompson, 2000, p. 17). The hypothalamus is also located near and has influence over what Olds and Milner (1954) dubbed the brain's **pleasure centers**.

Exploring the Limbic System

The limbic system is a series of brain structures that help us attach emotional meaning to sensory stimulation. In some systems of classification the limbic system is associated with the diencephalon, and in others it is associated with the telencephalon. The limbic system includes the amygdala (Latin for "almond," which it resembles), the septum (Latin for "dividing wall" or "enclosure"), the hippocampus (Latin for "seahorse" and based on resemblance), and portions of the thalamus. Bear in mind that many of the structures we are discussing are actually two—one on each side of the brain so technically you have two "amygdalae" but for sake of ease we refer to these in the singular. The amygdala integrates and directs emotional behavior, attaches emotional significance to what the senses signal, and mediates defensive aggressive behavior. Damage here can produce **Kluver-Bucy syndrome**, which is characterized by diminished fear and aggression as well as amnesia and hypersexuality. The septum inhibits emotionality, as evidenced by the fact that lesions in the septum produce septal rage syndrome. In this syndrome, damage to the septum leads to uninhibited emotional expression, particularly the expression of anger and aggression. The septum is also part of the pleasure centers of the brain. The hippocampus is a curved ridge in the limbic system, involved in moving signals from short-term memory to long-term memory.

Exploring the Telencephalon

The **telencephalon** consists of the right and left halves of the cerebrum (*tel* is a variation of the Greek *tele*, meaning "end" or "complete," so the translation is "end of the brain" or "completion of the brain"). The outer portion of the cerebrum is the cerebral cortex. This is the brain's outermost layer, the image you are probably familiar with from pictures of the human brain. This cortex is divided into four lobes (roundish projections) by sulci (deep grooves in the surface). The four lobes are named for the bones of the skull covering them

(see Figure 2.3) (Carlson, 2012). This part of the brain is correlated with the functions related to self-awareness or sentience that make humans unique in the animal kingdom. The tissue in the lobes can generally be mapped according to function, although in many cases, if an area is damaged another part of the brain may pick up that function. For most functions, their expression is contralateral ("opposite-sided"), meaning that an area on the right side of the brain controls something on the left side of the body. Next we summarize the four main lobes and some of their general functions.

The frontal lobes of the cerebral cortex are generally involved in motor behavior, expressive language, concentration, orientation (time, place, and person) thinking, and reasoning. These lobes contain the pyramidal system that is involved in fine, intricate movements. The left frontal lobe contains **Broca's area**, which is involved in speech production, and damage to this area can produce the experience of *expressive* aphasia (a self-conscious deficit in the ability to articulate or express language). The temporal lobes (located near the areas of your head called the "temples") are related to receptive language, memory, and emotion. These lobes contain **Wernicke's area**, which is involved in comprehending language. Damage to this area can produce *receptive* aphasia. The parietal lobes are located under the skull on the top of your head and contain the primary **somatosensory cortex**. This area receives and identifies sensory information from tactile receptors and processes visual and auditory sensations. Damage to the parietal lobes can produce Gertsmann's syndrome, which includes agraphia (inability to write), acalculia (difficulty with mathematical calculation), and right–left confusion. As you can imagine, researchers are trying to link what *DSM-5* calls Specific Learning Disorders to these areas of the brain (e.g., impairment in mathematics is related to problems in the parietal lobe). Finally, the occipital lobes (at the back of your head at the base of the skull) are largely associated with the **visual cortex**. Damage to the occipital lobes produces visual agnosia (the inability to recognize familiar objects on sight).

Under the cortex lie the smaller areas of the telencephalon (Bloom et al., 2005). The basal ganglia lie at the central regions of the cerebral hemispheres and are systems of cell **nuclei** that effect voluntary movement. They form the primary part of the extrapyramidal motor system (described earlier). Next we focus on the nerve cells in these structures and their function, so that we can begin to explain the mechanisms of action in psychotropic medications.

Review Questions

- How would you generally describe the functions of the brain stem, midbrain, and neocortex?
- What part of the midbrain is likely indicated in anxiety symptoms?
- What is the relationship of the cerebral cortex to the cerebrum?

SECTION THREE: AN OVERVIEW OF NEURONS AND GLIAL CELLS

"Neurons do not define the essence of people, nor do deficiencies in neurotransmitters explain mental disorders" (Kay, 2009, p. 288).

Learning Objectives

- Be able to discuss how neurons differ from other cells in the body.
- Be able to draw a simplistic picture of a neuron and label the soma, nucleus, axon, terminal button, synaptic vesicles, dendrites, and receptors.
- Know why the blood–brain barrier is important to designers of psychotropic medications.
- Understand our revised science of what glial cells do.

The brain weighs about 3 pounds and has a volume of about 3 pints. It contains a lot of **neurons**. Accounts vary on to how many neurons the brain contains: for example, Churchland (1995) and Cozolino (2010) estimate about 100 billion while Barlow and Durand (2002) estimated about 140 billion. Most recently Advokat et al. (2014) estimated

90 billion. Perhaps we are best off estimating "many billions of neurons in every human brain" (Thompson, 2000, p. 29) (or as Carl Sagan might have put it, "billions and billions"). As cells, neurons are unique in that they are created before we are born and have the capacity to live as long as we do. Up until the beginning of the 21st century, scientists commonly believed that at birth human beings had all the neurons they were ever going to have. This view is changing, as researchers now confirm that neurogenesis (the growth of new neurons) occurs in adult mammals (Martino, Butti, & Bacigaluppi, 2014; Shors et al., 2001; Van Praag, Christie, Sejnowski, & Gage, 1999) and correlates with the learning of new tasks (Gould, Beylin, Panapat, Reeves, & Shors, 1999).

Although all human cells renew themselves, not all cells divide regularly. One reason that neurons may not divide as regularly as other types of cells is that they form essential functional units in brains. As Thompson (2000) pointed out, everything people are or do has correlates in the sequencing of neurons and their interconnections. If neurons had to keep dividing to replace themselves, valuable sequences and interconnections might not form.

Although neurogenesis research continues to explore questions about how new neurons form, most knowledge about the correlation of neuronal function concerns the growth of axons and dendrites from existing neurons. This growth (called **arborization**) is prolific in the first few years of life. Moreover, you may have heard the saying "Size doesn't matter," and this is particularly true of the brain. Whales and dolphins have larger brains than humans, and although these mammals are no slouches intellectually, they do not match the human brain capacity for representational power. Nor do the *number* of neurons matter; it is the number of connections between the neurons that is important.

The neurons of the human brain have an enormous representational capacity. By way of analogy, Churchland (1995) compares this capacity to a standard 17-inch television screen. Such a screen has a representational capacity of about 200,000 pixels (a pixel is the smallest element of an image that can be processed). To get enough pixels to match the representational power of your brain, you would have had to cover all four sides of the Sears Tower in Chicago with such screens—and you have it all between your ears, as the saying goes. Such is the representational power of the brain.

THE BASIC ANATOMY OF A NEURON

Figure 2.4 is a simplistic rendering of a neuron. Actual neurons vary in length from a few millimeters up to about a meter and may have several thousand synaptic connections with other neurons (Julien, Advokate, & Comaty, 2014). Neurons come in many different types and shapes, but they all have structures similar to the ones in the figure. It is important to learn a simplistic version of a neuron first so that you can learn the story of neurotransmission. Then you can learn how medications interfere with the sequence of events in that story (or in other words how medications change the story of neurotransmission). Once you've learned that, you have a basic sense of the mechanisms of drug action. The importance of learning the basic parts of the neuron will become clear as we discuss the mechanisms of action of psychotropic medications. Using Figure 2.4 as your guide, let us begin by discussing the soma or cell body of the neuron. The dark spot on the figure of the soma is the cell nucleus, which contains the genetic material of the

cell. The soma contains the **mitochondria**, which are structures that provide energy for the neuron. Extending from the soma in one direction are **dendrites**, which are structures that receive inputs or messages from other cells through receptors. The receptors are typically pictured as located on the ends of the dendrites but can occur anywhere on the neuron. Receptors are basically chains of proteins that act as communication devices, allowing neurotransmitters (chemical messengers) to bind to them.

In our illustration, extending in the other direction from the soma is the axon. Many elements made in the soma (such as enzymes and receptors), as well as the "raw materials" for these elements, are transported up and down the axon. The axon also transmits electrical signals that can cause the cell to "fire." When a cell "fires," it releases neurotransmitter molecules from its terminal button. In our illustration at the far end of the axon are the terminal buttons. The terminal buttons contain sacks (called *synaptic vesicles*) of neurotransmitter molecules. When the electrical signal causes the cell to "fire," these sacks merge with the **permeable** membrane of the terminal button and the neurotransmitters are released into the synaptic cleft or synapse (the space between the terminal button and the neighboring receptors to which the neurotransmitter will bind). Although there is a universe of activity in each cell, this glance at the general

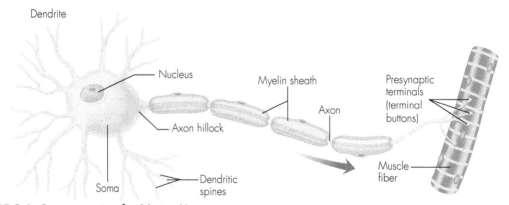

FIGURE 2.4 Components of a Motor Neuron

Source: From *Biological Psychology*, 7th ed., p. 32, by J. W. Kalat.

components will suffice until later in the chapter, when we discuss neurotransmission in more detail.

Now, we say that chemical neurotransmission occurs at the **synapses**, which Stahl (2000) defines as "specialized sites that connect two neurons" (p. 1). Neurons send synaptic information through firing and releasing neurotransmitter molecules. They receive synaptic information through their receptors. The number of synapses (points of connection between a neuron and neighboring neurons) on each neuron varies from around 5000 on a mammalian motor neuron to some 90,000 on a single Purkinje cell in the cerebral cortex. (This type of cell, named after the Czech physiologist who first charted its function, is related to the contraction of the heart.)

When the body is resting, the brain, which accounts for only about 2% of the body's mass, consumes about 20% of the body's oxygen. This is a lavish consumption of energy! The brain needs all this energy to maintain ionic gradient essential to receiving and sending information via the synapses. An ionic gradient is a form of potential energy that keeps the chemistry inside a cell different than the chemistry outside the cell so it can be thought of as a charged signal (an electrical charge). You can think of this charge as a rate of change in relation to the distance of the axon. There is a structure on the axon called the axon hillock. It is the last site in the soma or cell body where incoming signaling is summed and if it surpasses a particular threshold, the action potential (charge) is initiated down the axon toward the terminal button. As the electrical charge travels down the axon it may be facilitated by the influx of positively charged ions (e.g., sodium) or inhibited by an influx of negatively charged ions (e.g., chloride). When the action potential is facilitated all the way across the axon to the terminal button the cell fires, or releases, its neurotransmitter. As noted, to carry an electrical charge down an axon, positive ions must flow into the axon. Once the charge is carried down the axon, these positive ions are pumped back out of the cell (this is sometimes referred to as the *sodium potassium pump*). As you will see, these ionic gradients play the key role in determining whether or not neurons fire. Imagine: A single neuron handles a thousand signals in the space of a second, and it may fire several hundred times a second, so its energy consumption must be lavish.

GLIAL CELLS

Once thought to be an energy-saving device, glial cells have turned out to be much more. Myelin (pictured in Figure 2.4) is peculiar to vertebrates, although not all neurons in vertebrates are myelinated. For example, phylogenetically older fibers such as the C-fibers that innervate the skin and carry information about pain are less myelinated. If you have ever been pounding a nail and the hammer slipped, smashing your finger, you may recall having that split-second knowledge that it is going to hurt in a few milliseconds. With more myelin, you wouldn't have those milliseconds to anticipate the coming pain. Myelin is made of glial cells (particularly Schwann cells and oligodendroglia) but as you proceed up the evolutionary ladder, a particular type of glial cell called astrocytes increase in size and number.[1] In the 20th century, it was believed that myelin acted like the insulation on electrical wiring. This is one function of myelin. The more myelinated an axon is, the better insulated it is and the faster it can conduct a signal. When you see a person with a disease that degrades the myelin (such as multiple sclerosis), you see that he or she has difficulty moving, because the nerves coordinating the signals for the movement cannot send the electrical signals efficiently.

The conduction velocity depends on the diameter and myelination of the axon. A well-myelinated axon in a human motor neuron can conduct an impulse as fast as 130 meters per second (equivalent to approximately 300 miles per hour), whereas an unmyelinated fiber conducts at about 0.5 meters per second (a little over 1 mph). Events in the world of silicon chips happen in the nanosecond (a one-billionth of a second), whereas events in the

---

[1]There are three types of glial cells: astrocytes, Schwann cells, and oligodendroglia. Astrocytes move neurotransmitters, food, and waste. Schwann cells and oligodendroglia wrap around neurons like sheaths.

world of neurons happen in the millisecond (a one-thousandth of a second). Brain events are quite slow in comparison to computer events, but in complex tasks such as recognition, brains leave computers "in the dust," because brains accomplish recognition more quickly. In addition, all computers must put information through a central processing unit (CPU) whereas brains have enormous redundancy in the system so that if a signal does not get from point A to point B, the same signal can be sent from point C to point D or from point E to point F. Neurons are plastic and dynamic. Their information-relevant parts grow and shrink. The axons and dendrites are constantly changing, establishing new connections and removing old connections. This "arborization" is an important concept in psychopharmacology, because many drugs exert an influence to change the information-relevant parts of the neurons. Neurogenesis research findings are so new that speculations on the implications for pharmacology have just begun.

Myelin is made from a type of cell called a "glial cell." "Glial" means "glue," and glial cells form different types of protective barriers (sheaths) around neurons (of which myelin is one). In the late 19th century, when Ramon Santiago Cajal was doing work with neurons, his brother Pedro set forth a theory that glial cells were simply "support cells" for neurons. Cajal accepted his brother's theory and this led to the "neuron doctrine," which posited that neurons alone were responsible for our thought and mental processes. Glial cells usually outnumber neurons by a ratio of 10:1 making up 85–90% of the brain. Under the influence of the neuron doctrine, 20th century laypeople came to believe that we only used 10–15% of our brain power (because of course 85–90% of the cells were glial cells).

In different parts of the body, glial cells have different names that reflect the person who discovered them or their function. In the peripheral nervous system, Schwann cells perform the myelinating function; in the central nervous system, oligodendrocytes perform the same function. A third glial cell type, astrocytes, function as fences and filters for the blood–brain barrier and more importantly move neurotransmitters, food, and waste around the brain. A fourth type, microglia, function as scavengers cleaning up dead neurons and other disintegrated material (Fields, 2008, 2011). We'll take another look at the blood–brain barrier shortly.

Another important finding about astrocytes is that we learned that they can communicate to themselves with calcium waves. Astrocytes have hundreds of "endfeet" that spread out from their body toward blood vessels, other astrocytes, and neuronal synapses. Calcium released from internal stores can spread from astrocytes to areas hundreds of times larger than the original astrocyte. These calcium waves can also cause neurons to fire (Koob, 2009). This could radically alter our understanding of the electro-chemical processes in the brain. The implications are huge as we add the impact from 85% of the brain's cells, which previously have been more or less ignored in our efforts to understand the brain. This might be akin to thinking you know football as a game where a team must move the ball 100 yards to score a touchdown. Then you learn that actually it is 350 yards and the ball moves not just because of the teams but also in response to the volume of the crowd and how their cheers bounce off cars in the parking lot. It looks as if taking glial cells into the equation is literally a "whole new ball game."

THE BLOOD–BRAIN BARRIER

Over 100 years ago, Paul Ehrlich discovered that if blue dye is injected into an animal's bloodstream, all the tissues are tinted blue *except* the brain. You must inject the dye into the brain ventricles to get that tissue to turn blue. Although Ehrlich was working for a dye company on a different project, he thus unwittingly discovered the blood–brain barrier. In most of the body, the cells that form the capillaries are not spaced tightly together, so substances can move from blood plasma to the tissue.

In the central nervous system, the capillary cells do not have the same gaps, because they are filled by the astrocytes that make up the blood–brain barrier. This barrier blocks many substances from entering the central nervous system. In some areas, the barrier is weaker than others, to allow specific functions that have developed through evolution. One example of such an area is the *area postrema*, which signals vomiting. The barrier is weak here, so toxins in the blood can be detected. Once it detects toxins, the brain triggers the vomiting response to preserve the organism.

The blood–brain barrier serves an important survival function by keeping foreign elements such as toxins out of the brain. But what about things such as nutrients? Nutrients such as glucose must be transported through the capillary walls by special proteins. This is very important, because to exert their effects all current psychotropic medications must reach the central nervous system. To do so, they must pass through the blood–brain barrier. The glial cells that make up the blood–brain barrier have a high fat content. The myelination of the brain in infancy is one reason babies need a lot of fat in their diet. We refer to fatty cells as fat soluble (the technical term for this is **lipophilicitous**— another great cocktail party word). Thus, to pass through the blood–brain barrier, a molecule also must be highly fat soluble. Almost all psychotropic medication molecules are fat soluble, with perhaps the sole exception of lithium, which must be carried across the blood–brain barrier by other means.

Review Questions

- How do neurons differ from other cells in the body?
- Draw a simplistic picture of a neuron and label the soma, nucleus, axon, terminal button, synaptic vesicles, dendrites, and receptors. Explain why it is "simplistic."
- What is the function of the blood–brain barrier and why is it important to designers of psychotropic medications?
- How has our understanding of glial cells progressed in the 21st century?

SECTION FOUR: TYPES OF NEUROTRANSMITTERS

Learning Objectives

- Generally understand what makes a ligand a neurotransmitter.
- Be able to identify both excitatory and inhibitory neurotransmitters.
- Be able to describe the difference between polypharmacy and co-treatment.

The brain has literally dozens of known or suspected neurotransmitters. Scientists may discover many more. To be considered a neurotransmitter, a substance must (1) be synthesized in the **presynaptic** neuron, (2) be released from the presynaptic terminal, (3) cause excitatory or inhibitory signals, and (4) have some mechanism for removing it from the site of action (Churchland, 1995). Despite the number of existing neurotransmitters, only a fraction of those we know of are affected directly by the psychotropic medications we discuss in this book. Table 2.1 lists neurotransmitters commonly involved in the actions of psychotropic medications.

Neurotransmitters are made from **precursor compounds** in the neuron. You can think of precursors as the "raw materials" with which

TABLE 2.1 Neurotransmitters Involved in Psychotropic Medications and Their Abbreviations

Glutamate	Glu
Gamma-aminobutyric acid	GABA
Acetylcholine	Ach
Dopamine	DA
Norepinephrine	NE
Epinephrine	Epi
Serotonin	5-HT

© Cengage Learning®

neurotransmitters are made. These compounds include amino acids, glucose, and certain amines such as choline. You take many of these precursors into your body through the foods you eat. Think of neurotransmitters as chemical messengers in the nervous system. As we explain later, when a cell fires and releases neurotransmitters, these same transmitters bind to receptors on other neurons, conveying information and further exciting or inhibiting neighboring neurons.

Now we provide an overview of the primary neurotransmitters. Become generally acquainted with them, so that when we discuss mechanisms of action in drugs you can recognize the primary neurotransmitters involved. Although scientists generally think that typically neurons only produce one type of neurotransmitter, each neuron may be outfitted with receptors for multiple neurotransmitters. Thus, although typically a neuron that produces only dopamine releases only dopamine (there are always exceptions though), it can be affected by changes in available serotonin, norepinephrine, acetylcholine, and so on. This multiple sensitivity produces a "ripple effect": Using a drug to affect the levels of only one neurotransmitter may end up affecting the levels of many neurotransmitters.

GLUTAMATE (GLU)

Glutamate (also called *glutamic acid*) is one of the non-essential amino acids, meaning it is synthesized in the body and you do not have to acquire it in your diet. One of the main sources of glutamate in the body is the breakdown of **glucose**. Most neurons have glutamate receptors. Glutamate generally serves an excitatory function, encouraging neurons to fire, and plays a key role in sensory functions and in some brain structures we have discussed in this chapter, including the pyramidal and extrapyramidal nervous systems, the hippocampus, and the cerebellum. Glutamate may be the dominant excitatory neurotransmitter in our brains. Julien et al. (2014) noted that a newer drug for narcolepsy actually works by augmenting glutamate neurotransmission (as opposed to drugs such as amphetamines that augment dopamine neurotransmission). Researchers hope that a drug augmenting glutamate transmission will not show the dependence-inducing properties that amphetamines have. In addition, drugs that modulate glutamate have been recently targeted as a possible intervention for Schizophrenia (Hasimoto, Malchow, Falkai, & Schmitt, 2013). This is difficult because too much glutamate can trigger seizures or kill brain cells while too little can cause comas (Locke, 2008).

GAMMA-AMINOBUTYRIC ACID (GABA)

Gamma-aminobutyric acid (GABA) is one of the amino acid neurotransmitters and occurs almost exclusively in the brain. GABA reduces the firing of neurons and may be the predominant inhibitory neurotransmitter of the brain. Paradoxically, glutamate is a precursor for GABA, but whereas glutamate is excitatory, GABA is inhibitory. GABA is so common in the central nervous system that neurologists believe a full one-third of synapses are receptive to it (Zillman, Spiers, & Culbertson, 2007). Although GABA is inhibitory, it is important not to oversimplify this into the erroneous belief that all GABA transmission "mellows you out." For example, some areas of your brain (such as your sleep centers), when stimulated, calm you down. If GABA molecules inhibit these areas, then the end result is the *opposite* of calming you down. GABA-ergic areas of the brain also help people control motor behavior. People with **Huntington's chorea** have difficulty controlling their motor behaviors, and physiologists believe this is caused by losing GABA-ergic neurons (Zillman et al., 2007).

ACETYLCHOLINE (ACH)

Acetylcholine was the first major neurotransmitter to be identified in the 1920s. (Epinephrine was discovered in 1904 but is less important in psychopharmacology.) Acetylcholine is prominent in the peripheral and central nervous systems. It is present peripherally at the muscle–nerve connection for all voluntary muscles and at many involuntary nervous system synapses. The exact role of acetylcholine neurons is becoming clearer with research. Generally, they are believed to be involved in alertness, attention, and memory. Acetylcholine is made from choline (an amine and one of the B-complex vitamins) and **acetate**. Choline is supplied by foods such as kidneys, egg yolk, seeds, vegetables, and legumes. Acetylcholine has been linked to cognitive functioning, because Alzheimer's-type dementia is correlated with the degeneration of acetylcholine-rich tissues in the brain. Many drugs that temporarily slow the progression of Alzheimer's do so almost exclusively by enhancing the action of acetylcholine in the brain.

MONOAMINE NEUROTRANSMITTERS

Monoamine neurotransmitters are a class of neurotransmitters that share similar **molecular structures**. The monoamines include dopamine, norepinephrine, epinephrine, and serotonin. A subclass of monoamines is the catecholamines. The three catecholamine neurotransmitters are dopamine, norepinephrine (in the central nervous system), and epinephrine in the peripheral nervous system. The first two play important roles in both legal and illegal psychotropic compounds.

DOPAMINE (DA)

Dopamine was discovered in 1958. Dopamine is a major transmitter in the **corpus striatum** (cerebrum), regulating motor behavior and playing a large role in the so-called pleasure or reward centers. It is derived from tyrosine, which is an amino acid in our diets. The dopamine pathways in the frontal cortex, **nucleus accumbens**, and **ventral tegmental area** (VTA) underlie the pleasure centers. The firing of dopamine neurons in these areas is augmented by certain drugs, which seems to lead some people to use these drugs in ways that are described as "abuse" and that may induce psychological or physical dependence. We look at primary dopamine tracts when we discuss antipsychotic drugs in Chapter Seven.

NOREPINEPHRINE (NE)

In the 1930s, the neurotransmitter norepinephrine was found in both the central and peripheral nervous systems and in the sympathetic nerves of the autonomic nervous system (governing heart rate, blood pressure, bronchial dilation, and so forth). Norepinephrine is derived from tyrosine (an amino acid), and the cell bodies of most norepinephrine neurons are located in the brain stem in the locus coeruleus. From this area, norepinephrine neurons project widely throughout the brain and are involved in many responses, including feelings of reward, pain relief, mood, memory, and hormonal functioning.

"It's Greek to Me"

A few notes on terms: The word *norepinephrine* is synonymous with *noradrenaline*. Norepinephrine is similar to epinephrine, which is a hormone produced by the adrenal medulla (the core of the adrenal gland). *Epinephrine* is synonymous with *adrenaline*. You may ask (as we did), "Why are there two words for both norepinephrine and epinephrine?" Good question, and we don't have an answer, but here is a little background.

Basically, one word is derived from the Greek language and the other from Latin. *Epinephrine* is derived from Greek (*epi*, "on"; *nephron*, "kidney"). *Adrenal* is derived from Latin (*ad*, "toward"; *renal*, "kidney"). The prefix "*nor*" indicates that norepinephrine is a precursor to epinephrine. So to say a drug is "noradrenergic" means it enhances the action of noradrenaline/norepinephrine.

SEROTONIN (5-HT)

Serotonin is distributed throughout the body. Researchers in the 1950s initially investigated it as a central nervous system transmitter, because of its similarity in structure to **lysergic acid diethylamide (LSD)**. In the central nervous system, serotonin is the primary transmitter of the raphe nuclei, the group of neurons in the medulla and pons. From there, these neurons project throughout the cerebral cortex, hippocampus, hypothalamus, and limbic system (Julien, 2001). Serotonin is heavily involved in the sleep–wake cycle as well as in sexuality, mood, and emotion. This is why side effects from serotonergic drugs often include sleep and sexual side effects. Serotonin is derived from tryptophan, an essential amino acid that people must obtain through diet. Although depriving people of tryptophan is correlated with depressive symptoms in some but not all study participants, adding extra tryptophan does nothing to alleviate depressive symptoms (Hansen et al., 2011; Jacobson, Medvedev, & Caron, 2012; Parker & Brotchie, 2011).

REALITY IS COMPLEX AND ...

It is important to understand that each neurotransmitter may have a number of different receptors to which it can bind. These subfamilies of receptors may play varying roles in mental/emotional disorders. For example, there are numerous serotonin (5-HT) receptors, variously referred to by numeric labels (5-HT1, 5-HT2, 5-HT3, and so on) (Bloom et al., 2005).

Julien et al. (2014) have noted that researchers think neurotransmitters fit various receptors much like a key fits a particular lock. As Sopolsky (2005) noted, this is a time-worn and almost cliché way of teaching the relation between receptors and neurotransmitters but it has persisted because it communicates the basic idea. Thus, a drug that mimics the action of serotonin by binding to serotonin receptors may interact differently with different receptor subfamilies. This also has implications for the number of side effects a drug may have. Drugs described as "dirty" affect several receptors and subfamilies of receptors and have more side effects. The "cleaner" the drug is, the more focused its action and the fewer its side effects.

Another complexity is important here. Although researchers once hoped that certain neurochemicals would be specific to certain brain sites, they aren't. Moreover, there is no sharp distinction between chemicals found in the brain and hormones found in rest of the body. Hormones once thought unique to the rest of the body have been found in the brain, and chemicals once thought unique to the brain have been found in the rest of the body. In addition, neurotransmitters may work with other peptides (chain-links of amino acids), forming co-transmitter pairs. For example, dopamine works with enkephalin (a naturally occurring protein with morphine-like properties). Researchers are beginning to see that to influence neurotransmission, pharmacologists may need multiple drug actions. This area in the leading edge of psychopharmacology is also known as **polypharmacy**, which is the use of multiple psychotropic medications to bring about symptom relief. This practice may result in a person being placed on numerous drugs because of the presumed interactions among the drugs. Thus, you may hear of a drug such as methylphenidate/Ritalin "potentiating" fluoxetine/Prozac. In that instance, the methylphenidate/Ritalin enhances the action of the fluoxetine/Prozac. Polypharmacy has also led to the practice of combining two medications in a formulation for a single dose. An example is one of the newest mood-stabilizing medications olanzapine and fluoxetine/Symbyax, which combines an antipsychotic medication (olanzapine) and an antidepressant (fluoxetine). When such a combination has been tested in double-blind, placebo controlled, multi-site studies and found statistically significant, we no longer call it polypharmacy but rather co-therapy. This change in label means it has been tested and works better than a single drug alone. One problem with polypharmacy is that it is too easy for a client to end up on more than one medication while no one really knows which med is doing what and whether they are all necessary (see http://www.tedxcle.com/dr-elliott-ingersoll/).

Review Questions

- What sorts of classifications make something a neurotransmitter?
- Provide one example of an excitatory and inhibitory neurotransmitter.
- What is the story between polypharmacy and co-therapy?

SECTION FIVE: THE STORY OF NEUROTRANSMISSION

Learning Objectives

- Understand the "wires and soup" metaphor.
- Be able to outline the relationship between DNA, RNA, and mRNA.
- Understand basic functions of transporters and enzymes.
- Generally outline the story of neurotransmission including first and second messenger effects, neuronal firing, and the binding and reuptake/ breakdown of neurotransmitters.

Most psychopharmacology is the story of how different medications interfere with neurotransmission. If you become fluent in the language of neurotransmission, you can begin to understand the actions of medications on the brain. Stahl (2000) has offered two similes to help us understand neurotransmission: "wires" and "soup." In some respects, the nervous system is like an electrical system (wires) in the sense that connections between neurons are like millions of phone wires within thousands of cables. The big difference is that, unlike a phone or electrical system, neurotransmission is not all electrical. The impulse from the receptor of a cell to the terminal button is electrical. After the cell fires, the neuron sends neurotransmitters out into the extracellular fluid (the chemical "soup"), where the chemical messengers (the neurotransmitters) bind to receptors on other neurons. So neurotransmission is both electrical and chemical. Psychotropic medications can exert effects on both dimensions of neurotransmission. Stahl also discusses the notion of time and neurotransmission. Some neurotransmitter signals are fast (such as GABA or glutamate signals that occur in milliseconds), whereas others are slower (such as norepinephrine, with a signal lasting up to several seconds).

NEUROTRANSMISSION: THE TEAM PLAYERS

We now introduce some of the key players in neurotransmission. After this we present the entire process of neurotransmission, and then the ways psychotropic drugs interfere with the key players and the process to exert their influence on the nervous system.

Deoxyribonucleic Acid (DNA)

Deoxyribonucleic acid (DNA) is a **macromolecule**, a very large molecule consisting of hundreds or thousands of atoms, housed in the nucleus of the neuron that has two interconnected helical strands (the well-known double-helix shape). These strands and associated proteins make up the chromosomes that contain the organism's genetic code. When DNA is active, it makes ribonucleic acid (RNA) and gives RNA the genetic code. The messenger RNA then leaves the cell nucleus and attaches to ribosomes (protein structures that serve as the site of protein production) to create more proteins that serve as the basis for building other structures in the cell. Basically, the DNA acts as a template for messenger RNA synthesis; mRNA is a template for protein synthesis. DNA and RNA govern the production of enzymes, receptors, transporters, and other chemical supplies in and around the neuron's nucleus. DNA is still an uncharted frontier. Although the Human Genome Project has led to advances in understanding DNA, approximately 97% of DNA sequences are noncoding sequences and are still not understood (Flam, 1994; Suurkula, 1996).

Transporters

Transporters are just what the name sounds like— they move things around inside the neuron, outside the neuron, and in and out of the neuron. In terms of neurotransmitters, transporters create a type of recycling program: First the cell fires neurotransmitters into the synaptic cleft. Then the neurotransmitter binds to a receptor. When it eventually unbinds, it is then picked up by this transporter, taken back inside the cell, and stored for future use. Some transporters move enzymes around the neuron so they can carry out their functions.

Enzymes

Enzymes have multiple functions in the neuron, but typically they put together substances such as neurotransmitters in some areas, whereas they may dismantle neurotransmitters at other areas. Enzymes are also transported (by transporters) outside the cell where they break down neurotransmitters in the synaptic cleft. The enzymes and other elements are then transported down the axon. Enzymes also provide the energy for the transporters to "recycle" the neurotransmitter in the synaptic cleft. Two examples of psychotropic drugs that act by inhibiting enzymes are donzepil/Aricept and tranylcypromine/Parnate. The enzyme acetylcholinesterase (AChE) breaks down acetylcholine (Ach) and the enzyme monoamine oxidase (MAO) breaks down monoamine neurotransmitters. Donzepil/Aricept inhibits AChE causing more Ach in the synapses which can help mild to moderate symptoms of Alzheimer's type dementia. Drugs like tranylcypromine/Parnate inhibit MAO allowing more norepinephrine (NE) to be available in the synapses which can help symptoms of depression.

Receptors

Receptors are large molecules that are proteins (chains of amino acids) created in the soma (cell body) and transported by transporter molecules to different parts of the neuron. There are hundreds of types of receptors with specified functions. Receptors are inserted through the neuronal membrane by enzymes to perform these functions in neurotransmission. Receptors weave in and out of the cell membrane (often in a circular fashion), so part of them is outside the cell (extracellular) and part of them is inside the cell (intracellular). The binding site for the neurotransmitter is typically extracellular (outside the cell). There are many receptor subtypes. For example there are about a dozen serotonin receptor subtypes.

Many different proteins may serve as receptors, there are some primary types worth mentioning. **Ion channel receptors** (ionotropic receptors) function as **ion channels**. As Advokat et al. (2014) note these form a sort of pore that enlarges when certain neurotransmitters (and drugs) attach to them. This allows flow of a certain ion that could be positively (e.g., sodium) or negatively (e.g., chloride) charged. As we noted, an influx of positively charged ions will be excitatory to the cell and an influx of negatively charged ions will inhibit the cell. G-Protein-Coupled Receptors (GPCRs) are also called metabotropic receptors. Activating these receptors releases an intracellular guanosine-nucleotide binding protein (called a "G" protein for short) that controls enzyme functions in the **postsynaptic** neuron. Basically GPCRs change extracellular stimuli like drugs or neurotransmitters into intracellular signals (Advokat et al., 2014) through direct and indirect effects that will be discussed in the different drug classes covered in this book. Finally, carrier proteins are receptors that transport ligands such as neurotransmitters across cell membranes.

BACK TO NEUROTRANSMITTERS

As we have already noted, enzymes in the cell make neurotransmitter molecules. The enzymes then package the neurotransmitter into synaptic vesicles that are transported to the terminal button for storage. The synaptic vesicles protect the neurotransmitter from other enzymes that break down the neurotransmitter.

IONS

Ions are atoms or groups of atoms electrically charged by loss or gain of electrons. Cations are positively charged. Examples of cations are sodium (Na from the Latin *natrium*) and potassium (K, from the Latin *kalium*). Anions are negatively charged ions. Chloride (Cl) is an example of an anion. Ions flow in and out of neurons, increasing or decreasing the electrical charge. If the charge is positive enough, the neuron fires. If the charge is negative enough, the neuron resists firing.

ION CHANNELS

As noted above, ion channels are types of receptors that form channels or pores across the neuron membrane. They can open to allow positively or negatively charged ions into the channels, increasing or decreasing the chance that the neuron will fire depending on what sort of ion was let in. These channels can also remain closed. A cell in its **resting state** has anions intracellularly (inside the cell) and cations extracellularly (outside the cell). In this state the cell is *polarized*, with the positively charged ions on the outside and the negatively charged ions on the perimeter of the inside. If cellular events increase this state by resisting opening the ion channels or by letting in only negatively charged ions, the cell is *hyperpolarized*, decreasing the chance it will fire. If ion channels open the cell to positively charged ions, it then becomes *depolarized*, increasing the likelihood of firing.

A VIEW WITHIN THE CELL

You can think of the cell as a little "universe." In this universe, the DNA and mRNA are initiating protein synthesis in the ribosomes and those proteins are then used to create everything from enzymes to transporter molecules. The transporter molecules are busy transporting elements up and down the neuron axon, to and from the cell body, and moving in and out of the cell with other elements. The enzymes at some points are busy creating neurotransmitters from precursors, at other points dismantling neurotransmitters that have been fired, and at still other points providing energy for various functions of the cell.

Some readers may find a manufacturing metaphor useful. In the metaphor, the DNA and mRNA are the "brains" behind the outfit, providing parts lists and plans about how each element will function. The enzymes and transporters are like workers with different functions. One of the primary products is the neurotransmitter, and it is packaged in the synaptic vesicles (much like workers producing cell phones may package them in a plastic container for shipping). The transporters are like tractor-trailer rigs that take care of transportation and shipping needs for the business.

THE PROCESS OF NEUROTRANSMISSION

Now we describe a general sequence of events in neurotransmission. Again, remember that if you generally understand this sequence you will be able to understand how particular drugs interfere with the sequence and exert some of their effects. In this process, we talk about presynaptic neurons and postsynaptic neurons. These are really relative terms. To understand this, draw an image of three neurons side by side, using the image in Figure 2.4 as a guide. Make sure each neuron you draw has a cell body (soma), dendrites with receptors, and a terminal button. Label the three neurons "A," "B," and "C."

In doing this, you can see that the terminal button of neuron A is next to the dendrites for neuron B. The terminal button for neuron B is next to the dendrites of neuron C, and so on. Although this figure is oversimplified, it communicates the basic details. Remember that a synapse is the point where neurons communicate with each other and the synaptic cleft is merely the slight space between these two points. So with regard to the synaptic cleft between neuron A and B, A is the presynaptic neuron and neuron B is the postsynaptic neuron. With regard to the synaptic cleft between neuron B and C, neuron B is the presynaptic neuron and neuron C is the postsynaptic neuron. The labels merely reflect the position of each neuron with respect to a particular synaptic cleft. So in one sense, every neuron is a presynaptic neuron to some other neuron and a postsynaptic neuron with respect to still others. Similarly, when you are driving on a crowded freeway, you are in front of some driver and behind some other driver.

FIRST-MESSENGER EFFECTS

With the notion of presynaptic and postsynaptic neurons in mind, let's begin with the example. Note that when a cell "fires" (sends neurotransmitters out into the synaptic cleft), we call this *exocytosis* ("exo," outside; "cytosis," cell—outside the cell). So, in our example, neuron A fires and sends its chemical messengers (the neurotransmitters) out into the synaptic cleft. There some of them bind to receptors on neuron B. This initial binding is called a **"first-messenger effect."** The effect can be an excitatory effect (depolarizing the cell to increase the likelihood of firing) or an inhibitory effect (hyperpolarizing the cell to decrease likelihood of firing). The effect is not tied so much to the neurotransmitter that is binding but to what ion channels the receptors it is binding to control. In some presentations, the excitatory or inhibitory effect is labeled with reference to the synapse. Figure 2.5, from Kalat (2001), shows an example.

Remember that the resting state of the cell is called the *polarized state.* If the receptors open ion channels that allow only negatively charged ions to filter into the cell, then the cell becomes hyperpolarized or less likely to fire. In this scenario, the first messenger effect is inhibitory. If the receptors to which neurotransmitters are binding open ion channels that let positively charged ions into the cell, then the cell becomes depolarized or more likely to fire. In this scenario, the first-messenger effect is excitatory.

Remember, although part of the receptor is outside of the cell, the receptor also goes through the cell membrane into the cell. The chemical neurotransmitter binding at an excitatory synapse can initiate an electrical impulse that is carried through the receptor into the neuron. That signal may be strong enough to pass the axon hillock and to open ion channels that allow positively charged ions to enter the cell. The positively charged ions further facilitate the electrical signal, letting it continue down the axon to the terminal button. When a charge of sufficient intensity reaches the terminal button,

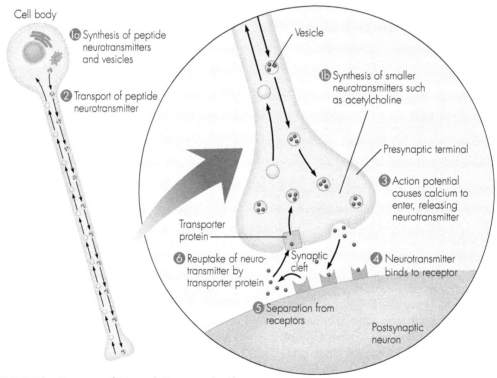

FIGURE 2.5 The Process of Neural Communication

Source: From *Biological Psychology,* 7th ed., p. 32, by J. W. Kalat.

the cell "fires" and the synaptic vesicle merges with the terminal button wall, letting neurotransmitter molecules flow out of the neuron.

Once outside the neuron, the neurotransmitters are in the chemical soup (extracellular fluid). There they gravitate toward receptors and, if they fit the receptors in question, bind to them. Once bound, they may exert an agonist or antagonist effect on other cells, and the process continues. Remember that there are billions of neurons, with trillions of synapses where each may communicate with the others.

Once fired from the neuron, neurotransmitters cannot just stay in the synaptic cleft indefinitely. They also do not bind forever to receptors but bind and release or are displaced by other molecules (drug or natural) that then bind to the receptor. The neurotransmitters are then either "recycled" by transporter molecules that carry them back into the cell for future use (reuptake), or they are deactivated by enzymes in the extracellular fluid and their constituent parts are either destroyed or recycled as precursors. Precursors derived from used neurotransmitter or from dietary intake are carried into the cell and then used to create the various elements we have been discussing here.

SECOND-MESSENGER EFFECTS

If the first messenger is the neurotransmitter, there are then **second-messengers** that cause second-messenger effects. These take more time than first-messenger effects, are more complicated, but also have a profound impact on neurotransmission. For example if a neurotransmitter attaches to a receptor it changes the shape of the receptor. Next it activates a "G" protein (discussed above) inside the cell membrane. The released element can then directly activate things like ion channels or indirectly activate enzymes like adenylyl cyclase. In this case the adenylyl cyclase then activates cyclic adenosine monophosphate (cyclic AMP) which is called the second messenger. The second messenger can have farther reaching effects like opening ion channels, changing enzymatic activities, or even affecting gene expression (Advokat et al., 2014). Compared with first-messenger effects, these second-messenger effects take longer to occur and last longer after they occur. The benefit of second-messenger effects is that they provide the cell with an efficient way to extend and amplify the cell's response to the transmitter (Bloom et al., 2005).

These first- and second-messenger effects may seem hard to imagine at first, but bear in mind that we are really just reviewing a sequence of events that affect the way the cell functions. Understanding of these events is still in the embryonic stage and will likely change a great deal over the next few years. Just remember that it is important to generally understand the sequence of neuronal events so you can understand (1) how psychotropic medications interfere with those events and (2) what effects are then correlated with specific types of interference. It is interesting to note that researchers hypothesize that second-messenger events can reach all the way back to the cell nucleus, where they may decrease the creation of receptors, reducing the sensitivity of the neuron. This effect, called **downregulation**, is one of the effects in a chain of events correlated with antidepressant-induced improvement in symptoms of depression. We return to this effect in Chapter Five. A second-messenger effect can also increase the synthesis of receptors, increasing the sensitivity of the neuron. This is called **upregulation**. Obviously not all these effects are necessarily good or therapeutic effects. These unwanted effects are called *side effects*, and one example caused by upregulation is **tardive dyskinesia**, an involuntary movement disorder. This is a side effect of older antipsychotic medications to which we return in Chapter Seven. We do want to note here that the further away from a first-messenger effect, the less well understood are the mechanisms of action.

A QUICK REVIEW

Let's review this information: A neuron gets a chemical impulse from a neurotransmitter that (via a first- or second-messenger system) may open ion channels or keep them closed. Depending on which channels are open, this leads the neuron to fire or not fire (exocytosis).

Firing causes the release of stored neurotransmitter and related events (exocytosis). The neurotransmitters shoot across the neuronal synapse to bind to receptors. Neurotransmitter binding to receptor is analogous to a key fitting into a lock. If the neurotransmitter in question (key) does not fit into the receptor structure (lock), binding does not occur there. If the fit is good enough, however, the chemical signal is changed into another electrical signal, and the process goes on.

WHAT HAPPENS WHEN NEUROTRANSMITTERS BIND TO RECEPTORS?

The neurotransmitter binding to the receptor is the first messenger. It may trigger changes alone or in the cell through second messengers. As a first messenger (quick signal), the neurotransmitter may alter the neuron's ionic gradient to make it fire, releasing more neurotransmitter. Depending on what type of receptor the neurotransmitter is binding to, it may inhibit the cell, preventing exocytosis.

The second messenger (slow signal) is an intracellular chain reaction created by the first-messenger neurotransmitter occupying the receptor. As noted, in second-messenger systems the neurotransmitter may change the shape of the intracellular part of the receptor. This change then triggers release of a portion of a G protein to either open ion channels or to bind intracellularly to an enzyme that may then cause subsequent changes inside the cell.

WHAT HAPPENS TO THE RELEASED NEUROTRANSMITTER?

The released neurotransmitter may be recycled and taken back into the cell by transporter molecules to be used later, it may be broken down by enzymes and its precursors reused by the cell at some point, or it may be broken down and metabolized.

This sequence of events can be altered by introducing psychotropic medications into the body, but as Stahl (2000) reminds us, that does not mean

researchers have even begun to understand these events or all the effects of psychotropic medications on these events (let alone why any of the latter would decrease the symptoms of mental or emotional disorders). As Stahl wrote, most of these events are still mysteries to neuroscientists. It is important to note there are nonchemical means of altering this sequence of events, such as aerobic exercise and meditation. We say more about such means later in the book.

Review Questions

- What is the wire-soup metaphor regarding brain functioning?
- What generally is the relationship between DNA, RNA, and mRNA?
- What are some basic functions of transporter molecules and enzymes in the brain?
- Give a rough outline of the "story" of neurotransmission.

SECTION SIX: PHARMACODYNAMICS OR HOW PSYCHOTROPIC MEDICATIONS AFFECT NEUROTRANSMISSION

Learning Objectives

- Be able to discuss what "agonism" and "antagonism" mean with regard to a drugs effects on the brain.
- Describe three broad mechanisms of how drugs interfere with the process of neurotransmission.

As we noted, we want you to understand the events of neurotransmission so that you can better understand how drugs interfere with those events and how the interference correlates with effects on symptoms. You have perhaps noticed that we keep avoiding the phrase "how drugs decrease symptoms of mental and emotional disorders." We are consciously avoiding it because, in most cases, scientists simply don't know how drugs specifically decrease symptoms. We want you to keep that in mind. This is one of the most compelling reasons for teaching psychopharmacology from multiple perspectives.

What scientists do know a good deal about is pharmacodynamics, defined as how drugs act (or try to act) in and on the body. Although this is a broad area, for our purposes we focus on 11 general mechanisms of drug action, with an example of each. Bear in mind that psychotropic drugs do not use all these mechanisms of action and may also exert more than one mechanism.

AGONISM AND ANTAGONISM

When discussing agonism and antagonism, we refer to the various mechanisms as causing agonist or antagonist effects. The easiest way to think of agonist or antagonist effects is in terms of what the cell would do naturally. Something that assists or facilitates a cell's functions is an agonist. An agonist facilitates an action. Something that interferes with an action is an antagonist. Because most cells fire naturally, anything that decreases the probability of this happening can be said to be an antagonist. Anything that increases the probability of this happening is an agonist. As usual, reality is more complex than this. This literature specifies not just agonism and antagonism but partial agonism, inverse agonism, partial inverse agonism, partial antagonism, inverse antagonism, and partial inverse antagonism. Although these concepts are much more exact, for this book the two broad categories of agonism and antagonism are enough.

MECHANISMS OF ACTION WITH EFFECTS ON PRODUCTION

Drugs can affect the intracellular production of various elements. Earlier we noted that transporters and other proteins carry into the neuron precursors from which things such as neurotransmitter are created. Drugs can interfere with this process by acting like precursors and thus increasing the amount of precursor material available. One such drug is levodopa/Sinemet. This drug basically functions as a precursor

to dopamine, allowing more dopamine to be made than normal. This is particularly important in Parkinson's disease, because the disease causes the degeneration of dopamine neurons and thus decreases available dopamine. The drug, at least for a while, corrects the shortage caused by degeneration of dopamine neurons. Levodopa/Sinemet is an example of a drug exerting an agonist action, because its end result is to help the cells do what they would naturally do.

Drugs can also inactivate enzymes whose job it is to create neurotransmitters. In this case, such a drug artificially decreases the levels of neurotransmitter in a cell by inactivating the enzymes that put the neurotransmitters together in the first place. Such a drug has an antagonist action, because it is stopping a cell from doing what it would do naturally. An example of a drug that acts in this manner is para-chlorophenylalanine/Fenclonine (PCPA). In addition to being a mouthful to say, this drug inactivates enzymes that create serotonin. Because the release of serotonin is necessary for inducing sleep, such a drug causes insomnia. Interestingly, it may also be one of the few aphrodisiacs in existence. Because serotonin is also related to subduing sexual response, animal studies have correlated hypersexuality with its artificial decrease from taking PCPA.

In our story of neurotransmission, we discussed transporters in and outside the cell that have various functions. One such function is the storage of newly created neurotransmitter molecules in the synaptic vesicles that protect them. The vesicles protect them from other enzymes whose job it is to break down neurotransmitter molecules. Thus, a drug that inactivates the transporter that carried the neurotransmitter into the synaptic vesicle leaves the neurotransmitter vulnerable to enzymatic breakdown. Such a drug, by interfering with this crucial storage, ultimately acts as an antagonist. Drugs using this mechanism of action also inactivate the proteins that help with exocytosis. A good example of a drug using these mechanisms of action is reserpine/Serpasil. Reserpine/Serapsil is no longer in the market, because it had unacceptable side effects, but its main mechanism of action affected acetylcholine, dopamine, norepinephrine, and serotonin.

It was used to investigate depression because it caused a depressogenic (depression–inducing) response in animals. In the 1950s, physicians also used reserpine as an antipsychotic.

Another mechanism of action that affects neurotransmitter production has to do with a special type of receptor called an *autoreceptor*. Autoreceptors seem to monitor levels of neurotransmitter in the synaptic cleft. For example, if there is enough dopamine in the synaptic cleft to bind to an autoreceptor, the autoreceptor sends a signal back into the neuron that basically says, "Slow down the synthesis and release of neurotransmitter." When an autoreceptor is open, production continues as normal. Thus, two mechanisms of action here may affect neuronal production of neurotransmitter. The first is a drug that blocks an autoreceptor antagonistically (sending no signal for the cell to slow down production of neurotransmitter). Such a blockage in fact results in more neurotransmitter being produced and released, because the mechanism to signal a decrease has been effectively disabled. Clonidine/Catapres works in this manner. The other mechanism is to introduce a drug that mimics the endogenous neurotransmitter and increases the signals going into the cell to slow down production and release of neurotransmitter.

MECHANISMS OF ACTION WITH EFFECTS ON RELEASE OF NEUROTRANSMITTER

As noted, the key element in exocytosis is the release of neurotransmitter into the synaptic cleft. Drugs may have mechanisms of action that can inhibit or facilitate this element. For example, drugs can stimulate the release of neurotransmitter from the terminal button. Such drugs act as agonists. Now here, remember our mantra. Students often assume that an agonist ultimately stimulates the nervous system, but this is clearly not true. We noted that the neurotransmitter GABA has an overall inhibiting influence on the nervous system, so if a drug facilitates the release of GABA that drug is still an agonist, whereas the end result of the

GABA release is ultimately inhibitory. Two substances that work by stimulating the release of neurotransmitter from the terminal button are black widow spider venom and sea anemone toxin. Both substances pierce the membranes of the neuron and synaptic vesicles, causing the neurotransmitter to leak out. In the case of the human central nervous system, after the human has been bitten by a black widow spider, the venom causes acetylcholine to leak out. Although most bites from a black widow spider are not usually lethal because the spider injects minute amounts of toxin when biting, the venom itself is 15 times as toxic as the venom from a prairie rattlesnake.

A substance that prevents the release of neurotransmitter from the neuron is botulinum toxin. This toxin has been anxiously discussed in the early 21st century as concerns about chemical warfare grow worldwide. Researchers estimate that one teaspoonful of pure botulinum toxin could kill the entire world's population (Carlson, 2001). This poison works by preventing the release of acetylcholine, which can paralyze muscles (including those used to breathe) and cause death. Oddly enough, diluted botulinum toxin is used dermatologically. Injected locally into wrinkled skin, it paralyzes the area, locally giving the skin a smoother appearance. The drug is available under the brand name Botox.

Another way that a drug can affect the release of neurotransmitter from the neuron is by imitating a first messenger. Nicotine is an excellent example. There are two subtypes of acetylcholine receptors: nicotinic and muscarinic. Acetylcholine binds to both types. Nicotine is structurally similar enough to acetylcholine to bind to the nicotinic receptors. Once there, it causes a release of the neurotransmitters in the neurons it binds to. This release is associated with the reinforcing properties of the drug. The body responds to the presence of nicotine by increasing the number of nicotinic receptors, resulting in the person needing more nicotine to get the desired effect (tolerance to the drug). This is why nicotine is associated with withdrawal symptoms. Although the number of nicotinic receptors eventually returns to the prenicotine state, this can take time, up to several months.

Drugs can also interfere with first-messenger effects by blocking receptors. In this instance, they block the receptor and exert no action; thus such drugs are antagonists. Older antipsychotics act in this fashion by blocking dopamine receptors and not allowing dopamine to bind. Curare also acts in this way by blocking acetylcholine receptors. As you may recall, acetylcholine is the neurotransmitter at most muscle–nerve junctions, so blocking the receptors in this area causes the paralysis for which curare is so well known.

MECHANISMS OF ACTION TARGETING NEUROTRANSMITTER DEACTIVATION

The two final mechanisms of action we outline are particularly known in antidepressants. They are both agonists in that they facilitate the action and duration of neurotransmitters in the synaptic cleft. The first is enzyme deactivation. As you may recall, once neurotransmitters are released into the synaptic cleft, enzymes that are also in the extracellular fluid can deactivate the neurotransmitters. By deactivating the enzymes that deactivate the neurotransmitters, a drug can artificially lengthen the amount of time the neurotransmitters can exert their influence in the synaptic cleft. Antidepressants called *monoamine oxidase inhibitors (MAO inhibitors)* work in this manner. The second mechanism of action that targets neurotransmitter deactivation is called *reuptake inhibition*. You will also recall that when neurotransmitters are in the synaptic cleft, they can be picked up by proteins called *transporter molecules* and taken back into the cell to be recycled. If a drug disables or slows down these transporter molecules, this drug effectively increases the length of time the neurotransmitters can exert their influence. Almost every antidepressant on the market uses this mechanism in some manner (except for MAO inhibitors).

Remember that a drug can use more than one of these mechanisms of action. It is also important to remember scientists simply do not know all the mechanisms of action for many drugs. It is hoped that future research will help map these mechanisms more effectively.

Review Questions

- Define "agonism" and "antagonism" with regard to the effects of drugs on the brain.
- Describe three broad mechanisms that drugs can use to interfere with neurotransmission.

SUMMARY

Although an integrative study of psychopharmacology involves more than physiology, physiology forms the base knowledge in the field. This knowledge base focuses on how psychotropic medications affect the central nervous system, which includes the brain and spinal cord. Medications can also impact the peripheral nervous system, including the sympathetic and parasympathetic nervous systems.

Understanding the story of neurotransmission is also crucial to understanding how psychotropic medication works. This understanding begins with learning about the structure of neurons, neurotransmitters, and their functions and interactions. The story of neurotransmission includes how neurotransmitters bind to receptors on neurons and the effects of this binding. Psychotropic medications can mimic or block binding, producing effects on the central nervous system. Once you understand the story of neurotransmission, you will better understand how psychotropic medications interfere with neurotransmission to produce various effects (some desired, some not).

This chapter has covered what we believe to be the most pertinent material on psychopharmacology from the medical model perspective. A basic understanding of the brain structures as well as the events involved in neurotransmission will facilitate mastering the subsequent material in the book on specific types of medications. We cannot overemphasize the importance of this, and we encourage the reader to work (in groups or individually) with the following Study Questions and Exercises.

CASE OF COLLEEN

Colleen is a 45-year-old single woman who has suffered from depression for 15 years. She has gotten relief from many SSRIs, but their effectiveness diminishes over time. She and her psychiatrist have tried fluoxetine, paroxetine, sertraline, and currently escitalopram oxalate. Colleen continues to complain of depressive mood, anhedonia at times, and a general lack of direction in her life. Her psychiatrist first considered a course of a low dose of valproate, a mood stabilizer, to ease her symptoms, but then remembered the six studies indicating that there is efficacy in combining aripiprazole, an atypical antipsychotic, in a very low dose with an SSRI.

Colleen agreed to try aripiprazole at 2 mg to determine if it could assist her. After eight days on the aripiprazole, Colleen noticed that she was agitated all the time and even very angry. This was not like her and she called her psychiatrist and, after a short discussion, he told Colleen to stop taking the aripiprazole immediately. In less than 36 hours, Colleen felt less agitated and angry. She continues to work with her psychiatrist and therapist on her depression.

Questions About the Case of Colleen

1. This case serves to introduce you to some of the dilemmas of psychopharmacology. Carefully discuss each concern with your instructor as each will serve as an advance organizer for a unit of the course. Almost every sentence stimulates a potential dilemma.

2. It appears that the use of aripiprazole triggered a negative pharmacodynamic reaction with Colleen. Speculate as to what you think might have happened?

CLASS EXERCISE: THE PSYCHODRAMATIC NEURON

Using placards that students can hang around their necks, label the primary parts in the story of neurotransmission. You will need cards to assign the following parts:

- Three receptors
- Three synaptic vesicles
- One transporter molecule
- One electrical charge
- Two enzymes
- Two ion channels

Mark off an area in your classroom to create a psychodramatic neuron. You can use a table or desk for the synaptic cleft. On one side, line up the synaptic vesicles (in the terminal button) of the presynaptic neuron. On the other side, line up the receptors. One enzyme stands at the end of the row opposite the makeshift cleft. This enzyme is going to put a neurotransmitter together from precursors. The other enzyme and one transporter molecule stand at the side of the table representing the cleft. These will compete for the neurotransmitter once it has bound to and released from the receptors. The person playing the electrical charge stands at the end of the row opposite the makeshift cleft. The people playing the ion channels stand outside the row; one holds a sign indicating a positive electrical charge whereas the other holds a sign indicating a negative electrical charge. Use Lego-type pieces for the neurotransmitter—about four pieces per neurotransmitter.

The action starts with each synaptic vesicle holding three neurotransmitters (each made of at least four Lego pieces). The electrical charge moves down the axon (the row). If the negative ion channel sign is in the row, the charge must stop and return to the top of the row. If the positive ion channel sign is in the row, the charge can proceed to the end, tapping the synaptic vesicles, which is their cue to "fire" the neurotransmitter into the cleft (set the Lego pieces on the table). The receptors should then pick up the neurotransmitter, one per hand only, count to five, then set them back down on the table. At this point, the enzyme and transporter compete for the released neurotransmitter. The transporter hands the neurotransmitter intact back to the synaptic vesicle, or the enzyme takes the neurotransmitter apart and carries the parts back to the enzyme near the soma, who puts them back together and carries them down the axon to the synaptic vesicles. The instructor should direct the action, stopping to interview the various parts, asking them what they are doing, what they will do next, and so on. As different drugs are introduced throughout the course, you can write them into the script of the psychodramatic neuron to show how they interfere with the action and exert their influences.

Although this exercise may seem odd, it really helps conceptualize the story of neurotransmission. The first author went to a Halloween party (come as your favorite neuron part) where the game was played well into the night.

STUDY QUESTIONS AND EXERCISES

1. Define the following terms: *psychopharmacology and pharmacodynamics.*

2. Describe the anatomy of a neuron. Include a definition of synapses and their critical importance in the process.

3. Discuss the importance of the blood–brain barrier and the qualities necessary for a psychotropic medication to cross this barrier.

4. Identify at least five primary neurotransmitters. Describe how each is thought to influence brain activity.

5. Outline the steps in the process of neurotransmission from exocytosis in the presynaptic neuron to reuptake and enzymatic breakdown of the released neurotransmitter.

6. Discuss the difference between an agonist and an antagonist, in the context of neurotransmission.

7. Discuss the various mechanisms of action through which psychotropic medications can interfere with neurotransmission.

CHAPTER THREE

Pharmacokinetics: How the Body Acts on Psychotropic Medications

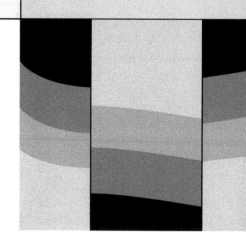

Pharmacokinetics is what your body does with a drug once you ingest it. Pharmacokinetics are the processes by which drugs are absorbed by the body, distributed within the body, and then metabolized, and excreted (Carlson, 2012). Obviously, to be effective a drug must reach its intended site of action. For psychotropic drugs, this intended site is the central nervous system, so the primary barrier that a drug must somehow get across is the blood–brain barrier. Pharmacokinetics also involves understanding the time course of a drug's effects (the intensity of the drug effect on the body across time). Understanding how a drug moves through the body and the length of time it takes to exert therapeutic effects can help clinicians understand what the client can and cannot expect from the drug. It is also important to understand that there is more than the drug involved in pharmacokinetics. For example, most of us know that grapefruit juice interferes with a large number of drugs making them less effective if they are taken around the same time as the grapefruit juice (Kiani & Imam, 2007; Marchetti & Schellens, 2007).

This chapter is divided into five sections. Section One discusses how drugs are absorbed into the body and the various routes of administration. Section Two covers what happens when drug molecules get to the bloodstream. In Section Three, we discuss drug distribution and important concepts like half-life and maintenance dose. In Section Four, we introduce drug binding and the various types of drug tolerance that one may develop. Finally in Section Five, we give an overview of how drugs are eliminated from the body.

SECTION ONE: DRUG ABSORPTION

Learning Objectives

- Be able to describe the various routes of drug administration.
- Understand why some methods of administration may be optimal for particular clients.
- Understand the concept of Lipophilicity.

How a drug gets into the bloodstream and is distributed throughout the body is referred to as **drug absorption**. In psychopharmacology, the primary aim is for drugs to get across the blood–brain barrier and into the central nervous system, the brain specifically. How do we determine how fast a drug gets to the brain? How do we know how much of the drug ingested reaches the brain? The answers to these questions depend on multiple variables (Ettinger, 2011). Some of the answers are found by examining routes of administration.

Routes of Administration

What is the first thing you must do with a drug for it to have its desired effect? Take it, of course. There are several ways you can do this that we call routes of administration, although not all are commonly used for administering psychotropic medications. The most common route is oral. For a drug to be taken orally, the drug must be capable of being dissolved (soluble) and must retain its integrity in the stomach fluids. This is one reason there are no psychopharmacologically effective nicotine products one swallows. Nicotine cannot withstand stomach fluids and breaks down before it can get to the central nervous system to exert its effects. So if you hear of an energy drink advertising nicotine for the "extra jolt," save your money. The closest to an oral administration one can get with nicotine is through gum, dissolving tabs or mouth spray (Bolliger, van Biljon, & Axelsson, 2007). The speed with which a substance moves from the site of administration to the bloodstream is called absorption and this rate varies depending on the route of administration. Following are summaries of the more common routes of administration some of which will not be as relevant to psychopharmacology but which we include here for the sake of thoroughness.[1]

Oral Administration

The most common route of drug administration for psychotropic medications is oral administration. Drugs taken orally can be in the form of tablets, capsules, liquid, and other types of pills. Some of the delivery systems are designed to be time-released (such as capsules for time-released methylphenidate/*Concerta/Focalin*). These drugs have to dissolve in stomach fluid and pass through the walls of the digestive tract to reach capillaries. Then the molecules enter the bloodstream and will eventually cross the blood–brain barrier. Obviously the drug must also be able to withstand stomach acids and other substances that break down food. Many drugs are not fully absorbed until they reach the small intestine. How quickly the contents of the stomach move into the small intestine depends on whether food is fatty (fatty foods slow movement), the amount of food in the system, the amount of physical activity the person engages in all make it difficult to predict how long it will take for an orally administered drug to reach its intended site of action (Meyer & Quenzer, 2005). Advantages of oral administration include safety and ease-of-use. Disadvantages include being a slower

route with different rates of absorption based on the body type, age, sex of the client and of course gastrointestinal side effects.

The fat solubility of the drug molecule also plays a role. **Lipophilicity** (think: "liposuction") refers to the fat solubility of a compound. Because the walls of the intestines, blood vessels, and neurons are composed of fats called **lipids**. The more fat soluble a drug is, the more easily it crosses these barriers. Some drugs, such as lithium, are not at all fat soluble (lipophilicitous) and must attach to another molecule and be carried across the barriers.

Inhalation

Inhalation is a predictable and direct route of administration with many applications. Inhalation is a fast and efficient delivery system because the lungs (part of the **pulmonary system**) constitute a large surface for absorption that is rich with capillaries that send substances directly to the brain without going through the heart first (Meyer & Quenzer, 2005). Recreational drug users such as cigarette smokers learn early on how efficient and rewarding this delivery system can be. Although we know of no psychotropic compounds taken by inhaler (other than experimental nicotine mouth sprays), cannabis (which has psychotropic properties) inhalers have been examined by the United Kingdom and Canada for administration of medical marijuana through vaporization. Vaporizers like the "Volcano" seem to be able to deliver cannabis with fewer harmful toxins like carbon monoxide, benzene, and other known carcinogens (Frood, 2007a). At the time of this writing, the states of Washington and Colorado decriminalized marijuana although federal laws still prohibit its use. Time will tell if this drug will make its way into the licit psychotropic substances (Frood, 2007b).

Injection

There are several types of injection: Subcutaneous, intramuscular, intravenous, and epidural. Subcutaneous is an injection just below the skin. The absorption depends on the rate of blood flow to the area of injection but the absorption rate is usually slow and prolonged. Drugs that are injected subcutaneously include hormones, birth control

---

[1]Some less common methods include intracranial (into the brain) and intraperitoneal (into the cavity surrounding the abdominal organs) which are not used for psychotropic medications.

drugs, and drugs for migraine headaches like Suma-triptan/Imitrex. Intramuscular injections are slow acting but produce more even absorption. Depending on the injection site and the blood flow to that area absorption usually occurs within an hour. Drugs can be mixed with substances (e.g., oils) that can slow the absorption. Many antipsychotics are now administered intramuscularly because disorders such as Schizophrenia frequently disrupt cognitive functions and interfere with routines and remembering to take medications. Intravenous injections are directly into the bloodstream and are the most rapid and precise ways to administer a drug (Ettinger, 2011). In this method, the drug does not pass through the lungs or digestive system. The downside to intravenous administration is that complications can prove lethal because the drug is getting into the system so quickly and directly. Epidural injections are used primarily for spinal anesthetics. In these cases, the drugs are administered directly into the cerebrospinal fluid surrounding the spinal cord bypassing the blood–brain barrier. The most common use of these is for facilitating analgesia in childbirth but no psychotropic medications are administered in this manner.

Transdermal Administration

Transdermal administration is done through a "patch" technology where the drug to be administered is on a patch that is then attached via adhesive to the skin. Because the skin is resistant to water passing through but allows fat soluble molecules through this can be a useful formulation. Nicotine patches, opioids for pain, and contraceptives are all examples of drugs that may be administered this way. Recently, (Azzaro, Ziemniak, Kemper, Campbell, & VanDenBerg, 2007) the antidepressant selegiline (an MAO inhibitor) was approved in a transdermal formulation. Although transdermal administration is a way to get controlled rates of absorption, it can cause skin irritation in some clients.

Rectal Administration

Rectal administration is less efficient than oral or inhaler administrations but can be useful for patients who have digestive tract difficulties. Again, we know of no rectally administered psychotropic medications. Although this route of administration would be faster acting than oral, the disadvantages are obvious to most people.

Mucus Membrane (transmucosal) Administration

Drugs can be administered via the mucus membranes (mouth or nose), which result in fairly direct absorption into the bloodstream. Drugs commonly administered this way include nicotine (gum), decongestants, and nitroglycerine for cardiac patients (Advocat, Comaty, & Julien 2014). This can be advantageous for clients like children who have trouble swallowing pills.

Review Questions

- Explain three routes of drug administration and some advantages and disadvantages of each.
- What route of administration would be good for a client who suffers from cognitive symptoms and why?
- Why is it important that psychotropic medications be highly fat soluble?

SECTION TWO: GETTING TO THE BLOODSTREAM

Learning Objectives

- Understand what a protein transporter is and the role it could play in medications getting to their intended site of action.
- Be able to describe the process of drug diffusion.
- Be able to describe the blood–brain barrier, its function and how drugs pass through it.

Cell Membrane Permeability

Once administered, a drug must pass through multiple membranes to reach the site of action which for psychotropic medications is the brain. The route of administration will determine which membranes the drug must pass through. Regardless of the route of administration, the cells lining the stomach, lungs, and the cells making up skin, muscle, and fat cells are composed of a **phospholipid biolayer** (two layers of lipid molecules that form a polar membrane). Phospholipids are the major components of cell membranes (so named because they contain an organic molecule from the phosphate group). Remember that lipids are molecules including fats and it is fats that we are interested in here. As written above, the drug molecules must be fat-soluble enough to pass through these membranes. The head of a phospholipid is positively charged and the tail negatively charged (thus "polar" membrane). Although the head attracts water, the tails repel water and prevent water-soluble elements from getting through. Embedded in these phospholipid molecules are proteins that act as transporters. For something to pass through the cell membrane, they must be carried through by the transporter or be fat soluble, which, as stated, most psychotropic medications are (Ettinger, 2011).

Drugs must also pass in and out of capillaries which are a route into the bloodstream. They are made of a single layer of cells that, though tightly packed, have gaps in them. Drug molecules can move through these gaps in a process called **diffusion**. This is how organisms exchange food, waste, gasses, and heat with their surroundings. The rate of diffusion is represented by Fick's law, which states that diffusive flux goes from regions of high concentration to regions of low concentration. This is affected by the thickness of the membrane through which molecules are diffusing, the surface area for gas exchange, and the mass and fat solubility of the molecule. Movement across membranes is in the direction from higher to lower concentrations. The larger the concentration gradient (the difference between levels of the molecule between the two sides of the membrane) the more rapid the diffusion. Drugs that are lipid soluble move through cell membranes via passive diffusion, which leaves the water in the blood or stomach and moves into the membrane (Meyer & Quenzer, 2005).

As noted in Chapter Two, psychotropic medications must also cross the blood–brain barrier. The brain requires more protection from foreign substances than other organs so the capillary walls do not have gaps. The gaps are surrounded by a type of glial cell called an **astrocyte**. These make up the blood–brain barrier. Over 100 years ago, Paul Ehrlich discovered that if blue dye is injected into an animal's bloodstream (in his case a rabbit's bloodstream), all the tissues are tinted blue *except* the brain. You must inject the dye into the brain ventricles to get that tissue to turn blue. Although Ehrlich was working for a dye company on a different project, he thus unwittingly discovered the blood–brain barrier. This barrier blocks many substances from entering the central nervous system. In some areas, the barrier is weaker than others, to allow specific functions that have developed through evolution. One example of such an area is the *area postrema*, which signals vomiting. The barrier is weak here, so toxins in the blood can be detected. Once it detects toxins, the brain triggers the vomiting response to preserve the organism.

The blood–brain barrier serves an important survival function by keeping foreign elements such as toxins out of the brain. But what about things such as nutrients? Nutrients such as glucose must be transported through the capillary walls by special proteins. This is very important, because to exert their effects all current psychotropic medications must reach the central nervous system. To do so, they must pass through the blood–brain barrier. The glial cells that make up the blood–brain barrier have a high fat content. The myelination of the brain in infancy is one reason babies need a lot of fat in their diet.

Drugs will also cross the placental barrier. The placental barrier allows nutrients and oxygen from the mother's blood to cross into the baby's blood. Mothers taking medications are also passing some of those medications on to the baby. The evidence on psychotropic medications used during breastfeeding is at the time of this writing limited for most drugs but particularly antipsychotics, hypnotics, and anxiolytics. Because we cannot formulate any generalizations about the use of these medications due to the dearth of data there is inherent risk for breast-feeding mothers who choose to use psychotropics. Fortinguerra, Clavenna, and Bonati (2014) analyzed 183 peer-reviewed papers that studied 62 psychotropic drugs. Of these only 30% were thought to be safe during lactation according to an evidence-based approach. Genung (2013) concluded that "medications have the same, though exaggerated, targets and side effects on infants as on adults. Therefore, each prescribed medication must be researched individually. Even small amounts of medications can accumulate to toxic amounts in breastfed infants" (p. 217).

Review Questions

- What is the role of transporters in drugs getting to the brain?
- What is the process of drug diffusion?
- Describe the blood–brain barrier, its function, what it is made of, and how it affects psychotropic medications.

SECTION THREE: DRUG DISTRIBUTION

Learning Objectives

- Be able to describe the concepts of half-life and steady state.
- Understand what the cytochrome P450 enzyme system is and why it is important for drug metabolism.
- Be able to describe what titration and a maintenance dose are.

Once a drug is absorbed into the bloodstream it is distributed through the body in the circulating blood. In many cases most of the drug will not reach the intended site (in the case of psychotropic medications the receptors in the brain) but is active in other parts of the body. Advokat, Comaty, and Julien (2014) note that most of any dose of a psychoactive drug is circulating outside the brain and is not contributing directly to the pharmacological effects. This widespread distribution may contribute to side effects, for example, antidepressants causing

nausea by their effects on the serotonin receptors in the digestive tract.

Your entire blood volume circulates through your body approximately once per minute. Usually within this minute the drug taken is distributed throughout the bloodstream. The route of administration will affect how much of the drug actually makes it into the bloodstream. For example, after oral administration the drug is reduced by enzymes in the digestive tract. Then veins leading away from the digestive tract flow through the liver further metabolizing part of the drug. This is called **first-pass metabolism** and may require that more of the drug be administered than if it were given intravenously (Advokat et al., 2014).

A drug's half-life tells us how long it stays in the body. The half-life is what the words sound like— the length of time it takes for the blood level of a drug to fall by half. So at one half-life, 50% of the initial dose is out of the bloodstream (much of it redistributed to the tissues of the body). At two half-lives, 75% of the initial dose is out of the bloodstream. At three half-lives, 87.5% of the drug is out of the bloodstream. So for each half-life, half of the drug remaining is redistributed out of the bloodstream. Advokat et al. (2014) estimate that the drug persists at low levels for at least six half-life cycles. Even though a drug half-life can be estimated it can vary person to person. Elderly people are going to take longer to metabolize a drug than a young person in their 20s. Half-life only applies to blood plasma levels, not the presence of the drug in other places like the central nervous system.

Half-life is also used to gauge what is called the steady state of the drug in the patient's body. This is roughly the amount of the drug in the patient's blood with regular dosing. The goal is to match a particular level of the drug with therapeutic results and then match dosing to achieve that level. This latter then becomes the maintenance dose, the dose needed to maintain levels of the drug linked to therapeutic response. The process of arriving at an optimal maintenance dose is called titration. When a doctor increases or decreases the amount of the drug to maximize therapeutic response we say she is titrating the dose up or down.

TABLE 3.1 Five Important Pharmacokinetic Terms

Half-life	Amount of time required for plasma concentration of a drug to decrease by 50% after a person stops taking it.
Steady state	The state when the concentrations of a drug in a person's bloodstream reach a plateau so that the amount being taken in each dose is roughly equivalent to the amount being eliminated.
Loading dose	An initial dose of drug that is higher than subsequent doses, given for the purpose of achieving therapeutic levels rapidly.
Maintenance dose	The regular dose of the medication that maintains the steady-state plasma concentration in the therapeutic range.
Titration	The art and science of balancing a drug dose against the patient's symptoms. Upward titration is gradually increasing the dose, and downward titration is gradually decreasing the dose.

© Cengage Learning®

Whenever you put a drug into your system, your body begins metabolizing it and trying to get rid of it. Drugs leave the body through the urine, perspiration, and exhalation. The hepatic system (liver) is one of the main metabolizers of drugs. Enzymes break down the drugs and the most common enzyme family is the **Cytochrome P450 enzyme system** about which more will be said later. The liver enzymes turn the drug into less active or inactive water soluble metabolites that are then sent to the renal system and filtered out by the kidneys. There are some terms related to drug metabolism that are helpful to know. The first is **elimination half-life**. The drug's half-life is the amount of time it takes for half of the drug's initial blood level to decrease by half or 50%. A drug's half-life may range from hours to days. The prescribing doctor's goal is to prescribe a dose of the drug that, based on the half-life, will result in a steady blood level of the drug sometimes called **steady state**.

Table 3.1 defines concepts related to pharmacokinetics: half-life, steady state, loading dose, maintenance dose, and titration. These terms are frequently used in medical practice and may be confusing to the layperson. Clients often ask questions about these terms. One client mistakenly thought he could stop taking medication after the loading dose because he interpreted "loading" in a manner akin to computer software—once loaded, no further loading needed. The half-life is particularly important in understanding how long it takes a drug to clear out of a person's system. This concept is helpful in explaining to clients why they are still experiencing side effects days after discontinuing medication.

Review Questions

- What is the relationship between a drug half-life and a steady state of the same drug?
- Describe the function of the cytochrome P450 enzyme system and its affects on psychotropic medications.
- What is meant by a maintenance dose?

SECTION FOUR: DRUG BINDING AND TYPES OF TOLERANCE

Learning Objectives

- Be able to recite the primary flaws in the theory that mental disorders were caused by a chemical imbalance in the brain.
- Understand depot binding and the effects on the plasma levels of medications.
- Be able to describe the types of drug tolerance.

Once in the blood plasma, drugs then are redistributed to various tissues including the central nervous system (a process labeled redistribution). The molecules then bind to particular target sites. In the case of psychopharmacology, these sites have typically been neurotransmitter receptor sites. As we will illustrate throughout this book, in the 20th century it was long believed (and the belief was perpetuated by billions of dollars in advertising and planned publications from pharmaceutical companies) that mental disorders were caused by a chemical imbalance in the brain. *We now have enough evidence to know that, in fact, is not the case and the idea has been falsified.* The fact that a chemical intervention alleviates or decreases symptoms in no way means the chemicals affected by the intervention were imbalanced to begin with anymore than if someone feels better after smoking marijuana it means they have a cannabinoid imbalance.

In the past few years, pharmaceutical companies are closing their neuroscience research facilities (Greenberg, 2013). In part this has been because *despite* the belief that psychotropic medications corrected a chemical imbalance, the success rate of many of these drugs is modest at best. [For example, meta-analyses suggest antidepressants are only better than placebo 50% of the time (Khan, Leventahl, Khan, & Brown, 2002).] Another problem has been a steep increase in the number of lawsuits and amounts in settlements where companies were fined for questionable practices linked to psychotropic medications. In 2012 alone, companies paid over $5 billion in fines related to allegations of fraud including misleading claims about drug safety (Associated Press, 2009; Isaacs, 2013). That said, it remains to be seen how much new research will be done on pharmacological interventions because we know that mental and emotional disorders are more complex than brain chemistry. Certainly current medications that target receptors sites will be used for symptom control so understanding binding is still important. Until we can understand the etiology of mental disorders, symptom control may be the best we can do.

Although we know from Chapter Two that drugs bind to receptors to cause main effects, it is important to note that drugs may also bind at sites where there appear to be no measurable effects. These sites are called drug depots and they include plasma protein, fat and muscle. Depot binding does effect drug action in that it decreases the concentration of the drug at sites of action because only freely circulating drugs can pass across membranes. Also because these molecules will eventually unbind and re-enter bloodstream it can lead to higher-than-expected plasma levels and in some cases drug overdose (Meyer & Quenzer, 2005).

Types of Tolerance

It is important to generally understand the types of tolerance clients can develop to drugs. Please note that in this book we avoid using the word "addiction." The emotional hysteria around this word, and the lack of operational definitions, make it too inexact to be helpful. Physical dependence is linked with the term *addiction* and implies that withdrawal signs are "bad" and only linked to drugs of abuse. This is far from the truth because severe withdrawal signs can follow cessation of such therapeutic drugs such as SSRI antidepressants.

Instead, we discuss types of tolerance and dependence. Advokat et al. (2014) define **tolerance** as the state of reduced responsiveness to the same dose of a drug. This can be produced by a variety of mechanisms, all of which result in the person needing increased doses of the drug to achieve the effects previously provided by lower doses. **Dependence** is defined as a physical tolerance produced by repeated administration of a drug and a concomitant withdrawal syndrome when the drug is discontinued. Julien outlines three primary types of tolerance: metabolic, cellular, and behavioral conditioning processes.

Metabolic tolerance is an increase in the enzymes that metabolize a drug, an increase caused by the presence of that or similarly acting drug. The most common enzyme system for metabolizing drugs is the **cytochrome P450 enzyme** family. These enzymes, produced in the liver, have evolved over 3.5 billion years to accomplish the detoxification (metabolism) of ingested elements such as chemicals and food toxins. There are several families of these enzymes, some more specific to certain substances than others. Thus, metabolic tolerance begins when you take a drug that is broken down by any one of these families. If you take the drug consistently, your body responds by elevating the level of enzymes needed to break the substance down. The elevated enzyme level breaks down the drug more efficiently, leading to the need for a larger dosage; thus the cycle begins. The drug, the amount taken, and the individual body's response to it, all determine the pattern of metabolic tolerance. This pattern does not inevitably spiral out of control to the point where the drug cannot be used. For example, many people take benzodiazepines such as Valium or Xanax on an "as needed" (p.r.n., from the Latin *pro re nata*, meaning "as needed") basis. Such a person may only take 0.25 mg of Xanax once or twice a week. Such a low dose is unlikely to produce any problems with metabolic tolerance. This raises another important point, though, namely that similar drugs can produce **cross-tolerance**. For example, if the same person who took one dose of alprazolam (brand name Xanax) once or twice a week was in the habit of drinking two to three alcoholic beverages each day, probably he or she would not get as much response from the Xanax as someone who only drank two to three alcoholic beverages per week. The person drinking alcohol daily has likely developed some metabolic tolerance to it, and the families of enzymes that break down alcohol are also involved in breaking down Xanax, thus diminishing the effect of the latter. For the record, anyone taking a benzodiazepine such as Xanax or Valium should not drink alcohol.

Cellular tolerance, which is more related to pharmacodynamics, occurs when receptors in the brain adapt to the continued presence of a drug. Two common forms of cellular adaptation are downregulation and upregulation. In downregulation, neurons decrease the number and/or sensitivity of receptors because of the presence of a drug. In upregulation, neurons *increase* the number of receptors. Another type of tolerance is **associative tolerance**. This is where one would display tolerance to a drug in some but not all settings. What seems to be the case is that contextual cues associated with drug onset act as conditioned stimuli that can bring about tolerance (Ettinger, 2011). This is one reason that if someone addicted to drugs returns to the same context they may have a higher chance of relapse. Finally, **behavioral tolerance** is similar to **state-dependent** learning. When animals are given intoxicating doses of alcohol before a learning task, they subsequently tend to perform that particular task better when under the influence of alcohol than when sober. This is behavioral tolerance.

Review Questions

- Why did people believe mental disorders were caused by chemical imbalances in the brain and what is the main weakness in that idea?
- What is depot binding?
- List and describe the different types of drug tolerance.

SECTION FIVE: ELIMINATION OF DRUGS

Learning Objectives

- Understand the role and relationship between the kidneys and liver in drug metabolism.
- Understand the promise and obstacles of pharmacogenetics.

The phrase "termination of drug action" refers primarily to the routes through which a drug leaves the body. These include bile (the fluid produced by the liver), the kidneys, lungs, and the skin. The majority of drugs are excreted by the kidneys and thus have to be transformed into more water soluble compounds (remember that psychotropic drugs typically begin as fat-soluble agents). In most cases, these transformations make the drugs less active as well. In this section, we will discuss the role of the kidneys and liver in drug elimination as well as other factors that may affect elimination.

The Renal System

The renal or urinary system consists of two kidneys, ureters (tubes that propel urine from the kidneys to the bladder), bladder, and urethra, which connects the bladder to the genitals for removal of urine. Like the brain kidneys are amazing organs. They constitute about 1% of our body weight and (similar to the brain) receive about 20% of the blood supplied by each heart beat. The kidneys excrete the majority of body metabolism products using functional units called nephrons, which number anywhere between 800,000 and 1.5 million. Nephrons consist of a "knot" of capillaries. Our blood enters these capillaries from the renal artery. Nephrons maintain concentrations of water in the blood; regulate blood volume, blood pressure, and the blood's acidity (ph); and process secretion and reabsorption of things like ions, carbohydrates, and amino acids. The fluids filtered out of the capillaries are held in a chamber called "Bowman's Capsule" from which they collect in ducts and are passed into the bladder. Drugs that are fat soluble (lipophilicitous) can easily cross the membranes of the renal system. Because most psychotropic drugs have to be fat soluble to cross the blood–brain barrier, they are readily reabsorbed from the renal system and back into the bloodstream making the kidneys only one system through which psychotropic medications exit the body.

The Liver and Drug Metabolism

Because the kidneys do not totally break down psychotropic medications, another system is necessary to effect their elimination from the body. The liver provides many functions including protein synthesis, production of enzymes for digestion and detoxification. The main tissue of the liver is made of hepatocytes and it is these that pick up reabsorbed psychotropic medications and transform them with enzymes that make them less fat soluble and more likely to be excreted in the urine. There are several enzyme systems or families in the liver but the most referenced in regard to pharmacokinetics is the cytochrome P450 enzyme system. According to Advokat et al. (2014), the genes involved in the development of this system originated over 3 billion years ago for the purpose of metabolizing and detoxifying elements from the

environment that find their way into our system. The P450 enzyme family is frequently mentioned in package inserts and other information about drugs citing the effects of the drug on the P450 system.

Other Factors Affecting Pharmacokinetics

We have learned a great deal in the late 20th and early 21st centuries about variables that can affect a drug's effects on the body. There are genes that can affect pharmacokinetics and the study of such factors is coming to be called pharmacogenetics (Perlis, 2007). One example is a gene labeled ABCB1 that is responsible for a protein (P-Glycoprotein) that regulates absorption and elimination of many psychotropic (and other) drugs. Variations of this gene can act as predictors of treatment outcome as well as the effects of polypharmacy (Akamine, Yasui-Furukori, Ieiri, & Uno, 2012). Advokat et al. (2014) wrote that as genetic testing becomes more common and affordable, testing will be accessible to determine how a person metabolizes certain drugs anywhere on a continuum from slow to fast. It should be noted that substantial ethical and financial obstacles must be dealt with before this is going to be a widespread practice (Morley & Hall, 2004; Mutsatsa & Currid, 2013).

Another field that has grown in the 21st century is **ethnopharmacotherapy** (now more frequently referred to as ethnopsychopharmacology) that explores differences in the way different groups are affected by medications. Although we each share over 99% of our genes with all other humans, small differences linked to race and ethnicity may play roles in how particular people respond to a medication. For example, studies have supported the idea that pharmacokinetics may vary in people of Asian descent resulting in different dosing requirements and side-effect profiles (Wong, 2012). A similar area is the growing discipline of developmental pharmacology. One of the great gaps of knowledge in psychotropic medication use is the long-term effects of medications in pediatric populations. The Clinton administration passed one of the first bills to offer incentives to companies for running more trials with children and adolescents but our knowledge is still far from complete. Currently, we know that there are significant developmental differences in changes in drug absorption, distribution, metabolism, and elimination. There are also developmental differences in the development of enzymes to break down drugs (van den Anker, 2010). At the other end of the developmental spectrum we need more data on how psychotropic medications affect elderly clients. The same issues that are relevant in pediatric populations arise at the other end of the lifespan spectrum. Concerns about impaired absorption, factors slowing distribution and variables interfering with metabolism are all important aspects of what is coming to be called geriatric psychopharmacology (Grossberg, 2010; Howland, 2009b).

Review Questions

- What is the relationship between the liver and the kidneys in metabolizing and excreting drugs?
- What is pharmacogenetics? What are some of the promises and obstacles of this new field?

CASE

Learning Objectives

- Apply an understanding of pharmacokinetics to the case of a person.
- Understand how changes in the body or inputs to the body can impact how the body handles the medication.

A 53-year-old female is on a regimen of lithium (mood stabilizer) and an atypical antipsychotic, Seroquel, for Bipolar I Disorder. For six months, she was stable and asymptomatic. Although she had significant side effects including weight gain and sedation, she resolved to stay on the medications as long as they reduced her symptoms. Unexpectedly, she developed confusion, tremor and agitation. When her lithium level was measured, it showed a toxic concentration level of 2.4. When the patient's medication regimen was analyzed, it turned out that one week before the confusion she started taking over the counter Tylenol 650 mg three times a day. She did not inform her counselor or the prescribing physician of the over-the-counter use of Tylenol. According to the physician, the Tylenol was reducing urinary clearance of lithium raising lithium plasma levels leading to toxicity. Although she had been warned not to use over-the-counter medications without her doctor's approval, her symptoms and mental functioning are such that she claims (and we believed her) that she forgot about the warning.

Questions About the Case

1. Does this case represent an example of pharmacokinetics? Why?

2. In your own words try to describe what happened to this patient/client once she began taking the Tylenol?

3. How could a nonmedical mental health professional assist this client with remembering restrictions related to her medication?

CHAPTER FOUR

Psychological, Social, and Cultural Issues in Psychopharmacology

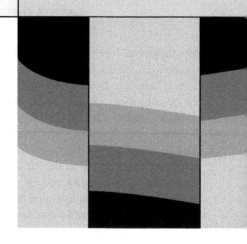

This chapter is divided into four sections. Section One provides an overview of issues surrounding adherence and compliance with medication prescriptions. Section Two addresses how to speak with clients about medications. Section Three covers the new subdiscipline of ethnopharmacotherapy and Section Four provides an overview of how institutions like pharmaceutical companies are impacting mental health practice.

SECTION ONE: ADHERENCE AND COMPLIANCE WITH MEDICATION REGIMENS

Learning Objectives

- Understand the difference between compliance and adherence.
- Be able to discuss the different ways clients conceptualize their symptoms.
- Be able to discuss common reasons people do not comply with medication regimens.
- Know the predictors of noncompliance and therapeutic ways to work through them with clients.

Many psychological issues that clients have related to psychotropic medications are illustrated in discussing **compliance** with medication. Even when a person suffers from terrible **ego-dystonic symptoms**, if taking medication is incongruent with the person's self-image, noncompliance or nonadherence may be

an issue. Compliance is the overall extent to which a client takes medication as prescribed. **Adherence** is more specific, referring to the extent that the client takes the prescribed medication at the exact time and in the correct dose (Demyttenaere, 2001). We include adherence in our general discussion of compliance.

We recall one client (Agnes) who interpreted taking a medication as a sign of weakness that she avoided thinking about. Agnes had lost her husband one month before she consulted a physician for her "nerves." Her physician was torn as to the best course of action. Under earlier diagnostic manuals (e.g., *DSM-IV-TR*, APA, 2000), she was experiencing uncomplicated bereavement, which is a developmentally normal event following loss of a loved one. However, she was not eating or sleeping, and met the *DSM-5* (American Psychiatric Association [APA], 2013) criteria for a Major Depressive Episode. *DSM-5* omitted the exclusion not to diagnose someone with depression if they had just lost a loved one [a move many in the field are critical of (Frances, 2013)].

Agnes asked if there were medication to "calm her nerves" but then became agitated stating that taking the medication would be a sign of weakness. The doctor wisely refrained from prescribing and connected Agnes with grief counseling. In the counseling sessions, Agnes revealed that the bottom line was "anyone who would take a pill for their mind is crazy." Her response was clearly related to her own perceptions of psychotropic medication, which reflected the cultural stigma attached to mental/emotional disorders, particularly for a woman in her 70s.

Understanding such stigma is an important variable in understanding clients who may resist or feel conflicted about taking medication (Knudsen, Hansen, Traulsen, & Eskildsen, 2002), but the stigma seems to vary from generation to generation; from culture to culture (Britten, 1998; Priest, Vize, Roberts, & Tylee, 1996). Mental health professionals must be willing to commit the time with clients to explore issues such as stigma. For Agnes, cognitive techniques helped her reframe and metabolize her grief but ultimately her mind was made up about psychotropic medication and, right or wrong, it was not of therapeutic value to challenge it.

CLIENT REACTIONS TO THE MEDICAL MODEL OF MENTAL ILLNESS

Some qualitative studies examine the way clients perceive the medical model description of their symptoms. In one study of women suffering from symptoms of schizophrenia (Sayre, 2000), most of the sample seemed to have been given a medical model explanation of their symptoms (e.g., "Schizophrenia is a brain disorder"). Client responses fell into six general categories. The members of one group more or less accepted the disease explanation and viewed their problems as related to some externally caused illness that could be treated with medication. The members of another group (labeled the "problem group") saw their symptoms as arising from personal qualities and behaviors that were the root causes. The members of a third group (the "crisis group") viewed their symptoms as a response to some crisis or other recent stressor. In a fourth group (the "ordination group"), the members saw their symptoms as a sign of special powers or responsibilities. Although this explanation is similar to tales of initiation told in shamanic traditions of many indigenous people, in this case the explanations were more consonant with the symptom profile than any spiritual crisis. In the fifth group (the "punishment group"), members saw their symptoms as punishment for past actions. In the final group (the "violation group"), members viewed their hospitalization as an attack on them by hospital staff and the idea that they had an illness an excuse for detaining them. In the case of schizophrenia, although there is strong support for a theory of biological etiology, the symptom presentation is still heterogeneous.

Even if a clinician believes the etiology of a disorder is more physical than mental (e.g., more brain than mind), it is important for the therapeutic relationship to consider the way a client makes meaning of his or her symptoms. Clearly, some perceptions of illness recorded in the Sayre (2000) study may reflect the illness more than they represent any personal or cultural aspects of the client. For example, **illusions** or **hallucinations** may be perceived as a sign of special powers (as in shamanic initiation) but also may reflect **megalomania**, which manifests in many people suffering from severe disorders such as schizophrenia or Bipolar I Disorder.

It is important to remember that some clients prefer to use the medical model perspective to explain their symptoms. In such cases, a psychological perspective can help counselors understand why some clients have this preference. Although ideally clients will become able to face all the variables related to their symptoms, this may take time. In some cases of depression, the medical model may provide a good explanation; however, where the depression is **overdetermined**, the medical model may serve as what Yalom (1995) called an "explanatory fiction"—an explanation that is more allegory than fact corresponding to some external truth. One client (let's call him James) had low **self-efficacy** and was actively suicidal. This followed a series of difficult life events, including the loss of a job, being dumped by a longtime girlfriend, and the death of his mother from pancreatic cancer. Clearly, these life experiences were strongly related to his depression but for James, the explanatory fiction of his depression as a medical illness made it easier to accept help in the form of counseling and antidepressant medication. James took the antidepressants for eight months while also engaging in counseling. After eight months, his doctor titrated him off the medication. James terminated the counseling relationship after one year, at which time he was functioning much better.

The medical model as explanatory fiction or useful metaphor is illustrated in the notion that alcoholism (or any substance dependence) is a "disease" with a biological etiology. This notion is not supported by science or logic (Ross & Pam, 1995), but rather on the agenda of the group defining it. The Veterans' Administration does not refer to alcohol dependence as a disease while the American Medical Association does. Defining alcohol-related problems as a "disease" can also steer us away from research supporting moderation management in some drinkers [e.g., some people can have an alcohol problem at one point in their life then return to moderate drinking (Hester, Delaney, & Campbell, 2011)]. On the constructive side, the metaphor of alcohol dependence as a disease has helped some clients avoid becoming crippled by guilt and self-recrimination so they can more fruitfully engage in treatment. Certainly the reverse holds true as well—some clients use the metaphor of alcoholism as a disease to avoid taking any responsibility for their drinking ("I can't help it—I have a disease"). Ethically, the clinician needs to know when the medical model perspective seems to be the best explanation for symptoms and when it seems the best metaphor to help the client engage in treatment. When metaphors are mistaken for facts, however, the potential exists for damaging word magic. One example is that in many polls, Americans believe that people who once have a problem with alcohol must abstain totally for the rest of their lives (Lillenfeld, Lynn, Ruscio, & Beyerstein, 2010) while more and more research supports that some (but not all) people can learn moderation management (Hester, Delaney, & Campbell, 2011).

Another example of metaphor gone wrong was a case of a fifth-grade student that I (Ingersoll) consulted on. The student was diagnosed with attention-deficit-hyperactivity disorder (ADHD), with an inattentive specifier (in *DSM-5* criteria). The school counselor and I learned that the diagnosis had been made in a physician's office without an assessment of the child's behavior across several settings. The child appeared inattentive because in school she would unpredictably stare off into space or get up and meander around the classroom. The physician told the parents that their child had a "chemical imbalance." They took this to mean that the medication (a stimulant in this case) would correct the problem. Although the medication seemed to help the daydreaming, it also seemed to exacerbate the behavior of getting out of her chair and wandering around the room. The school counselor and I referred the child to a specialist who helped children with mild to moderate symptoms of ADHD. The parents agreed, and the counselor worked with the student on learning how to concentrate and helped the parents and teacher at the school cue and reinforce appropriate behavior in the student. After six months, the child was able to be titrated off the medication. Had the parents continued under the assumption that their child had "a chemical imbalance," the child might not have received the help she needed or would have received it later than she did.

Even though a client may prefer a medical model explanation of symptoms because it is less threatening to his or her sense of self, mental health professionals must resist being caught up in the word magic of the medical model. We recall attending a presentation at a professional conference where the presenter lectured for three hours on the biological bases for mental disorders, without producing one reference or fact to support his thesis. He seemed far too mesmerized by the medical model to bother to provide factual support for his claims. Even though he was trained in psychosocial interventions, he did not mention the ones we know are effective for many of the disorders he covered (such as ADHD). In addition, this psychologist supported the movement to give psychologists the legal power to write prescriptions for psychotropic medications. As such, he was clearly biased. A better approach would have been to set his presentation in the context of his position that psychologists should be allowed to prescribe psychotropic medications.

A study of adolescents with mental/emotional disorders summarized their perceptions of treatment. These teenagers shared the common negative perception that staff relied too much on the medical model to explain depression. They reported that the staff seemed to just want to give them medication and to not talk to them about what was really bothering them (Buston, 2002). What was "really bothering them" in this case were psychological and cultural variables that they saw as related to their depression. These adolescents wanted to discuss their psychological perspectives with clinicians rather than just have their symptoms described as a disease process treatable with pills. More recent studies confirm that children and adolescents will often resist taking medication (Worley & McGuinness, 2010) many times for reasons that can be addressed in counseling like fearing personality changes, social stigma, and concerns about addiction (Hamlin, McCarthy, & Tyson, 2010).

COMPLIANCE AND ADHERENCE

Perhaps the best way to begin this section is to ask the reader a simple question. Have you ever (1) not taken a medication as directed, (2) taken more of a medication than prescribed, (3) taken less of a medication than prescribed, (4) stopped taking a medication before your doctor recommended it, (5) resumed taking a medication left over from an earlier prescription without checking with your doctor for the new episode? If you have done any of these, you have not followed—technically, you have been noncompliant with—a medication plan. (When we ask this question in class, 80 to 90% of our students raise their hands; we do, too.) Researchers estimate that only 50% of people on any prescription medication always take it as prescribed (Patterson, 1996).

Although there is no absolute way to predict which clients will be most compliant with medication regimens, some characteristics can be assessed. We have long known that adherence rates vary across racial/ethnic demographics (Cuffs et al., 2013; Diaz, Wood, & Rosenheck, 2005) with people of color reporting adherence rates between 66 and 77% while Caucasians report adherence rates around 90%. We also know that the younger the person taking the medication, the less adherence they exhibit (Worley & McGuinness, 2010). In general, people who follow medication plans are usually emotionally mature, in stable family situations, employed, and pay for their own or part of

their treatment. This profile implies that the further along a client is developmentally, the more likely he or she is to follow a medication plan. Although there are dozens of lines of development, some key lines such as cognitive, emotional, and ego development seem particularly germane here. When you talk to a client about medication, you must consider his or her developmental level as well as lifestyle to get a sense of how compliant that person is likely to be. Predictors of noncompliance include being male, being young, and experiencing severe side effects (Demyttenaere, 2001).

It is also important to examine the clinician's attitude toward compliance. Many interns go into a mental health field with the misconception that part of their job is to make sure the client stays on prescribed psychotropic medications. This is untrue and may reflect anything from unresolved power issues, to poor training, to the unresolved power issues of their supervisors in the field. It is not the job of a mental health professional to make sure clients stay on their medications. It is the job of a mental health professional to help clients weigh the benefits and risks of taking medications, to help clients process conscious and unconscious resistance to medication, and to work with any number of theories to explore the risks and benefits of medications and how the medications relate to the goals a client has set in counseling. In the end, it is always the client's choice whether or not to take medications, even when not doing so will likely result in incarceration or confinement in a more restrictive treatment setting.

REASONS THAT CLIENTS MAY NOT COMPLY

When the noncompliance issue arises, mental health professionals must explore it with clients. Noncompliance can be caused by many things, including cost of the treatment, forgetfulness, and client values and beliefs (Demyttenaere et al., 2001). Beck, Rush, Shaw, and Emery (1979), who initiated research on irrational beliefs that contributed to noncompliance, concluded that clients on antidepressants were often noncompliant because of irrational thoughts about their medications. These researchers found the following three irrational thoughts among the primary ones associated with medication noncompliance: "The medication won't work," "I should feel good right away," and "My depression is incurable."

The Medication Won't Work

Sometimes the client just thinks the drug will not work, without any evidence to support that notion. You may find the client has a pessimistic worldview—part of what Beck et al. (1979) called the *cognitive triad of depression*. Another possibility is that perhaps the client is involved in what is called a negative feedback loop. In a **negative feedback loop**, the client for some reason stopped getting reinforcers that up to a point were satisfying. An example is when a client suffers the breakup of a romantic relationship that he or she experienced as reinforcing. The result of losing these reinforcers was depression, but the depressive symptoms then began prompting reactions in other people, reactions that became reinforcing. In the latter example, assume the client then started getting more calls from friends who were concerned about him or her. Those calls then become reinforcing and, rather than seeking out another relationship, the client may come to rely on those calls. This pattern is colloquially referred to as "getting some secondary gain from the symptoms." In such cases, clients prefer to believe no drug will work for their symptoms, because if they lose the symptoms they lose the secondary gains.

I Should Feel Good Right Away

It would be ideal if all medications worked immediately. But that simply is not the case with most psychotropic medications, particularly antidepressants, that may take anywhere from two to six weeks for the full therapeutic effects to manifest (when they do work). Counselors and other therapists must help clients deal with the early onset of side effects and later onset of therapeutic effects. It is wise to let the client describe how he or she is feeling before the counselor asks direct questions about non-life-threatening side effects. In some instances (outlined by Greenberg & Fisher, 1997), side effects actually have some placebo value in that the client may interpret them as the medication "working."

My Depression Is Incurable

If a client seems to feel his or her depression is incurable, here again counselors should investigate what possible secondary gains the person may be getting from the symptoms (the negative feedback loop may be operating). This belief may also be a manifestation of one aspect of the **cognitive triad of depression**. Readers may recall that Aaron Beck stated that the cognitive triad of depression was comprised of negative feelings about self, the world, and the future. A third possibility is that the client actually has a subtle death wish and is mentally prepared to decompensate (decline in functioning) to the point where he or she may have the nerve to attempt suicide. A final possibility is that the client has engaged in several unsuccessful treatments and has come to believe there is no treatment for his or her condition. Taking a thorough treatment history is invaluable in identifying this last dynamic.

Patterson (1996) added that clients may not comply with their medication plan because of trouble with routines, or inconvenience; medication as evidence of an undesirable self; misinformation; and other issues.

Trouble with Routines, or Inconvenience

Trouble with routines, or inconvenience, is often a problem for clients with impaired cognitive functioning. The client may forget or become confused about the medication regimen, grow tired of taking the medication, or may not be able to afford the medication (or believes she or he can't afford it). Clients who do shift work, for example, may have changes in routine that hinder remembering when to take medication. This is one reason pharmaceutical companies try to develop medication formulations that allow once-daily doses or even intramuscular injections that let a client get the medications injected once a month.

Problems of inconvenience often relate to side effects. One client we treated felt lethargic and sedated when taking her medication. She worked in a university setting as a recruitment coordinator. Her job required enthusiastic presentations and campus tours throughout the day. This particular client felt the side effects made her job much more difficult. The extra effort to get through the workday was so inconvenient that she responded by stopping her medication.

Medication as Evidence of an Undesirable Self

The notion that taking medication shows undesirable personal traits is particularly important when considering the client's psychological perspective. Such a client may believe that requiring medication is a sign of weakness or indicates some flaw or stigma related to mental illness. The client may be embarrassed at the prospect of other people finding out about her or his taking medication. Other clients may say they feel they are not their "real selves" while on medication. Although this may in fact be true, it is also possible that the client has been experiencing symptoms for so long (as in **Persistent Depressive Disorder** [previously called **Dysthymia**] in *DSM-IV*) that he or she has included the symptoms in his or her definition of "real self." Generally speaking, clients who negatively interpret taking medication are concerned about losing control over their lives. They may feel their symptoms have taken control of their lives to some extent and that the medications further decrease their control. This resistance can be complicated by paranoia that is part of the client's symptom profile or that arises when the client (sometimes for good reasons) does not trust the therapist or prescribing physician.

In such cases, one excellent strategy is based on Rogers's (1957) six core conditions of constructive personality change. First, make sure the client is capable of making psychological contact. Clients with psychotic or manic symptoms may not be able or willing to make psychological contact. Second, if the client is able/willing to make psychological contact, Rogers's conditions posit that he or she is in a state of incongruence between ideal self and what he or she currently perceives as the self. In this situation, we assume that the lack of congruence is related to mental/emotional symptoms and the prospect of taking medication for those symptoms. Third, Rogers stipulates a therapist who is congruent, meaning that he or she is aware of both the client's ideal and current sense of self, how they overlap and where they may not. Fourth, the counselor experiences

unconditional positive regard for the client. In this case, unconditional positive regard includes a nonjudgmental acceptance of the client's conflicts about taking the medication, including an acceptance of extreme feelings (e.g., some clients say they would rather die than take medication). Fifth, the counselor experiences an empathic understanding of the client's perspective, and sixth, when the counselor experiences this empathic understanding of the client he or she conveys it to the client. When these conditions are met the stage is set, according to Rogers, for constructive personality change—in this case, dealing with medication issues. If you are using another model of counseling, remember that it is most helpful to clients to work with a counselor who is empathic and willing to talk with them about their fears related to psychotropic medications.

Misinformation

Misinformation can be an easily remedied reason for noncompliance. In some cases, fixing **misinformation** simply requires referring the client to a credible source of information or sharing that information in the counseling session. One problem is related to the labels categories of the medications have. One client, who was taking olanzapine (Zyprexa) to control his symptoms of Bipolar I Disorder, heard that the medication was an "antipsychotic" and promptly replied, "Well, I'm not psychotic, so that must be the wrong medicine." A good part of an entire session was spent discussing how such medicine categories are labeled and how they really do not relate well to different uses with different clients. To the notion of misinformation we add the idea of disinformation contamination. **Disinformation** is the intentional spreading of information that is patently untrue, for political or other purposes. When disinformation concerning drugs (such as "All drugs cause addiction") contaminates a client's consciousness, it is possible that person may then assume any drug, even one that could help, is more dangerous than it actually is. The U.S. government's "war on drugs" has been built on disinformation for political purposes, such as labeling marijuana and heroin "narcotics," which gives the impression that they are similar substances (they are not). Another example is when the government sponsored researchers who claimed their studies showed that the drug 3,4-methylenedioxy-*N*-methylamphetamine (MDMA) caused literal holes in the brain (Ricaurte, Yuan, Hatzidimitriou, Cord, & McCann, 2002). When his conclusions could not be replicated and were challenged Ricaurte claimed that the facility that dispensed the drug for his study gave him methamphetamine instead of MDMA (a labeling error he claimed). He later retracted the paper (Ricaurte, 2003). Disinformation like this only makes citizens more mistrustful of government spokespeople. Until the government accepts a reasonable policy on drug use and tells the truth about what we do know, disinformation will continue to contaminate the thoughts of the public regarding all medications.

Other Issues

Sometimes, when symptoms are controlled, a client believes she or he is cured (as with an antibiotic) and stops taking the medication. This is another illustration of how different psychiatry is from other branches of medicine. In the **allopathic treatment model**, symptom cessation often means the condition has in fact been cured. This is not necessarily so with the many mental/emotional disorders where "cure" is not possible yet or not necessarily due to medications. Clients suffering from depression that appears psychological in origin may take medications such as antidepressants for six months and engage in counseling at the same time. For many such clients, the medication provides a chemical window of opportunity wherein they get the energy to deal with the psychological issues related to the depression. Once they have resolved some of the psychological issues, their doctors can titrate them off the medicine. Other clients may suffer from psychological symptoms that seem to have a strong biological component (such as symptoms of Bipolar I Disorder). These clients may be facing years or a lifetime of some medication regimen and face different issues from those who need medication for only a short period.

At the other end of the spectrum is the client who stops taking the medication after a short period because she or he does not notice any effect. As we emphasize throughout this book, many of these medications may take weeks before their therapeutic effects begin. In addition, some clients who discontinue their medication do so because they do not like the side effects. Our experience is that such clients would do better to contact their prescribing professional to see if there is a different medication they may be better able to tolerate. Although mental health clinicians cannot make specific recommendations about medications, they can refer clients back to their doctors when necessary.

Patterson (1996) also noted that some clients believe their medications are not working because they have unrealistic expectations for the medication. One client we recall who was taking an antidepressant was astonished at how sad she became at the funeral of a beloved aunt. She had a history of being overwhelmed by powerful depressive episodes and had developed a defense of warding off strong feelings, assuming that if she could do that, she could maintain emotional control. She said she sobbed throughout the funeral as if she hadn't cried for years (and in fact she hadn't). This client had an unrealistic expectation that the medications were akin to a vaccine against sadness. With her counselor, the client came to see her emotional expression at the funeral as a personal victory in that she expressed her true feelings and was able to grieve with loved ones but wasn't overwhelmed by the grief. Whether this victory was the result of the therapy, the antidepressant, or both could not be differentiated, but it was one of the first signs of improvement in quality of life for this client.

Another problem (although not as common as supposed) is clients who abuse their prescription medication because they like the effects or get a "high" from the medication. Of greatest concern among the psychotropic medications are the benzodiazepines and amphetamines, which can be abused to induce an altered state of consciousness and can potentially induce dependence. Although this is a concern for a minority of clients, most clients on these medications do not abuse them and once government disinformation is sifted out, the risk is relatively minor.

Perhaps the most problematic situation is when the medication seems to work for the client but it is precisely these therapeutic effects that the client does not want. This may be the case particularly when the symptoms are pleasant or somehow reinforcing for the client. We recall one client (Jacob) who suffered from Bipolar I Disorder and who really missed the manic "highs." When Jacob suffered from mania his "highs" eventually became incapacitating, leading him to high-risk behaviors that twice ended with his incarceration. He said that although the medication seemed to preclude the mania, it made him feel "normal." For Jacob, "normal" was not as good as he felt in a manic phase. The client tried three times to titrate off his medication over a period of five years. Each time he relapsed within eight months. This was truly frustrating for him, because his manic episodes always ended with him incarcerated or in an inpatient treatment facility. In cases such as Jacob's, an existential counseling approach is very helpful. Such approaches help clients develop a sense of meaning in the middle of difficult or even unacceptable existential givens (such as illness, infirmity, and mortality). John Brent's (1998) article on time-sensitive existential treatment is an excellent synopsis of an approach that can be used with clients such as Jacob. In Jacob's case, he had to work through the difficult reality that every time his doctor titrated him off his medication, he relapsed within one year. The existential givens for Jacob included a nervous system that seemed to require medical intervention for Jacob to be able to function in Western society.

Review Questions

- What is the difference between compliance and adherence?
- What are four different ways clients may conceptualize their symptoms?
- What are common reasons clients do not comply with medication regimens?
- What are predictors on noncompliance? What are some therapeutic ways to work through them with clients?

SECTION TWO: TALKING TO CLIENTS ABOUT MEDICATIONS: KNOW AND EDUCATE THYSELF

Learning Objectives

- Be willing to examine your own personal and countertransference issues regarding medication.
- Be able to discuss supervision issues that arise in assessing and monitoring clients taking psychotropic medications.
- Understand the important advocacy role mental health professionals play.
- Assess your own willingness to be an advocate for your client.

The variation on the **Delphic motto** ("Know thyself") in the subheading for this section is another good mantra for any mental health professional in training. Your own attitudes about and past experiences with psychotropic medication can seriously affect your work with clients. It is of the utmost importance that all mental health counselors be aware of their own psychological issues with medication to preclude countertransference reactions. Recall that countertransference occurs when a client's issue triggers unresolved issues in the therapist, which the therapist may not be aware of. If left unaddressed, these can then render the therapist less effective with the client.

One counseling student we worked with had been an excellent student and had done equally well in her internship until she got her first client being treated with mood-stabilizing medication (lithium). She felt the client should stop taking the medication because of the severe side effects and almost went so far as to say that in a session with the client. This intern, who was normally open, interested, and very present in counseling and supervision sessions, became emotionally "closed off." In supervision, it turned out she had had a sister who suffered from schizophrenia and had committed suicide. The intern had experienced a great deal of anguish in watching the effects of the medication on her older sister and to some extent blamed the low quality of her sister's life—and her eventual suicide—on the medication. Although the counselor's sister had been on a different medication (haloperidol/Haldol), the issues the counselor's client was dealing with were similar enough to trigger the counselor's own unresolved issues related to psychotropic medication.

If your client is on medication, take a minute to check in each session with the client about therapeutic effects, side effects, and compliance. If there seem to be problems with compliance, shift the focus of the session to that. Remember, however, that the aim of counseling or psychotherapy is not to make sure your client stays on his or her medication. Clients have a legal right to refuse medication and some studies suggest counseling is the most common response to medication refusal even in inpatient settings (Carey, Jones, & O'Toole, 2013). Your client is another human being who has a right to make choices about her or his life and the treatment of his or her symptoms. Many beginning therapists are so consumed with worry over their client's compliance with a medication regimen that they cannot be present—attentive—for the client in the session. Some researchers have found that even clients with severe mental disorders can learn to assume responsibility for their medication management (Dubyna & Quinn, 1996; Mitchell, 2007). We will discuss adherence issues when children and adolescents are taking psychotropic medications in the chapter devoted to children and adolescent issues. The issues related to adherence are even more complex where children and adolescents are involved party because most psychotropic medications do not have on-label approval for pediatric use (Dean, Witham, & McGuire, 2009).

When mental health therapists are talking to clients about medication education is a critical component (American Academy of Child & Adolescent Psychiatry, 2009; Patterson, 1996). As indicated by many of the irrational thoughts about psychotropic medication just described, most people are not aware of what such medications can and cannot do for them. Patterson points out that the therapist must emphasize that these medications are treatments, not cures, and that the client ultimately

must manage his or her own life. Understanding the main effects, the side effects, and how the medication is supposed to alleviate the symptoms is important knowledge for the client. Patterson also recommends, when talking to clients, using the word *medications* rather than *drugs*, because the latter term may be confused with drugs of abuse—about which very few people actually have good information, as we noted earlier in the chapter.

Ingersoll (2001) noted that the mental health clinician is in the role of "information broker," which requires some real work. To be a good information broker, you must first be able to differentiate good information from bad information. For our purposes, good information draws from clinical case summaries, peer-reviewed literature, and one's own clinical observations. The biggest problem with peer-reviewed literature is that it may be biased toward the medical model, for reasons we discuss later in the book such as being funded by the pharmaceutical company making the drug. Because of this bias, peer-reviewed literature should also be complemented with clinical case observations published in medical journals and newsletters on psychopharmacology. In addition, it is always important to read the sections of peer-reviewed articles that describe who funded the research. Research funded by a pharmaceutical company may be biased toward that company's products. Obviously, to be a good information broker, you also need at least an adequate understanding of research design. This enables you to see the difference between a study that truly supports the efficacy of a drug and a study design that merely supports a particular *view* of a drug.

SPECIFIC SUPERVISION ISSUES

The student intern case discussed in the last section gives one example of how supervision plays an important role in dealing with clients who take psychotropic medication. In all supervision, the key is assuring quality treatment for clients. For clinicians in nonmedical fields such as counseling and psychology, supervisors are there to monitor client welfare by assuring that clinicians comply with legal and ethical standards as well as standards of good practice. An important component of supervising mental health clinicians is discussing medications that clients are taking and how the clinician is talking about these with clients. As stated earlier, there are no clear prohibitions against nonmedical mental health professionals discussing psychotropic medications with clients, and codes of ethics and standards in counseling, psychology and school psychology state that clinicians should be competent including knowledgeable about treatment options that clients may encounter. Buelow, Herbert, and Buelow (2000) note, legal problems are currently more likely to arise from mental health clinicians *not* learning about psychotropic medications than from discussing them. The types of supervision issues will vary depending on the mental health professional and the setting. Of the nonmedical mental health professionals, psychologists have the broadest practice guidelines (depending on training) and thus will have more complex supervision issues. The American Psychological Association [APA] (2011) set forth guidelines for psychologists practicing at three points on a continuum regarding psychotropic medication. The first point is for those rare psychologists who have prescribing privileges. The second is for psychologists actively collaborating in medication decisions. The third and most common is when psychologists provide information that may be relevant to prescribing professionals. That is the practice point we focus on here as it is most common for psychologists and social workers, school psychologists, counselors, and other nonmedical mental health professionals.

What are some of the important supervision issues relevant to psychopharmacology? Berardinelli and Mostade (2003) have listed the following categories of responsibilities, which include activities for supervisors and supervisees: assessment, monitoring, and advocacy.

ASSESSMENT

In the assessment phase of a counseling relationship, the mental health clinician needs to learn what current medications clients are taking, including dosage, frequency, and formulation. In addition, clinicians need to assess the client's use of other licit or illicit recreational drugs. Fulfilling this responsibility assumes some knowledge of the categories, effects, and side effects of psychotropic medications on the part of the supervisor and the supervisee. As Ingersoll (2001) notes, this is where training in psychopharmacology becomes important, particularly for supervisors. The APA has created curricula for three levels of training in psychopharmacology, and the first level (or its curricular equivalent) (APA, 1995) should be required for supervisors of mental health professionals.

The assessment phase should include getting a signed release from the client to view copies of the file on the client kept by the prescribing professional. Many large providers like hospitals are using electronic note systems like Epic and Avatar. Each of the charts in these systems have sections on client medication but sometimes they are broken into current medications and all previous medications. Obviously it is important to know when clients started and stopped medications so you can understand what has worked and what has not for each client. Assessment may also include (with client permission) contacting the prescribing professional for consultation and to let her or him know (again, only with the client's release) what you are treating the client for, and ask about the professional's sense of how the medication is working for the client (along with any other questions you may have). This is an opportunity to at least establish a connection with the prescribing professional, learn about his or her prescribing style, and make a good first impression. With that in mind, you should know what symptoms the prescribing professional has prescribed the psychotropic medications to treat and be familiar with the medications prescribed. While prescribers may speak in terms of diagnoses, always try to get them to specify particular symptoms because clients with the same diagnosis can present quite differently. Supervisors will want to make sure the supervisee is following these guidelines and adequately understands the topics relevant to his or her clients at each stage of assessment.

Berardinelli and Mostade (2003) also noted that supervisors should monitor exactly how supervisees are discussing medication side effects with clients. Although it is important to make sure the client is aware of potential side effects, we must avoid leading questions that elicit complaints of side effects (e.g., "are you having headaches with this medication?"). There is clearly more art than science to this. The initial topic can be discussed with open-ended questions about how the client is feeling, whether he or she has followed the medication prescription, and how he or she thinks the medication is working. Depending on the client, opening a session with specific questions that list side effects such as "Are you experiencing any sexual side effects, headaches, dizziness, or nausea?" may not be the best strategy unless there are compelling reasons to take this approach. Some clinical judgment is necessary here. Clients who are more prone to obsessively worrying about side effects may respond to such concrete questions as a list of things they then imagine they are experiencing. However, clients who are functioning at a concrete intellectual level may need direct questions to share side effects that are occurring. Unless you feel direct questions are necessary (as in the case of clients who are concrete thinkers), you can begin asking open-ended questions to elicit the client's thoughts about how the medication seems to be working.

MONITORING

Monitoring is an important component of the therapeutic relationship and supervision. Supervisors should make sure supervisees are checking in with clients at each session about medication, updating medication information as it changes, and keeping records of medication compliance as well as the client's response to medications. The last item is particularly important, especially for clients who do not see the same prescribing professional on a regular basis or for clients who have not given the clinician permission to contact their prescribing professional. The record of client responses to medication is also important in relation to the record of what is happening with the client psychologically.

For example, in one case we treated, the client suffered from Bipolar I Disorder and seemed to show subtle signs of improvement just before the onset of manic symptoms. This happened twice, with two different medications the client was on. The first time the therapist took the shift as a signal of improvement in mood, but the second time the therapist saw it as the first sign of approaching manic symptoms. The client learned in this case the difference between mood stabilization and the onset of manic symptoms. Genuine improvement in this client appeared similar but was followed by increasing insight and unimpaired reality testing.

In another case, the client's perceptions of how helpful the medication was correlated with how events were unfolding in her personal life. When her personal life was going the way she wanted, she felt the medication (in this case an antianxiety medication) was helping. When events in her personal life were not going well, she complained that all she got from the medication were side effects. In tracking this relationship, the issue of locus of control emerged as important in counseling. The client came to realize that she had, over a period of years, established the medication as an external locus of control and that the medication now provided a convenient target when things weren't going well. After six months of work on this locus-of-control issue, this particular client asked her doctor to titrate her off the medication. After a year she was still functioning well without it.

ADVOCACY

Advocacy is actively supporting the client to make sure she or he is getting the best service possible. Where medication is concerned, supervisors must make sure their supervisees' efforts at advocacy do not cross the line between support and actually recommending medication. Although mental health professionals do not recommend medications, they can ask prescribing professionals questions on the client's behalf (e.g., "My client is taking an older antipsychotic with severe side effects. Do you think she would benefit from one of the newer antipsychotic medications?") According to Berardinelli and Mostade (2003), advocacy issues include recognizing client needs and the particular needs of certain client populations, integrating medication issues into counseling, and knowing when to refer clients for case management and other services. Advocacy in this sense requires that supervisors and supervisees be familiar with community resources, including medication programs and trials, and programs that help clients pay the cost of medications and provide education to significant others and employers when necessary and when desired by the client.

An interesting question is whether mental health professionals should suggest to prescribing professionals that a particular client may benefit from a particular medication. The short answer is no. In the most conservative sense, in this situation the mental health clinician is assuming he or she has the same level of knowledge of psychotropic medications as the prescribing professional. Although this is possible, the most conservative interpretation of such action could be that the mental health professional is practicing medicine without a license. Obviously, cases in which mental health professionals have the proper training and legal mandate to prescribe (as in certain states and territories where psychologists have the right to prescribe psychotropic medications) do not apply here. The long answer is that because reality is complex we must look at the context of the situation and how the clinician approaches the prescribing professional. Ingersoll (2001) noted that much can be accomplished by assuming the "one down" position and approaching the prescribing professional with the attitude of requesting education. For example, if a client is prescribed carbamazepine/Tegretol for Bipolar I Disorder and still relapsing, the mental health clinician may wonder if new antipsychotics have been tried for the manic symptoms. Certainly carbamazepine/Tegretol has efficacy for some clients but if the client is relapsing the question may be worth asking. In this example the clinician may ask, "I've heard that some clients with this disorder take atypicals in addition to other mood stabilizing agents. How do you feel this client would respond to such a combination in treating Bipolar I symptoms?" If a clinician seriously questions the work of a medical professional, there are several possible approaches. If the work of the clinician appears to constitute malpractice, a report to the prescribing professional's licensing board is in order. If the questions simply revolve around whether the best medication was selected for the client, the clinician can reinforce the client's right to ask the prescribing professional questions or seek a second opinion if that is an option. We emphasize that this advocacy issue is grey and clinicians would do best to exercise conservative judgment here.

Review Questions

- What personal beliefs do you bring to the profession about psychotropic medications?
- What are key issues in assessment and monitoring for supervisors of mental health professionals who treat clients taking psychotropic medications?
- Discuss the extent to which you feel comfortable advocating for a client. If a senior clinician told a client incorrect information about a medication what would you do?

SUMMARY

Many psychological issues arise in our clients when either psychotropic medication is recommended or taken. Clients use several strategies to avoid medication, including irrational beliefs about medications, secondary gains from symptoms, and difficulty with routines.

Multiple truths and realities govern the way clients respond to a course of psychotropic medication. Therapists need to recognize how clients accept psychotropic medications into their intrapsychic and unconscious worlds. It is helpful to talk to our clients about the strengths and limitations of both medications and conventional therapy. In addition, mental health clinicians need to know how to collaborate with medical professionals as well as how to review medication issues in supervision sessions.

SECTION THREE: ETHNO-PSYCHOPHARMACOLOGY: GROUP DIFFERENCES IN RESPONSE TO PSYCHOTROPIC AGENTS

Learning Objectives

- Be able to give a general definition of ethnopharma-cotherapy and its main concerns.
- Discuss the role of sex and race in how pharmaceuti-cals affect people.
- Understand the effects of discrimination and oppres-sion on people's view of prescription drugs.
- Be able to articulate ethical concerns that arise when dealing with prescribing professionals.

Ethno-psychopharmacology, a relatively new subdiscipline of psychopharmacology, explores eth-nic and racial differences in response to medica-tions, differences that appear to be physiologically based (Ng, Lin, Singh, & Chiu, 2008). Scientists have known for years that people of different racial and ethnic backgrounds may have genuine physical differences that make them more or less sensitive to certain drugs or medications. Alcohol has always been a quintessential case in point (Westermeyer, 1989). People of Asian descent and women have less of the enzyme that breaks down alcohol (alco-hol dehydrogenase). This makes these groups more susceptible to the effects of alcohol (Gordis, 2000; Julien, Advocate, & Comady, 2011). This does not mean they are more likely to develop patterns of abuse or dependence, just that they are more sensi-tive to the effects. If such differences exist across groups regarding alcohol, many researchers began wondering whether such differences also exist for psychotropic medication, and in fact they do. These physiological differences can also be further accen-tuated by cultural differences in diet; use of sub-stances such as herbs, alcohol, and caffeine; and the extent of environmental pollutants (Bhugra & Bhui, 2001; Malik, Lake, Lawson, & Joshi, 2010). Ethno-psychopharmacology is now being viewed through the discipline of pharmacogenetics.

As genomic sequencing becomes more accessible some researchers like Ng and Castle (2010) believe we will be able to link racial and ethnic genetic differences to differential responses to medications. While this is still in the future, the possibility is intriguing (Jones & Perlis, 2006).

SEX DIFFERENCES

After some stark initial findings, scientists now agree that extensive work is needed to explore sex differences in response to psychotropic medication (Jensvold, Halbreich, & Hamilton, 1996; Marazziti et al., 2013). Strong evidence shows that males and females respond differently to medication, but little research is devoted to understanding this difference. Robinson (2002) has documented that although women are the primary consumers of most types of psychotropic medication, and although sex dif-ferences appear in the absorption, metabolism, and excretion of many medications, little attention has been paid to these differences in research. This gap implies an ethical imperative for pharmaceutical companies. If they target women in direct-to-consumer advertising (Petersen, 2009), then they must conduct research supporting the safety and efficacy of these medications for women. Until such a research database is built, clinicians must advocate for clients by keeping up-to-date on the research that exists on psychotropic medica-tions and responses of females. In addition, there are sex differences in symptom profiles. For example, women are more likely to have atypical symptoms of depression, comorbid anxiety and attempt sui-cide (Gorman, 2006).

Differences in absorption exist between premen-opausal women and men, with premenopausal women moving material more slowly through their digestive tract. This delays peak levels and low-ers blood concentrations of medications. Women also typically weigh less than men, have less total blood volume than men, and carry a higher percent-age of body fat than men. For example, women may initially have low blood levels of a compound, but if the compound is stored in fat cells then levels may rise overall, eventually providing women with higher levels of the compound than men would have. The fact that women clear drugs more slowly than men means that optimal doses for males may be too high for females. Robinson (2002) notes that this may be why women experience side effects from psychotropic compounds about twice as often as men. Along these lines, Hamilton (1986) found that women taking older antipsychotic medications have higher rates of tardive dyskinesia (a disorder of abnormal, late-appearing, involuntary movement) than do men taking the same medications. In addition to these differences, women's physiology changes through the menstrual cycle. Premenstrual changes include a slowed rate of gastric emptying and decreased gastric acid secretion. Both these changes tend to raise blood serum levels of psychotropic medication before menstruation.

It is important to know that many psychotropic medications appear to interfere with fertility. Psychotropic medications (and particularly mood stabilizers and antipsychotics) have been shown to have adverse reproductive and gynecologic effects (Talib & Alderman, 2013). If a client on psychotropic medications is trying to become pregnant, she should discuss this decision with her physician, who can help her weigh the risks. This is an area where female clients may need the support and advocacy of mental health professionals. Many clients still believe they cannot question their doctors and cannot participate in treatment decisions.

Several psychotropic medications have also been linked to **teratogenesis** (the development of birth defects). Obviously, if a woman is pregnant, she should, if possible, refrain from taking any psychotropic medications. Although this is not always possible, the risks to the unborn child must be weighed against potential risks to the mother should she stop taking a particular medication. In other cases medications have documented dangers to the neurodevelopmental health of the fetus (Galbally et al., 2010; Gentile, 2010). Such decisions are typically difficult. One client whom I (Ingersoll) treated in the late 1980s was taking mood-stabilizing medications that had been shown to put the fetus at risk (lithium/Lithobid, which causes a heart valve defect called Epstein's Anomaly). She chose to go off the medication during her pregnancy, which resulted in her decompensation and the need for a more restrictive treatment setting (an inpatient facility, in this case). Although we may never know the impact of her emotional suffering (as a result of relapse related to going off medication) on her child, we do know that going off the medication decreased the child's risk of heart malformation associated with the medication the mother was taking.

The Food and Drug Administration (FDA) requires that prescription medications that may cause harm to the developing fetus be classified according to one of five categories (A, B, C, D, X). Category A includes medications for which controlled studies in women fail to show risks to the fetus in the first trimester and the risk of harm appears low. Category B includes medications for which animal studies have not shown fetal risk but there are no controlled studies in pregnant women or for which a risk shown in animal studies was confirmed in studies with women. Category C includes medications for which either studies with animals have shown teratogenic effects or there are simply no animal or women's studies. Category D includes medications for which there is positive evidence of human fetal risk. Such medications have warning sections in their labeling. Category D medications may still be used if the risk–benefit analysis shows that more harm may come to the mother if the medication is *not* used. Category X includes medications for which studies in animals or humans clearly link the medication to fetal abnormalities and the use is unacceptable (e.g., all formulations of lithium has a rating of "X"). This information is listed in the **contraindications** section of the label.

Robinson (2002) has summarized some of the literature on teratogenic effects (causing malformations) of particular medications. Most of these effects are due to antimanic drugs and are risks primarily in the first trimester. These are summarized in Table 4.1. Please note that this is not an exhaustive list. Although many medications have teratogenic properties, scientists are not sure about many other medications yet. One good source of information is the Pregnancy Teratogens Healthline at http://www.healthline.com/health/pregnancy/teratogens.

TABLE 4.1 Examples of Antimanic Medications and Teratogenic Risks

Medication	Risk	Citation
Lithium	Ebstein's anomaly	Altshuler, Burt, McMullen, & Hendrick, 1995
Carbamazepine	Craniofacial defects Neural tube defects	Jones, Lacro, Johnson, & Adams, 1989; Rosa, 1991
Valproic acid	Neural tube defects	Koren & Kennedy, 1995
Antidepressants	Neonate CNS depression and urinary retention	Preston, O'Neal, & Talaga, 2002

© Cengage Learning®

Many states have set up their own websites dealing with teratogenic information. For example, the FDA has an informational PDF at http://depts.washington.edu/druginfo/Formulary/Pregnancy.pdf. Discussing the prospect of psychotropic medication for pregnant women, Preston, O'Neal, and Talaga (2002) comment, "It is important to remember that absolute data in this area is disturbingly incomplete" (p. 229). As noted in Chapter Three the same holds true for breast-feeding on psychotropic medication (Fortinguerra, Clavenna, & Bonati, 2009). Therefore, the mental health professional concerned with client advocacy must keep up with the literature in the area and be willing to help the client (and/or guardians) weigh the risks of particular medications.

In addition to teratogenesis (malformation of the fetus), psychotropic medications may affect the developing fetus, the newborn, the actual process of birth, and breast-fed infants. Psychotropic medications may result in behavioral problems in the child who is exposed to these drugs in utero. Finally, because pregnancy induces so many changes in a woman's body, these changes can radically alter the action of psychotropic medications (Preston, O'Neal, & Talaga, 2002).

RACIAL DIFFERENCES

In addition to cultural differences in attitudes and trust toward psychotropic medication and the doctors who prescribe them, scientists are now learning that psychotropic medications affect people with different racial backgrounds in significantly different objective ways. Here is a summary of a few of the racial differences that researchers have found in physiological responses to psychotropic medications:

- Some studies have found that African Americans taking older antipsychotic medications are more likely to develop tardive dyskinesia than Caucasians taking the same medications (Glazer, Morgenstern, & Doucette, 1994; Morgenstern & Glazer, 1993). This may also be related to the fact that many studies have consistently found that African Americans are more likely to be diagnosed with severe mental disorders and receive higher doses of the medications to treat them (Netjek, 2012; Strickland, Lin, Fu, Anderson, & Zheng, 1995) or to reasons that may be related to racism. In a recent study reviewing prescription trends by racial group, Daumit and colleagues (2003) found that African Americans were still more likely to receive older antipsychotics as opposed to the newer, supposedly more effective, **atypical antipsychotics**. Also, African Americans are more likely to be treated with polypharmacy strategies than Caucasians (Garver et al., 2006).
- Compared with Caucasians, nearly all minority groups have lower odds of adequate antidepressant use (Quinones et al., 2014). African Americans are also far less likely to adhere to antidepressant treatment later in life than Caucasians (Kales et al., 2013). Some of this seems to be an effect of systematic oppression leading to a mistrust of mainstream medicine.

- Asians and Asian Americans report more adverse effects from antipsychotic and tricyclic medications than do Caucasians. They also show higher plasma levels than do Caucasians at the same dosage (Bond, 1990; Bowden, 1995; Pi, Gutierrez, & Gray, 1993). This evidence tends to point toward the need for lower doses for these clients.
- African Americans appear to be more sensitive to tricyclic medications than are Caucasians in terms of both therapeutic and side effects (Lin & Poland, 1995).
- There are disparities on Medicaid expenditures on psychotropic medications for maltreated children. In a sample of over 4000 children, children of color received substantially less Medicaid support for psychotropic medications (Raghavan et al., 2014). African American children received $292 less on average per year than Caucasian children and Hispanic children received $144 less per year. These findings demonstrate that policy makers need to pay more attention to the needs of children of color.
- There are also racial disparities in the monitoring of patients on chronic opioid therapy. There are disparities in prescribing habits (Tait & Chibnall, 2014) as well as in monitoring patients with African Americans being less likely to be prescribed opioid pain medication and more likely to be subjected to more drug tests than Caucasian peers. Compared to Caucasian patients, African American patients are more likely to be referred to a substance abuse specialist than a pain specialist (Hausmann, Gao, Lee, & Kwoh, 2013).
- Also, African Americans seem to have a host of different influences affecting their rates and expression of depression, compared to other racial groups in the United States (Meyers, 1993) though they are less likely to take antidepressants (Paulose-Ram, Safran, Jonas, Gu, & Orwig, 2007).
- Recall that the cytochrome P450 enzyme system governs metabolism of, among other things, psychotropic medication. The differences outlined in the following studies seem to be based on racial differences in this important enzyme system (Lawson, 1999; Lin, Poland, & Anderson,

1995; McGraw, 2012; Wood, 2001). These differences may vary for genetic and environmental reasons. Various enzymes vary dramatically across different racial groups (Lin, Poland, & Nakasaki, 1993). This same mechanism may also partly cause the increased risk of **hypertension** in African Americans (Strickland et al., 1995).

In comparing data from across different societies, one confounding factor is that average daily dose of medication or minimum effective dose frequently varies from one society to the next. For example, minimum effective dosage of a medication is often higher in the United States than in other countries (Bhugra & Bhui, 2001). Also note that much research on racial group differences in adverse effects focuses on older medications (tricyclic antidepressants, older antipsychotics) that are slowly being phased out with the arrival of newer agents with better side effect profiles. Even though newer medications ostensibly have fewer side effects, the data on older medications point to differences between groups that will likely also have implications for newer compounds. In addition, because many minorities live in lower socioeconomic brackets, they may be prescribed older psychotropic medication that is available in less expensive, generic form because the patent has expired.

What should the nonmedical mental health therapist do with this information? First, we hope this information makes clinicians better information brokers, as we mentioned earlier. For better or worse, prescribing professionals may fail to take racial/ethnic differences into account and mental health clinicians need to raise these relevant points for the well-being of the client. This is particularly true in clinic settings where prescribing professionals (doctors and psychiatrists) are so overwhelmed with work that they may only get 10 or 15 minutes with clients. Doctors report racial and ethnic differences in comfort discussing things like medication cost with the prescriber and the time limitations only exacerbate such problems (Dalawari et al., 2013). In situations like these, clinicians must be willing to advocate for their clients. Later in this

TABLE 4.2 Important Cultural Dimensions Related to Psychotropic Medications

The client's diet
Any dietary restrictions
Relevant religious taboos
Alcohol, caffeine, and nicotine intake

© Cengage Learning®

chapter, we offer one model on how to collaborate with prescribing professionals. In monitoring the therapeutic and side effects of medications on their clients, therapists need to be alert to the differences we have discussed. As a starting point, Bhugra and Bhui (2001) recommend screening the items in Table 4.2 for clients receiving psychotropic medication.

As noted, there has been little research on ethnopharmacotherapy. Although a small number of committed researchers are making important contributions in this area, the nonmedical mental health clinician must regularly review the literature, because these studies are frequently not included in books on psychotropic medications.

A FOCUS ON THE CULTURAL PERSPECTIVE

Recall that what we call the *cultural perspective* describes subjective, shared experience and beliefs. It is the dimension that describes phenomenological aspects of groups. In this sense, *culture* can refer to shared worldviews and beliefs clustering around race, ethnicity, socioeconomic status, sexual orientation, spiritual tradition, sex, gender, ability/disability, or age. Culture can also refer to shared worldviews and beliefs clustering around one's professional identification. Thus one can speak of the culture of the pharmaceutical industry, the culture of the counseling profession, and the culture of the psychiatric profession.

Because a mental health professional's main tool is the therapeutic encounter, the impact of culture on

that encounter must be figured in. The therapeutic encounter is supposed to improve the interpersonal functioning and the subjective comfort of the client. This necessarily implies defining "normal" and "abnormal" behavior, and cultural milieu determines to a large extent whether a person's behavior or emotional state is considered "normal" or "abnormal." Students in the mental health professions have increasingly addressed cultural variables with regard to mental health diagnosis and treatment (Labruzza, 1997; Malik et al., 2010), but how does culture relate to psychopharmacology? There are two dimensions to this relationship: the shared beliefs of cultural groups, and group differences in response to medications. We already explored the latter through the social perspective. We now address what scientists know about those factors relating to the shared worldviews and beliefs of groups. As Lin (1996) noted, psychopharmacologists simply do not know much about how cultural or ethnic factors affect whether or not a particular medication will be helpful for a particular condition.

Shared Belief Systems Regarding Psychopharmacology: Multicultural Variables

Human beings in the 21st century are still grappling with the challenges presented by diversity in the species. For example just think of how human universals vary culture to culture. Although the human body generally has a universal structure, it is adorned and altered differently across cultures and even subcultures (witness the current increase in tattooing in U.S. culture). Although many personal developmental sequences occur across cultures, cultures label and facilitate them differently (Gardiner & Kosmitzki, 2001).

Many aspects of culture may make Western forms of mental health work challenging. Consider, for example, an Arabic student who is suffering from symptoms of depression and who comes to a college counseling center at the urging of his roommate. Also consider that for this client, sharing intimate personal information outside the family may be anathema. Further, consider that this client also may view taking psychotropic medication as a sign of weakness. True, this client shares the structures of a triune brain and the accompanying nervous system however, without understanding and attempting to accommodate this client's cultural background, a therapist is unlikely to succeed in treatment.

Discrimination and Oppression

The cultural perspective also provides a vehicle to explore shared worldviews that stem from a history of discrimination and oppression. Many African American clients with whom we have worked approach counseling and psychotherapy with a great deal of suspicion. Without understanding the shared worldview that underlies this suspicion, mental health professionals may misinterpret it as paranoia or resistance. There is ample justification for African Americans to mistrust mental health treatment systems. Flaherty and Meagher (1980) documented that in mental health systems, African Americans tend to receive less desirable treatments (Puyat et al., 2013). In addition, many researchers have noted that African Americans have been more likely to be hospitalized (Lawson, Hepler, Holladay, & Cuffel, 1994), involuntarily committed, and placed in restraints than members of other ethnic groups (Lawson, 1999). In addition, as Lawson (1999) explained, mental health providers are often not African American and may have views of treatment very different from the views of African Americans.

Many clients of African American and Hispanic background may share a suspicion of mental health counseling and psychotropic medication, believing that basically these interventions are tools of oppression and to be avoided. Moreover, until very recently psychotropic medication trials were conducted largely with Caucasian, male samples and then assumed to generalize to other cultural groups. Again, to interpret this as symptomatically significant paranoia only exacerbates the misunderstanding. African American resistance to participation in the mental health treatment system occurs in light of the Tuskegee study sponsored by the U.S. government in the 1930s. It is now widely known that

in this study, treatment was withheld from African American men with syphilis. The study continued for some 40 years before it was ended by a newspaper exposé. The federal government finally acknowledged the study officially in the 1990s, under then-president Bill Clinton. I (Ingersoll) worked with a granddaughter of one man in the Tuskegee experiment, in a sociodramatic recreation of the devastation wrought by the study. This gave me a firsthand understanding of how "paranoia" regarding medical interventions was a healthy defense for members of this family.

A substantial body of literature supports the charge that minority clients with mental and emotional disorders have often been misdiagnosed, which has led to incorrect treatment (Lawson, 1999). Strickland et al. (1995) demonstrated that African Americans and Hispanics are overdiagnosed with schizophrenia and more likely to be given antipsychotics when such medications are not needed. Bell and Mehta (1980, 1981) made a strong case that African Americans suffering from Bipolar I Disorder (and showing excellent lithium response) were often initially diagnosed with schizophrenia and therefore given antipsychotic medication. Stratkowski, McElroy, Keck, and West (1996) have also demonstrated that African Americans with mood disorders are more likely to have psychotic symptoms associated with these disorders. Their conclusion was that this required more careful differential diagnosis so that African American males who were really suffering from Bipolar I Disorder were not mistakenly diagnosed with schizophrenia. As Lawson (1999) noted, this evidence is especially problematic because there is also evidence that African Americans are more likely to develop tardive dyskinesia in response to antipsychotic medications.

Ideally, in the first encounter with culturally different clients the counselor or prescribing professional will be aware of these issues and (if psychological contact permits) will explore them with clients who appear highly guarded or suspicious. In many cases, frank discussion of the issues is the best approach. Generally speaking, the professional should also note that stress plays an important role in shaping compliance with a medication regimen and in the patient's response to the medication. Many culturally different people are under enormous amounts of stress including financial stress, stress related to relocation, and stress resulting from isolation when they move to a new country and leave family and community supports. Prescribing professionals need to consider the possibility of these stressors for such clients (Bhugra & Bhui, 2001).

CASE STUDY: THE CASE OF RAFAEL

Rafael, a 57-year-old married Mexican man, came to counseling at a mental health center because he complained of hearing many voices. He visited his priest, who was unable to assist him and who referred him to the mental health center. The staff psychiatrist evaluated Rafael and prescribed Loxitane (loxapine), an antipsychotic for his hallucinations and disorganized thinking. He told Rafael to take his medication daily and assigned him to an agency counselor.

Each week Rafael reported to his counselor that he took his medication, but this puzzled her, because he seemed ever more psychotic and disorganized. However, he reported compliance. Rafael became so confused and impaired that he could no longer drive to his appointments, so his wife brought him. After one very perplexing session, the counselor asked his wife if Rafael was taking his medications. She looked away and said quietly, "Only on the days he comes to see you. On all the other days he prays to the Blessed Virgin for his health with his men friends." The counselor learned that Rafael encountered great resistance about medications from his cohort of friends, who urged him not to take his medication but to pray for sanity and health to the Blessed Virgin. So the only times he took Loxitane were on the days he had an appointment with his counselor. Fortunately his counselor was able to seek the assistance of the Latina counselor on staff and Rafael's priest to intervene with Rafael and his wife and prevent further decompensation and possible hospitalization.

Obviously, it is an error to prescribe psychotropic medications with the assumption that all people from all cultures will receive support and understanding of the process in their homes. People from many cultures have various rules, rituals, and ideas about the danger of "pills for the mind," and the levels of resistance are legion.

The astute reader may have a question at this point that goes something like this: "So in reality, all Rafael's prayer did not cure his psychosis, but the Loxitane seemed to help. Doesn't this validate the importance of the medical model intervention (medication) over the prescribed cultural cure (prayer)?" Certainly Rafael's symptoms seemed to benefit from the medication, but that intervention needed to be complemented with the support from his prayer time with friends. Without seeing a way to integrate these two things, Rafael simply stopped taking the medication. In this case, the counselor also consulted with Rafael's priest, who met with Rafael to discuss the difference between praying for healing and praying for a cure. When Rafael was able to engage in this dialogue, he came to understand that although his prayers to the Blessed Virgin did not produce a "cure" per se, he did receive "healing" of sorts in the form of comfort and the strength to eventually go on the medication despite the opinions of his friends. Here, the prayer and the medication served as different tools that brought about different types of healing.

CASE

Mr. Liao is 75-year-old citizen who came to the United States 50 years ago from mainland China. Currently he suffers from a very rare autoimmune disorder of the liver that is not stable with medication. He is also seriously depressed. His life partner of 40 years is trying desperately to take him to a psychiatrist for an evaluation. Mr. Liao knows that if his partner is successful it will confirm the Chinese communities' suspicions that they are gay and they will be ostracized from their cultural group. He insists that acupuncture and Chinese herbal medicine will help him more than western antidepressants. His partner insists that he is wrong and hires a private ambulance to take Mr. Liao to the community psychiatrist. The psychiatrist evaluates him puts him on a course of citalopram and buspirone and refers him to the culturally sensitive counselor at the agency. He also refers Mr. Liao's partner.

Questions About the Case

1. What are the salient cultural concerns in this case?

2. Speak to the potential conflict between western and eastern approaches to medicine.

3. Discuss what happens to people in cultures where the gay and lesbian lifestyle is either forbidden by religious practice or rejected by cultural norms.

4. How did the psychiatrist respond to Mr. Liao's concerns?

A MEETING OF SUBCULTURES: COLLABORATION WITH PRESCRIBING PROFESSIONALS

Cultural variables can also be interactions between professional subcultures such as counseling and psychiatry or, more generally, between prescribing professionals and nonmedical mental health therapists. Western culture shares a belief in a hierarchy among health professionals, with doctors at the top. The mental health hierarchy has psychiatrists at the top. Neal and Calarco (1999) noted that in the past medical training always emphasized that the doctor is in charge in any team approach to treatment and that some doctors, having internalized this belief, can be quite authoritarian even when they have not studied and do not understand psychotherapeutic approaches. Although one can certainly deconstruct this, place it in nested contexts, or argue that it is a "patriarchal hangover," it still exists as a shared belief with which nonmedical mental health clinicians must deal.

Ingersoll (2001) noted that the nonmedical therapist's approach depends on the attitude of the prescribing professional toward psychotherapy. If a psychiatrist does not value psychotherapeutic approaches, the mental health professional may find a "one down" approach helpful. In this approach the nonmedical therapist presents him- or herself as willing to learn

about medications from the prescribing professional. This approach can begin the alliance-building process between the medical and nonmedical members of a treatment team and can give the mental health professional an opportunity to practice equanimity.

At the time of this writing, there are some problematic trends that could create a larger divide between medical and nonmedical mental health professionals. First more and more people with mental health problems are going to their general practitioners rather than a psychiatrist (Olfson, Kroenke, Wang, & Blanco, 2014). Although nonmedical mental health professionals can certainly collaborate with general practitioners, they often do not have extensive training in mental health issues. They do their best to help clients alleviate symptoms with medications but may not be aware of the overdetermined nature of some disorders. Another reason for this shift may be that increasingly fewer psychiatrists are accepting new patients with noncapitated insurance, Medicaid and Medicare compared to physicians in other specializations and in general practice. Acceptance rates for all types of insurance were significantly lower for psychiatrists than physicians in other specialties and this may pose barriers to mental health service (Bishop, Keyhani, & Pincus, 2014).

In collaborating with prescribing professionals, mental health clinicians can benefit from a judicious combination of equanimity and what we would colloquially call "people skills." Centuries ago, Buddhism introduced equanimity as one of the four sublime states (the other three being love, compassion, and sympathetic joy). **Equanimity** is the practice of approaching an interaction with respect and caring while remaining unattached to how the interaction unfolds and how you are treated (Gunaratana, 2002). Although this approach can be challenging, it is possible. Reflecting on the good that could come to the client you share with the prescribing professional can be enough to foster the equanimity you need. Also, if a particular prescribing professional thinks poorly of mental health professionals in general, you are not likely to change his or her mind in one interaction.

Next, use good interpersonal skills. This is obvious, but worth noting because people can forget these skills in the press of a crisis or busy day. Most prescribing professionals are equally busy and well intentioned. Reminding ourselves of this can serve as a cue to enter the interaction in a courteous manner regardless of how frantic the setting or your mind-set may be. Ideally both professionals approach the relationship with some mutual respect, because this inevitably helps the client, who would likely be disadvantaged by friction between providers. As Balon (1999) points out, good collaboration is important because the team approach is an economic necessity and likely to remain so.

How the collaboration is set up is important. In agency work, therapists do not have much choice about which doctors they are going to work with. In private practice there is more choice, depending on which practitioner can be persuaded to collaborate. Evidence is growing that a good therapist–prescriber relationship is correlated with more positive client outcomes (Neal & Calarco, 1999). Next we discuss some important elements of collaboration.

Conditions of the Relationship

Each professional should know the credentials of all other collaborating professionals as well as the areas of specialization and populations each party has worked with. As noted, mental health professionals want to know the medical practitioner's attitude toward counseling and psychotherapy, because a negative attitude can diffuse the therapeutic alliance. Also, it is important to define the role (if any) the mental health clinician plays in giving feedback to the medical practitioner (and whether the professional will welcome or resist feedback).

Confidentiality Issues

Regardless of whom the client met first (doctor or mental health professional), the recommendation for either therapy or medication presupposes that the client's case will be fully disclosed to the prescriber and that appropriate documentation and releases must be obtained. This is even more important since the enactment of the Health Insurance Portability and Accountability Act of 1996 (HIPAA).

Confrontation Issues

At times, clients either decompensate in reaction to a psychotropic medication or quickly develop adverse effects to the medications. The treating medical professional may be either oblivious to the changes or may insist that the medications are correct for this client. To prepare for such conditions, the mental health clinician must develop assertive and appropriate confrontation skills to advocate well for the client.

Transference and Countertransference Issues

Finally, transference and countertransference issues must be addressed when they arise, and a vehicle must be set in place for addressing them. To avoid triangulation, which will likely undermine the treatment plan, each professional must be aware of his or her transference and countertransference relationships with the client and with each other. Whenever a third party is brought to the relationship, the impact on the client must be assessed.

SECTION FOUR: SOCIAL INSTITUTIONS AND THEIR IMPACT ON PSYCHOTROPIC MEDICATIONS

Learning Objectives

- Be able to discuss the supposed risks and benefits of direct-to-consumer (DTC) advertising of psychotropic medications.
- Understand how financial conflicts of interest in pharmaceutical research can harm your clients.
- Understand the five schedules used for categorizing drugs by the Drug Enforcement Agency (DEA).

Although many social institutions could be examined here, we focus on the FDA and on pharmaceutical companies in general, because they have the most profound impact on psychotropic medications.

It would be nice if mental health professionals could operate in a vacuum unaware of what the FDA and pharmaceutical companies were doing, but responsible advocacy requires at least a general understanding of these two forces.

The Food and Drug Administration

The FDA is the federal U.S. government agency charged with overseeing drug testing and development, approving new drugs and compounds, and monitoring approved drugs and compounds. Currently, the FDA has nine different centers or offices, performing a variety of functions. In the early 20th century, the FDA was part of the U.S. Department of Agriculture. As recently as 1929, consumers got all but 5% of their medications directly from pharmacists, with no prescription from doctors necessary (Temin, 1980). This changed with the passage of the 1938 Food, Drug, and Cosmetic Act, which was amended in 1962. The FDA has historically addressed three distinct (and at times antithetical) risks:

1. The risk of overpaying for a drug (because of diluted form or low quality)
2. The risk of an adverse drug reaction
3. The risk of failing to recover after taking a drug as prescribed

These risks receive different emphasis at different times in history, but the results have largely been of the "good news/bad news" type (Temin, 1980). The good news is that although regulation has not eradicated risk, it has decreased some risks by requiring standards of dosage, potency, and proof of efficacy. The bad news is that the result has been to further remove the power of choice from the consumer and from the prescribing professional. These results take on a surreal quality today, when, as psychologist Robert Anton Wilson (2002) noted, there is no "war on drugs," only a war on *some* drugs. Although tens of thousands of citizens are denied access to medical marijuana because it is allegedly "addictive," millions are prescribed legal antidepressants that are clearly "addictive" and that in many studies perform no better than placebo.

Review Questions

- What is ethnopharmacotherapy and what concerns does it try to address?
- What are some differences in response to medications that have been noted across the sexes and persons of different races?
- How can a history of discrimination and oppression affect peoples' views of psychotropic medication?
- What is the best strategy for approaching prescribing professionals with questions?
- What confidentiality issues can arise when consulting with prescribing professionals?

PHARMACOECONOMICS

Pharmacoeconomics is an interdisciplinary field where clinical outcomes overlap with health economics (Makhinova & Rascati, 2013). It began in the late 20th century as research on the economic evaluation of pharmaceutical products. Most importantly, it was to help clinicians make choices about new pharmaceutical products and helping clients get access to new medication (Schulman & Linas, 1997). Because of the economic pressure on health care systems worldwide this has developed into a thriving subdiscipline in schools of pharmacy that grant PhDs in Pharmacoeconomics (Slejko, Libby, Nair, Valuck, & Campbell, 2013). Ultimately we want to know if newer treatments that cost more are more effective. As in the case of antidepressants, it seems that they all have an efficacy hovering around 50% and newer ones do not noticeably outperform older ones. Another variable that Pharmacoeconomics must include is the power of pharmaceutical companies.

The Power of Pharmaceutical Companies

Drug companies have enormous power in all Western economies, and their power is also growing in Eastern economies. They were among the few companies to survive the Great Depression with little negative impact (Healy, 1997). Because they have enormous economic power, they also have important responsibilities once a given drug is released and important ethical considerations regarding their relationships with medical schools and other researchers (Schowalter, 2008). In many schools, Human Research Ethics Committees are reluctant to regulate potential conflicts of interest between researchers and pharmaceutical sponsors (Newcombe & Kerridge, 2007). In a survey of U.S. medical schools, only a minority of them had comprehensive conflict of interest policies (Chimos, Evarts, Littlehale, & Rothman, 2013; Chimos, Patterson, Raveis, & Rothman, 2011). The problem is not confined to the United States. In a Canadian study on conflict of interest parameters, researchers concluded only about 23% of schools polled had strong conflict of interest policies (Canadian Medical Association, 2013). Brubaker (2012) summarized conflicts of interest in three elements:

1. Main Interest: Promoting and protecting the integrity of research, patient safety and the quality of medical education.
2. Secondary Interests: Financial gain and desire for professional advancement.
3. The conflict itself wherein the main interests are sacrificed in pursuit of the secondary interests.

Brubaker (2012) suggests that all disclosures should be mandatory and should be labeled so that there is no doubt that they are mandatory. She feels that professional associations and licensure boards are well-suited to enforce such changes. Certainly changes in medical education can have an impact. Epstein, Busch, Busch, Asch, and Barry (2013) examined psychiatric residents' prescribing of antidepressants before and after a mandatory conflict of interest training. The residents who had the training were significantly less likely to prescribe the most heavily promoted antidepressants. Reviewing similar studies, Korn and Carlat (2013) conclude that strongly enforced conflict of interest policies do affect prescribing behavior.

Pharmaceutical Company–Sponsored Research

A problem recently explored in medical journals concerns pharmaceutical companies contracting with medical colleges to conduct research on company compounds. Researchers have raised the problems of conflict of interest (Boyd & Bero, 2000), publication bias (Rivara & Cummings, 2002) and what appear to be influences in effect size (Djulbegovic et al., 2000). Djulbegovic and colleagues found that industry sponsored studies were far more statistically likely to have higher quality scores than government funded studies. Although these specific areas are indeed problematic, recently the focus has shifted to overall bias in industry-sponsored research. The bias includes the sponsor's role in the study design, investigators' access to data, and control over publication (Schulman et al., 2002). The conflict-of-interest biases were addressed by the Association of American Medical Colleges guidelines on the management of financial interests related to biomedical research (Task Force on Financial Conflicts of Interest in Clinical Research, 2001). The International Committee of Medical Journal Editors (ICMJE) also revised guidelines requiring full disclosure of the sponsor's role in the research as well as requiring that investigators be independent of the sponsor, be fully accountable for the study design, have access to all study data, and have control of all editorial and publication decisions (International Committee of Medical Journal Editors [ICMJE], 2001). Recently, the ICMJE (which includes editors from the *New England Journal of Medicine* and *JAMA*, the *Journal of the American Medical Association*) adopted a policy that requires studies on medications be listed on a public registry before enrollment of human subjects. The committee felt this would give the public access to many of the studies with negative findings that pharmaceutical companies frequently keep private. This policy was adopted in the wake of unpublished data linking some antidepressants with suicidal behavior in children (Tanner, 2004).

Although these seem reasonable guidelines to safeguard the research process, the question remains, are the guidelines adhered to? In a national study of

U.S. medical school agreements to conduct research for pharmaceutical companies, Schulman et al. (2002) found that the ICMJE guidelines were rarely followed. The authors gathered results from 108 of 122 medical colleges. The median number of site agreements per college per year was 103. The researchers found that agreements between pharmaceutical companies and medical colleges rarely required an independent committee or monitoring board as a condition of the agreement. Agreements rarely addressed collection or monitoring of data, or analysis and interpretation of results. Only in 17 cases of 108 did institutional review boards routinely review agreements. In addition, most colleges got low compliance scores for access to data and power over publishing results. The authors conclude, "A reevaluation of the process of contracting for clinical research is urgently needed" (p. 1340).

Nonmedical mental health clinicians may wonder what this has to do with them. The short answer is that an overview of the influence of pharmaceutical companies seems to call into question how much clinicians can rely on published research to give a sense of the efficacy and safety of psychotropic medications. It is also important for client advocates to think critically about prescription medications. Although pharmaceutical companies certainly have improved the quality of life for many, they are among the wealthiest companies in the United States and, as such, have enormous political influence. This requires oversight and monitoring by the government, consumer groups, and those who advocate for consumers—including mental health clinicians. Those who have power rarely give it up willingly, so it must be monitored by those under its influence. However, having too much government regulation may also block a person who wants/needs a particular compound from getting it.

Pharmaceutical Companies and Direct-to-Consumer Advertising

The economic power of the pharmaceutical industry is enhanced by its direct link to the consumer through advertising. Pharmaceutical companies are now allowed to advertise directly to consumers via print and media campaigns for medications. This is called direct-to-consumer (DTC) advertising or sometimes direct-to-consumer-pharmaceutical advertising (DTCPA). DTC advertising can be defined as efforts by pharmaceutical companies to promote prescription medication directly to consumers (patients) rather than doctors. DTC advertising is now the most prominent sort of health information that the public encounters (Ventola, 2011). It is only legal in the United States and New Zealand although Canada allows ads that mention either the product or its use but not both. Pharmaceutical companies have put a major effort into overturning DTC bans in Canada and the European Union (Ventola, 2011).

Before the ban on such advertising was lifted in the late 1980s, pharmaceutical companies spent approximately $12 million a year on drug advertisements, mostly aimed at prescribing professionals. Since DTC advertising has been allowed, companies spent $600 million on such advertising in 1996 and $900 million in 1998 (Hollon, 1999). Further loosening of restrictions in 1997 (especially regarding television ads) led to DTC advertising to be a multi-billion dollar industry with $4.51 billion being spent between 2008 and 2009 (Avery, Eisenberg, & Simon, 2012). Antidepressants are the second largest prescribed drug class in the United States and DTC ads have significant impact on the sales of antidepressants (Avery, Eisenberg, & Simon, 2012a). Companies are currently including psychotropic compounds for children in their marketing strategies for those few drugs (such as stimulants) that do carry FDA on-label approval.

Advocates of the DTC movement note that it can be an excellent way of providing educational information to the consumer including new drug treatments and awareness of symptoms (Hollon, 1999; Womack, 2013). Critics note the considerable profit margins correlated with advertising and suggest that, without medical oversight, whatever quality information is available will get lost in the race for profits (Hollon, 1999; Womack, 2013). In a recent analysis Avery, Eisenberg, and

Simon (2012b) concluded that less attention in ads is given to risks of medications, ad content favors communication of benefits though they feel the balance is getting better.

Many advertisements for psychotropic medication make a point of stating that the psychological disorder (whichever is being targeted in the ad) is a "medical illness," thus seeking to capitalize on the association with allopathic models for treating disease processes such as bacterial infections. Taken literally, this could severely affect mental health professionals. Imagine if the relevant regulatory bodies agreed that mental/emotional disorders were strictly "medical illnesses." If this stricture were taken to the logical extreme, we could all be accused of practicing medicine without a license. DTC advertising is correlated with significantly larger profits. In the year 2000, the most advertised drugs saw increases in sales of 32% (Express Scripts, 2001). This trend, for better or worse, will certainly drive pharmaceutical companies to get FDA on-label approval for as-yet-untapped markets such as children and adolescents. As noted

these take time. See the FDA approval process detailed in Table 4.3. While the debate on DTC advertising rages on (Ross & Kravitz, 2013), studies increasingly conclude it can lead to needless and potentially harmful overprescribing (Niederdeppe, Byrne, Avery, & Cantor, 2013).

The Subculture of the Pharmaceutical Industry

A culture is a group of people with a shared belief system or worldview, and each pharmaceutical company, as well as the industry as a whole, develops its own subculture. With the repeal of laws banning DTC advertising, pharmaceutical companies have more opportunities than ever to portray themselves to the public. In many commercials, pharmaceutical companies portray themselves in almost heroic fashion as being on the front lines of battle against some disease or on the brink of some discovery that will revolutionize medicine. At the same time, critics have had more opportunities than ever to point to the tactics underlying DTC advertising and to what they

---

TABLE 4.3 Phases of the FDA Approval Process

Preclinical research and development using animal models (can last up to six years).

Filing and approval of Investigational New Drug Application.

After approval of Investigational New Drug Application, FDA has 30 days to decide if clinical trials will be allowed.

Phase 1: If the drug is approved, clinical trials begin with a small number of healthy volunteers (lasts about 18 months).

Phase 2: Phase 2 clinical trials include patients who might benefit from the drug (lasts about two years).

Phase 3: Phase 3 clinical trials proceed with a large number of patients where the drug is tested against placebo. This phase must yield at least two "pivotal" trials with statistically significant results. Trials typically last 4 to 6 weeks (entire phase requires about 18 months).

When Phase 3 is over, the company files a New Drug Application summarizing data.

The FDA then has 24 months to approve or not.

If the New Drug Application summarizing data is approved, the FDA then must approve the label for the drug.

Finally, after approval of label and after marketing begins, the drug must be monitored in the market for newly discovered problems.

feel are misrepresentations of facts about medicine and medical science. As MacDonald (2001) pointed out, such ads are more designed to sell the medications in question than to inform the public. Although both perspectives may have merits, the truth probably lies somewhere in the middle. The culture of pharmaceutical companies exists in the semi-free-market economy (one dynamic that prevents a purely free-market system is the granting of huge government subsidies to large corporations), and the bottom line is that the companies must make profits. How much profit they should make has been a point of contention since Estes Kefauver opened his hearings on the drug industry in the late 1950s.

The culture of pharmaceutical companies cannot be divorced from the fact that they are among the wealthiest and most powerful industries in the world. Critics such as Ariana Huffington (2000) note that the prescription drug industry cloaks its "self-interest in language about pharmaceutical research and the public good" (p. 169). Huffington chronicled the efforts of several pharmaceutical companies to stop production of inexpensive AIDS drugs in South Africa. The companies wanted South Africans to pay U.S. prices for the drugs, but the U.S. price of $500 a week equaled the annual per capita income of sub-Saharan Africa. Three companies sued South Africa to keep the South African law allowing access to these medications from taking effect. The companies also lobbied for severe trade sanctions against South Africa. Huffington raises serious questions about the ethics of an industry that makes among the largest profits in the world, neglecting research on lethal diseases in favor of developing yet more antidepressant medications or pharmaceuticals for pets (pet pharmaceuticals gross about $1 billion annually in the United States).

On the other side of the argument, commentator Thomas Sowell (2002) notes that the costs of medications reflect years of research and development, as we have seen in reviewing the FDA process. He also notes that although other countries have scientists and facilities capable of developing new medicines, economic and political situations in those countries discourage companies from investing as hugely as U.S. pharmaceutical companies do in developing new products. Sowell makes the case that the U.S. patent laws allow the company to recoup its investment and make a profit. Other countries often ignore or evade U.S. patent laws to get medications more cheaply. He also adds that the United States produces a disproportionate share of the life-saving drugs in the world.

When we ask doctors what they feel the main impact of DTC advertising is, they say it increases the numbers of patients who come in asking for some medication they saw advertised. These doctors also add that rarely do the clients fully understand what the medication can actually do for them and what the possible adverse effects are. Mental health clinicians therefore need to be aware of the connection between the way pharmaceutical companies portray themselves and those companies' economic interests, because clinicians must bridge the information gap for their clients. Students in mental health areas may feel it is hard enough keeping track of all the new medications, let alone understanding other integrative variables such as the FDA and the culture of the pharmaceutical companies. But education that is only utilitarian in nature is incomplete and potentially dangerous. The clients whom mental health professionals are pledged to serve deserve clinicians who can help them navigate complex reality by weighing the claims made for any medication in the given social and cultural environment.

The Drug Enforcement Agency

The federal Drug Enforcement Agency (DEA) is another agency that has enormous power in the United States. Reports conflict regarding the extent to which the DEA uses this power wisely, the extent to which it abuses this power (see, e.g., Szasz, 1992), and the extent to which it actually violates civil rights (Wilson, 2002). The DEA is in charge of defining and enforcing the federal drug schedules, Schedule I through Schedule V. We discuss these categories because it is important to understand that these drug categories are set up for law enforcement purposes rather than pharmacological clarity. The closer to Schedule I, the more closely monitored the drug. In many instances, the DEA guidelines refer to substances by names that

TABLE 4.4 Summary of Drug Enforcement Agency Drug Schedules

Schedule	Drugs Defined as Having ...	Examples
I	A high potential for abuse and no accepted medical use	Marijuana, heroin, mescaline
II	High abuse potential and liability for dependence. Prescriptions cannot be phoned in or renewed	Morphine, amphetamine
III	Some potential for abuse but less than drugs in the first two categories	Some stimulants and CNS depressants; lower-dose opioids
IV	Lower potential for abuse than those in Schedules I to III	Valium, antidepressants
V	The lowest potential for abuse	Drugs that contain small amounts of narcotics for antidiarrheal purposes

© Cengage Learning®

are pharmacologically incorrect (e.g., calling marijuana or LSD "narcotics"). In addition, Schedule I drugs supposedly have no medical benefit, but this is often debated, as in the case of medical marijuana.

Table 4.4 summarizes the five drug schedules. Although very few psychotropic medications described here are in the first two schedules, a few, such as methylphenidate (Ritalin), are on Schedule II. Readers can review the relevant laws and drug schedules on the DEA website at www.usdoj.gov/dea/.

Review Questions

- What are the supposed risks and benefits of DTC advertising?
- How could a conflict of financial interest in a study on a particular medication, actually harm your client if they are taking that medication?
- List and describe the five federal drug schedules. What are the weaknesses of this system?

CONCLUSION

We have covered a broad spectrum of issues in this chapter that are not normally addressed in books on psychopharmacology, yet all can have profound effects on clients. The primary activity that unites the diverse elements covered here is advocacy. Different professionals approach advocacy differently. Some mental health professionals such as counselors and social workers give a great deal of attention to client advocacy in their training and enter the field expecting to advocate for their clients in a variety of ways. Others, such as psychiatrists, may not really reflect on advocacy much while training but may develop a passionate commitment to it in the field. Moreover, different treatment settings deal with advocacy in different ways. We authors have both worked in agencies that used a treatment team approach, where the division of labor included advocacy in the job descriptions of some team members but not all. However advocacy issues are approached, it is important that the material introduced in this chapter be considered, because, as noted earlier in this chapter, the stakes for the client are very high.

Many readers who previewed this material told us it was easy to feel overwhelmed by the enormity and number of issues to consider. Here are some suggestions on ways that counselors and other mental health therapists can begin to integrate the issues in their practice:

- Consider practicing Integral diagnosis of the type suggested by Ingersoll (2002). This source gives a framework for evaluating clients with respect to social and cultural variables in addition to the standard five-axis *DSM* diagnosis. This complementary model to standard *DSM* diagnosis requires that clinicians review physical, behavioral, psychological, cultural, and social factors relevant to the client. In addition, before a diagnosis is made, the model requires that clinicians consider relevant lines of development in the client's case.

- Talk to your clients about the issues raised in this chapter and get their perspectives. Often clients know much more about their conflicts and cultural mores than you do and can teach you about their perspectives. Asking your clients to teach you about their culture can be rewarding and also contribute to the therapeutic process.
- Address cultural and social issues in your supervision, or form a special supervision group around cultural and social issues.
- Whether you work in private practice or at an agency, consider developing a website of peer-reviewed journal articles on topics such as ethnopharmacotherapy. If you have a supervision group, perhaps everyone could commit to reviewing one article per month and posting the review or abstract with the full reference on the website.
- As an exercise in professional development, have staff consider a case with and without the cultural/social variables and then discuss how adding these variables to the case summary may enrich treatment possibilities.
- Keep an anonymous file in Excel or some other database program for your clients on medication. List diagnosis, medication, dosage, race, gender, age, and ethnicity if known. If you work in an agency where you may see hundreds of clients per year, such records can reveal interesting patterns.

SUMMARY

Perhaps more than any other, this chapter illustrates how an integrative view of psychopharmacology expands the things we consider. Although generations of psychotropic medications were tested on Caucasian adult males, only recently has the subdiscipline of ethnopharmacotherapy questioned the legitimacy of generalizing from such studies to people of different sexes, races, and ethnic backgrounds. Further, mental health clinicians need to understand the cultures that their clients identify with so that they can better understand how culture may impact the way a client reacts to the idea of taking a psychotropic medication.

Although culture, sex, race, and ethnicity are important factors to consider in psychopharmacology, the impact and power of social institutions must also be considered. Institutions such as the FDA, the DEA, and the pharmaceutical industry hold enormous power that must be held accountable to checks and balances. Along the lines of culture and the impact of social institutions on clients, mental health clinicians must be prepared to advocate for clients when necessary.

STUDY QUESTIONS AND EXERCISES

1. When recommending to female clients that they be evaluated for psychotropic medication, several unique issues and concerns arise. Discuss in detail these problems, and develop a strategy of how you will address them.

2. How do you perceive the FDA and the pharmaceutical industry to be relating to clients who take psychotropic medications? Give examples.

3. How might you try to influence outcomes relevant to the FDA or pharmaceutical companies that concern you?

4. Do you support DTC advertising? Why or why not?

5. Generally discuss your perspective on free-market economies and whether or not indigent clients should have access to expensive medications. How do you support your views? If you support both free-market economic theory and access to medical treatment for the poor, how do you reconcile these two positions?

6. Are there any psychotropic prescription medications that you think should be over the counter? Explain your rationale.

7. From your personal or professional experience and the examples cited in this chapter, develop a strategy for talking with a client from a culture other than your own about taking psychotropic medication.

8. How would you deal with a Mexican man who refused medication because he believes his symptoms are a message from God telling him that he is one of the chosen few?

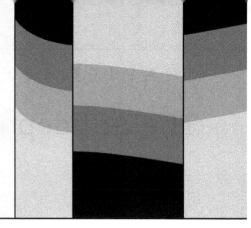

PART TWO

Introduction

This second part of the book contains four chapters covering classes of commonly prescribed psychotropic drugs used to treat depression, anxiety, psychosis, mood symptoms like mania, and a host of other conditions. Each chapter includes some history on the discovery and use of each category of drugs. This history provides the context that informs the four perspectives we comment on in each chapter. In addition to the history, we present medical model theories of how the drugs work and cover common drugs in each category including their side effects.

Each chapter includes relevant material from the psychological, cultural, and social perspectives. As we have in previous chapters, we will note both the generic and brand names of medications (e.g., fluoxetine/Prozac) each time we mention them. Our students have shared that this repetition helps them learn the names. The *PDR,* the *Physicians' Desk Reference,* is the standard reference book on drug names, both generic names and brands. It is available both at the reference desk of most public libraries and online.

CHAPTER FIVE

The Antidepressant Era

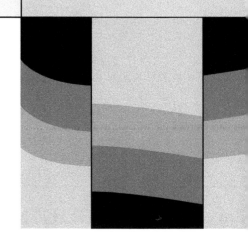

The title of this chapter derives from a book of the same title by David Healy (1997). Healy points out the important but overlooked fact that depression proper (what the *DSM-5* calls Major Depressive Disorder) [American Psychiatric Association (APA), 2013] was basically unheard of as recently as 50 years ago. For Healy, the antidepressant era unfolded against a backdrop of battles within the psychiatric profession (people endorsing the medical model perspective battling those endorsing models emphasizing a psychological perspective), regulatory agencies such as the Food and Drug Administration (FDA), and the pharmaceutical industry. Antidepressant medications are among the medications most advertised directly to consumers and evidence is mounting that this does not in fact increase consumer knowledge about depression and antidepressants but rather increases misperceptions like the discredited chemical imbalance theory of depression (Park, 2013).

This chapter is divided into seven sections. Section One provides an overview of the current impact of antidepressants and Major Depressive Disorder. Section Two describes early theories of antidepressant action. Section Three covers the neurotrophic/plasticity theory of antidepressant action and other newer findings. Section Four begins coverage of the classes of antidepressant medications with what are called first generation antidepressants. Section Five is devoted to selective serotonin reuptake inhibitors (second generation antidepressants). Section Six covers third-generation antidepressants like bupriopion and duloxetine and experimental drugs

like ketamine. Section Seven covers important psychological, cultural, and social perspectives on antidepressants including the concerns about violent behavior being correlated with antidepressant therapy.

SECTION ONE: THE CURRENT IMPACT OF ANTIDEPRESSANTS

Learning Objectives

- Know what the point and lifetime prevalence of Major Depressive Disorder is.
- Understand the conditions that are often comorbid with depression.
- Be able to articulate sex differences in reported rates of depression.
- Know what meta-analytic studies note as the overall efficacy of antidepressants.

A television commercial features a grimacing young man with his face against a wall. The commercial's narrator lists several symptoms of fear and anxiety related to Social Anxiety Disorder (previously Social Phobia in *DSM-IV*). The last scene in the commercial shows the same young man smiling, rising from a table in a crowded room apparently to receive acclaim for some accomplishment. The ad ends by repeating the name of the medication and informing the viewer, "Your life is waiting." As we noted in Chapter Four, there is vigorous debate as to whether such ads are a valuable source of information or prey on the misconceptions many people have about such drugs being "magic potions" to change their lives.

At this writing, antidepressants are still one of the most advertised and prescribed psychotropic medications. Over $11 billion is spent annually for antidepressants and it is estimated that between 17 million (Ross, 2012) and 22 million Americans (IMS Health, 2014) take them. In the late-20th century prescriptions for antidepressants for children increased at an exponential rate (Bostic, Wilens, Spencer, & Biederman, 1997) despite scant evidence to support their use for children and growing evidence that these drugs may exacerbate symptoms such as suicidal ideation in child and adolescents. In 2003, the FDA issued a public health advisory about the risk of suicidality in children taking SSRI antidepressants, which led to the "black box warning" on antidepressants. After this point prescription rates for children and adolescents declined (Libby et al., 2007). About 65% of antidepressants are prescribed for depression and about 16% for anxiety disorders (Mark, 2010). In the early part of the 21st century, meta-analytic studies began suggesting that the efficacy of antidepressants is about the same as the placebo, in other words 50%. The efficacy increases as the severity of depression in the subjects increases but there does not seem to be any difference in efficacy between the antidepressant drugs (Del Ra, Spielmans, Fluckiger, & Wampold, 2013; Kirsch & Low, 2013). Some chalk this up to methodological problems (Petkova, Tarpey, Huang, & Deng, 2012) but it is clear there is a strong placebo response in studies on antidepressants that needs further exploration.

Antidepressants are used both on and off label for numerous disorders. When antidepressant medications were introduced in the mid-20th century, physicians primarily used them to treat depression. Currently, antidepressants are used to treat a variety of disorders, including a number of anxiety disorders, impulsive aggression, and even chronic pain. Although antidepressants may help people with a variety of depressive symptoms, most studies on antidepressants examine their use in treating Major Depressive Disorder as defined by *DSM-5*. Thus, before discussing the history of antidepressants, let's review Major Depressive Disorder proper.

MAJOR DEPRESSIVE DISORDER (MDD)

The 12-month prevalence of MDD is approximately 7% with significant differences across age groups. For example, the prevalence in 18–29 year olds is three times higher than in people 60 years or older. It seems that male children are more prone to depression than female children but after puberty, females have a 1.5–3 fold higher reported rate than males (American Psychiatric Association, 2013).

MDD is diagnosed when a person meets five criteria from a list of nine in *DSM-5*. Practitioners using the International Classification of Diseases Mental and Behavioral Disorders (WHO, 1992) can choose from specifiers of severity based on the number of symptoms a client has. Symptoms in both manuals include vegetative symptoms like increase or decrease in ability to sleep, increased or decreased eating and weight changes, decreased sex drive, difficulty concentrating, and anhedonia (loss of pleasure in things the person used to enjoy). The depressed person may also have inappropriate guilt, recurrent thoughts of death, fatigue most of the day, and feelings of worthlessness. It is important to note that we have no clear understanding of why the antidepressant drugs covered in this chapter would directly reduce the symptoms listed. There are different theories but we have yet to understand why people get depressed and, when medication helps them, why it helps them. That said though, we know that the more vegetative symptoms a client with depression has, the better candidate they are for an antidepressant. We should note that it is important to add that depression is also part of the symptom profile in *many* disorders including Bipolar I Disorder, Bipolar II Disorder, Persistent Depressive Disorder (previously Dysthymia in *DSM-IV*), Schizoaffective Disorder, Cyclothymia, and Substance Use Disorders.

COMORBIDITY OF DEPRESSION AND ANXIETY

Depression and anxiety, two of the most common symptom types seen by mental health professionals, are often comorbid (occur together) in adults as well as children. This is so much the case that the study groups for *DSM-5* considered a Mixed Anxiety and Depression diagnosis though it did not appear in the final draft. This highlights the importance of an accurate diagnosis, because a client may suffer from depression with some secondary anxiety, anxiety with some secondary depression, or from both an anxiety disorder as well as a mood disorder. Even when a client's symptoms fall into one diagnostic cluster at the time of intake, such a client may later show symptoms outside that cluster. Diagnosis is a process that continues throughout the therapeutic relationship and goes well beyond the limited categories of the *DSM*. Although we focus mainly on depression and antidepressants in this chapter and on anxiety and anxiolytics in Chapter Six, these are rather artificial distinctions we use for instructive purposes. Just as students must learn the "laws" of Newtonian physics before they can understand the exceptions to those laws that occur in particle physics, they must also learn how classes of medications evolved around diagnostic categories and how market and clinical forces exploit the permeable nature of these classes. In the next section, we discuss theories of antidepressant action from the medical model perspective.

ANTIDEPRESSANT EFFICACY

When an antidepressant "works," what does that mean and *how* does it work? The drug "working" usually means is some but not all symptoms decrease or go into remission. How the drug works is a harder question to answer. The simple answer is "we don't know." We have theories but we don't know. It is interesting that when we were writing the first edition of this book, published reports of antidepressant efficacy estimated the drugs worked approximately 65%. This figure came from analyzing published results; however, as became known in the late 20th century, when pharmaceutical companies started paying to have research done on their own medications, they often retained the rights to all results and in many cases chose to suppress unfavorable results and redesign the study to increase the probability of favorable results (Petersen, 2009). That was when the debate began about true efficacy. Researchers began analyzing not just published studies but all studies logged in the FDA database. Based on this initial findings were that efficacy rates seemed closer to 50% (Armstrong & Winstein, 2008). As noted, the debate on efficacy is ongoing but there is a robust placebo response seen in antidepressant studies that you do not see in studies treating disorders like Schizophrenia. This may be because depression is overdetermined, meaning there are many ways one could get depressed (Ingersoll & Marquis, 2014) whereas Schizophrenia (though we still don't know its etiology) seems more rooted in the brain and nervous system.

Review Questions

- What are the point and lifetime prevalences for Major Depressive Disorder?
- What conditions are most commonly comorbid with Major Depressive Disorder?
- What are the sex differences in reported rates of depression?
- What do meta-analyses suggest the overall efficacy of antidepressants to be?

SECTION TWO: THEORIES OF ANTIDEPRESSANT ACTION

Learning Objectives

- Be able to describe the amine, reuptake inhibition and downregulation theories as they relate to antidepressant action.
- Understand how each of these theories built on its predecessor.
- Understand the barriers and failed attempts at measuring levels of neurotransmitters in the brain.

Researchers have sought to delineate profiles of clients with depression, to gauge the degree to which a particular client's depression is biological in nature. They have assumed that clients with depression that was more biological in nature would be better candidates for antidepressant medications, whereas clients whose depression was more psychological in nature would be better candidates for counseling or psychotherapy. As Stahl (2000) concluded, however, "The search for any biological markers of depression, let alone those that might be predictive of antidepressant responsiveness, has been disappointing" (p. 145). Today, the field of pharmacogenetics aims to match antidepressant response to idiosyncrasies of client's genomes but this research has just begun and it remains to be seen if it will bear results that are applicable (Jones & Perlis, 2006).

How do antidepressants work? Various theories from the medical model perspective are proposed to explain antidepressant action. Each tends to build on its predecessors. In this sense, these theories actually demonstrate one of the ideals of scientific method—new theories ideally are built on older theories. However, although these theories do build on one another, scientists still do not understand why antidepressants alter mood. Perhaps Healy (2002) captured the ultimate usefulness of theories when he stated, "[H]aving a theory is scientifically useful primarily because having a theory leads to action" (p. 118). In this case, the action depends on the theory. From an integrative perspective, we will see that even rigorous theories of how antidepressants work only correlate the drug mechanisms of action with symptom relief. It must be noted, however, that this correlation is not causation. In the case of depression, many times the theories about medications *lead to* diagnoses rather than the other way around. This has been emphasized both by psychiatrists with knowledge of pharmacology (such as Healy) and by laypeople such as Elizabeth Wurtzel. In her memoir of suffering from depression, Wurtzel (1994) commented that once she was prescribed Prozac, she had a diagnosis. She wrote,

> Rather than defining my disease as a way to lead us to fluoxetine, the invention of this drug has brought us to my disease. Which seems backward,

but … this is a typical course of events in psychiatry, that the discovery of a drug to treat, say, schizophrenia, will tend to result in many more patients being diagnosed as schizophrenics. This is strictly Marxian psychopharmacology, where the material—or rather, pharmaceutical—means determine the way an individual's case history is interpreted. (p. 265)

Amine Theory

The amine theory of depression began as the **catecholaminergic hypothesis of depression** proposed by Ernst Albert Zeller and his research team (Zeller, Barsky, Fouts, Kirchheimer, Van Orden, 1952). Catecholamines are organic compounds derived from the amino acid tyrosine and include the neurotransmitters norepinephrine (NE), dopamine (DA), and epinephrine (Epi). A broader chemical class is the amines that are compounds derived from ammonia by replacing one or more hydrogen atoms with organic groups. The neurotransmitters serotonin (5-HT), DA, NE, Epi, and acetylcholine (Ach) are all amines. Thus, as soon as researchers began to suspect serotonin (5-HT) played a role in depression the catecholamine hypothesis was made broader into the amine hypothesis.

The **amine hypothesis** began with researchers observing the effects of antidepressants on norepinephrine. Simply put, the amine hypothesis *proposed* that people who suffered from depression did not have enough amines, particularly NE, in their synapses, and if you could increase the NE then they would not be depressed. It was a parsimonious theory and, as with most parsimonious theories, it did not address the complexity of the situation. It is important to note though that researchers in the mid-20th century can be forgiven for adhering to the overly simple amine hypothesis because at that point all they knew about the drugs was that they somehow increased amines.

The first step in the amine hypothesis is credited to Ernst Albert Zeller (mentioned above) who was working as a biochemist at Northwestern University in the 1950s. Zeller and his research team had discovered that one function of the enzyme monoamine oxidase (MAO) was to disable neuro-transmitters after they had been fired from the terminal button (Zeller et al., 1952). This made sense because scientists knew neurotransmitters did not just float in the synapse forever and that the body must have a way to disable them. While screening chemicals for this disabling ability, Zeller found that iproniazid/Marsilid (the antitubercular drug Nathan Klein used as an antidepressant) was a powerful inhibitor of MAO (thus the name *MAO inhibitor*) (Snyder, 1996). Further research confirmed that iproniazid/Marsilid, by disabling MAO, did indeed raise NE levels in the synapse. In 1957, Udenfriend, Weissback, and Bogdanski (1957) observed that iproniazid/Marsilid also increased the release of serotonin (5-HT) in the brain.

It is widely believed that scientists at the time used a drug called reserpine/Serpalan to deplete the brain of amines and cause an animal model of depression. The story is that researchers gave both reserpine/Serpalan and iproniazid/Marsilid to monkeys. First the reserpine/Serpalan made them appear lethargic and fatigued (the animal model of depression) and then the iproniazid/Marsilid led the monkeys to become highly animated. This then led to the notion that perhaps iproniazid/Marsilid was a **psychic energizer** (Snyder, 1996) or what the reserpine research team called a "marsilizer" referring to the trade name of the compound (Lopez-Munoz & Alamo, 2009). This was found to be more speculation than fact on the part of Nathan Klein (1970) who popularized the MAO Inhibitors for their antidepressant properties (Baumeister, Hawkins, & Uzelac, 2003).

Researchers later discovered that reserpine/Serpalan did cause both norepinephrine and serotonin to leak out of the synaptic vesicles into the synaptic cleft, where MAO disables it. Thus, disabling MAO greatly increases the newly leaked norepinephrine and serotonin in the synaptic cleft, allowing more binding to area receptors than does an undrugged state. These discoveries (exaggerated though they seem to have been) were the primary support for the amine theory. Historical review of the reserpine/Serpalan studies revealed that in actuality only a subset of patients developed depressive

symptoms while on reserpine/Serpalan (Akiskal & McKinney, 1973). Again, to clarify, the amine theory of depression was that people who are depressed do not have enough amines (such as nor-epinephrine) in the synapses between important neurons. Drugs that increased the amines thus alleviated depression.

To this point, this first MAO inhibitor (iproniazid/Marsilid) had only been used to treat tuberculosis. It was noticed that the drug also had power to stimulate the CNS in patients being treated. This was initially thought to be a side effect (Selikoff, Robit-zek, & Ornstein, 1952). This then led Jackson Smith (1953) to try the drug on depressed patients. They noted improvement in 2 of the 11 in the group and other studies followed [it is thought that one of the later researchers, Max Lurie, coined the term antidepressant (Lopez-Munoz & Alamo, 2009)]. Nathan Klein carried out the same procedures on subjects and reported that 70% showed substantial improvement (Loomer, Saudners, & Kline, 1958). Given that the response rate in Smith's study was only 18%, it is curious that response rates in Klein's studies rocketed to 70%. To date we are not aware of any re-analysis of this early work. Be that as it may, iproniazid/Marsilid, was on the map as an antidepressant.

Tricyclic antidepressants evolved in Europe through the work of Roland Kuhn (1958) about the same time MAO inhibitors were developing in the United States. Given the MAO research, Kuhn and his colleagues thought tricyclics worked in the same way, by disabling MAO or some related enzyme and increasing NE in the synaptic cleft. The clinical actions of both drugs, after all, were quite similar. This assumption soon ran into problems, however, when researchers discovered that much of the MAO in the nervous system exists inside the cells rather than in the synaptic cleft. Also, all antidepressants seemed to have a time lag of at least two weeks before they took effect. This didn't make sense, because MAO began to inhibit iproniazid within hours after the patient took the first dose.

As noted, the amine theory proved too parsimonious. For one thing, the idea of depressed clients being deficient in a neurotransmitter should correlate with lower levels of the metabolite for the neurotransmitter they are supposed to be lacking. Although some subjects in studies show this correlation, others do not. Stahl (2000) noted that when the metabolite for serotonin (5-HT) is low, it is more likely correlated with impulsive behavior than with depression proper. Plus, the amine theory did not explain why it took the antidepressants four to six weeks to work.

The Discovery of Reuptake Inhibition

The next researcher to make important discoveries in this area was Arvid Carlsson who discovered how tricyclics blocked reuptake of serotonin at the brain level (Carlsson, Fuxe, & Ungerstedt, 1968). After this discovery, Izyaslav Lapin and Gregory Oxenkrug (1969) postulated the serotonergic theory of depression, similar to the amine theory only focusing on serotonin rather than norepinephrine. In the 1950s, working at the National Institutes of Health in Bethesda, Maryland, Julius Axelrod discovered that with tricyclic antidepressants, norepinephrine was increased in the synaptic cleft when the drug inhibited the reuptake mechanism discovered by Carlsson. The mechanism works like this: When norepinephrine is released into the synaptic cleft, it has a period of time to bind to receptors. After this period, it is either broken down by MAO or a transporter molecule attaches to the NE neurotransmitter and takes it back inside the cell that released it in the first place, where enzymes store it in synaptic vesicles so it can be released again. In this way, the transporter molecule provides something like a recycling service.

Other researchers have identified a similar mechanism for most other neurotransmitters, with the exception of acetylcholine, which is deactivated by the enzyme acetylcholinesterase (just as norepinephrine can be deactivated by monoamine oxidase). This discovery only served to reinforce the amine theory of depression, because researchers eventually discovered that drugs such as tricyclic antidepressants work by inhibiting this reuptake mechanism and thus allowing released neurotransmitters to stay

longer in the synaptic cleft. For his work in this area, Axelrod shared the 1970 Nobel Prize in Medicine with Ulf von Euler and Sir Bernard Katz. (It is one of the few Nobel prizes awarded for work related to psychotropic medications because most discoveries in the area of psychotropic medications are more luck and serendipity than the result of carefully crafted hypotheses).

Nevertheless, the same time lag noted for MAO inhibitors existed with tricyclic antidepressant drugs that inhibited reuptake. For example, about an hour after the person takes a tricyclic antidepressant the reuptake inhibition begins and the amount of neurotransmitter in the synaptic cleft increases, but symptoms do not abate for between two and four weeks (maybe even as long as six weeks). So, despite making important contributions to the understanding of reuptake inhibition, Axelrod had not solved the riddle of how tricyclic antidepressants actually *work* to change mood.

Downregulation Theory

Although enzyme deactivation and reuptake inhibition are important elements in most antidepressants' mechanism of action, they still don't account for the two- to six-week lag of the antidepressant effect. The reuptake properties of tricyclic antidepressants and selective serotonin reuptake inhibitors begin increasing levels of neurotransmitters within an hour of someone's taking the medicine. Another problem is that other drugs that dramatically boost the levels of similar neurotransmitters (cocaine) do not act as antidepressants. Although they may induce euphoria, they also cause an emotional "crash" when the drug wears off. This knowledge contributed to the development of postsynaptic receptor desensitization (downregulation) theory as a complement to the amine theory. This theory proposes that initially the receptors in the depressed person are hypersensitive to neurotransmitter because depressed people have less of that neurotransmitter (remember these are just theories that were partially but not totally accurate). Because there was supposedly less neurotransmitter, the researchers hypothesized that receptors act as if they are "starved" for it, so they upregulate (increase in number). (Remember, this is a theory using metaphors—not concrete truths. In the metaphor used to explain this theory, receptors are not really "starved" for a neurotransmitter but if they had human qualities one might say they would act as if they were. Such **anthropomorphizing** of things like neurons is replete with ways it can be misunderstood). With antidepressant treatment, as more neurotransmitter becomes available, the receptors get more neurotransmitter than is needed because they previously increased in number (upregulated) to make use of the available neurotransmitter in the synaptic cleft. At this point, the cell gets bombarded with neurotransmitter, because the increased levels of neurotransmitter are now binding with the increased numbers of receptors. The theory suggested that the cells then *adjust* by decreasing the number and sensitivity of receptors, because more neurotransmitter is available. Theoretically, this normalizes transmission or provides the "balance" that is correlated with decrease of symptoms. So according to downregulation theory, the antidepressant effect is the result of two mechanisms. The first is the increase of neurotransmitter released into the synapse (accomplished through reuptake inhibition or enzymatic inhibition), and the second is the downregulation of receptors to a "normal" level of responsiveness (to adapt to the increased levels of neurotransmitter). The time frame required for neurons to decrease the number of receptors correlates closely with the lag time between taking a drug and experiencing the antidepressant effect (two to six weeks depending on the client and dosage of medication) (Stahl, Hauger, Rausch, Flieshaker, & Hubbell-Alberts, 1993).

The downregulation theory led researchers to consider the role of receptor sensitivity in mental/emotional disorders. This combination of the amine theory and downregulation theory was used to account for the action of antidepressants until very recently. Remember, these were and still are just theories. Researchers never had conclusive evidence that the theories fully explained the function

of antidepressants nor that there was any "chemical imbalance" that caused depression. To be clear, there is no direct way to measure an extracellular level of any neurotransmitter in the human brain. Some postmortem studies on the brains of people who committed suicide suggested there were low levels of 5-HT in the brain stem tissue but without a baseline it is not possible to say what is "low." Also the amount of 5-HT in tissue is not necessarily reflective of extracellular amounts (amounts in the synapse) (Jacobson, Medvedev, & Caron, 2012). For decades, researchers have probed the brain with indirect measures looking for biomarkers of 5-HT. Cerebrospinal fluid (CSF) levels of the 5-HT metabolite 5 hydroxyindoleacetic acid (5-HIAA) have been thought to reflect brain levels of 5-HT but the correlations between lower levels of this metabolite are more consistent with things like aggression, suicidality and impulsivity than depression (Placidi et al., 2001).

There have been so-called challenge methods where 5-HT in the central nervous system is challenged with another agent and the resulting changes in things *linked to* 5-HT have been observed. For example, fenfluramine/Pondimin has been used in depressed subjects in this manner. Fenfluramine/Pondimin stimulates 5-HT to trigger secretion of prolactin. The prolactin is measured and a blunted response was thought to reflect low 5-HT level and a robust prolactin response to reflect a high 5-HT level (Mann, McBride, Malone, DeMeo, & Keilp, 1995). The problem with this is that the triggering of prolactin secretion is a complex process involving not just 5-HT but gamma-amino-butyric acid (GABA), peptides, and oxytocin (Emiliano & Fudge, 2004). As these examples illustrate, "... the association of 5-HT deficiency, or any other singular biochemical anomaly, with major depression as the all-encompassing syndrome is inconclusive" (Jacobson et al., 2012).

Variations on these theories were proposed, such as the permissive theory, which restated the amine hypothesis but included serotonin rather than exclusively focusing on norepinephrine. The permissive theory also tried to explain the role of serotonin in regulating levels of norepinephrine and dopamine. Although all these theories expanded available data on antidepressant action, none fully accounted for antidepressant effects or the strong placebo responses in many studies of antidepressants (we return to these later). The latest hypothesis to explain antidepressant effects takes the discussion deeper into the mysteries of the cells called *neurons,* as we describe next.

Neurotransmitter Receptor Hypothesis

The neurotransmitter receptor hypothesis asserts that in depression, something is wrong with particular receptors for monoamine neurotransmitters. Researchers think this "something wrong" leads to depression. It is also related to the upregulation of receptors discussed earlier. Because this hypothesis focuses on the receptors and because receptors are a function of gene expression, this hypothesis also considers that depression may relate to some function (or malfunction) of gene expression. Certainly this is a possibility; however, where genetics is concerned it is important to state hypotheses tentatively and concisely to avoid lapsing into word magic. Although admitting that direct evidence to support the genetic hypothesis is lacking, Stahl (2000) discusses the previously outlined postmortem studies of the brains of suicide victims where test results show that the tissue in parts of these brains have increased numbers of 5-HT2 receptors. He concludes that further research may support a genetic variation of the neurotransmitter receptor hypothesis.

Review Questions

- What are the theories of amine theory, reuptake inhibition, and downregulation, and how do they relate to antidepressant action?
- How did each of the theories in question (1) build on each other?
- What efforts have been made to measure neurotransmitter levels in the brain? Why have these failed?

SECTION THREE: THE NEUROTROPHIC/ PLASTICITY HYPOTHESIS AND NEW THEORIES OF ANTIDEPRESSANT ACTION

Learning Objectives

- Be able to articulate the basic steps in the neurotrophic/plasticity theory of depression and antidepressant actions.
- Have a general understanding of signaling pathways in cells and how they may figure into antidepressant action.
- Be able to give an overview of the neuropsychological theory of antidepressant action and re-learning in recovery from depression.

The **neurotrophic/plasticity hypothesis** began as the **cellular/molecular theory of antidepressant action** (Duman, Heninger, & Nestler, 1997). This required advances in medical technology that allowed scientists to peer inside neurons. The result is a theory that transcends the other theories outlined so far. At the outset, we want to stress that this is unlikely to be the final word on the biological theories of depression, because it also leaves many questions unanswered.

The cellular/molecular theory of depression was first outlined by Duman et al. (1997). In a sense it is a metatheory, in that it encompasses and transcends its predecessor theories in a way that it is a theory about the previous theories. The authors begin by summarizing the complementarity of amine theory and downregulation theory, noting that these theories accurately outline certain actions of antidepressants but fail to explain why such actions would improve mood. They then assert that increases in the levels of available neurotransmitters and the resulting downregulation are merely the beginning of antidepressant action. Next they document intracellular changes in response to someone taking antidepressant medications. Note that these authors maintain that once a person takes an antidepressant medication, these intracellular changes occur *after* the drug increases the neurotransmitter levels and persist after downregulation. These authors explain that within the cell, antidepressants cause an increase in cyclic adenosine monophosphate (cyclic AMP or cAMP). Cyclic AMP is a second messenger molecule with many functions. Some of these functions are activating enzymes in the neuron, amplifying the effects of hormones and neurotransmitters, and providing other vital functions in the cell. The cAMP levels raised by taking antidepressants apparently do not return to lower levels as the person adjusts to the presence of the drug. Interestingly, cAMP governs the production and processing of neurotrophins called *brain-derived neurotrophic factors (BDNFs)*. BDNF is a neurotrophin in the brain that plays an important role in regulating neurogenesis (creation of new neurons), differentiating neural pathways during neurodevelopment, and modulating synaptic plasticity as well as dendritic growth.

So after administration of antidepressants, as cAMP increases in response to the antidepressant medication, these neurotrophins (BDNF) also increase. You can think of the neurotrophins as akin to brain cell nutrients in that they trigger changes associated with neurogenesis and maintenance of existing neurons. Many of the changes following antidepressant treatment occur in the hippocampus, which is part of the limbic system.

Without unpacking all the molecular biology involved, let's say the basic idea is that the cell goes through many changes after an antidepressant is introduced into the system and that the increase in neurotrophins (cell nutrients) may be one of the most important. The developers of the cellular/molecular theory of depression are proposing that stress and disease processes cause neurological atrophy ranging from reversible to irreversible. One manifestation of this hypothesized atrophy is depression. Such damage may be reversed by an increase in cell nutrients that is one of the many results of taking an antidepressant medication. Brain-derived neurotrophic factor holds promise for treating degenerative brain disorders such as Parkinson's disease. In a recent study in the United Kingdom, researchers injected neurotrophic factor directly into the brain of patients

suffering from Parkinson's disease. These patients experienced dramatic decreases in their symptoms (Schorr, 2004). It has also been shown that infusion of BDNF into the hippocampus of rats produced what appeared to be antidepressant effects (Hurley et al., 2013). Such work may hold promise for mental and emotional disorders that have clear biological correlates, but those correlates must be conclusively determined.

The following flow chart summarizes these theories of depression and how each one builds on previous ones.

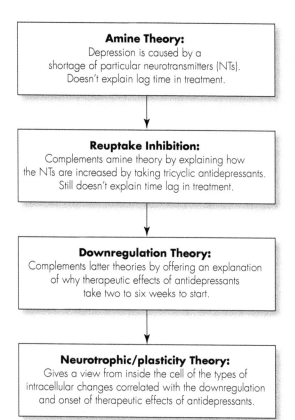

Not only does the neurotrophic/plasticity theory of depression hold promise for providing a fuller understanding of how antidepressants work, it also promises a fuller understanding of nonpharmacologic approaches to treating depression. Scientists have known for some time that physical exercise is effective in reducing depressive symptoms (De Melo Coelho et al., 2013; Salmon, 2001). Researchers have already documented that general physical exercise rapidly increases brain-derived neurotrophic factors (Russo-Neustadt, Beard, & Cotman, 1999). In studies using brain scan technology, depressed participants taking an antidepressant medication and depressed participants engaging in interpersonal therapy showed similar changes in their brain scans as their depression improved. Although the therapy group took longer to manifest these changes, they were as significant as the changes in the group taking the antidepressant (Brody et al., 2001). Apparently exercise and counseling/psychotherapy may induce the same types of intracellular changes as antidepressants. If future research supports this hypothesis, it is important for counselors and other mental health professionals to understand, because this radically expands a client's treatment options. This is also why we emphasize an integrative openness regarding the mind–brain issue in this book: Mind—intention, attention, and awareness—may well be as effective—or more effective—than pharmacologic interventions.

NEWER HYPOTHESES AND THEORIES

Since the advent of the neurotrophic/plasticity theory, researchers have learned many new things about how antidepressants seem to work in the brain. First, BDNF has been traced to genes. The gene for BDNF is on chromosome 11 and is about 1300 letters long. In most animals, letter 192 is "G" (for guanine) but in some it is "C" (cytosine). This causes a slightly different protein to be built with methioline rather than valine at the 66th position. Thus, with regard to the gene for BDNF there are three types of people in the world:

1. Val-vals
2. Val-mets
3. Met-mets

   In research on the five-factor model of personality, the most neurotic to least neurotic are supposedly val-vals (most neurotic), val-mets, and met-mets (least neurotic). Thus, building BDNF proteins with methioline *may* serve a protective factor from things

like depression and anxiety (Kourmouli et al., 2013). This is the type of research necessary to address the complexity of how genes may contribute to developing symptoms like depression.

The Emerging Science of the Role of Signaling Pathways in Depression

We have already noted that antidepressants seem to increase cAMP, which then increases BDNF. We have further learned that there is signaling pathway for cAMP that may be pivotal in therapeutic response to antidepressants. We noted that cAMP is a second messenger that has many functions including transferring into cells the effects of hormones that cannot pass through the cell membrane. There are also multiple signaling pathways used by cells to regulate cellular processes. cAMP also qualifies as one of these. In the cAMP pathway, cAMP activates molecules called effectors that bind to proteins to regulate their biological activity.

   One effector that may play a role in antidepressant effects is protein kinase and in particular on family of enzymes labeled protein kinase A (PKA). It seems that PKA activity is increased after four to six weeks of antidepressant treatment. PKA activity in turn activates the cAMP response element binding protein (CREB), which is a transcription factor (a protein that binds to specific DNA sequences). This in turn affects the expression of several genes involved in cell survival, neuroplasticity, and cognition. Again we can see that the more current theories of antidepressant action are increasingly sophisticated regarding how complex the human nervous system is compared to earlier theories like the amine theory. CREB has been implicated in both depression and antidepressant treatments (Pilar-Cuellar et al., 2013). The implication is that things that affect cAMP and BDNF have ripples far down the signaling pathway increasing the variables that may play a role in alleviating depression whether the client is involved in antidepressant therapy, exercise, or psychotherapy or all of the above.

   The next pathway that may play a role in antidepressant response is called the Wnt/B-Catenin pathway (Wnt). The Wingless-type family of proteins play key roles during neurodevelopment like neural differentiation, formation of the hippocampus, dendritic arborization, axon guidance, and formation of synapses. On a larger scale, this family of proteins plays a role in memory and spatial learning (Pilar-Cuellar et al., 2013). Wnt is also implicated in the etiology and treatment of depression (Hernandez, Nido, Avila, & Villanueva, 2009). In the absence of Wnt signaling, important functions in the cell are blocked by glycogen synthase kinase-3 and other ligands. This "blocking" seems undone in some (but not all) clients with antidepressant and so-called mood-stabilizing medications (Jope & Bijur, 2002).

A third pathway that may be important in antidepressant treatment is called the mTOR pathway and is related to rampamycin genes. Thus, the abbreviation mTOR is derived from the original name for this pathway "mammalian target of rampamycin." This pathway is important in apoptosis (cell death) and has mainly been studied in cancer, and a number of neurological diseases like Alzheimer's-type dementia. Recent studies associate mTOR signaling in depression because of the fast-acting effects of ketamine (discussed below) as an antidepressant (Mathew, Keegan, & Smith, 2005).

Reviewing physiological theories of how antidepressants work can be dizzying as well as impressive. The key is to not forget that although these theories encompass truths about antidepressants and depression, they are only partial truths. These theories give us important truths from the medical model perspective. However, they are only partial truths; resist the temptation to simplify the complexity of something such as recovering from depression with word magic claiming that antidepressants corrected a "chemical imbalance." When clients respond to antidepressants, that response is only partial in some cases. As Ross (1995) pointed out, even in those studies up to 30% of the clients may respond to placebo, but this finding is never systematically followed up. Finally, Stahl (2000) noted that in terms of recovery, follow-up studies of depressed clients after one year of treatment indicate that approximately 40% still meet the criteria for the same diagnosis and 20% never recover fully or meet the criteria for dysthymia (low-grade depression). Further, Stahl notes that in

18-month follow-ups, many clients who respond to antidepressants report that the antidepressants stop working. This is given the highly technical name "pooping out." The percentage of clients whose antidepressants "poop out" after 18 months is as high as 20 to 30% in some studies.

TOWARD AN INTEGRATIVE THEORY OF ANTIDEPRESSANT ACTION

It seems that as our technologies improve, we are peering deeper and deeper into the brain, the neurons, glial cells, and the universe within each cell. At some point, it is reasonable to ask how far down this path we can go and get results. At some point, we will reach the subatomic level and will we yet have a complete picture of depression and antidepressant action? Some theorists are positing an integrative approach that moves from the top down and the bottom up. The "bottom up" part is the theories of antidepressants that we have covered thus far. The "top down" is a new theory called the cognitive neuropsychological theory of antidepressant action.

This theory was laid out in the context of selective serotonin reuptake inhibitors (SSRIs) but can be generalized across antidepressants. The basis of the theory is this: that depression comes with a negative cognitive bias and antidepressants, even after only one day of treatment, are correlated with a decrease in negative bias and an increase in positive bias (Harmer & Cowen, 2013). This theory can be traced back to Crews and Harrison (1995). The essence of the idea is that people who are depressed show a negative emotional bias that has sometimes been called "depressive realism" because they are more accurate at picking out negative realities than "healthy" controls (Kronbrot, Msetfi, & Grimwood, 2013; Moore & Fresco, 2012). The neuropsychological theory of antidepressant action suggests that the time lag for therapeutic effect (two to six weeks) may be as much a function of time spent "re-learning" how to interpret life events as much as a physiological process. There are studies comparing depressed people with normal controls and testing their interpretations of faces they are shown. The depressed people are more likely to judge a facial expression negatively than the controls (Beck, 2008).

Interestingly, even in studies where nondepressed controls are given antidepressants, a statistically significant percentage have an increase in expressed positive bias (Harmer et al., 2003). This seems to be the case except when the antidepressant is administered intravenously. Because we know antidepressants promote synaptic plasticity in animal models, it may be that the antidepressants are providing a chemical "window of opportunity" for the clients to rewire their experience through experiencing a more positive bias. This raises more ethically tricky questions like would drugs that seem relatively harmless like cannabis and induce positive mental states also function as antidepressants?

Review Questions

- Describe the additions of the neurotrophic/plasticity theory to amine, reuptake and downregulation theories—specifically—describe what happens with cAMP and BDNF.

- What is the healthiest genetic combination for hearty BDNF?

- Describe how the neuropsychological theory of antidepressants could bring the best of the pharmacological and psychotherapeutic worlds together.

SECTION FOUR: OVERVIEW OF FIRST-GENERATION ANTIDEPRESSANT MEDICATIONS

Learning Objectives

- Understand how vegetative symptoms are important to gauge therapeutic response.
- Be able to describe the primary mechanisms of action for MAO Inhibitors and Tricyclic Antidepressants.
- Know the potential side effects for MAOIs and TCIs.

In this section of the chapter, we convey a more standard presentation of the antidepressants. It is difficult to make global statements about the efficacy of antidepressants in general; however, the literature does seem to agree that all the different classes of antidepressants are about equally effective. Stahl (2000) summarized this agreement, noting it is a "good news/bad news" scenario. The good news is that 50–60% of depressed clients on any antidepressant respond positively to it, and even more may respond if tried on several different compounds. Half of these responders may progress into full remission within six months of treatment. In addition, antidepressants seem to significantly reduce relapses as well. The bad news is that many responders never reach full remission and that in 20 to 30% of the people who respond at all to antidepressants, the effects tend to "poop out" or wear off after about 18 months.

Although Stahl emphasizes the medical model perspective of depression, equating it with diabetes or hypertension, the "bad news" merely means that in some cases biological interventions are time limited. This is only truly "bad news" if in fact there are no other treatments for depression, which is not the case. Given that many people don't maintain their response to antidepressants, it makes sense to view a response as a time-limited window of opportunity within which to employ an integrative approach to treatment. An integrative approach uses all the perspectives we have been discussing in this book.

The Role of Vegetative Symptoms

In the treatment of MDD, note that the more **vegetative symptoms** a client suffers from, the better candidate the person is for antidepressant medication, because these symptoms are most affected by the medication. Maybe because depression is overdetermined (meaning it may be caused by biological, psychological, cultural, social, and perhaps even spiritual factors), a preponderance of vegetative symptoms point toward a stronger biological component in etiology. Table 5.1 contains a list of common vegetative symptoms for MDD.

TABLE 5.1 Common Vegetative Symptoms in Major Depressive Disorder

Sleep disturbance (early morning waking, frequent awakening, occasional hypersomnia)

Appetite disturbance (decreased or increased appetite with accompanying weight fluctuations)

General fatigue

Decreased sex drive

Restlessness, agitation, or psychomotor retardation

Diurnal variations in mood (usually feeling worse in the morning)

Impaired concentration and forgetfulness

Pronounced anhedonia (loss of pleasure in most or all things)

© Cengage Learning®

Monoamine Oxidase (MAO) Inhibitors

We noted that the first MAO inhibitor was iproniazid/Marsilid, but this compound fell into disfavor because some physicians reported hepatotoxicity (liver toxicity). The drug seemed to cause a type of cell death in the liver. Less toxic MAOIs such as isocarboxazid/Marplan and phenelzine/Nardil have been introduced. To review the mechanism of action, MAOIs inhibit the enzyme (MAO) that breaks down neurotransmitters thought to be related to depression (specifically norepinephrine). When the drugs inhibit this enzyme, more NE is in the synaptic cleft to bind to receptors. This binding then presumably causes downregulation of receptors and the cellular/molecular changes described earlier though those effects are studied more specifically with SSRIs. When this chain of events occurs, the person's depressive symptoms tend to improve.

MAO inhibitors are not specific to any type of MAO, so they inhibit all types of MAO throughout the body and not just in specified areas thought related to depressive symptoms. In addition, the effects of older MAOIs are irreversible; such irreversible effects are rare in psychopharmacology.

TABLE 5.2 Examples of MAO Inhibitor Antidepressants and Common Daily Dosage Ranges

Generic Name	Brand Name	Common Daily Dosage Range
Selegiline	L-Deprenyl	10 mg
Isocarboxazid	Marplan	20–50 mg
Moclobemide	Manerix	150–500 mg (available in Canada)
Phenelzine	Nardil	30–75 mg
Tranylcypromine	Parnate	20–40 mg

© Cengage Learning®

Thus, the chemical bond of the MAO inhibitor with the MAO cannot be broken and enzyme function returns to normal only when the body creates new enzymes. This attribute has earned MAO inhibitors the nickname "suicide inhibitors," because their binding to MAO is irreversible meaning that the MAO molecule "suicidally" binds and "goes down with the ship." Further, there are two types of MAO in the body, labeled MAO A and MAO B. Both forms are inhibited by the older, original MAO inhibitors, which are nonselective. The MAO A form metabolizes the neurotransmitters most closely linked to depression (serotonin and norepinephrine). The MAO B form is thought to convert some ligands (called *prototoxins*) into toxins that cause cell damage. Researchers have linked MAO B inhibition to prevention of neurodegenerative processes such as those in Parkinson's disease (Finberg, 2014). Table 5.2 lists some available MAO inhibitors by brand and generic names and dosage range. Please note that the dosage ranges are those common in the United States and that dosage range, as well as minimum effective dose, changes from nation to nation.

Common Side Effects of MAOIs

The side effects of MAOIs are more severe and more frequent than those of other antidepressants. Most are related to the increased activity of norepinephrine,

TABLE 5.3 Common Side Effects of MAO Inhibitors

Orthostatic hypotension (a drop in blood pressure that results in dizziness on standing)

Nighttime insomnia, daytime sedation

Headache

Muscle cramps

Weight gain

Difficulty urinating

Tyramine intolerance

© Cengage Learning®

TABLE 5.4 Examples of Foods High in Tyramine Content to Avoid When Taking MAOIs

Cheeses (cream cheese, such as the common Philadelphia brand, and cottage cheese are safe)

Chicken liver and beef liver

Yeast preparations (avoid brewer's yeast, and powdered and caked yeast as sold in health food stores)

Broad beans and fava beans

Herring

Beer, sherry, ale, red wine, liqueurs

Canned figs

Protein extracts (such as soup cubes and commercial gravies)

© Cengage Learning®

but some are related to the enzyme inhibition that causes the NE increases. Table 5.3 lists common side effects of MAOIs.

Inhibition of MAO A and Tyramine Intolerance

One of the most dangerous side effects of traditional MAO inhibitors is tyramine intolerance. We noted that MAO A metabolizes neurotransmitters that are linked to depression. By slowing down this metabolism, the neurotransmitters remain active longer and this sets in motion the events correlated with symptom improvement. MAO A also metabolizes tyramine, a dietary amine. If the MAO A is not there to break it down, this amine can build up and cause the release of norepinephrine and other sympathomimetic amines, raising blood pressure. In severe reactions, the blood pressure elevation can cause hemorrhage and death. The side effect is easily controlled with a diet low in tyramine-containing foods. Table 5.4 lists examples of foods to avoid when taking MAO inhibitors. A physician should give a complete list to the clients for whom they prescribe these medications.

Obviously, because most MAOIs bind irreversibly, there is no specific antagonist that people can take if they accidentally ingest a food high in tyramine while taking their MAOIs. In such a situation, clients are usually advised not to lie down as this will exacerbate the increase in blood pressure. Clients are

usually directed to go to an emergency room for treatment. Treatment may include taking a calcium-channel blocker such as nifedipine that can lower blood pressure to avert a hypertensive crisis. A note on discontinuation: If MAOIs are stopped, the client should maintain dietary restrictions for about two weeks. That's how long it takes to build up an adequate level of monoamine oxidase. The same holds for making a transition from an MAO inhibitor to another antidepressant medication.

In general, MAOIs are used to treat depression that has been resistant to treatment with other types of antidepressants. This is more due to the side effect profile than to questions of efficacy, because this MAOI class of antidepressants is just as effective as the other classes. In addition to being used against depression, MAO inhibitors have been used with mixed results in treating Bulimia Nervosa, Social Anxiety Disorder, migraine headaches, neurodermatitis, Borderline Personality Disorder, and Panic Disorder.

Contraindications for MAOI Therapy

Clients with a history of liver disease, congestive heart failure, recreational drug use/abuse/dependence, hypertension, or uncontrollable tyramine consumption are not good candidates for MAOI therapy.

In addition, clients who, for whatever reason, are unlikely to abide by the dietary restrictions are also poor candidates for this type of therapy.

Newer MAO Inhibitors

We briefly want to note two developments in MAO inhibitors. The latest efforts of pharmaceutical companies have resulted in MAO inhibitors that form *reversible* bonds with MAO. These are called *RIMAs* (*reversible inhibitors of MAO*). Their mechanism of action is precluding the breakdown of NE, 5-HT, and DA. Also, certain MAO inhibitors are selective for A and B. One new drug that offers both developments is selegiline/Eldepryl and L-Deprenyl. This drug is metabolized to an amphetamine molecule, which slows dopamine reuptake. It is reversible, and in low doses (5 to 10 mg a day) it affects only MAO B. At low doses, no dietary restrictions seem necessary. It does not act as an antidepressant at low doses, however. The prescribing professional must raise the dosage to get an antidepressant effect, and at this level the drug affects both MAO A and MAO B. At this level, although still reversible, dietary restrictions are necessary. Other RIMAs are being developed, one that would focus on MAO-A and still aim for an antidepressant effect (Fowler et al., 2010).

Although MAO inhibitors are rarely the medication of first choice, they may be used after other medications have failed to provide results. The following case illustrates that dynamic while also illustrating the inadequacy of strictly viewing a client's symptoms through the medical model perspective.

The Case of Allan

Allan, a 54-year-old lower-middle-class Caucasian male of Baptist faith, was referred for treatment as part of coordinated services at a mental health agency. Ten years prior to referral he was diagnosed as severely depressed and prescribed a tricyclic antidepressant (TCA) (imiprimine/Tofranil) that he took for about 10 weeks. During this period he was hospitalized twice, more for his complaints about his reactions to the medication than his depression. After the second hospitalization, he was prescribed an SSRI (fluoxetine/Prozac) for his ongoing depression and buspirone/BuSpar for his bouts of anxiety. At no time in the record of his assessment was there any mention of personality impairment or disorder.

Within two weeks of beginning fluoxetine/Prozac, Allan became very agitated, anxious, and paranoid, and had to be hospitalized a third time. The treatment team felt Allan might be suffering from an Atypical Depression, and he was taken off the fluoxetine/Prozac and put on an MAOI (tranylcypromine/Parnate). Allan was advised about the important dietary restrictions he had to follow while on tranylcypromine/Parnate. Soon after, his condition did improve and some of the depressive symptoms lifted. A month later, Allan was transferred to a different case manager because his current one left the agency. Within two weeks he was hospitalized a fourth time for a severe allergy reaction. It was soon determined that Allan had deliberately eaten some cheese because he was in a rage about losing his case manager. By the time Allan was discharged and assigned to a counselor, he was threatening suicide almost daily and refusing to come to counseling. Eventually, however, he began to attend counseling.

The treatment was very challenging, and because of Allan's feelings and suspicions about his care he basically did all he could to undermine his counselor's efforts. Gradually the counselor learned three very important facts about Allan and his life. The first was his enormous fear and then absolute rage about being abandoned and then turned over to someone else for care. The second was his great skill and talent as an electrician and his very fragile self-appraisal of his skills. The third was his gradual discovery of his homosexuality and deep attraction to his male therapist.

The therapist developed a treatment plan to address all three themes. He and Allan planned better for therapeutic interruptions by improving backup support, he referred Allan to a vocational rehabilitation office for additional training in electronics, and he helped Allan talk more concerning his feelings of homosexuality. Gradually Allan stopped taking all medications and worked on his issues in therapy. Here is an example of a case where the client masked severe issues in both psychological and cultural realms and presented a picture of a complex clinical depression. It took time, a great deal of disruption, medication changes, hospitalizations, and careful listening to get a more accurate therapeutic focus on Allan. Being alert only to a client's depressive symptoms with the sole intent of administering psychotropic medications would inevitably have missed the important integrative aspects of Alan's dilemmas. Overall, Allan's MAOI treatment stabilized him for several years. He continued with the medication in conjunction with bimonthly psychotherapy until he was 62. Then he was titrated off the MAOI and saw his therapist only on an as-needed basis. He continues to work as an apartment superintendent 40 hours a week in his neighborhood.

TRICYCLIC ANTIDEPRESSANTS

As noted, the word *tricyclic* in "tricyclic antidepressants" refers to the three-ring molecular core of the drugs in this class of compounds. According to Stahl (2000), the term "tricyclic antidepressant" is outdated by the standards of current psychopharmacology. Newer and similar agents can have more than three rings to their structure, and these agents are used on-label for a variety of disorders other than depression. Nevertheless, for instructional purposes we use the term *tricyclic antidepressants,* or *TCAs.* As noted in the history section in the introduction to Part Two, the TCAs were unexpectedly born from chlorpromazine, the first antipsychotic, also known as a *neuroleptic.* TCAs were created because drug companies were seeking compounds with fewer side effects and with application to other disorders. Table 5.5 lists commonly prescribed TCAs by their brand and generic names and the typical dosage range for each compound.

The primary mechanism of action in all TCAs is inhibition of the reuptake norepinephrine and serotonin (and to a slight extent dopamine). As the cellular theory of depression described earlier suggests, researchers assume that other changes in the affected neurons are related to the reuptake

TABLE 5.5 Examples of Tricyclic Antidepressants and Common Daily Dosage Ranges

Generic Name	Brand Name	Common Daily Dosage Range
Amitriptyline	Elavil	75–250 mg
Amoxapine	Asendin	200–300 mg
Clomipramine	Anafranil	50–200 mg
Doxepin	Sinequan, Adapin	75–250 mg
Imipramine	Tofranil	75–250 mg
Nortriptyline	Pamelor	50—100 mg
Maprotiline	Ludiomil	50–200 mg

© Cengage Learning®

inhibition. In addition, all tricyclic compounds block receptors on acetylcholine, histamine, and epinephrine neurons. These additional mechanisms of action have no therapeutic effects for depression and cause most of the side effects of taking TCAs.

Side Effects of TCAs

We have listed the side effects of TCAs in Table 5.6 by class. As noted, the side effects come from the drug molecules binding to certain receptors and blocking them. In Chapter Two we described this "blocking" as an antagonist effect, meaning the molecule binds, does not initiate an effect on the neuron,

TABLE 5.6 Common TCA Side Effects Listed by Class

Class	Description of Side Effect
Anticholinergic	Dry mouth, dizziness, constipation, difficulty urinating, blurred vision
Adrenergic	Sexual dysfunction, sweating, orthostatic hypotension
Antihistaminic	Sedation and weight gain

© Cengage Learning®

and prevents other ligands from binding and exerting their effect. Because this is an antagonistic action, we use the prefix "anti-" when describing the side effect. For example, a TCA molecule blocking an acetylcholine receptor exerts an "anticholinergic" effect. A TCA molecule blocking a histamine receptor exerts an "antihistaminic" effect. Conversely, if a drug molecule has an agonist action we do not use the "anti-" prefix and we simply say the drug had a cholinergic or histaminic effect. Table 5.6 is just a general introduction to possible side effects, not an exhaustive list. Please note that not every TCA drug produces every side effect and that effects also vary depending on the specific responses of the individual taking the drug.

TCAs also have potent effects on the peripheral nervous system. Especially in combination with other medications, they can cause cardiac depression and increased electrical activity that results in arrhythmia. Both can lead to heart failure.

For a prescribing professional, choosing the right TCA seems to be a matter of preference based on matching the TCA to the client's symptoms. It does appear that because more safety risks come with TCAs (e.g., cardiac arrhythmia) they require closer therapeutic drug monitoring than other classes of antidepressants (Ostad, Heimke, & Pfuhlmann, 2012). Some TCAs are more sedating (Elavil), others are more stimulating (Norpramin). Pointing out the contrast to some of the other classes of antidepressants, Schatzberg and Nemeroff (1998) have argued that if a client does not respond to one TCA, it is unlikely that he or she will respond to any other TCA and the prescribing professional is best advised to try another class of antidepressants. Note that some other medications can significantly raise or lower a client's TCA plasma level. For example, SSRI antidepressants or stimulants such as methylphenidate (Ritalin) can increase TCA plasma levels as much as eightfold, whereas substances such as carbamazepine (Tegretol) and nicotine can significantly lower TCA plasma levels. This simply indicates that clients need quality care from the professional prescribing the medications. Medical professionals are trained to be alert to drug–drug interactions, which is becoming a crucial aspect of

psychopharmacology as more and more compounds come to market. TCAs are indicated for depression and are approved by the FDA for childhood enuresis, and Obsessive-Compulsive Disorder (OCD). Off-label uses include insomnia, Panic Disorder, PTSD, Generalized Anxiety Disorder (GAD), chronic pain (all classes of antidepressants have been tested as analgesics for chronic pain and frequently are more effective than placebo), and Bulimia Nervosa.

Tricyclic Derivatives

There is a subclass of antidepressants derived from TCAs that is referred to by several labels, including "secondary amines," "second-generation antidepressants," or "atypical" antidepressants. The numerous labels are unfortunate because they make it hard to tell what is being referred to, because some of the labels (such as "second-generation antidepressants") are also used to refer to totally different classes of drugs. To avoid confusion, we call these compounds *tricyclic derivatives*. Most have a two-ring molecular structure and have been discovered from metabolites of the tricyclic antidepressants (which is a common practice as we will see in examining other drugs). One strategy for creating marketable compounds is to examine the metabolites of a parent compound. The metabolites can be found in the urine of people taking the parent compound. If the metabolites are active, they can be synthesized into a similar agent that acts like the parent compound but is possibly weaker in therapeutic and side effects. As such, these compounds may still produce the desired therapeutic effect with lower levels of side effects. Table 5.7 lists some examples of TCA derivatives. Note how the generic name is similar to the parent compound.

TABLE 5.7 Examples of TCA Derivatives and Their Parent Compounds

TCA Derivative Generic Name	Parent Compound Generic Name	Dosage Range
Nortriptyline	Amitriptyline	50–100 mg
Desipramine	Imipramine	75–250 mg

© Cengage Learning®

Benefits and Drawbacks to TCAs and TCA Derivatives: A Summary

As you have read this chapter, you probably have already guessed what the benefits and drawbacks of TCAs and TCA derivatives are. The benefits center around two things. First, these drugs are among the most extensively studied psychotropic medications on the market. This is largely because they have been on the market almost 60 years. When TCAs were put on the market, their only competition was MAO inhibitors. Because MAOIs had the potentially dangerous "cheese effect" related to tyramine intolerance, they were quickly displaced by the TCAs, which did not require a focused dietary regimen (other than avoiding alcohol and other drugs that may interact). Thus, TCAs became the drug of first choice for depression and remained so well into the 1980s, when Prozac was introduced. Once established as a drug of first choice, they then provided the baseline against which all other newer antidepressants were measured. The result is a wealth of information on the TCAs, a situation that makes even conservative medical practitioners comfortable prescribing them to patients. Although the SSRIs (which we discuss next) are currently thought of as the drug of first choice for people with depression, no one disputes that far more data are available on the TCAs. The other advantage to TCAs is their lower cost. After a pharmaceutical company is approved to sell a drug for a given purpose and if the patent was applied for after 1995, the company can get patent rights to the compound for up to 20 years. After this time, other companies can produce the drug generically and sell it for a lower price. In 2010 American pharmaceutical companies had an unprecedented number of medications go generic. This was referred to as the "patent cliff." In total, patents on drugs worth $12 billion expired in 2011 and in 2012 the figure was closer to $30 billion (DeRuiter & Holston, 2012). Many companies release metabolite compounds at the end of such patent cycles like desvenlafaxine/Prestiq is a metabolite of venlafaxine/Effexor (Wegman, 2009). The result is that clients with no insurance and little income will likely be able to afford a generic drug as opposed to one that has not yet "gone generic." For example, in 2000 a common wholesale price for a nongeneric SSRI was approximately $150 for a 30-day supply. By contrast, the same supply of generic Elavil (amitriptyline) was approximately $5. Of course, now most SSRI drugs are available in generic form and are often the drug of first choice because of their safety profile. It is logical to imagine that after several newer antidepressant compounds become available in less expensive generic formulations, the use of TCAs will continue to decrease. That is what is happening in the early 21st century with exceptions of treatment resistant symptoms (Pitchot, Scantamburlo, & Ansseau, 2011). The following case demonstrates how TCA medication played an important role in the treatment of one client.

The Case of Rita

Rita, 31, sought counseling for several years in the late 1980s for generalized sadness, some hopelessness, lack of energy, great worry, a loss of a genuine sense of pleasure, and a recurrent sense of loneliness. Although she went to several mental health professionals during this period, not one suggested assessment for depression. Rita experienced almost no relief, as evidenced by her therapist shopping. She complained to her few friends, "They are all good listeners, but I don't feel I'm getting any help. Maybe that's just my lot in life." About this time she stopped all therapy and began a very aggressive program of exercise and vitamin therapy. Also, she began to see a massage therapist for body massage twice a month and she began to meditate every morning. She felt some relief and improvement, but those feelings were short-lived. In November of the same year she became despondent with great personal anguish, had plaguing suicidal thoughts, and isolated herself from friends and family. Living single, she told one friend, "I might as well not live, no one will ever love me and I'm not lovable." After a terrible period of two weeks, one of her friends took her to a local emergency room. There the attending physician diagnosed MDD;

prescribed imipramine/Tofranil, which is a TCA as well as one of the most commonly used antidepressants at that time; and referred her to a female psychiatrist for follow-up. Gradually Rita improved. She followed up three times with the psychiatrist and continued on imipramine as prescribed for six months.

In the middle of this six-month period, Rita met a man whom she began to date. Rita quickly became attached, which seemed to frighten her companion and he abruptly ended the brief relationship. This termination triggered a severe suicidal depression in Rita, and she slit her wrists. Her landlord found her, and she was rushed to a local hospital and admitted to the psychiatric ward. After two weeks in the hospital, the treating team noted almost no improvement in Rita. She remained on suicidal precaution (being monitored closely for suicidal ideation), and she was sleeping poorly. The team decided to titrate her off the imipramine and began a course of nortriptyline/Pamelor, a different type of TCA, as soon as possible. The team also introduced a low dosage of diazepam/Valium, an anxiolytic, to address her sleep and anxiety problems.

Rita was hospitalized for nine weeks, and the medication change and the milieu of in-patient therapies assisted her recovery. After discharge, Rita remained on diazepam/Valium for an additional two months and on nortriptyline/Pamelor for an additional 15 months. She also began treatment with a skilled licensed counselor who was very knowledgeable about psychopharmacology. Rita remained in therapy until two months after titrating off nortriptyline/Pamelor. Five years later she remained stable, with no recurrence of her major depressive episode with an attempted suicide.

Most of Rita's treatment was in the medical model realm through the introduction of TCAs. It was not uncommon during the 1970s, when Rita received treatment, for psychiatrists to try different TCAs with a patient who demonstrated little response with one type. Also, it was not uncommon to add an anxiolytic in conjunction with a TCA to address symptoms of anxiety and sleeplessness. It is clear from the case material that Rita's earlier attempts with psychotherapy, in the psychological

realm, were very unsuccessful and the therapists seemed naive to the importance of medication assessment because of Rita's chronic symptoms. We believe Rita's recovery after discharge resulted from careful interventions in both the medical model and psychological perspectives.

Review Questions

- How can monitoring vegetative symptoms give you a sense of the client's response to antidepressants?
- What are the primary mechanisms of action for MAOIs and TCAs?
- What are the primary side effects of MAOIs and TCAs?

SECTION FIVE: SECOND GENERATION ANTIDEPRESSANTS: SELECTIVE SEROTONIN REUPTAKE INHIBITORS

Learning Objectives

- Understand the benefits and potential risks of SSRI medications.
- Be able to describe the primary mechanism of action in SSRIs and how it relates to the neurotrophic/plasticity theory of antidepressant action.
- Understand the controversy over SSRI-related violence and who is at risk.

Although we noted that TCA derivatives were sometimes referred to as "second-generation" antidepressants, the label more accurately belongs with the SSRIs (Olver, Burrows, & Norman, 2001). We begin the story returning to some historical high points.

A Bit More History

We noted in the beginning of this chapter that the amine theory was expanded to include the effects of serotonin on mood. This opened up a line of research looking at the effects on depression of drugs that made more serotonin available in the central nervous system. The first such agent trazodone/Desyrel had been released in 1981, but because of a rare but problematic side effect (priapism—prolonged and painful erection in males), it failed to gain widespread use although it is still used at lower doses as a sleep aid. In the early 1970s, a research team at Eli Lilly (Byron Malloy, David Wong, & Ray Fuller) had synthesized an agent labeled LY86032. Healy (1997) notes that the team created the compound in a series of "moonlighting experiments" and finally decided it was an inhibitor of serotonin reuptake. Following their discovery, they conducted several meetings to explore uses for the new compound. Ironically, when someone first suggested that the drug be tested as an antidepressant, the response was that it would not likely be useful in treating depression and that there was not much of a market for antidepressants anyway (Coppen & Healy, 1996).

Because serotonin is widely distributed in the body, any agent that affects its action is likely to have numerous effects. Research teams initially decided that fluoxetine/Prozac might be an antihypertensive agent, partially because in the 1970s the antihypertensive market was larger than the antidepressant market. In 1981, Marie Asberg and Lil Traskman (1981) demonstrated that serotonin metabolites were significantly decreased in the cerebrospinal fluid of suicidally depressed people. This led to speculation about the role of serotonin in depression. According to Healy (1997), this development and the ever expanding antidepressant market of the early 1980s led to clinical trials of fluoxetine/Prozac as an antidepressant, and the first evidence to support this hypothesis became available in 1985. Fluoxetine/Prozac was licensed in the United States in 1987. Several other compounds were made available at this time, including SmithKline and Beecham's paroxetine/Paxil. Paroxetine/Paxil hit the U.S. market in 1993, delayed by SmithKline and Beecham's skepticism about the market. In an effort to distinguish its compound, SmithKline and Beecham created the category *SSRI,* and the label "stuck" as the category in which all similar agents were grouped.

The SSRIs seemed to have treatment effects similar to those of TCAs with different side effects. It should be noted here that efficacy of all classes of antidepressants appear to be generally equal but some people respond better to one than another. Meta-analytic studies that suggested there were consistent differences in efficacy across compounds have been criticized for serious methodological problems (Del Ra et al., 2013).

Interestingly, whereas TCAs are molecularly similar across compounds, SSRIs are remarkably different in chemical structure. SSRI effects across the range of 5-HT receptor systems also vary. Thus, whereas Schatzberg and Nemeroff (1998) noted that if patients don't respond to one TCA it is unlikely they will respond to another, the situation is quite different with SSRIs and physicians may try patients on several agents before finding one that provides optimal symptom relief.

As Kramer (1993) has noted, no drug in the history of psychiatry has received more positive and negative attention than fluoxetine/Prozac. At the height of its popularity, sales of the drug topped $1.2 billion annually in the United States alone. This success, as has been the pattern, led to a plethora of SSRI agents being released in a short period of time. The SSRI compounds, and their general dosage range, are listed in Table 5.8.

TABLE 5.8 Examples of SSRI Antidepressants and Common Daily Dosage Ranges

Generic Name	Brand Name	Common Daily Dosage Range
Citalopram	Celexa	20–40 mg
Escitalopram oxalate	Lexapro	10–20 mg
Fluoxetine	Prozac	10–60 mg
Fluvoxamine	Luvox	50–250 mg
Paroxetine	Paxil	10–40 mg
Sertraline	Zoloft	50–200 mg

© Cengage Learning®

Mechanism of Action

As already noted, although SSRIs are classed together many clients may have very different reactions to the drugs. This is one reason we provide no charts on when certain clients should get particular drugs: There is no database of knowledge from which to create such a chart. Whereas fluoxetine/ Prozac may work for one client, another may respond only to citalopram/Celexa. A strictly medical model perspective offers no explanation for this, and although biological differences in client nervous systems may someday be found to underlie the phenomenon, we believe an integrative research approach to the problem may also yield useful hypotheses. A great deal of research has been done on SSRIs, and many authors now note that although more data on the TCAs are available, the SSRIs are really the drugs of first choice for depression. This is due in large part to a less severe profile of side effects and the difficulty of overdosing on the drugs. As Stahl (2000) explained, taking a two-week supply of a TCA would be lethal to many clients, whereas SSRIs rarely cause death in overdose unless combined with other agents (Fitzgerald, & Bronstein, 2013). In fact, McKenzie and McFarland (2007) examined trends in antidepressant overdoses. They found a dramatic rise in the United States in antidepressant overdoses between 1983 and 2003. These are not reported as fatalities because the drugs involved were mostly SSRI antidepressants. They noted that had TCAs been used, it would have tripled the death rate from overdose. One exception is citalopram/Celexa as it is more dangerous than other SSRIs because it causes QTc prolongation (Flanagan, 2008). While we will discuss this in great detail in Chapter Seven, suffice to say here that the QTc interval is the measure of time between the start of what is called a "Q" wave and the end of what is called a "T" wave in the heart's electrical cycle. If this interval gets too long cardiac problems and even death can result.

As the name *selective serotonin reuptake inhibitor* suggests, the primary mechanism of action is the inhibition of reuptake of serotonin back into the neuron.

However, researchers have learned over the past decade that a great deal more is going on than this. Once taken, the drug inhibits the reuptake of serotonin so more serotonin molecules are near the cell body area. Whereas researchers used to think that the increase was immediate, in the synapses it appears that the increase is first felt near the dendrites on the cell body, and scientists currently believe this increase produces many of the side effects. Over time, the increase of serotonin in this area causes the autoreceptors to decrease in number (to downregulate) as well as to become desensitized. Recall that autoreceptors are specialized receptors that, when triggered, signal the cell to decrease the production of neurotransmitter. So if SSRI medications cause the downregulation of autoreceptors, it stands to reason the cell will produce more serotonin than it normally would. Researchers believe this information is communicated to the cell's nucleus, where the genome (via signaling pathways) sends out instructions to cause these same receptors to become less sensitive over time. Note that this hypothesis regarding genetic expression still requires more research. In addition, if medications do affect gene expression researchers need to investigate whether nonpharmacologic elements may also affect gene expression in the same manner.

Scientists now believe that as well as downregulating, the postsynaptic neurons also desensitize over time in the same way as autoreceptors on the presynaptic neuron do. This is a *ripple effect,* or what Stahl calls a *cascade effect,* wherein SSRIs affect the brain.

Common Side Effects

Another advantage to SSRI antidepressants is that, unlike TCAs, they have far fewer anticholinergic or antihistaminic side effects. The side effects listed in Table 5.9 are due almost exclusively to the selective serotonin reuptake inhibition. There are many serotonin receptor systems throughout the central and peripheral nervous systems, and SSRIs can significantly affect them. Also there are multiple serotonin receptor systems and different SSRI compounds have different effects across these families.

TABLE 5.9 Common SSRI Side Effects

Headache

Nausea

Nervousness

Diarrhea

Insomnia

Weight gain

Sexual dysfunction

© Cengage Learning®

These side effects often decrease or cease after therapeutic effects take hold, with the exception of sexual dysfunction. As we stated earlier in the chapter, SSRIs have a variety of on-label and off-label uses. Currently, different SSRIs have on-label uses approved for Major Depressive Disorder, Persistent Depressive Disorder (Dysthymia previous to *DSM-5*), Social Anxiety Disorder (Social Phobia prior to *DSM-5*), Post-Traumatic Stress Disorder, and Obsessive-Compulsive Disorder. Off-label uses have included Panic Disorder, Generalized Anxiety Disorder, premature ejaculation, migraine headaches (as prophylactic), diabetic neuropathy, fibromyalgia, and neurocardiogenic syncope (Stone, Viera, & Parman, 2003). In 2013, the FDA approved the marketing of a low dose of paroxetine/Paxil (repackaged under the commercial name Brisdelle) as a nonhormonal treatment for menopausal symptoms (Toftegard, Voigt, Rosenberg, & Gogenur, 2013). This has caused concern because paroxetine/Paxil is one drug that has a weak estrogenic effect that could promote the growth of breast tumors in women because 70% of breast cancers in women are estrogen-sensitive (Healy, 2014).

Antidepressant-Induced Sexual Dysfunction

A particularly troubling side effect for many people is antidepressant-induced sexual dysfunction (AISD). This has been a problem for many clients taking a wide range of antidepressants, and the earliest documentation of it dates back to the early 1960s (Healy, 1997). Initially researchers found it hard to determine how much of the problem was due to the drugs and how much to the depression, because decreased libido is one of the vegetative signs of depression. George Beaumont (1973), who published one of the first papers on the topic, noticed that clients treated with clomipramine/Anafranil, a TCA with stronger effects on serotonin, had delayed orgasm. Beaumont learned that varying the client's dosage could somewhat control the problem. Also in the case of clomipramine/Anafranil, an orgasm rebound apparently could result when the drug was discontinued. Healy (1997) recounts the story of a nun who experienced three days of spontaneous orgasms when withdrawing from clomipramine/Anafranil.

With serotonin-related AISD, apparently the drug's stimulation of serotonin receptors in the spinal cord can inhibit the spinal reflexes, orgasm, and ejaculation (Stahl, 2000). Although early market research with SSRIs reported that approximately 4% of patients taking them would experience this side effect, Healy (1997) states that the number is now confirmed to be well over 50% and may be higher. There are multiple approaches to treating this side effect, and it is worth discussing, because this problem is often why clients stop taking the medication. From the psychological perspective, it is important that counselors tune into clients' comfort in discussing sexual issues. Many clients are uncomfortable with the topic, and this seems to have contributed to under-reporting of the side effect when SSRIs were first released. It is above all important to communicate to clients that prescribing professionals can do many things to decrease or ameliorate this side effect, including switching the client to another medication, supplementing the SSRI with a second medication, or altering the dosage.

The only antidepressant not associated with some sexual dysfunction is bupropion/Wellbutrin (Demyttenaere & Jaspers, 2008) and in studies exploring AISD mirtazapine/Remeron was a distant second correlated with AISD about 30% of the time (Segraves & Balon, 2013). In a large-scale examination of interventions for AISD, females seemed to respond well to augmentation with high doses of bupropion/Wellbutrin where males more often responded to augmentation with sildenafil/Viagra and tadalafil/Cialis (Taylor et al., 2013).

Do Antidepressants Induce Dependence?

The simple answer to the politically delicate question "Do antidepressants induce dependence?" is yes. We are deliberately using the word "dependence" rather than "addiction," because colloquial overuse of the latter has attached a great deal of emotional baggage to it. This baggage has rendered it almost meaningless except when one wants to elicit strong emotional reactions from readers. We prefer the construct of dependence, defined as a physical tolerance produced by repeated administration of a drug and a concomitant withdrawal syndrome (Stahl, 2000). Given this definition of dependence, we can state that SSRI antidepressants can induce what seem to be tolerance and dependence. As Advokat, Comaty, and Julien (2014) stated, "a discontinuation occurs in perhaps 60% of SSRI-treated patients following abrupt cessation of drug intake … onset of the syndrome is usually within a few days and persists perhaps 3 to 4 weeks" (pp. 406–407). Table 5.10 lists a more complete list of discontinuation syndrome symptoms.

TABLE 5.10 Symptoms of Serotonin Withdrawal

Lethargy

Fatigue

Gastrointestinal disturbance (nausea, vomiting, diarrhea)

Paresthesias (numbness or tingling in extremities)

Insomnia

Agitation/anxiety

Schatzberg, Cole, and DeBattista (1997) offered the first definition of what they called "serotonin reuptake inhibitor discontinuation syndrome." They noted that the syndrome typically consisted of physical and psychological symptoms. Their list of physical symptoms include disequilibrium; gastrointestinal symptoms such as nausea, vomiting, and diarrhea; flulike symptoms including lethargy, fatigue, and chills; sensory disturbances such as paresthesia; and sleep disturbances such as insomnia. Their list of psychological symptoms may include anxiety, agitation, and crying spells. Using the acronym "FINISH" Advokat et al. (2014) list discontinuation syndrome symptoms as Flu-like, Insomnia, Nausea, Imbalance, Sensory disturbances, and Hyperarousal. One important distinction between dependence on SSRI antidepressants and dependence on a drug that, for example, induces a "high" or euphoria (such as heroin) is that it appears a person who has developed physiological dependence on an SSRI antidepressant does not experience a "craving" for the drug as does someone dependent on heroin (or other opioids). This is why there is little abuse potential for antidepressants and no real "street value" for the drugs.

Another type of dependence is psychological dependence. In this syndrome, a person comes to believe he or she cannot function without a particular drug. In such cases we would say the person in question is psychologically dependent on the drug. Although there may not be physiological tolerance and withdrawal, psychological dependence can be every bit as difficult to deal with as physical dependence. Certainly a client could develop psychological dependence on SSRI antidepressants (or any medication, for that matter). Prescribing professionals and mental health professionals must help clients understand their relationship to the medication. It is important for clients to understand what the medication can do for them, and what they must do for themselves. In our opinion, the people least likely to develop psychological dependence on antidepressants are those who undergo counseling while they are taking the medication. In the counseling relationship, clients learn to differentiate their role from the role played by medications.

PSYCHOLOGICAL AND CULTURAL ISSUES WITH SSRIS

In the late 1980s and early 1990s, a backlash arose against SSRIs in general and Prozac in particular. We briefly review this episode here, because it was the first public outcry about possible dangers of antidepressants. These issues still come up in dialogue with clients and there are some serious concerns about using SSRIs with children and adolescents. The concern at the center of the backlash was whether SSRIs and other antidepressants could in fact instill violent, suicidal behaviors in people. The Church of Scientology launched the attack against Prozac in 1989. It should be clearly understood that Scientology holds as a doctrine a model of the mind falsified many times over and because of this misguided model, Scientologists believe contemporary mental health interventions to be useless and even harmful (e.g., the idea that your brain records everything that happens to you even if you are unconscious and forms "engrams" that can disturb you psychologically. We know of course that this is not true.). Psychiatry is at the top of the list for Scientologists in what the group calls the evils of mental health treatment (Church of Scientology, 1994).

Scientology's main ammunition in the initial attack on antidepressants appeared to be a 1990 (February) *American Journal of Psychiatry* article (Teicher, Glod, & Cole, 1990) reporting that after two to seven weeks on Prozac, six patients became preoccupied with obsessive, violent suicidal thoughts. These patients had not been responsive to other drugs, but four of the six were also on other medications. Although this was a small sample of cases, the authors were concerned because, as they wrote, "None of these patients had ever experienced a similar state during treatment with any other psychotropic drug" (p. 207).

Because some links appear between serotonin and aggression, there was concern that Prozac might trigger aggression or even sociopathy. Scientologists cited the case of Joseph Wesbecker, who in 1989 attacked his coworkers with an assault rifle, killing 8, wounding 12, and then killing himself.

Scientologists blamed Prozac; however, the case history and witnesses indicate that he had a history of violent preoccupation before taking Prozac. At the time (1991), the FDA announced that Prozac and other antidepressants do not cause suicide or violent behavior and actually tend to reduce them. Although Scientology's claims about antidepressants (and psychotropic medications in general) are not all substantiated, their concerns should not be completely discarded. It is interesting that in 2004 the FDA issued a public warning about possible connections between adolescent suicides and SSRI medication. Scientologists must be given credit for questioning some of the word magic from extreme proponents of the medical model perspective. The FDA has required that SSRI antidepressants come with a warning on the label (called a "black box warning," because the warning is situated in a black box on the label) that SSRIs can sometimes spur suicidal behavior in children and adolescents (Neergaard, 2004). The warning states that "anxiety, agitation, panic attacks, insomnia, irritability, hostility, aggressiveness, impulsivity, akathisia (psychomotor restlessness), hypomania and mania have been reported in adult and pediatric patients being treated with antidepressants for major depressive disorder as well as for other indications, both psychiatric and non-psychiatric" (quoted in Healy, Herxheimer, & Menkes, 2007, p. 18).

In clinical trials, aggression and violence are coded under the term "hostility." This includes homicide, homicidal acts, homicidal ideation, aggressive events, suicide, and conduct disorders. In trials on paroxetine/Paxil, there were 60 events from a sample of 9219 subjects. In the placebo condition, there were 20 events from a sample of 6455 subjects. In healthy volunteer trials, there were 3 hostile events in 271 volunteers taking paroxetine and none in the 138 taking placebo (Healy et al., 2007). Kauffman (2009) reports even more startling data noting that in a controlled trial of paroxetine/Paxil 75% of subjects had an adverse effect, 21% experienced a severe adverse effect and 13% (one in eight) committed a suicidal act. Part of the discrepancy in data is that not all studies get reported. In 53 healthy volunteer studies on sertraline/Zoloft, the results of only 14 were reported. In the unreported trials, there were high dropout rates due to side effects like akathisia (motor restlessness) (Kauffman, 2009) and akathisia is hypothesized to be related to hostile behavior (Healy et al., 2007).

The problem is not limited to SSRI antidepressants. In pediatric trials of venlafaxine/Effexor (a NE and 5-HT reuptake inhibitor discussed below) 2% of children dropped out because of hostility—more than twice the dropout rate in the placebo group (Kuslak, 2003). Healy et al. (2007) noted that this issue will continue to cause problems not just in treatment but what the legal ramifications are between medication and violence. This is all the more problematic because we now have evidence that the "… trial designs were devised by SSRI makers to prevent reports of suicides, by eliminating subjects with the slightest trace of suicidal tendencies" (Kauffman, 2009, p. 7).

When Eli Lilly denied links of suicidal behavior to the drug fluoxetine/Prozac, they cited a sponsored meta-analysis in the *British Medical Journal*. This study included only 3067 patients of the 26,000 in clinical trials and some of these had been rejected by the FDA in the United States. Also, "… no mention was made that Lilly had had benzodiazepines co-prescribed to minimize the agitation that had been recognized with fluoxetine/Prozac alone" (Kauffman, 2009, p. 9).

Cases Involving SSRI Medication

In the following two cases, SSRI medication proved helpful, but not a panacea. We recommend an exercise with these cases. In both cases, assign elements of the case to the four perspectives of our integrative model. This can increase your awareness of how medication can be a helpful, if only partial, component of treatment.

The Case of Linda

Linda, a 39-year-old Latina, came to therapy after a painful and difficult divorce. She had three children, ages 6, 8, and 11. Her concerns were focused on family survival; she had great worries about the children and feelings of worthlessness. The process of divorce was very difficult, and there were many terrible moments with her ex-husband, some of which the children witnessed. Linda quickly established a therapeutic relationship and began to put her life back together. Around the time of what would have been her 14th wedding anniversary, Linda showed signs of slipping into a clinical depression. After discussing these symptoms and changes with her therapist, she agreed to consult a psychiatrist, who recommended a course of treatment using sertraline/Zoloft.

Linda reluctantly agreed and began taking the medication. Her therapist was aware of the necessity of sertraline/Zoloft at this time for her and spoke to her in every session about its impact in her life. Linda experienced relatively few side effects, with some general nervousness at the beginning of treatment and a mild loss of sexual excitement, about which she talked in therapy. Linda's clinical symptoms lifted after four months and she was titrated off the sertraline/Zoloft.

Linda worked with her therapist for 17 months and made several changes to improve her life and inner attitude. The combining of talk therapy with psychiatric medication was crucial to the success of the overall treatment. Her therapist recognized Linda's serious depressive signs, referred her to a psychiatrist, and continued to see her during this period. Without the medication Linda's condition would likely have deteriorated, with little hope for progress in therapy. The success of this treatment depended on a well-trained therapist who, recognizing the severity of Linda's depression, referred her for medical evaluation in a timely and appropriate manner.

The Case of Jack

Jack, a 29-year-old single bisexual man, came to therapy ostensibly to sort out issues of great career ambivalence. Raised in a strict religious family, Jack lost his mother at age 20 and his father at 12. During his teenage years he was isolated, rebellious, and naive. He completed high school but never quite settled on college. After high school he had sustained heterosexual and homosexual relationships. He was brilliant, with an IQ over 155 and a great capacity to synthesize complex material. Recently, he had ended a five-year homosexual relationship, had made peace with an older sister who supported him, and had applied and been accepted to a prestigious East Coast college to study philosophy.

As the treatment unfolded, very complex material and conflicts entered into the work with Jack. He suffered greatly from the losses of both parents and seemed unable to grieve for them and move on. He expressed a great deal of excitement for female companionship, yet remained constantly disappointed in these relationships. In the transference he was meek and dependent, challenging and demanding, and rebellious and attacking. He sought to find from therapy quick-fix solutions to his historical problems and current dilemmas. He loved to philosophize and gossip. During moments of his greatest anguish and chaos, he identified with the antigovernment types of Montana who felt totally trapped by the rules of living in a democracy. About a year into the treatment he became seriously depressed and was referred to a psychiatrist who, after an evaluation, prescribed paroxetine/Paxil. Jack took the medication as ordered for about six months, and he reported relief from many of his depressive symptoms.

Gradually he then became disenchanted with the paroxetine/Paxil. He said he had all but lost his sexual drive and desire and wondered if the medication was a method to modify or control his radical thinking about some of the absurdities of American culture. At first it seemed he was expressing symptoms of paranoia, but when therapy explored the meanings, it appeared his feelings and meanings were rooted in a genuine disagreement with much of the fabric of American life. He identified with groups and cultures that deeply questioned the rules and values of Western culture. Jack's experiences were particularly poignant because of the many hateful reactions he encountered from society when he lived openly with his partner. Some of his agony was rooted in life experiences that were discriminatory and threatening. Although the medication was temporarily helpful, it could not address issues and conflicts he

experienced as a result of internal group identifications. Understanding these dilemmas in his life allowed exploration of many alternative options for his present and future life choices. He gradually came off the paroxetine/Paxil in consultation with his psychiatrist.

In this case, we can see how a psychopharmacological intervention was helpful temporarily and that its limited effectiveness led to a deepened understanding of the client's struggles and therapeutic interventions. In this case, we see the paroxetine/Paxil as a bridge to more critical unfolding of Jack's psychic and political life.

Review Questions

- What are the benefits and risks of SSRI medications?
- What is the primary mechanism of SSRI medications and how does it relate to the neurotrophic/plasticity theory of antidepressant action?
- What is the controversy over SSRI-related violence and who is most at risk for this?

SECTION SIX: THIRD-GENERATION ANTIDEPRESSANTS

Learning Objectives

- Be able to describe how many third-generation antidepressants are really variations on existing compounds.
- Understand the mechanisms of action for third-generation antidepressants.
- Have a sense of the promises and pitfalls of ketamine as an antidepressant.

SSRIs constituted the second generation of antidepressants; there is now a third generation of antidepressants that includes drugs with diverse properties and that were chemically inspired by the development of the SSRIs (Olver et al., 2001). This category of

TABLE 5.11 Current Third-Generation Antidepressants

Generic Name	Brand Name	Common Daily Dosage Range
Bupropion	Wellbutrin	200–450 mg daily
Remeron	Mirtazapine	15–45 mg daily
Venlafaxine	Effexor	75–375 mg daily
Reboxetine	Edronax, Vestra	4–8 mg daily
Duloxetine	Cymbalta	40–60 mg daily
Desvenlafaxine	Prestiq	50 mg once daily

© Cengage Learning®

drugs has a variety of actions that may include, but are not confined to, serotonin reuptake inhibition. Like the second-generation SSRIs, these drugs are supposed to have better side effect profiles and more safety than MAO Inhibitors and TCAs. However, despite much initial speculation that they might be more effective than SSRIs, they seem, at most, to be only equally effective and subject to the same "pooping out" problems as SSRIs.

The third-generation antidepressants include such drugs as bupropion/Wellbutrin, mirtazapine/Remeron, venlafaxine/Effexor, duloxetine/Cymbalta, and reboxetine/Edronax. In addition there is a new drug desvenlafaxine/Prestiq that is made from the metabolites of venlafaxine/Effexor. At the time of this writing, another third-generation antidepressant (nefazodone/Serzone) was taken off the market by manufacturer Bristol Myers Squibb because of rare but lethal side effects related to liver failure. Table 5.11 summarizes the current third-generation antidepressants.

Bupropion/Wellbutrin: A Norepinephrine-Dopamine Reuptake Inhibitor

The mechanism of action for bupropion/Wellbutrin was unclear for some time. Although it at first seemed to have potent reuptake inhibition properties for NE and DA, the drug itself was actually a weak inhibitor of these reuptake processes. Researchers recently discovered that when taken into the body, the drug goes through an anabolic metabolism, which means that as the drug is metabolized, initially it becomes more potent. This is why psychopharmacologists sometimes call it a "prodrug," meaning a drug that acts like a precursor and then becomes activated through the body's metabolic processes. From the psychological perspective, clients report that bupropion/Wellbutrin is somewhat stimulating and (from the medical model perspective) is not associated with AISD, which makes it an alternative for clients who are troubled by AISD. Some clients even report an increase in libido (though bupropion/Wellbutrin should not be thought of as an "aphrodisiac"). Interestingly, bupropion was initially marketed with two different brand names for two different purposes: Wellbutrin as an antidepressant and Zyban as a smoking cessation aid. These distinctions are less relevant now that it is available in generic formulations. Bupropion/Wellbutrin seems to decrease the craving sensations associated with nicotine withdrawal (Warner & Shoaib, 2005).

Bupropion/Wellbutrin is available in an extended-release (XR) formulation that requires one dose per day. The dosage range for bupropion is from 150 to 450 mg daily. Side effects can include insomnia, gastrointestinal distress, and treatment-emergent hypertension. Bupropion/Wellbutrin has been shown to reduce the seizure threshold and is contraindicated for people who suffer from a seizure disorder, a head injury, or an eating disorder. Alcohol use is also contraindicated while taking bupropion, because it also lowers the seizure threshold. Overall bupropion compares favorably with other antidepressants (Maneeton, Maneeton, Eurviryanukul, & Srisurapanant, 2013) and may be preferable due to not causing weight gain or sexual dysfunction.

In 2012, the FDA recalled one 300 mg generic version of bupropion/Wellbutrin made by Watson pharmaceuticals. In testing the generic versions of four drug makers, Watson's version of the drug was not therapeutically equivalent to the brand name (FDA, 2013).

Mirtazapine/Remeron: A Serotonin-Norepinephrine Antagonist

Mirtazapine/Remeron is a drug that increases both serotonin (5-HT) and norepinephrine r (NE) release by blocking the appropriate autoreceptors (in this case the alpha-2 autoreceptors on both the NE and 5-HT neurons). Recall that autoreceptors help neurons regulate their output of whatever neurotransmitter the neurons happen to produce. Artificially blocking these with the mirtazapine/Remeron molecule so they cannot be naturally stimulated to give the slow-down signal the neuron is "fooled" into increasing its release of neurotransmitter. This increase then theoretically causes the same ripple effect in the central nervous system that we summarized in discussing the molecular/cellular theory of depression. Stahl (2000) offers the analogy that this mechanism of action is like "cutting the brake cable" (p. 251) and thus increasing neurotransmitter release. Mirtazapine/Remeron also blocks adrenergic receptors on terminal button of serotonin neurons. When these are blocked it causes the neurons to release more serotonin. Finally the increased release of serotonin stimulates 5-HT1 receptors while 5-HT2 and 5-HT3 receptors are blocked by mirtazapine/Remeron. Like all drugs, mirtazapine has side effects. It also blocks various serotonin and histamine receptors, resulting in sedation and weight gain. The typical dosage range for mirtazapine is 15 to 45 mg daily. It is also available in an orally dissolving "Soltab" formulation (Organon, 2003). Mirtazapine/Remeron compares favorably with SSRI antidepressants but seems to have better efficacy with mixed anxiety and depression (Kim et al., 2011).

VenlafaxineEffexor: A Serotonin-Norepinephrine Reuptake Inhibitor

Venlafaxine/Effexor has earned the label "dual reuptake inhibitor," because it combines the SSRI mechanism of action with potent reuptake inhibition of norepinephrine. It is currently available in an extended-release formulation and can be taken once daily. Researchers consider this once-daily administration significantly reduces side effects. Stahl (2000) asks, "Are two antidepressant mechanisms better than one?" Because reality is complex, the answer is "It depends." For some clients who have not responded to more specific, single-action agents (such as SSRIs), additional mechanisms of action can result in enhanced efficacy. From an integrative perspective we must note that the question presupposes a clear medical model etiology to depression, and this hypothesis has not been confirmed. Common side effects associated with venlafaxine/Effexor include gastrointestinal distress and insomnia. The common dosage range for venlafaxine/Effexor is 75 to 300 mg per day. A recent meta-analysis suggests that venlafaxine/Effexor is superior to SSRI antidepressants but has a significantly higher dropout rate due to adverse events (side effects) (de Silva & Hanwella, 2012).

DESVENLAFAXINE/PRESTIQ

In 2008, the FDA approved desvenlafaxine/Prestiq for the treatment of depression. It is designed from a metabolite of venlafaxine/Effexor and is a serotonin-norepinephrine reuptake inhibitor. Despite being a metabolite of venlafaxine, it appears desvenlafaxine has a different binding profile at both NE and 5-HT receptors. This leads to more adrenergic activity in desvenlafaxine which may account for the increase in cardiovascular side effects like heightened blood pressure. The parent compound (venlafaxine) only shows increased NE activity at higher doses but desvenlafaxine shows this at doses below the minimum therapeutic dose of 50 mg (Kamath & Handratta, 2008). Anything less than the minimum effective dose of 50 mg per day fails to show any difference from placebo (Liebowitz, Tourian, Huang, Mele, & for the Study 3362 Investigators, 2013; Rosenthal, Boyer, Vialet, Hwang, & Tourian, 2013). In comparisons between desvenlafaxine and its parent compound venlafaxine there appear to be few differences either in efficacy or tolerability that are significant enough to warrant a new drug. It has been suggested that desvenlafaxine was created and released about the same time as venlafaxine went generic and that this drug may be more about pharmaceutical profits (a "me too drug") than about clinical utility (Sopko, Ehret, & Grgas, 2008).

Reboxetine/Edronax: A Selective Noradrenergic Reuptake Inhibitor

First recall that *noradrenaline* is synonymous with *norepinephrine* (the difference being that the latter term is derived from the Latin and the former from Greek). Thus, reboxetine/Edronax is a selective inhibitor of norepinephrine reuptake. You may think this sounds like a tricyclic antidepressant, and that is correct. The difference is that reboxetine/Edronax supposedly does not have the "dirty" quality of binding to histamine and acetylcholine receptors (which cause many of the side effects associated with the TCAs). As such, reboxetine/Edronax was supposed to be useful for patients who respond better to NE reuptake inhibition or as a complement to SSRI therapy where response has been partial. The initial efficacy of reboxetine/Edronax seemed to be equal to the TCAs and the SSRIs (Messer, Schmauss, & Lambert-Bauman, 2005).

Side effects may include tremor, agitation, and changes in heart rate and blood pressure. Stahl (2000) also describes a milder set of side effects, similar to TCA anticholinergic side effects (dry mouth, constipation, and urine retention). He noted that these effects are milder and shorter in duration, because they do not result from direct blockage of acetylcholine receptors. These effects are more a result of reboxetine's effects on the sympathetic and parasympathetic nervous systems, both of which are highly populated with norepinephrine receptors.

The problem turned out that reboxetine/Edronax does not seem to have efficacy for depression. It was never FDA approved for use in the United States, which is telling. More recently a meta-analysis published in the *British Medical Journal* (Eyding et al., 2010) revealed, once again, some very biased information from the company that produced reboxetine/Edronax. Reboxetine/Edronax was compared to SSRI and placebos across 13 clinical trials involving over 4000 patients. The maker of reboxetine/Edronax (Pfizer) never published data on 75% of those patients, which inflated the drug's effectiveness over placebo by 115% (Szalavitz, 2010). In 2007 the United States passed a law to make all data—positive and negative—from clinical trials on drugs regulated by the FDA public. What Eyding et al. (2010) found was that the partial presentation of data inflated the drug's effectiveness and greatly underestimated potential harm from adverse events. This particular drug highlights the important of access to positive and negative data as well as published and unpublished trials.

BRINTELLIX/VORTIOXETINE

Vortioxetine/Brintellix is being labeled an atypical antidepressant. It was FDA approved in late 2013 for MDD but there is much confusion over its mechanism of action; the maker (Takeda Pharmaceuticals) claims it is a 5-HT1d antagonist and a 5-HT1b partial agonist. It also binds on 5-HT1a, 5-HT3, 5-HT1d, and 5-HT7. The pharmacy information card (Takeda Pharmaceuticals, 2013) states with regard to the binding "the clinical relevance of this is unknown" and "the mechanism of the antidepressant effect of vortioxetine is not fully understood …" (p. 1). Gibb and Deeks stated that "vortioxetine is a bis-aryl-suphanyl amine compound that combines serotonin (5-HT) reuptake inhibition with other characteristics, including receptor activity modulation" (p. 135). Boulenger, Lundbeck, Loft, and Olsen (2014) concluded that the treatment has similar adverse effects as SSRI and SNRI; nausea, headache, diarrhea, dry mouth, and dizziness. They found it superior to placebo. Pearce and Murphy (2014) compared the significance of vortioxetine compared to other antidepressants and concluded "… vortioxetine is an effective agent for the treatment of MDD, but it does not have any clear advantages over other available treatments" (p. 1542). Similarly, Dubovsky (2014) concluded that the "advantages of vortioxetine over existing antidepressants are not yet clear."

MILNACIPRAN/SAVELLA

Milnacipran/Savella is a drug that blocks adrenergic and serotonergic reuptake and is FDA approved for the treatment of fibromyalgia. Fibromyalgia is characterized by pain and sensitivity to pressure (allodynia). It can also cause fatigue, stiffness, bowel and bladder problems, and numbness or tingling (Wolfe, 1989). There is some speculation that the genes responsible for fibromyalgia also play a role in Major Depressive Disorder (Buskila & Sarzi-Puttini, 2006). Kohno et al. (2012) noted that it is possible that Milnacipran/Savella blocks NMDA receptors in the spinal cord contribute to analgesia. This may be the case though only in combination with reuptake inhibition of monoamines.

Duloxetine/Cymbalta: A Newer Serotonin-Norepinephrine Reuptake Inhibitor

Duloxetine/Cymbalta is a serotonin-norepinephrine reuptake inhibitor (SNRI) approved by the FDA in 2004 for depression, Generalized Anxiety Disorder, fibromyalgia, and some types of neuropathic pain (it was approved for generic versions in 2013). Duloxetine/Cymbalta seems to have a similar same side effect profile as do SSRI medications and is no more effective in alleviating depression than SSRI medications of venlafaxine/Effexor (Cipriani et al., 2012). When compared to escitalopram/Lexepro or venlafaxine/Effexor duloxetine dropout rates due to adverse events were higher.

In addition to the modest efficacy of antidepressants, another problem was confirmed in the Sequenced Treatment Alternatives to Relieve Depression trial (STAR★D) conducted in 2006 (Warden, Rush, Trivedi, Fava, & Wisniewski, 2007). This was the largest prospective, randomized treatment study at that time aimed at helping outpatients who had not had adequate benefit to their first antidepressant. Switching medications or trying to augment the medications the patients started on showed no significant differences in remission rates or times to remission. Participants who required increasing numbers of steps (adding, changing or augmenting medications) experienced great depressive symptoms and greater relapse rates (Warden et al., 2007). Thus it seems that we need a new direction for antidepressant research and novel agents that are perhaps even radically different from existing compounds. Ketamine may be just such an agent.

INTO THE FUTURE: KETAMINE

As early as 2000, researchers were learning that ketamine, a glutamatergic *N*-methyl-D-aspartate receptor (NMDA-R) antagonist, produced rapid and sustained antidepressant action in people suffering from severe depression that in many cases was treatment-resistant (Berman et al., 2000; Cornwell et al., 2012). These effects are immediate, last several days and appear to be linked to glutamatergic neuronal system as well as the mTOR signaling pathway discussed above (Naughton, Clarke, O'Leary, Cryan, & Dinan, 2014). Although some researchers feel there is evidence that the serotonin neuronal system is involved in the therapeutic response (Gigliucci et al., 2013) that is not yet clear. The evidence of therapeutic mechanism now seems focused on the glutamate system.

Glutamate is a major mediator of excitatory synaptic transmission in the human brain. It has important roles in synaptic plasticity, learning, and memory. Glutamate's possible role in depression was hypothesized in the late-20th century (Skolnick et al., 1996). The research had suggested that antagonizing NMDA receptors could be a viable treatment option in depressed clients. It took over 15 years of studies to validate this hypothesis.

Ketamine is an anesthetic agent for diagnostic and surgical procedures in humans and in veterinary medicine. It is perhaps better known as a drug of abuse called *Special K* on the streets. Ketamine can produce a dissociative state that many find pleasurable. Ironically this effect was pioneered by the son of the founder of Eli Lilly Pharmaceuticals, John Lilly (1996, 2006). John Lilly was trained in both neuroscience and psychoanalysis and he is best known as an explorer of altered states of consciousness. Working at the National Institute of Mental

Health in the 1950s, Lilly wanted to isolate the brain from external stimuli. Toward this end, he invented the sensory deprivation tank, which was a dark, soundproof tank filled with body-temperature salt water in which subjects could float for hours (1956). In his own explorations with the tank he took doses of ketamine and claimed to experience what felt like out-of-body (OOB) experiences that took him to different levels of consciousness (Lilly, 1977, 1997).

As is often the case, any form of hallucinogenic experience is quickly labeled "psychotomimetic" by mainstream psychiatry (Browne & Lucki, 2013). Although politically incorrect to state, it may in fact be that the ketamine experience is an altered state that is not mimicking psychosis. Side effects include dizziness and perceptual disturbances but why these are supposedly "psychotomimetic" is not explained. Also listed among the "adverse effects" are euphoria and increased libido (Murrough, Perez, & Stern, 2013). We will let the reader judge if those should in any way qualify as adverse. Regardless the "adverse effects" reported returned to baseline within two hours of dosing. Although any drug that may induce altered states should be avoided by people with a vulnerability to mental disorders, there is growing evidence that drugs such as LSD, psilocybin, MDMA, and ketamine can be powerful therapeutic tools in the right hands and under the proper restrictions (Roberts & Winkleman, 2007). We will discuss this further in the upcoming chapter on the topic. One of the problems with ketamine as an antidepressant is that it must be given intravenously and the effects only seem to last a few days. For those reasons, it may do better to use it as a model for other drugs that can affect NMDA receptors in a similar manner but have therapeutic effects that last longer and are possible to get in an oral formulation.

The neurobiological mechanisms underlying the antidepressant actions of ketamine are more complicated than simple antagonism (blocking) of NMDA receptors. 30–40 minutes after administration of a low dose subjects experience dissociative effects. After this, antidepressant effects begin approximately 110 minutes into the experience and are sustained for up to seven days (Zarate, Singh, & Carlson, 2006). Ketamine seems to initiate a cascade or chain reaction of events that results in rapid response. These may include effects on NMDR receptors, BDNF translation, mTOR activation, increased synaptic proteins, and increased synaptic plasticity. It is surprising that the psychological effects of a dissociated state of wellbeing reported by so-called abusers of ketamine (Zarate et al., 2010) is not considered a therapeutic mechanism yet. Most recently attention has been given to BDNF. In a recent study, ketamine significantly increased markers of BDNF in subjects whose depression responded to ketamine treatment (Haile et al., 2014). Hopefully further research will clarify what else contributes to the therapeutic effects.

Review Questions

- In what way are third-generation antidepressants like venlafaxine/Effexor similar to SSRI and TCA compounds?
- Describe the primary mechanisms of action in bupropion/Wellbutrin, duloxetine/Cymbalta, and mirtazapine/Remeron.
- What are the potential gains and drawbacks of ketamine as an antidepressant?

SUMMARY POINTS ABOUT ANTIDEPRESSANTS

We end this section of the chapter with a few key points to communicate to clients about antidepressants. These are paraphrased from Julien, Advokat, and Comaty (2011):

- Onset of clinical action for all antidepressants may take from two to six weeks.
- Symptomatic improvement is usually most seen in physiological symptoms. Many other symptoms may respond only partially to the drugs.
- Although these medications may improve mood, they do not erase all sadness or one's ability to experience the full range of emotions.

- The best indication of medical response includes improved sleep, less daytime fatigue, and some improvement in emotional control, and mental clarity.
- There may be side effects, but these can often be managed by dosage adjustment, augmentation, or switching to another antidepressant.
- Length of treatment varies with the client. It takes four to eight weeks for symptoms to subside, and if you quit at this point the relapse rate can be as high as 80%. A general guideline is to continue for six months and then gradually decrease.
- SSRI antidepressants (and possibly other types) do induce a type of dependence. They do induce a tolerance effect that can result in a withdrawal syndrome, which can be pronounced if clients do not appropriately go off the medication under their doctor's supervision.

CASE OF JOSHUA

Joshua is a 36-year-old African American businessman who recently came to counseling because of many changes in his life, including sleeplessness, loss of energy, feelings of hopelessness, lack of concentration, and difficulties with his relationships at home and at work. After a three-session assessment, which included an evaluation of Joshua's thoughts and feelings, he reluctantly agreed to see a psychiatrist for an evaluation to determine his need for an antidepressant medication. The psychiatrist recommended that Joshua begin a course of treatment with fluoxetine/Prozac. A week later, he began taking the fluoxetine/Prozac while continuing weekly therapy with his counselor. Almost immediately Joshua complained of sleeplessness, irritability, and nervousness. His therapist encouraged him to give the fluoxetine/Prozac time, at least three weeks, which he did. However, the side effects did not subside. In fact, Joshua reported that they worsened.

Throughout this period, Joshua continued to attend his weekly sessions to talk both about his depression and his reaction to the medication. Both the counselor and Joshua felt that their work together deepened. After four weeks on the fluoxetine/Prozac, Joshua decided to talk over his problem with the psychiatrist. The counselor and Joshua prepared for this meeting, which went well, and as a result, Joshua was titrated off the Prozac. The psychiatrist prescribed a course of venlafaxine/Effexor, an SNRI for Joshua.

Joshua took the venlafaxine/Effexor as prescribed, and after about 25 days on the medication reported to his counselor that he was feeling better. It is clear from the medical model perspective that the fluoxetine/Prozac was not helping Joshua, and it was equally clear that venlafaxine/Effexor began to alleviate some of his symptoms. What is more difficult to ascertain is the impact of the emerging counseling relationship and how Joshua's growing trust in his counselor also contributed to his psychological relief. Joshua continued the venlafaxine/Effexor and the counseling for nine months and made almost a complete recovery. Although the technical aspects of this case are clear, it is most difficult to tease out the impact of the authentic counseling relationship on Joshua's movement back to health.

ANTIDEPRESSANTS IN OLDER CLIENTS

Depression in elderly people is thought to be underreported (Satlin & Wasserman, 1997). Elderly people compose 12% of the population and account for approximately 20% of all suicides. Men account for 81% of suicides in those 65 and older. Risk factors for later life depression include female gender, unmarried status, stressful life events, lack of social support, and concurrent medical illness.

Satlin and Wasserman (1997) have noted that the literature is an imperfect guide to pharmacologic treatment of the elderly for several reasons.

- Published antidepressant trials use clients 55 to 65, whereas antidepressants are being prescribed for people considerably older.
- Participants in studies are atypical in that they are often free from medical illness. Although this makes it easier to see the relationship of the

drug under study to the symptoms, it does not mirror the reality that many older clients with depression have complicating medical conditions.

- Most studies include only those clients with moderate depression.
- Therapeutic response is measured only by the decline on depression scales, thus many people who showed "therapeutic response" have significant residual symptoms that continue to interfere with quality of life.
- With elderly clients it is important to screen for substance abuse, current nonpsychotropic medications, and general medical conditions. SSRIs are primary drugs of choice, starting at half-dose. Julien (2001) advises prescribers to start with a lower dose and titrate slowly. In addition, apparently bupropion and venlafaxine are promising treatments. Low doses of stimulant medication have also been used to improve mild dysphoric states (Satlin & Wasserman, 1997). We devote Chapter Thirteen to an overview of geriatric psychiatry.

SECTION SEVEN: FOCUS ON PSYCHOLOGICAL, CULTURAL, AND SOCIAL PERSPECTIVES

Learning Objectives

- Understand why it is important to talk to clients about how they feel about taking antidepressants.
- Be able to describe the placebo problem and the difference between active and inert placebos.
- Be able to discuss some nonpharmacologic treatments for depression.

In this section, we return to exploring antidepressants through psychological, cultural, and social perspectives—several issues concerning antidepressants that are rarely mentioned in standard psychopharmacology texts. As we noted in the cases for this chapter, the various quadrants offer us important perspective on these issues.

PSYCHOLOGICAL PERSPECTIVES

What does it mean to someone to take an antidepressant? As with many things in life, the meaning varies from person to person. Researchers working from the medical model perspective have tried to determine whether a given depressive episode was biological or psychological in etiology (Stahl, 2000). From an integrative perspective, this does not go far enough, because in the psychological realm alone many variations of psychological responses to stress or trauma can be delineated. John Teasdale (Teasdale, Segal, & Williams, 1999; Teasdale et al., 2000) hypothesized that even if biological mechanisms in some people allowed sadness to slide into depression, these same people could learn to stop that series of events through psychological, nonpharmacologic means. Using a variation of awareness meditation (described in Chapter Three) Teasdale was able to help clients disidentify from their thoughts to the point where they could preclude depressive episodes that likely would otherwise have followed periods of normal stress or sadness.

Another perspective regarding the variety of psychological experiences of depression views the subjective experience of depression in relation to a client's level of development. Human development can progress far beyond the stage of having a healthy ego. Most people have the capacity for growth beyond the levels of healthy ego development (Alexander & Langer, 1990). This further development is referred to as "transpersonal," meaning "going beyond" or "including and transcending" the personal (Walsh & Vaughan, 1980). On the personal level of development, the subjective experience of depression is qualitatively different from that on the transpersonal level. Moving from personal to transpersonal frequently includes an existential component wherein the person feels a sense of meaninglessness and horror when confronted with the existential givens of the world (aging, illness, death, human cruelty). After passing such a developmental milestone, people who have stabilized ego functioning may experience the world without benefit of the filters the ego puts in place. This experience calls on such people to develop a deeper and broader philosophy or "big picture" in order to continue living and growing. Sometimes the spiritual personages considered saints in both Eastern and Western traditions report an experience called "dark night of the senses," which qualitatively resembles anhedonia (a loss of joy or pleasure in all things). The dark night of the senses is a period of desolation where one no longer finds joy in life. Rather, one confronts the stark pain inherent in human existence and seeks a way to deal with that pain. Far from being a chemical imbalance of the brain, such a state is frequently a prelude to a more expanded state of spiritual understanding. We realize that in a society that values materialistic explanations, it is hard enough to accept various psychological theories for things such as depression, let alone to consider a worldview that, for lack of a better term, is spiritual in nature. Yet an integrative exploration of any topic must be broad enough to include a place for such worldviews. With these worldviews come technologies such as meditation that have rich potential for treating symptoms such as those seen in depressed clients.

DIFFERENT PERSPECTIVES ON THE PLACEBO PROBLEM

Placebo responses are common, according to researchers such as Fisher and Greenberg (1997) and practitioners such as Colbert (2002). These professionals begin by claiming that the evidence of efficacy of counseling and psychotherapy (from the psychological perspective) is not given equal weight with the evidence supporting pharmacologic interventions (medical model perspective). They then note that although medical research on psychotropic medication is lavishly funded by the pharmaceutical companies, research on counseling and psychotherapy struggles, because it has far fewer resources (when was the last commercial you saw for counseling?). Finally, many have claimed that many research results from the medical model perspective that do not distinguish between placebo and drug never get published and are not as accessible to the public as the published studies that support the efficacy of the drugs over placebo.

For example, Khan, Leventhal, Khan, and Brown (2002) demonstrated that in over 50% of the trials on antidepressants in the FDA database, researchers found no significant difference between active placebo and the drug being tested. Many of these studies are never published in peer-reviewed journals, because they are less likely to be published than studies that showed significant differences between placebo and drug. Another scenario is that when pharmaceutical companies sponsor studies, they may include clauses that allow them to "hold" results for a period of time before releasing them back to the researchers, who may then try to publish them. Bodenheimer (2000) has documented cases where companies prevented important research findings from being published because the results were not favorable regarding the compound being tested.

From the cultural perspective, one question is how far the culture of the pharmaceutical industry may go in protecting its interests. Although more research needs to be done regarding client responses to placebos (Naudet et al., 2013), it is unlikely the companies themselves would carry out such research. Government is more likely to fund it with tax dollars targeted for such research, but again, how will politicians who receive financial support from pharmaceutical companies view such research?

Pomerantz (2003) offers another perspective on antidepressants and placebo effects. Summarizing prescription trends, he notes that spending for antidepressants increased 600% during the 1990s and that in 2000 alone over $7 billion was spent on SSRI medications. He then cites studies from the United States and Italy suggesting that a significant percentage of clients stop taking the SSRIs after one or two months. He reminds us that off-label uses for SSRI antidepressants keep growing despite little evidence to support such uses. This practice includes using SSRIs for mild depression, for which SSRIs are no more effective than placebo in many studies. Pomerantz contends that in cases where SSRIs are being used off label, this use is akin to using them as active placebos. Because most clients feel *something* on beginning the medication, they assume something is working to help them, without realizing they are just feeling drug effects that may be unrelated to their problem. Because Streator and Moss (1997) have demonstrated that large numbers of patients are taking SSRIs for off-label uses, Pomerantz concluded this is simply very expensive (wastefully so) placebo therapy.

OTHER TREATMENTS FOR DEPRESSION

You can see that the systematic use of RCTs and the standardization of categorical psychiatry rely predominantly on the medical model perspective. Despite the dominance of the medical model perspective, many people seek out alternative and/or complementary treatments (herbs, and so forth), which we discuss more thoroughly in Chapter Ten. One battle in mental health treatment is between the proponents of the psychological perspective, who point to successful psychosocial treatments for mood and anxiety disorders, and proponents strictly adhering to the medical model perspective, which reduces mental disorders to biochemical entities ignoring their social, cultural, and personal meaning. More studies are now showing the efficacy of the psychosocial methods. Two studies have even documented through brain scans that the neurological changes attributed to antidepressants also occur with psychotherapy (Brody et al., 2001; Martin, Martin, Rai, Richardson, & Royall, 2001).

Nevertheless, U.S. trends show an increased number of people given medication for depression, a decreased number receiving counseling or psychotherapy, and a lowered percentage of treatment costs covered by insurance (Olfson et al., 2002). In addition to the standard psychosocial interventions, an increasing number of studies show that exercise is effective in alleviating symptoms of depression (Babyak et al., 2000; Leppamaki, Partonen, Hurme, Haukka, & Lonnqvist, 2002; Salmon, 2001), as are yoga postures and breathing exercises (Jorm, Christensen, Griffiths, & Rodgers, 2002; Nyer et al., 2013; Ray et al., 2001). There is also a growing literature on nutrition and depression (Recheneberg & Humphries, 2013). Continued research on these nonpharmacologic treatment options is important. The case of Alex illustrates

some problems when doctors may prescribe potential drugs of abuse ostensibly for depression.

A PROBLEM CASE: THE CASE OF ALEX

Alex, age 27, has been treated for his depression with dextroamphetamine/Adderall for the past five years. Recently, his psychiatrist lost his license to practice for prescribing addictive medications to patients who then sold the drugs on the street. Criminal charges against him are pending. When mental health professionals attempted to refer Alex to another psychiatrist, he indicated that he would only go to one that would give him dextroamphetamine/Adderall for his depression and withdrawal. No psychiatrist in the community would agree to that drug for Alex. After several months of suffering, Alex agreed to see a psychiatrist who recommended a course of bupropion/Wellbutrin for him. The psychiatrist cautioned about the dangers of long-term use of dextroamphetamine/Adderall and explained the potential proactive effects of bupropion. After a long discussion/argument, Alex agreed to give the bupropion/Wellbutrin a try. Six months later the psychiatrist added 50 mg of sertraline to the bupropion. In the last five to six years, psychiatrists have found this combination to be very effective with long-term depression. Alex continues to refuse to attend counseling for his depression.

Questions About the Case of Alex

1. Discuss the impact of Adderall on depression. Why did Alex refuse to switch medications?

2. What do you do when the patient/client attempts to control the treatment?

3. Do you believe Alex will ever try counseling? Why? or Why not?

When to Recommend Medication Evaluation

For mental health therapists, all these considerations raise the question "When should I recommend a medication evaluation?" As the cases in this chapter illustrate, antidepressant medication ideally provides a chemical window of opportunity for clients to gather the energy for making changes through counseling and psychotherapy. When to recommend this "window of opportunity" depends primarily on client factors: in particular, the severity of the depression and the associated risks to the client (or others) such as suicidal thinking or failing to meet caregiving responsibilities. Ideally, the counselor can develop some alliance with the client and work through the question with him or her. Clients who resist the idea of medication can use this resistance to apply themselves to counseling. Clients at risk for harming themselves or others by omission or commission require a more aggressive intervention to stabilize them.

The Culture of Pharmaceutical Companies: Are Newer Antidepressants Medical Innovations or "One-Trick Ponies"?

The issue of whether the newer antidepressants are just "one-trick ponies" relates directly to the culture of pharmaceutical companies and the legal-economic aspects of drug development in the United States. When pharmaceutical companies find a mechanism of action that seems effective, they focus research on finding as many permutations of that mechanism as possible. There are likely several reasons for doing so. Certainly one is that by fully exploiting the mechanism they may break through to advances that will help clients. The other reason may be less noble and more related to the amount of time and money it takes to really develop new compounds. Consider the FDA regulations we discussed in Chapter Four. There we noted that the FDA requires companies to show through randomized, double-blind, placebo-controlled studies that their medication treats the symptoms of some disorder. These regulations are objectively built into this society through the authority of the FDA and related laws passed by state and federal legislators. Given these structures, it costs millions of dollars just to begin the long journey toward FDA approval. This increases the probability that once a single company has cleared part of the path to FDA approval, other companies will follow in that wake.

Recall that the first company to break SSRIs into the market was Eli Lilly, with fluoxetine/Prozac, and that after this, numerous other companies spent a great deal of money putting similar and equally effective SSRI compounds on the market (fluvoxamine/Luvox, sertraline/Zoloft, paroxetine/Paxil, citalopram/Celexa, escitalopram/Lexapro, etc.). These compounds were similar but different enough to garner FDA approval and be able to compete in the marketplace. The National Institute for Health Care Management (NIHCM) (2002) reported that approximately two-thirds of the medications the FDA approved in the 1990s were merely modified versions of existing drugs. Only 15% were for drugs containing new active ingredients.

Companies often seek to extend their patent rights over an existing compound either by bringing out a slightly different version of the compound or by seeking FDA approval for a new use for the existing compound. About a year before its patent ran out for fluoxetine/Prozac, Eli Lilly brought out fluoxetine under a new name (Sarafem) and received FDA approval for its use for Pre-Menstrual Dysphoric Disorder (PDD). This is curious, because the latter was technically not a *DSM* category at the time and only a condition for which further research was needed. It has been included in the Depressive Disorders in *DSM-5*.

At the same time, rival companies are constantly seeking ways to bring out generic versions of compounds other companies have patented. For example, in 1998, Apotex Corporation filed for approval of a generic form of paroxetine/Paxil. Paroxetine/Paxil was worth $2.1 billion in 2001, and the company with the patent rights (GlaxoSmithKline) sued Apotex for patent infringement. In 2003, a court ruled in favor of Apotex and GlaxoSmithKline stock fell sharply (Sipkoff, 2003). The companies filed an agreement in settlement in 2007 but as of 2012 there were still court cases dragging on as appeals are filed and as both companies assert the other was not abiding by the settlement. Critics thus question whether enough energy is going into the study of new compounds or whether pharmaceutical companies are relying on "one-trick ponies" for guaranteed profits, and such ponies tend to pay off a great deal. So what begins as serendipity, the possibility that a drug may have other uses with varied disorders, becomes a corporate strategy to fully support a new diagnostic category without the necessary research.

These issues have been summarized as the Matthew effect (Merton, 1968) and the Luke effect (Healy, 1997). Both paraphrase quotations from the biblical texts bearing these proper names. Merton summarized the Matthew effect as "To him who has, more shall be given, and from him who has not, even more shall be taken away." He noted that the survival of ideas depends on how effective they are. In addition, Healy (1997) added that whose interests the ideas coincide with and the degree to which they have commercial application for brand name recognition also influence how much effort and energy is put into them. Thus, SSRIs in general and the outdated theories about why they work (for example, the "chemical imbalance" theory) garner a great deal of support and name recognition, and any company with a similar compound can "jump on the bandwagon" for an increased probability of success. Conversely, Healy noted that this effect may reduce the chance that different (and thus financially riskier) ideas will not get funded by pharmaceutical companies.

Based on this logic, Healy proposed the Luke effect, which followed the biblical parable that when a sower sows seed, some will fall on thorny ground and wither, some will fall on fertile ground and be choked by weeds, and some will fall on fertile ground and flourish. Thus, the now-outdated metaphor of "chemical imbalance" provides fertile ground on which to sow the seeds of compounds that work like others that correct this hypothetical "imbalance." Healy concludes, "This parable ends with an exhortation to those who have ears to listen, which I will argue is what drug companies do very successfully, as part of the business of bringing the development of their compounds to fruition" (p. 180).

We want to emphasize that we are not raising these issues to condemn pharmaceutical companies for seeking to make profits. Again from the social perspective, the principles of the free market and how those principles are implemented through laws are an integrative part of our society. This does not mean, however, that they should evade inspection, commentary, and a system of checks and balances.

Review Questions

- Why is it important to discuss how clients feel about taking medication?
- What is the placebo problem and what is the difference between active and inert placebo?
- What are some nonpharmacologic treatments for depression?

SUMMARY

Antidepressants have a huge presence in our culture, not all of which is well deserved. Although there are several theories of how antidepressants work from the medical model perspective, depressive symptoms are highly overdetermined and biological variables are only one group of many related to the development and resolution of depression. We noted in Chapter One that an integrative model requires consideration of lines and levels of development. The current concern over the extent to which antidepressant medications may induce or exacerbate suicidal thinking in children and adolescents points to the importance of developmental studies on the effects of all psychotropic medications. Although antidepressants have efficacy in treating depression, research indicates that depressed clients also respond well to counseling or psychotherapy, exercise, and perhaps even activities such as yoga and meditation. Whereas antidepressants are an important component of treatment for some clients, mental health professionals will benefit from an integrative overview of depression and how the intrapsychic, cultural, and social perspectives can complement what antidepressants can offer.

STUDY QUESTIONS AND EXERCISES

1. Describe your understanding of the placebo effect and your sense of the current state of effectiveness of antidepressants (TCAs, MAOIs, and SSRIs).

2. Discuss vegetative symptoms and your understanding of how antidepressants work in general to relieve these symptoms. Demonstrate how the medical model theories in psychopharmacology build on one another.

3. Discuss the impact of Prozac (fluoxetine) on the antidepressant model, and in your response focus on its significance from the psychological, cultural, and social perspectives.

4. After reading this chapter, summarize your thoughts about how you could talk to your clients about beginning a course of antidepressant treatment and about the potential side effects of the medication.

5. Some might say the era of antidepressants was an "incidental" outcome of scientific research that fueled a range of diagnostic categories (*DSM IV-TR*). Discuss.

6. Detail the strengths and limitations of TCAs, MAOIs, and SSRIs.

7. From the chapter, what is your understanding of a serotonin–norepinephrine reuptake inhibitor? Identify one, give an example of a type of client for whom it could be prescribed, and explain why.

8. Discuss some potential multicultural problems with using antidepressants as the only mode of treatment with certain populations.

9. Identify several problems encountered with prescribing antidepressants to children.

10. What is your understanding of an SSRI and SNRI? Identify an SNRI, and give an example of a type of client for whom it could be prescribed.

11. Discuss some cultural problems with using antidepressants as the only mode of treatment.

12. Describe some ways that an informed counselor can speak to a client about the effectiveness and uses of antidepressants when the client is uncertain about the course of action he or she wants to take.

13. Based on your knowledge after reading this chapter, would you take an antidepressant that was recommended to you? Why or why not?

CHAPTER SIX

The Age of Anxiety

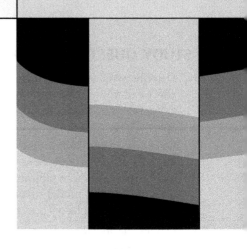

The multiple perspectives we have been using in this book are particularly useful in understanding the impact anxiety has on U.S. society. The word "anxiety" comes from a Latin root meaning to "choke or throttle" connoting a troubled state of mind (Tone, 2009). Anxiety disorders are believed to be the most common mental health problem in the United States. Two common measures are lifetime morbid risk (the theoretical risk of getting a disorder at any point in life) and 12-month prevalence (the proportion of the population thought to suffer from the disorder in any 12-month period). Baxter et al. (2013) conducted a meta-analysis of 87 studies from 44 countries between 1980 and 2009. They found that anxiety disorders are common across the globe with an estimated current prevalence of approximately as much as 28% of the global population. The prevalence of anxiety disorders in the United States is estimated for lifetime morbid risk/12-month prevalence as follows: Specific Phobia 18.4%/12.1%, Social Anxiety Disorder 13%/7.4%, Post Traumatic Stress Disorder (PTSD) 10.1%/3.7%, Generalized Anxiety Disorder 9%/2%, Separation Anxiety Disorder 8.7%/1.2%, and Panic Disorder, 6.8%/2.4%, (Kessler, Petukhova, Sampson, Zaslovsky, & Wittchen, 2012). Although anxiety disorders are prominent, it is important to realize that their incidence has remained steady over several decades despite pharmaceutically funded efforts to make the public think there is an epidemic that needs medicated (Baxter et al., 2014).

Although psychotropic medications are available for anxiety disorders, many psychological treatments also have excellent track records. Remember, from an integrative perspective it is not enough to describe anxiety symptoms, posit a biological explanation, then describe how certain drugs act biologically to (at least temporarily) decrease or eliminate these symptoms. With sentient beings, we have to look to the psychological, cultural and social variables that contribute to anxiety.

We recall a client (Elijah) who lived in what could be described as a "**toxic environment**." Elijah's urban residence was the regular scene of violence, and he himself had witnessed two shootings in his 23 years. He was court-ordered to receive treatment for an alcohol-related charge (drunk and disorderly conduct). Even after abstaining from all drugs for 60 days, Elijah was what could only be described as "a nervous wreck." He showed symptoms of both Panic Disorder and PTSD (the latter related to stimuli associated with the shootings he had witnessed). In consultation with a psychiatrist, who prescribed SSRI medication, Elijah asked why he had his symptoms, and the doctor replied, "Some people have a genetic predisposition to such things." As Charlie Brown would say, "Good grief!" In this client's case, genetic predisposition not withstanding, there were clearly psychological, cultural, and social contributors to his anxiety. His alcohol use was a classic example of self-medication. Although the SSRI medication provided a window of opportunity for Elijah, it was going to take far more to alleviate his anxiety. Tragically, Elijah was stabbed in a fight at his residence, and although he recovered from that, he never reentered treatment. As we have urged in previous chapters, mental health professionals must not lose sight of clients like Elijah nor surrender them to the partial truths of medical model explanations.

Although society has effective psychological interventions for anxiety, researchers estimate that only 30% of people suffering from an anxiety disorder seek treatment, although treatment is effective for 70 to 90% of those clients who seek it (Preston, O'Neal, & Talaga, 2002). Why is there so much anxiety in this population? It is not enough for mental health professionals to treat clients and refer them for psychiatric consultations. From an integrative perspective, we must wrestle with the question of why there are so many anxious people. Although moderate alcohol use can be perfectly appropriate, mental health professionals need to ask why there is so much abuse of alcohol in Western societies. When reflecting on cases like Elijah's, therapists must also remember that anxiety symptoms are just as prominent in people living in nontoxic environments. What are people so anxious about, and is medication really the best solution? Although mental health clinicians must know about medications that can provide relief for clients, they must also address these broader questions.

This chapter is divided into eight sections. Section One provides an overview of anxiolytic medications and the construct of anxiety. Section Two focuses on areas of the central nervous system pertinent to anxiety and its treatment. Section Three covers central nervous system depressants including barbiturates and benzodiazepines. Section Four covers nonbenzodiazepine alternatives in treating anxiety. Section Five introduces newer approaches to treating anxiety. Section Six covers antidepressants used as anxiolytics. Section Seven summarizes anxiolytic therapy by diagnosis and Section Eight returns to important psychological, cultural, and social considerations.

SECTION ONE: OVERVIEW OF ANXIOLYTIC MEDICATION AND THE CONSTRUCT OF ANXIETY

Learning Objectives

- Understand that there is a wide variety of anxiolytic drugs.
- Have a working definition of anxiety.

Thirty years ago, we would probably have titled this entire chapter "Central Nervous System (CNS) Depressants," because those were the primary compounds available for treating anxiety. Currently, psychotropic medications from numerous classes are used to treat anxiety symptoms, including CNS depressants, SSRI antidepressants, and unique compounds such as buspirone (BuSpar). There is currently research being done on developing different benzodiazepines (Trincavelli, Da Pozzo, Daniele, & Martini, 2012), anxiolytics from antibiotics (Johnstone et al., 2004) and from neurosteroids (Nothdurfter et al., 2011). In addition, more studies are examining melotonin (Ochoa-Sanchez et al., 2012) and kava (Alramadhan et al., 2012), which we discuss further in the chapter on herbaceuticals. In general, anxiolytics are the most commonly used psychotropic medications and general practitioners (nonpsychiatrists) prescribe the vast majority (less than 20% are prescribed by psychiatrists). This situation required us to structure this chapter differently from the others in this book. For this chapter, we begin with a general discussion of anxiety, then describe anxiety from the medical model perspective, and then describe the different classes of drugs for anxiety. In discussing each class of drugs, we outline some of the drug's history; mechanisms of action; side effects; and potential for tolerance, dependence, and overdose. Finally, we outline recommended pharmacologic approaches as well as other treatments for particular anxiety disorders from *DSM-5*. The treatment of anxiety in children and adolescents will be covered in a later chapter.

The Construct of Anxiety

Anxiety, in and of itself, is natural and adaptive. A moderate amount of anxiety enhances physical and intellectual performance. This is reflected in what is called the Yerkes-Dodson law (Yerkes & Dodson, 1908). Simply stated, it means people perform a little better when they are slightly anxious, but too much anxiety tends to impair performance and too little leaves them unmotivated to do their best (Barlow & Durand, 2002). You may have been initially anxious picking up this book. If you were moderately anxious, the anxiety likely helped you motivate yourself to get to this chapter. Readers who felt crippled with anxiety reading Chapter One probably didn't get this far.

Anxiety was instrumental in the birth of psychoanalysis and psychodynamic models of the mind. In *Inhibitions, Symptoms, and Anxiety* (Freud, 1925), Freud unfolded his thinking about anxiety and its relationship to the structural model of the mind: id, ego, and superego. In this seminal work, he developed the notion of anxiety neurosis and identified two forms. The first was a sense of worry or dread that originated in a repressed wish or thought that generated conscious and unconscious conflict and was curable through the psychological treatment he developed into psychoanalysis. The second was an overwhelming sense of *panic,* accompanied by autonomic nervous system arousal (sweating, increased heart rate, and diarrhea). This, he thought, resulted from a buildup of libido and required a sexual outlet. Freud viewed anxiety as a result of conflict between unconscious sexual or aggressive wishes in the id and the corresponding punishment (or threat of punishment) from the superego. Anxiety is thus seen as a signal of danger in the unconscious, which could then result in a dangerous behavior or in inhibition. In response to the signal, the ego mobilizes defense mechanisms to prevent unacceptable feelings from emerging into consciousness. If the signal fails, the anxiety just keeps getting more intense and becomes immobilizing.

As you can see from this summary, although his explanations were mostly wrong, Freud was correct in differentiating panic from anxiety and would not be the last to do so. Anxiety is often differentiated from panic and fear. Anxiety is defined as a future-oriented, negative mood state characterized by bodily symptoms of physical tension and by apprehension about the future. A key feature of the apprehension is related to the sense that the person cannot control upcoming events (Barlow & Durand, 2002). Anxiety itself can be seen in the 11 Anxiety Disorders listed in the *DSM-5,* in several of the Personality Disorders (Histrionic, Dependent, and Obsessive-Compulsive), Delirium, Delusional Disorder, Major Depressive Disorder, and Schizophrenia. Anxiety Disorders are commonly comorbid with Substance Use Disorders (Wolitsky-Taylor, Operskalski, Ries, Craske, & Roy-Byrne, 2011). Fear is an immediate alarm reaction to danger and is characterized by autonomic nervous system stimulation (e.g., increased heart rate and respiration). The autonomic nervous system stimulation is thought to help the person escape the feared stimulus. Panic, in contrast, is an abrupt onset of intense fear, usually accompanied by physical symptoms such as heart palpitations, shortness of breath, and dizziness. Barlow and Durand (2002) described panic as a fear response when there is nothing (apparently) to be afraid of (in other words, a false alarm).

The Case of Marcia

Marcia, a 36-year-old female teacher, married with two adolescent teenagers, has struggled with mental and emotional issues for the past 11 years. She has been diagnosed with (not at the same time) Major Depressive Disorder, Dysthymic Disorder, Seasonal Affective Disorder, Avoidant Personality Disorder, and Personality Disorder Not Otherwise Specified (NOS). During the course of her treatment, Marcia was a very compliant patient. She always took her medications, mostly TCAs, and seldom missed therapy sessions. During the 11 years of her treatment, she had cognitive-behavioral therapy with a feminist female therapist, gestalt therapy with a male therapist, and holistic therapy with another female, and she tried various workshops and techniques such as art therapy. Almost always, the intervention or theoretical approach was combined with a psychotropic medication. Marcia improved slightly, only to return to what appeared to be a depressed and irritable state.

In the 10th year, after much frustration, Marcia was referred to a psychoanalytically oriented psychotherapist who spent several sessions with her conducting an assessment. After this thorough and extensive evaluation period, he made the diagnosis of Generalized Anxiety Disorder (GAD) and began to speak with her about the ways anxiety and panic manifested in her life. She seemed to talk about being incurably worried, exhausted, and never able to relax. Marcia existed in a state of agitation. They also discovered together that the closer Marcia got to a performance, a test in graduate school, giving a party, or being at a party, the more she panicked and fretted. The therapist referred her to a psychiatrist for assessment for medications and she prescribed clorazepate/Tranxene for her anxious conditions. The combination of insight therapy and clorazepate/Tranxene was very beneficial. Marcia gradually decreased her irritability, learned more about the triggers and pressures on her life from inside herself, and appeared less depressed.

In the first session, Marcia said three things that helped the therapist clarify his diagnosis: (1) "As I get closer to an obligation or performance, I begin to worry, ruminate, fret, and feel totally overwhelmed"; (2) "I fight these terrible battles within myself, should I do this or should I do that? How can I ever find a peace of mind?"; and (3) "Most of the time I disagree with my other doctors and therapists that I have depression, it always felt like something else, not depression." Thus, from her own words and her various therapeutic journeys, it is evident that Marcia had a strong personal hunch that her previous diagnoses and treatments were not quite accurate. (We might say her intrapsychic intuition was working fine.) Marcia was most helped by a dynamic psychotherapy and a benzodiazepine, clorazepate/Tranxene. Although we have not delved into the social and cultural influences in Marcia's case, it illustrates a very common error in current diagnostic thinking, namely that many anxiety symptoms often get subsumed in a diagnosis of depression (as mentioned in Chapter Three). It is true that Marcia did get depressed and exhibited depressive symptoms, but her primary problem was anxiety, showing the importance of thorough diagnosis before any referral for medication.

THEORIES OF ANXIOLYTIC ACTION

As with depression, theories of anxiety rooted in the medical model hypothesize that some physiological process is deficient or impaired and that this deficiency or impairment results in a person having anxiety. Although some research supports this hypothesis, it is far from conclusive. As noted at the beginning of this chapter, there are more successful psychosocial interventions for anxiety than any other category of disorders. If anxiety were due solely to a physiological problem, why would psychological interventions be so successful? Even the most rigorous medical model theory of anxiety cannot dismiss the importance of the mind and of the type of knowledge available from a psychological perspective.

Review Questions

- What are some general types of anxiolytic drugs?
- What is your working definition of anxiety?

SECTION TWO: THE CENTRAL NERVOUS SYSTEM: ANXIETY, BRAIN CIRCUITS, BRAIN STRUCTURES, AND NEUROTRANSMITTERS

Learning Objectives

- Understand the role of the Behavioral Inhibition System in Anxiety.
- Be able to articulate what neurotransmitter systems seem to be important in treating anxiety.

In earlier chapters, we have described several brain structures and some of the neurotransmitters in the brain associated with the types of symptoms psychotropic medications are designed to treat. In this section, we return to this topic to summarize the more popular medical model explanations of anxiety. A primary brain circuit associated with anxiety is called the *behavioral inhibition system (BIS)* (Baskin-Somers, Wallace, MacCoon, Curtin, & Newman, 2010; Gray, 1987; McNaughton & Gray, 2000). This circuit leads from the limbic system to the frontal cortex and is triggered from the brain stem. In the limbic system, meaning attaches to incoming stimuli and the frontal cortex processes executive functions. The circuit is triggered by things such as unexpected events that act as signals for danger; for example, abrupt changes in bodily functioning or visual stimuli. In abrupt changes in body functioning, the signals arise from the brain stem, and in changes in visual stimuli they descend from the cortex. Either way, BIS activation leads the person to freeze, experience anxiety, and evaluate the situation for danger (Keough & O'Conner, 2014).

This brain circuit is hypothesized to underlie the type of anxiety seen in GAD (Maack, Tull, & Gratz, 2012) and creates effects that differ from the "fight or flight" circuit. The fight-or-flight circuit originates in the brain stem (associated with vital body processes such as heart rate and respiration) and proceeds through several limbic system structures. Stimulating this circuit produces an "alarm and escape response" that researchers believe manifests as panic such as that seen in Panic Disorder. In the panic response, the limbic system, hypothalamus, and pituitary gland release a cascade of neurotransmitters and hormones that prepare the body for action. Markarian, Pickett, Deveson, and Kanona (2013) have also noted that the BIS can trigger anxiety when "… decreased responsiveness to rewards and a heightened sensitivity to aversive stimuli may predispose for difficulties regulating emotions" (p. 285) suggesting a role for the BIS in personality disorders.

A Hypothesized Braking System

Preston et al. (2002) note that the brain does have a "brake system" of sorts. This brake system consists of the ion channels on most neurotransmitters that allow negative ions (particularly chloride) to flow into the neuron to decrease its excitability. Researchers hypothesize that an as-yet-undiscovered endogenous benzodiazepine molecule binds with receptors to allow this influx of chloride ions. The hypothesis basically states that a deficiency of this yet-to-be-discovered substance causes anxiety disorders. Like the amine theory of antidepressant action, this hypothesis is a convenient extrapolation from the minimal data available on these brain circuits but is hardly convincing when you consider all the environmental and psychological factors that can trigger anxiety. Much research on anxiety and brain structures points to action in the amygdalae. The amygdalae are almond-shaped structures (one on each side of the brain) in the limbic system that are involved in how we attach emotional meaning to incoming stimuli. Advokat, Comaty, and Julien (2014) have summarized research showing that electrical lesions of the amygdala result in an anxiolytic effect as well as research documenting amygdala abnormalities in patients with Panic Disorder. The latter two examples have a "chicken-and-egg" problem. Miller, Piasecki, Peabody, and Lonstein (2010) found that antagonism of GABAa in anxiety-resistant rats increased anxiety. GABA is a neurotransmitter that tends to function in the brain to calm the organism. As noted, although this research certainly supports the hypothesis that the amygdala plays a role in anxiety symptoms, it does not confirm that defects in the amygdala cause anxiety symptoms.

Neurotransmitters Involved in Anxiety

GABA has clearly been indicated as playing a role in relief from anxiety in that facilitation of GABA binding is one mechanism that decreases anxiety. For example, benzodiazepines facilitate the binding of GABA to GABA receptors but do not directly stimulate GABA. By binding to an adjacent receptor, they change the shape of the GABA receptor making it more receptive to GABA molecules. Less well understood are the roles of serotonin and norepinephrine. Currently, some medications prescribed for anxiety target either serotonin (e.g., SSRI antidepressants) and/or norepinephrine. Perhaps it is easier to understand how norepinephrine is involved in anxiety, because the fight-or-flight circuit includes large releases of norepinephrine via the locus coeruleus. The locus coeruleus ("blue disk") is a small brain structure (estimated to be about 10,000 neurons) whose neurons project to most other norepinephrine neurons in the brain. This structure can trigger the release of norepinephrine, stimulating the sympathetic nervous system, resulting in tachycardia, tremor, sweating, and anxiety. One medication (clonidine/Catapres) paradoxically treats such stimulation by releasing norepinephrine as an alpha adrenergic receptor agonist, and this fools the brain into thinking the NE levels are higher than they really are and thus overall lowering NE levels. Although this medication successfully reduces physiological symptoms associated with noradrenergic overactivity, it does not relieve the psychological aspects of anxiety.

Another neurotransmitter implicated in anxiety is serotonin. Although its role is still unclear, apparently several serotonin agonists are helpful with anxiety. One theory is that the brain structures implicated in fear and anxiety (the hippocampus, amygdala, septum, and dorsal raphe nucleus) are rich in 5-HT1a receptors. In animal models, mice bred without these receptors have heightened fear responses (Rambos et al., 1998) so the fact that SSRI drugs activated them through reuptake inhibition is thought to account for their anxiolytic quality in some clients.

In the last 20 years, researchers have made numerous advances in conceptualizing and treating anxiety disorders. Some may argue that the anxiety disorders are so heterogeneous that it is not accurate to include them all under one category, and there is much to support this assertion. *DSM-5* redesigned the anxiety disorder so that Obsessive Compulsive Disorder and PTSD were moved out of Anxiety Disorders and into their own categories (Obsessive Compulsive and related Disorders and Trauma and Stressor Related Disorders respectively) (APA, 2013).

Review Questions

- What is the role of the Behavioral Inhibition System?
- What neurotransmitter systems seem important in the treatment of anxiety disorders?

SECTION THREE: CENTRAL NERVOUS SYSTEM DEPRESSANTS

Learning Objectives

- Be able to state the differences between an anxiolytic and a hypnotic.
- Know what the mechanisms of action are for barbiturates and benzodiazepines.
- Be able to list the advantages of benzodiazepines over barbiturates including the risks of overdose and addiction.
- Understand how the early anxiolytics like meprobemate became the first celebrity psychotropics.

Central nervous system depressants are a group of medications with diverse chemical structures that induce behavioral depression. They produce many effects ranging from relief from anxiety and inhibitions, to inducing relaxation and sleep, to inducing unconsciousness, general anesthesia, and (in overdose) coma and death. The predominant tendency of all these drugs is to inhibit the excitability of neurons.

Unfortunately, several terms are used to refer to CNS depressants, including *sedatives, tranquilizers, hypnotics,* and *anxiolytics,* which can cause confusion when you are first learning this material. In the first half of the 20th century, anxiety was not a common construct and most patients were medicated with "sedatives" for "anxiety neuroses." These sedatives were usually **bromides** or barbiturates combined with everything from cannabis to digitalis. With refined diagnostic criteria, therapists would now say that many of these cases of "nerves" were actually depression and would be more likely to treat them with compounds described in Chapter Five (Healy, 2002).

The inducement of sleep is referred to as a "hypnotic effect." This is inaccurate, because sleep induction is actually very different from what happens (or doesn't happen) in hypnosis, but the term was coined at a time when people believed hypnosis induced a sleeplike trance. **Anxiolytics** are drugs used for treating anxiety. We prefer the term *anxiolytic* throughout this book. The inaccurate phrase "minor tranquilizers" is often used for anxiolytics but indicates only that these drugs treat milder symptoms than those treated by drugs labeled "major tranquilizers." As you will see in Chapter Seven, the phrase "major tranquilizer" is also sometimes misapplied to certain types of antipsychotic medication. So many poorly chosen words! At this point, the reader may conclude that the field of psychopharmacology could benefit from the services of a grammarian. Although we want readers to be familiar with all these terms, we encourage the use of the more accurate terms "anxiolytics" and "hypnotics." Anxiolytics are for decreasing anxiety and hypnotics are for inducing sleep. Next we discuss the CNS depressants that are currently (or historically have been) used to treat anxiety.

Barbiturates

The first barbiturates were created in the late 19th century and introduced to the United States in 1912, the first being phenobarbital. According to Julien et al. (2011) between 1912 and 1950, hundreds of barbiturates were tested and at least 50 were marketed. Although these medications are rarely used for anxiety now, they dominated the antianxiety market until about 1960, when their dangers and drawbacks became widely known. We discuss barbiturates in this book not so much because they are often used but because their undesirable qualities set the baseline for desirable qualities researchers wanted in the anxiolytic drugs they were trying to develop and that currently dominate the market. As Stahl (2000) points out, barbiturates do not really have a specific anxiolytic effect but merely reduce anxiety as a side effect of their overall sedating effects, much like drinking too much whisky might.

The name "barbiturate" is said to have been chosen *either* because the urine of a girl named Barbara was used to derive the compound *or* because it was synthesized on St. Barbara's Day (Snyder, 1996). For the curious minded, St. Barbara's Day is December 4 and she is the patroness of miners (and perhaps barbiturate users, for all we know). She was martyred in C.E. 235 or 238. As far as using urine to synthesize compounds is concerned, the curious minded might

also wonder what that is about. The answer is, as mentioned earlier, that drug companies examine the urine of subjects taking medications, to check for active metabolites of the drug. These active metabolites then provide the blueprint for synthesizing the compound or similar compounds. Barbiturates are derived from a parent compound barbituric acid that was first synthesized in 1864. It was marketed in the United States as Veronal in 1903 and because of loose guidelines governing pharmacy practice became a popular street drug known as "goofballs" or "the poor man's psychoanalysis" (Tone, 2009). There was also a combining of barbiturates with beer into a deadly concoction called a "Wild Geronimo" (Rasmussen, 2009).

Barbiturates have rapidly become the dinosaurs of drugs. As anxiolytics, they have been displaced by benzodiazepines. The effects of barbiturates are quite similar to those of alcohol, and their main advantage is that they are cheap because their patents have expired (although this is not really an advantage because most benzodiazepines are generic as well). Barbiturates differ from each other primarily in terms of how quickly they act and in the intensity and duration of their action. Half-lives range from three minutes to several days. The differences in these properties are the main consideration in deciding which barbiturate to use. The clinical use of these has declined because they are lethal in overdose, the therapeutic dose can be close to a toxic dose, they induce tolerance and dependence, and they interact dangerously with other drugs (Advokat et al., 2014).

Mechanisms of Action

Researchers once believed barbiturates caused a general decrease in neuron excitability throughout the nervous system. They believed the dominant action was to hyperpolarize many types of neurons (recall that "to hyperpolarize" means to increase the probability that a neuron will *not* fire). As with reality, the truth appears more complex than that. In Chapter Two, we wrote that glutamate tends to be a generally excitatory neurotransmitter and that GABA is generally an inhibitory neurotransmitter. Initial evidence in the late 20th century was that barbiturates may act as glutamate antagonists (Zhu, Cottrell, & Kass, 1997), as well as GABA agonists (Tomlin, Jenkins, Lieb, & Franks, 1999). Although there are still aspects of barbiturate action we do not understand, the primary mechanisms seem to be these. First barbiturates act to prolong and potentiate the actions of GABA. At higher doses, they bind to GABAa receptors acting directly on them. When a drug allows an influx of negatively charged ions into the neurons, it hyperpolarizes the neurons, decreasing the probability that they will fire. Barbiturates also block AMPA/kainite receptors (glutamate receptors) decreasing the excitability of neurons (Loscher & Rogawski, 2012). In addition to facilitating the binding of GABA, barbiturates allow the influx of chloride, a negatively charged ion, into the neurons. This effect accounts for the increased toxicity of barbiturates compared to benzodiazepines (Advokat et al., 2014). Table 6.1 summarizes these hypothesized mechanisms of action in barbiturates. You can imagine that combining all these mechanisms of action would have a potent inhibiting effect on the nervous system.

The neurons in the reticular activating system (RAS) are particularly sensitive to barbiturate drugs. The RAS is involved in sleep, and this is one reason why barbiturates have a hypnotic effect. In addition, sites of action include the cerebellar **pyramidal cells** (involved in fine movement), the substantia nigra (motor skills), and the thalamus (processing sensory information). Barbiturate action on these brain structures results in loss of coordination (ataxia), which increases with dosage. In terms of pharmacokinetics, barbiturates are rapidly absorbed and distributed to most body tissues. The ultra-short-acting barbiturates are lipid soluble, cross the blood–brain barrier quickly, and can induce sleep in seconds. As noted, barbiturates differ in their length of action. Table 6.2 lists commonly used barbiturates, duration of effect, and common uses.

Common Side Effects

Common side effects for barbiturates include behavioral depression, sleepiness and particularly disruption of REM sleep, motor and cognitive inhibition similar to those seen with alcohol, ataxia (loss of muscle coordination), and respiratory depression. Barbiturates are contraindicated in people with severe respiratory disease or liver impairment, or who are concomitantly using other CNS depressants. They are clearly contraindicated for people who may be experiencing suicidal ideation, because the drugs are so easy to overdose on.

Tolerance and Dependence

Barbiturates can induce both physical and psychological tolerance and dependence. Physical tolerance occurs via metabolic and cellular mechanisms. Metabolic tolerance is caused by an increase in the enzymes that metabolize barbiturates, resulting in a need for higher and higher doses. Cellular tolerance is the condition of

TABLE 6.1 Hypothesized Mechanisms of Action in Barbiturate Medications

Action	Result
First-messenger binding	Facilitates the actions of to GABA receptors (acts as a GABA agonist) at those receptor sites, decreasing neuronal activity
Antagonism of glutamate	Decreases neuronal activity
Facilitation of chloride conductance into neurons	Further hyperpolarizes neurons

© Cengage Learning®

TABLE 6.2 Examples of Barbiturate Drugs, Their Duration of Effect, and Common Uses

Name	Duration of Effect	Common Uses
Thiopental	15 minutes	Anesthetic
Secobarbital	30 minutes	Hypnotic
Pentobarbital	4 hours	Hypnotic
Phenobarbital	6 hours	Anticonvulsant

© Cengage Learning®

the neurons adapting to the presence of the drug. Physical dependence is usually manifested by sleep difficulties when withdrawing from barbiturates, but withdrawal from high doses may also be accompanied by hallucinations and lethal convulsions (Advokat et al., 2014). The psychological dependence results from the anxiolytic action. Depending on the individual and on the set and setting of barbiturate administration, some people may experience a euphoric response that is also linked to psychological dependence. The phrase "set and setting" refers to the mind-set of the person taking the drug and the physical place and context (setting) where the person is taking a drug.

Barbiturates and Overdose

Researchers estimate that barbiturates have been involved in nearly one third of drug-related deaths, including the deaths of several celebrities (Boston University Medical Center, 2002). Actresses Rachel Roberts and Carol Landis both committed suicide with barbiturates, and actresses Judy Garland and Marilyn Monroe are said to have died of barbiturate overdoses [although signs of overdose are still being disputed in Monroe's case (DiMaggio, 2006)]. Although many of these deaths appear to be intentional suicides, others are accidental or possibly murders. The effects of barbiturates can be so disorienting that a person may take one dose and then a second or third, having forgotten the previous doses. The toxicity of barbiturates is also apparent in their approval as euthanasia agents for lab animals. Partly in response to the toxicity of barbiturates and to their multiple uses, pharmaceutical companies in the early to mid 20th century began to seek out nonbarbiturate alternatives with all the efficacy of barbiturates but without their toxicity and dangers.

The Case of Francis

In the late 1990s, Francis, a 42-year-old unmarried stock broker working in a high-powered investment firm, found himself increasingly tense, edgy, and agitated, which he expressed in an aggressive temper with coworkers and friends. He remembered that his father in his 40s had taken some sort of "-barbital" to help him calm down. He

called his father, who even in his late 70s was very sharp. His father remembered that he had taken pentobarbital/Nembutal and it was very helpful in low doses. He even remembered the physician who had prescribed the medication and encouraged Francis to give him a call, because he was a friend and still in practice. Francis did, and the doctor, simply basing his decision on how helpful pentobarbital had been for his father, prescribed it for Francis. Francis did not seek assistance from therapy or a psychiatrist.

Francis began to use the sedative medication and found it very helpful. In fact, as time went on, he felt he needed more and more to get into the same calm and soothing state. He slept longer and deeper, but found waking up very difficult. Even though his physician warned him, Francis continued to need an ever greater supply of pentobarbital/ Nembutal. Colleagues and friends began to worry about Francis's unpredictable behavior, his barbiturate-induced stupors, and his impaired decision-making skills. Francis continued to deteriorate until one day he didn't come to work, nor did he call. One of his worried colleagues went to his home and found him in a deep sleep. He noticed the bottle of pentobarbital/Nembutal and immediately called for help from an emergency medical technician (EMT). Francis was taken to a nearby emergency clinic, revived and treated, and released with a referral to a psychiatrist who specialized in anxiety disorders. He never followed up.

We have not yet addressed a psychological factor crucial to this case: Sometimes adult children who have overidentified with their parents seek out treatments that were helpful to their parents, even if those treatments are outdated. Francis kept himself outside the appropriate treatment nucleus and found treatment for his anxiety in exactly the same manner that his father had 20 years earlier—and it was not effective.

Nonbarbiturate Alternatives: Mother's Little Helpers

The subtitle of this section, "Mother's Little Helpers," refers to the Rolling Stones song of the same name that was Keith Richards and Mick Jagger's attempt to write a song that highlighted that drug problems are not confined to rock stars. The song is about a woman's use of Valium to relieve the tedium of 1960s suburban life. Although Valium is a benzodiazepine, the benzodiazepine story begins with the search for nonbarbiturate alternatives to anxiolysis. The aim of nonbarbiturate alternatives was to make a drug that was safer but still reduced anxiety. Most of the nonbarbiturate alternatives were extremely similar to barbiturates in everything except molecular structure. Although each one was initially marketed with great fanfare as a safe alternative to barbiturates, most were equally dangerous and many were subsequently withdrawn from the market. The important result of research on nonbarbiturate alternatives is that it led to discovering the benzodiazepines, which we discuss shortly.

Meprobamate

In 1945, Czechoslovakian pharmacologist Frank Berger was attempting to develop antibacterial agents. In his research he stumbled onto a sedating compound that seemed to act like a barbiturate but did not induce sleep as readily. He noted it seemed to induce "tranquilization" without necessarily inducing sleep, and that term was used in marketing the new compound, to present it as different from barbiturates. The compound was marketed as *meprobamate/Miltown* in 1955 (Berger, 1970). Its primary success was that while reducing anxiety, it allowed people to remain awake. Like barbiturates, meprobamate/Miltown produced daytime sedation, relief from anxiety, and sometimes euphoria. Although not as toxic in overdose as barbiturates, meprobamate/Miltown seemed to induce tolerance and dependence to the same degree and appeared more teratogenic than barbiturates. Meprobamate is still prescribed under the trade names Miltown as well as Equanil.

Meprobamate/Miltown also signaled the beginning of the celebrity endorsement for drugs. Famous television star Milton Berle endorsed how well meprobamate/Miltown made him feel and that he took it. His frequent testimonials earned him the nickname "Uncle Miltown" by Time

magazine in February of 1957. According to Andrea Tone's research, in 1956 comedians made as many jokes about Miltown as they did about Elvis Presley (Tone, 2009, p. 65). Carter Wallace pharmaceuticals also commissioned artist Salvadore Dali to create a walk-though art work ("Crisalida") that represented a person's metamorphosis from the evils of nightmares to the divine dreams (all thanks to meprobamate/Miltown of course). By the mid-1960s, more people than ever were taking prescription anxiolytics.

It should be noted that Frank Berger, who developed meprobamate/Miltown in 1950, was a driving force against the popularization of medications in the media as well as the use of drug company representatives (called detail men in the 1950s) to educate physicians about medications. Because of the money he brought to Wallace Laboratories, he had enormous influence. Insisting that good sales pitch would never be good science, he insisted that no detail men be used and that only ads that are factual and educational should be released to doctors. This rule held until Berger retired in 1973 (Tone, 2009).

The Quaalude Years

Glutethimide/Doriden was introduced in 1954, and methaqualone/Quaalude in 1965. Both were hailed as nonbarbiturate alternatives but experience showed otherwise. In the 1970s and 1980s, methaqualone/Quaalude rivaled marijuana and alcohol in level of abuse in the United States. By 1972, the practice of mixing methaqualone/Quaalude with wine ("luding out") was widespread across college campuses. Far from being nonbarbiturate alternatives, glutethimide/Doriden and methaqualone/Quaalude induced tolerance and dependence syndromes, and methaqualone/Quaalude overdose proved even harder to treat than barbiturate overdose. Methaqualone/Quaalude was linked to numerous deaths, so it was banned from the U.S. market in 1984. When taken off the market, methaphalone/Quaalude was placed on federal drug Schedule I, glutethimide/Doriden was placed on Schedule II because of overdose deaths. Federal drug schedules are really a listing on five levels of drugs considered least to most dangerous. Schedule I is for drugs that are illicit and supposedly have no medical uses although, as we will discuss later, this classification is debatable. As with barbiturates, euphoria associated with methaqualone/Quaalude seemed dependent on the set and setting of the drug user. In addition to these drugs, carisaprodal/Soma was introduced and is technically a precursor to meprobemate/Miltown. This is still used as a muscle relaxant in the 21st century. A final note, chloral hydrate/Notec, which was synthesized in the 1800s, is still abused as a CNS depressant which when combined with alcohol is abused as a "date-rape" drug (sometimes called a Mickey Finn) (Julien et al., 2011). These stories point out one pervasive problem in psychopharmacology: once the "genii" is out of the bottle (e.g., a drug is out on the market) it is almost impossible to put it back even though it may be criminalized.

The Case of John

John, a 36-year-old waiter, ex-con, and entrepreneur, was a product of the late 1960s and early 1970s. He believed one should be mellow at all times and should not become stressed under any circumstances. He was in a methadone treatment program to overcome his longstanding addiction to heroin. With the pressures of new marriage and a child, John felt he was becoming tense, agitated, and anxious. He visited his primary care doctor and told him about everything except the methadone treatment. After a brief assessment, the doctor prescribed methaqualone/Quaalude for John. The year was 1979, and given this drug's street reputation John was pleased. He called it his "cool-down script." Soon it seemed to others that the "ludes" became John's substitute for his heroin addiction. He became a quasi-dealer for methaqualone/Quaalude and eventually became dependent on it. He deteriorated gradually but eventually lost his job and family as a result of this abuse/dependence. Fortunately, John had the inner resilience to request in-patient treatment and follow-up therapy to address his serious dependence.

Although scenarios such as John's are not common today, clinicians recognize that in the history of developing pharmaceuticals for mental and emotional disorders some drugs, if abused, are very dangerous.

BENZODIAZEPINES

Benzodiazepines are the prototypic anxiolytic medications. Over the past 40 years, barbiturates were replaced by benzodiazepines, which are less dependence inducing and have less abuse potential. Benzodiazepines are still the leading treatment for anxiety (Dell'osso & Lader, 2013) and currently account for 90% of the anxiolytic market. In the United States, benzodiazepines are among the most prescribed drugs (Baldwin, 2012). In a recent meta-analysis, Dell'osso and Lader (2013) found the most common psychiatric disorders benzodiazepines were prescribed for included GAD, Obsessive Compulsive Disorder, Social Anxiety Disorder, PTSD, Panic Disorder, Agoraphobia (Panic Disorder and Agoraphobia are stand-alone disorders in *DSM-5* as well as ICD-10), Sleep Disorders, Depressive Disorders, Alcohol Withdrawal (as a drug replacement strategy in Addiction Medicine), Delirium, Schizophrenia, and for side effects from neuroleptic medications (like haloperidol/Haldol or chlorpromazine/Thorazine). As you can see, they are used across a broad spectrum of disorders.

Some Anxiolytic History

Ever since Frank Berger had synthesized meprobamate, researchers had tried numerous combinations of muscle relaxers and sedatives to come up with an anxiolytic drug that would not totally sedate a person but would decrease anxiety significantly. Following up on research begun by Berger, Leo Sternbach, a Polish chemist working for Roche Drug Company in New Jersey, first synthesized chlordiazepoxide/Librium and diazepam/Valium. In trying to learn how meprobemate/Miltown acted at a molecular level, Sternbach and his colleague Earl Reeder were synthesizing chemicals called *quinazolines* and screening them for antianxiety properties. He screened 19 out of 20 compounds with no success, and moved on.

As the story goes (Snyder, 1996), a year and a half later, while cleaning his lab, he found the 20th compound and decided to have it screened. It turned out quite active. The final steps of its synthesis completely altered its chemical properties from a quinazoline to what we now call a *benzodiazepine*. The first benzodiazepine chlordiazepoxide/Librium was patented in 1959 and marketed as Librium in 1960. Research continued, and diazepam/Valium was released in 1963. Currently, 15 benzodiazepines (12 of which are commercially available in the United States) are on the market and listed in Table 6.3 (Julien et al., 2011). Benzodiazepines are

TABLE 6.3 Examples of Benzodiazepines

Brand Name	Generic Name	Mean Elimination Half-life (Range in Hours)
Valium	Diazepam	20–50
Librium	Chlordiazepoxide	50–100
Dalmane	Flurazepam	70–160
Paxipam	Halazepam	10–20
Centrax	Prazepam	30–200
Tranxene	Chlorazepate	20–170
Ativan	Lorazepam	10–24
Klonopin	Clonazepam	18–50
Ativan	Lorazepam	15
Dormalin	Quazepam	25–50
ProSom	Estazolam	13–35
Versed	Midazolam	1.5–4.5
Serax	Oxazepam	5–15
Restoril	Temazepam	8–35
Halcion	Triazolam	1.5–5
Xanax	Alprazolam	11–18

effective in reducing anxiety-related symptoms in 70 to 80% of people. This result must be considered in light of the fact that the symptoms vary considerably across time and go into remission with a placebo in 25 to 30% of clients. Benzodiazepines also serve as sedatives, muscle relaxants, intravenous anesthetics, and anticonvulsants.

Varieties of Benzodiazepine Compounds

The five families or subclasses of benzodiazepines vary in potency, duration of action, and amount of time they take to clear out of the body. The older compounds rely more heavily on the liver for metabolism. The more drug metabolism relies on the liver, the more the drug induces moderate metabolic tolerance. The names of the five families of benzodiazepines are related to their chemical properties.

2-Keto Compounds

Of the three types, 2-keto benzodiazepines are the oldest and most lipophilicitous. These compounds are oxidized primarily in the liver, a relatively slow process. As a result, these benzodiazepine compounds have the longest elimination half-lives (up to 60 hours). Many have multiple active metabolites, so it takes the body longer to clear them out of the system. An example of a 2-keto compound is diazepam/Valium. Diazepam/Valium (like many 2-keto compounds) is a prodrug, meaning (as noted earlier) it actually enters the body relatively inactive and becomes active as the body begins to metabolize it. The initial compound (diazepam) acts as a precursor for methyldiazepam, which is further metabolized to oxazepam/Serax. The 2-keto compounds are more likely to induce tolerance and dependence because of their potency. Because people taking these compounds still have active metabolites in their urine, pharmaceutical companies found they could synthesize less-potent compounds that would clear more quickly and still produce the desired anxiolytic effects.

7-Nitro Compounds

7-Nitro compounds (e.g., clonazepam/Klonopin) typically have shorter half-lives but by no means the shortest. As you can see from the overview of clonazepam/Klonopin in Table 6.3, the half-life is 18–30 hours—short compared to chlordiazepoxide/Librium but quite long compared to midazolam/Versed.

3-Hydroxy Compounds

The 3-hydroxy compounds are also metabolized through the liver, as well as through direct joining with endogenous compounds, which brings about more rapid oxidation (negative charging and water solubility) and thus a shorter half-life (10 to 15 hours). Examples of 3-hydroxy compound benzodiazepines include oxazepam/Serax, lorazepam/Ativan, and temazepam/Restoril. Although less likely to induce tolerance and dependence than the 2-keto compounds, these medications still possess these drawbacks and should not be used for long-term treatment of symptoms.

Triazolo Compounds

The triazolo benzodiazepine compounds are very similar to the 3-hydroxy compounds. They are more quickly oxidized, rely less on the liver to metabolize, and leave fewer active metabolites in the system than do the hydroxy compounds. They also have short half-lives (15 hours). An example of a triazolo compound is alprazolam/Xanax. The triazolo compounds have been the most frequently prescribed benzodiazepines for anxiety since the late 20th century (Ballenger, 1995).

Imidazo Compounds

The imidazo compounds (midazolam/Versed) are short-acting benzodiazepines developed by Hofman-LaRoche in the 1970s. They are used for seizures, insomnia, and inducing sedation and amnesia before surgical procedures. As can be seen from the overview of midazolam/Versed in Table 6.3, these compounds can have a half-life as short as 90 minutes. Imidazo compounds are more popular in veterinary medicine because of their water solubility.

Pharmacokinetics

All classes of benzodiazepines are well absorbed. The majority of shorter-acting benzodiazepines have no active metabolites and thus are excreted more quickly. The rest are metabolized first into active metabolites and then are further metabolized, taking longer to excrete from the body. Benzodiazepines come in parenteral and oral formulations.

Mechanisms of Action

Research continues to shed new light on mechanisms of action (summarized in Table 6.4) in the benzodiazepines. First and foremost, benzodiazepines are pure GABA agonists because they facilitate GABA binding at GABA receptors. GABA is 200–1000 times more abundant in the brain (depending on which part of the brain you study) than other neurotransmitters like serotonin and acetylcholine. The GABA binding facilitated by benzodiazepines then leads to opening of chloride channels, which further hyperpolarizes neurons (remember that chloride is a negatively charged ion) (Dell'osso & Lader, 2013; Wafford & Ebert, 2006). There are two types of GABA receptors in the brain; GABAa and GABAb. GABAa is the target of benzodiazepine drugs. GABAb receptors are also implicated in anxiety. Basically when they are stimulated, they exert an inhibitory influence by decreasing the amount of potassium ("K" from the Latin Kalium) in the cell. Recall that potassium is excitatory and decreasing it would tend to inhibit the cells. A good example of a GABAb agonist is Baclofen, which is a derivative of GABA. Baclofen/Kemstro has been shown effective in treating anxiety in PTSD, Panic Disorder, and alcohol withdrawal (Vinkers, Crayn, Olivier, & Groenink, 2010).

TABLE 6.4 Mechanisms of Action of Benzodiazepines

Facilitate the binding of GABA through binding at a benzodiazepine receptor

Facilitate the flow of chloride into the neuron to decrease its excitability

Block stress-induced increases in NE, 5-HT, and DA

© Cengage Learning®

Side Effects

The side effects of benzodiazepines are dose related and are extensions of their therapeutic effects. The side effects include sedation, lethargy, ataxia, motor and cognitive impairments, slurred speech, and amnesia (depending on the benzodiazepine used). Side effects may also include respiratory suppression, depression, and in some cases a paradoxical excitation/agitation (Pies & Rogers, 2005). Note that unlike barbiturates, benzodiazepines do not appear to significantly disrupt REM sleep. They do however decrease REM sleep throughout the night and REM rebound is a possibility if a person is withdrawing from benzodiazepines (Greenblatt, 1991). Although they may disrupt deeper, delta-wave sleep, these effects are experienced as less troublesome than disruption of REM sleep. Specifically focusing on adverse effects Martin et al. (2007) summarized the following problematic side effects:

- Cognitive effects include impairment of learning, psychomotor slowing and anterograde amnesia (inability to create new memories after whatever caused the amnesia).
- Psychomotor effects include some evidence that (depending on the dose) benzodiazepines may impair driving ability.
- There is still controversy over whether benzodiazepines have teratogenic effects. The general consensus is that teratogenicity is low but some studies have illustrated a low correlation between benzodiazepines and cleft palate (see also Howland, 2009a).
- Some studies note subjects have a paradoxical reaction where after taking the drug they experience excitability. The disinhibitory effects (similar to alcohol) could produce increased aggression, anxiety, and hyperactivity.
- Special consideration is required before prescribing these to elderly clients as they are more sensitive to the effects of benzodiazepines. Over sedation can create a pseudodementia and some users may develop hangovers due to their sensitivity.

- Tolerance and dependence are still problems although the studies reviewed indicate that the majority of people taking benzodiazepines take them as prescribed (do not abuse them).

Tolerance and Dependence

Benzodiazepines can induce physical tolerance and both psychological and physical dependence. Although the benzodiazepines do not induce as much metabolic tolerance as barbiturates, they do increase production of hepatic drug-metabolizing enzymes (e.g., cytochrome P450 system). They also cause cellular tolerance in the form of down-regulation or decreased sensitivity of the receptors. Patterns of dependence can develop even at therapeutic dosages if continued over a long-enough period of time. If benzodiazepines are taken short term or infrequently (e.g., p.r.n., for Latin *pro re nata,* "as circumstances require"), clients generally do not develop tolerance to the therapeutic effects of the medications. As we have mentioned, although a great deal of hysteria surrounds the abuse of drugs with reinforcing properties, only a minority of clients on benzodiazepines abuse them. Some researchers have used patient databases to identify things like "doctor shopping," which are highly correlated with abuse (Pradel, Delga, Rouby, Micallef, & Lapeyre-Mestre, 2010). The passage of laws to monitor prescriptions for drugs of abuse allow such patterns to be identified. In Ohio, where we work, there is an Ohio Reporting System (ORS) that is the state prescription monitoring program that is limited to health care professionals and law enforcement. There is still debate about the tension between things like the ORS database and confidentiality (Brushwood, 2003). When tolerance and dependence do occur, early withdrawal signs include insomnia, restlessness, and irritability, and the return of the anxiety for which the medication was being taken in the first place. The compounds with the highest affinity for receptors and the longest half-lives are more likely to induce tolerance and dependence. Most people taking benzodiazepines as prescribed do not develop tolerance but still experience the anxiolytic effects. Also note that any dependence that occurs is not associated with the types of craving experienced by people withdrawing from drugs such as cocaine or heroin. Acute benzodiazepine withdrawal lasts approximately 2–12 months but in some cases can last years at a lower grade level (Higgit, Lader, & Fonagy, 1985; Murphy & Tryer, 1991). It is hard to give concrete estimates because treatment depends on the type of benzodiazepine the client was taking. Short-acting benzodiazepines produce a more intense withdrawal than longer acting ones (Rickels, Schweizer, Case, & Greenblatt, 1991). Strategies to titrate clients down on the dosage of medication often result in craving and return to use so replacement and antagonist strategies are being developed (Hood, Norman, Hince, Meichar, & hulse, 2014).

Overdose Potential

Although the overdose potential of benzodiazepines is less than that of barbiturates, they are still toxic in overdose. Perry, Alexander, and Liskow (2006) report that doses of diazepam as high as 1355 milligrams have been reported without significant toxicity. Apparently when oral benzodiazepines are involved in overdoses, they are often only one of several substances ingested. Intravenous benzodiazepines, in contrast, have a high potential for toxic overdose, but of course the availability of these compounds is restricted. One of the more positive advances in this area is the development of a benzodiazepine antagonist (flumazenil). This compound binds to the same receptors as benzodiazepines but exerts no activity. It also competitively blocks these receptors, so it displaces benzodiazepines that have bound there. This drug can be used to treat a benzodiazepine overdose, although it may have to be injected multiple times, because its half-life is much shorter than the benzodiazepines it is intended to displace. In one 10-year review of benzodiazepine overdoses in adults treated with flumazenil, of the 904 cases treated, 13 developed seizures after administration and one death occurred. Although not a perfect record, many lives were saved with flumazenil that would have been lost without it (Kreshak, Cantrell, Clark, & Tomaszewski, 2012).

The Case of Jennifer

Jennifer, a 26-year-old ballet dancer, began to experience mild panic attacks prior to both rehearsal and performances. She developed powerful resistance to dancing, accompanied by tightness in her chest, rapid breathing, and sweaty palms. Until the recent attacks, Jennifer had been recognized as one of the premier young dancers in the ballet company. Now she could barely perform. The director of the company referred her to a panic/phobia specialist at a local teaching hospital. Jennifer went for an assessment and complete psychological and physical workup. As a result of the evaluation, he recommended group therapy and a regimen of prazepam/Centrax for Jennifer.

Jennifer expressed some reluctance to him about both treatments. She said her Eastern European culture frowned on sharing your deep personal problems in a group of people, and she was worried about the impact of the medication on her functioning and dancing. The psychiatrist addressed both issues (cultural and intrapsychic) with Jennifer and paid very close attention to her feelings about the panic and the treatment. Eventually Jennifer agreed to both treatments.

This treatment protocol was very successful for Jennifer. The prazepam gave her relief from her panic and agitation almost immediately and continued for her 12-week course of treatment. The 10-week group helped Jennifer talk about some of her fears and anxieties about professional dance, provided hope and support, and facilitated her catharsis with some rage issues that had been building in her. She was a willing and positive contributor to the group process, and she benefited from both treatment interventions.

We believe it is important to provide realistic cases about panic and anxiety with some that demonstrate improvement by the client. This well-designed treatment easily could have soured if Jennifer had become dependent on her prazepam and was not able to titrate off of it or if she had become overly dependent on her group.

The Case of Sherry

Sherry is a 46-year-old sexual abuse survivor with three children. She is divorced and works as an administrative assistant for a local accounting firm.

Sherry has been in treatment on and off for over 20 years with several therapists and group approaches. Sherry has tried many medications during this time: TCAs, SSRIs, antipsychotics, antimanics, and more recently, a short-half-life benzodiazepine, alprazolam/Xanax.

Sherry reported that most medications helped her only for brief periods during the course of her treatment. Eventually all were either ineffective or caused her some discomfort because of side effects. Most recently, Sherry felt her therapy was going well. She reported less agitation, fewer intrusive memories of her abuse, almost no nightmares, and far less panic. She also reported improved relationship with her children, as well as comfort and success at work, and she began to date again. Sherry attributed her improvement to her twice-a-week therapy with an eclectic female therapist and her ability to take alprazolam/Xanax p.r.n. when she felt mounting agitation or anxiety in herself. She has learned to self-monitor these feelings, often derived from her chronic sexual abuse by her father between age 5 and 9. Sherry has learned in therapy that at certain times in her daily life she needs the help of alprazolam/Xanax. This occurs about once or twice a week, and Sherry believes the alprazolam/Xanax is very helpful at these times. Sherry has been using alprazolam in this way for three and a half years. She is not dependent on it and uses it very appropriately. Both Sherry and her therapist have begun to talk about what her life would be like without the alprazolam/Xanax.

We believe there are many varied uses for the benzodiazepines and that clients, therapists, and physicians can discover their uses by a careful understanding of the client and/or by applying an integrative framework to the case.

The Case of William

William, a 27-year-old, African American firefighter, developed panic attacks after a very serious fire. Almost immediately, the department physician prescribed diazepam/Valium for him, which he began taking. William did not like the drowsy, stuporous feeling from taking diazepam/Valium. In fact, after a week he became more agitated by the medication.

His panic attacks worsened, and they got so intense that his supervisors recommended him for a disability leave because he could not function at work. William was distraught. He did not feel he had had an opportunity to talk with anyone about his panic and fears, and he detested the impact of the diazepam/Valium on him. Finally, William's minister recommended to him an African American therapist at a neighborhood mental health center.

Certainly many factors influence this case. From the medical model perspective, William was speedily administered diazepam/Valium for his panic, with no evaluation or other considerations. From a psychological perspective, William certainly had a reaction to the medication, and it is possible to hypothesize from the information presented that he also may have been very reluctant to take it. From a cultural perspective, William is an African American, and he seems to trust the counsel of his minister about his mental health concerns first.

In considering the social perspective, a few issues loom. One could assume that diazepam/Valium was the benzodiazepine of choice by the fire department physician. Certainly many social forces are at work in recommending William for leave, including the potential stigma against firefighters with mental health problems. None of William's spheres of experience or vantage points were explored in detail except by his minister.

William had several complex psychological issues that he discussed with his therapist. The first was his personal fear of medication, accompanied by a need to know more about the impact of the diazepam/Valium and its side effects. William was a Gulf War veteran, and elements of the fire that triggered his panic seemed reminiscent of some of the horrors he had witnessed in that war. Over a three-month therapy, William and his therapist worked on these issues, consulted with the staff psychiatrist, and developed a plan for him to return to work. Through some selective cognitive-behavioral therapy, William learned about his repressed fears by experiencing an all-engulfing fire that kills humans, and he gained some control over his panic. After a consult with the staff psychiatrist at the mental health center and a careful evaluation, they agreed to a course of oxazepam/Serax p.r.n. for times when William could not manage his growing panic. Oxazepam/Serax is from a different chemical family and is less potent than diazepam/Valium. The psychiatrist carefully explained all aspects of oxazepam/Serax to William and empowered him to take it only as needed. Together William and his therapist developed a strategy whereby he returned to work at full salary on "light" duty as a dispatcher, with the goal that he could request a return to regular duty. The minister initiated a treatment regimen that addressed William's issues from an integrative perspective, and assisted in his recovery. The diazepam/Valium was not helpful, but the combination of oxazepam/Serax and therapy was.

Review Questions

• What is the primary difference between an anxiolytic and a hypnotic medication?

• What are the known mechanisms of action for barbiturates and benzodiazepines?

• What are the advantages of benzodiazepines over barbiturates including the potential for overdose and addiction?

• How did meprobemate/Miltown become the first "celebrity drug"?

SECTION FOUR: NONBENZODIAZEPINE ALTERNATIVES

Learning Objectives

• Be able to state how nonbenzodiazepines are similar to and dissimilar from benzodiazepines.

• Understand why buspirone may be a good medication for people recovering from drug or alcohol use problems.

• Be able to generally describe two new approaches to anxiolytic medications.

Researchers have made numerous efforts in recent years to synthesize some nonbenzodiazepine compounds that have the therapeutic effects of benzodiazepines without the possibility of tolerance and dependence. We discuss some of these and then newer research directions for anxiolytics.

HYPNOTICS

Hypnotics are classes of drugs that help you to sleep. Although these are structurally dissimilar from benzodiazepines, they bind to the same receptors as benzodiazepines and exert an agonist effect. Zolpidem/Ambien was marketed in 1993 as a short-term hypnotic. It is classified as an imidazopyridine which are GABAa receptor agonists. Chemically, it is structurally different from a benzodiazepine but acts in much the same manner. It binds at the benzodiazepine receptor but tends to induce sleep far more than providing a wakeful anxiolytic effect. Initially, it was believed that zolpidem did not induce tolerance and dependence with continuous use (Harrison & Keating, 2005). However, recent case studies and analyses contradict this (Chapla, Gallucci, Trimzi, & Meier, 2013; Zammit, 2009). There have been many clinical anecdotes about people "sleep binge eating," "sleep driving," and having rages under the influence of zolpidem/Ambien. One of the more famous was that of REM guitarist Peter Buck who was charged with attacking British Airlines staff and ransacking the first class cabin after ingesting zolpidem/Ambien with wine. Buck had no recollection of the incident and was cleared on the grounds that the medication induced the behavior and the amnesia (BBC News, 2002). In 2007, the FDA released a bulletin asking all manufacturers of hypnotics to strengthen their labeling to include the risk of "sleep driving" and similar activities that people may engage in under the influence and then not recall (Zammit, 2009).

Zaleplon/Sonata, like zolpidem/Ambien, is also a pyrazolopyrimidine that is structurally dissimilar to benzodiazepines but functions in much the same manner. Interestingly, this class of drugs is being researched for their possible use as nonsedating anxiolytics. Released in 1999 as a hypnotic agent, Zaleplon/Sonata has a very short half-life (about one hour) and induces sleep fairly effectively.

A modified release of Zaleplon/Sonata was released in 2011 and seems more useful to treat middle-of-the-night awakening (Greenblatt et al., 2011). Zaleplon/Sonata is a selective agonist at the alpha1-3 subunits of the GABAa1 receptor and like zolpidem/Ambien, was first thought to have low abuse potential (Dooley & Plosker, 2000) but later studies found that to not be true (Paparrigo-poulos, Tzavellas, Karaiskos, & Llappas, 2008). At the time of this writing, an aerosol formulation of Zaleplon/Sonata is in development (Avram & Donnelley, 2013).

Eszopiclone/Lunesta is a short-acting hypnotic that belongs to a class of drugs called cyclopyrro-lones. Approved by the FDA in 2004, there were nearly 6 million prescriptions written for the drug by 2011 (Greenblatt et al., 2011). The mechanism of action for eszopiclone/Lunesta is still unknown but thought to result from the drugs interaction with GABA receptor complexes located near benzodiaze-pine receptors (Sonovion Pharmaceuticals, 2012). The results of meta-analyses done to establish the efficacy of nonbenzodiazepines as hypnotics have shown only modest efficacy of eszopiclone/Lunesta in treating insomnia (Huedo-Medina, Kirsch, Middlemas, Klonizakis, & Siriwardena, 2012). There are also adverse effects that can include hallucinations and aggression (Duggal, 2007). Eszopiclone/Lunesta can also cause residual sedation and impair driving ability in the early morning. One of the odder side effects is a bitter, metallic taste in the mouth.

BUSPIRONE: A UNIQUE ANXIOLYTIC

Davis Temple and Michael Eison of Bristol-Myers Company (now Bristol-Myers-Squibb) developed buspirone/BuSpar in 1968. Like so many other psychotropic medications, its development as an anxiolytic was serendipitous. The initial research goal for Temple and Eison was to develop an improved antipsychotic medication. Chemically, buspirone/BuSpar resembles butyrophenone anti-psychotics more than anxiolytics. It is classed as an azapirone, a class of drugs that differ in structure and uses in psychiatry (World Health Organization, 2004). Although ineffective in alleviating symptoms of psychosis, buspirone/BuSpar did seem to have antianxiety properties in humans and antiaggression properties in other primates (Schatzberg, Cole, & DeBattista, 1997). In 1986, the FDA approved it for the market, to treat anxiety. Buspirone/BuSpar is classed as an azaspirodecanedione. Buspirone/BuSpar was the first serotonergic drug that showed efficacy for treating anxiety and more specifically GAD (Mokhber, Azarpazhooh, Khajehdalueee, Velayati, & Hopwood, 2010). More recently, bus-pirone/BuSpar was tried to treat Attention-Deficit Hyperactivity Disorder (ADHD) but methylpheni-date/Ritalin was superior to buspirone/BuSpar in treating symptoms of inattention (Davari-Ashtiani et al., 2010). It is also being investigated for efficacy in treating menopausal syndromes (Shumilov & Touitou, 2010).

Although more will be said about buspirone/BuSpar later, we want to address a small detail that students invariably raise in our seminars. We are frequently asked, "Why is BuSpar (the brand name for buspirone) spelled with an upper case "S"? This is a good question for which we had no answer. Finally one of our students (personal communication, Barry Zabielinski, June 1999) tracked down an answer through numerous phone calls to the manufacturer. The manufacturer said there was no esoteric meaning underlying the odd spelling, but the marketing team wanted the brand name to stand out and so capitalized the first and third letters. Another insight into the culture of the phar-maceutical industry!

Mechanisms of Action

As noted, buspirone/BuSpar is unlike the anxiolytic compounds discussed thus far. Although the vast majority exert CNS depression by acting as GABA agonists, buspirone is actually a serotonin agonist and antagonist. Because serotonin is related to certain types of disinhibition of behavior and such disinhibition is also related to relief from anxi-ety, researchers have hypothesized since the 1980s that serotonin agonists may alleviate anxiety (Feld-man, Meyer, & Quenzer, 1997). Buspirone/BuSpar is believed to act as a serotonin antagonist at the 5-HT1a receptors. These receptors are found in parts of the brain associated with fear and anxiety responses including the amygdala, septum, and hippocampus. Readers may be pondering the phrase "serotonin agonist" and wondering if buspirone would be helpful for depression, given that most of the newer antidepressants discussed in Chapter Five are serotonin agonists. Buspirone/BuSpar also acts on the noradrenergic system to increase the firing of neurons in the locus coeruleus. Recall from Chapter Two that such neuronal firing would seem to increase anxiety, not decrease it. How do we account for the fact that in this case the stimulation of these neurons by buspirone/BuSpar is associated with an anxiolytic action? Perry et al. (2006) explain that buspirone's/Buspar's effects on the hippocampus and raphe nucleus seem to override this stimulation of the locus coeruleus.

Although not as powerful an agonist of serotonin as a drug such as fluoxetine/Prozac, buspirone has shown some efficacy for treating depression (Julien et al., 2011) but is more often used as a supplement to more conventional antidepressants (Stahl, 2000). Researchers have noted that buspirone/BuSpar may interact with dopamine as a weak agonist in some areas of the brain and as a weak antagonist in others. These effects are not considered clinically significant (Perry et al., 2006). Note that buspirone/BuSpar does not interact with GABA or benzodiazepine receptors, so it does not have significant sedative, muscle relaxant, or anticonvulsive properties.

Side Effects and Dosing

The side effects of buspirone/BuSpar primarily include headache, dizziness, GI upset, and sometimes anxiety and tension. Some patients taking buspirone/Buspar have reported restlessness or fidgeting. Patients suffering from Parkinson's disease may show a worsening of their Parkinsonian symptoms on buspirone/BuSpar. Buspirone/BuSpar is not recommended during pregnancy or while breastfeeding, mainly because researchers have no data about its effects on fetuses or neonates. Buspirone/BuSpar is not associated with tolerance, dependence, or overdose. Because the drug is not associated with any euphoric or other reinforcing effects, it is not likely to be abused.

Interestingly, buspirone/BuSpar has a more desirable side-effect profile than the benzodiazepines, because it does not impair motor performance to any great degree and does not show any negative interactions with alcohol. Buspirone/BuSpar may exacerbate psychotic symptoms in patients suffering from psychotic disorders because of its weak dopamine agonism. Given this favorable side effect profile, many clinicians have wondered why it is not more routinely prescribed, because it has FDA approval for GAD. Schatzberg et al. (1997) have recommended buspirone/BuSpar as the drug of choice for treating GAD, Social Anxiety Disorder, Mixed Anxiety, and other combinations of depression, and anxiety in patients with a history of substance abuse.

Schatzberg, Cole, and DeBattista point out that many psychiatrists and physicians assume buspirone/BuSpar is weaker and slower to work than benzodiazepines, particularly in patients who have a history of being treated with benzodiazepines. These authors note that if patients like the more immediate effects of sedation that follow the first dose of benzodiazepines, they may think buspirone/BuSpar is not working, because it lacks this effect. Both benzodiazepines and buspirone/BuSpar take two to four weeks before reaching maximum therapeutic effects, although the patient feels the impact of benzodiazepines within an hour of the first dose. Schatzberg and colleagues did not note that until going generic, buspirone/BuSpar was one of the most expensive anxiolytics on the market (Modell, 1995), which may have accounted for its less frequent use by prescribing professionals. Benzodiazepines can be problematic in that their withdrawal effects may be similar to (or worse than) the anxiety symptoms clients initially began taking them to dispel. Buspirone/BuSpar has little to no tolerance or withdrawal effects and therefore is a more flexible drug to use with such clients (Chodera, Nowakowska, & Bartczak, 1994).

Because buspirone/BuSpar does not interact with GABA receptors at all, it has some advantages over benzodiazepines. These are summarized in Table 6.5.

As Schatzberg et al. (1997) noted, though, buspirone/BuSpar does not give the immediate effect of

TABLE 6.5 Advantages of Buspirone Over Benzodiazepines

Lacks hypnotic, anticonvulsant, and muscle relaxant properties

Much less likely to induce drowsiness and fatigue

Does not impair psychomotor or cognitive function

Shows little potential for abuse and dependence

Does not induce tolerance

Has no synergistic effect with alcohol

Lacks affinity for GABA and benzodiazepine receptors

Is not cross-tolerant with benzodiazepines

© Cengage Learning®

drowsiness that is typically anxiolytic. Many people with anxiety who have taken benzodiazepines may mistake the lack of this effect for evidence that the buspirone/BuSpar is not working. Clients need to be informed that buspirone does work differently from benzodiazepines and should be told not to expect the same sensations when taking buspirone/BuSpar.

Although dosing is done by the prescribing professional, mental health clinicians should be aware some psychiatrists think that many clients go off buspirone/BuSpar because they do not believe it is working and that this in turn is related to not having a high-enough initial dose. Perry et al. (2006) advise that the usual dosage for anxiety is between 15 and 45 mg per day, given b.i.d or t.i.d. (from the Latin *bis in die,* "twice a day"; *ter in die,* "three times a day"), but this can be increased to as high as 60 mg per day.

Tolerance, Dependence, and Overdose

As noted in Table 6.5, some of the strongest arguments in favor of using buspirone/BuSpar are that it does not induce tolerance and dependence. In addition, it is highly unlikely that clients could overdose on buspirone. These effects seem minimal to nonexistent with buspirone, primarily because of its mechanisms of action, which are wholly different from those of

benzodiazepines. A note of caution should be added, though. Recall from Chapter Five that serotonergic antidepressants were once believed to not induce tolerance and dependence and that this has since been disproved (Schatzberg, 1997). Therefore, prescribers may do well to watch for a discontinuation syndrome in longer-term users of buspirone at higher doses.

Before discussing a case, let's summarize when buspirone/BuSpar may be better for a client than a benzodiazepine. Benzodiazepines are effective when used over short periods or infrequently (p.r.n.). Clients with fairly severe anxiety on a chronic basis are good candidates for trying buspirone/BuSpar. A review of studies indicated that buspirone/BuSpar may be helpful in clients with GAD. There are mixed results for buspirone's/BuSpar's effectiveness in other disorders (Perry et al., 2006). Thus clients would likely be taking something every day to treat their anxiety, so buspirone/BuSpar is attractive in that it has not been shown to induce tolerance or dependence. Generally speaking, many clinicians believe buspirone/BuSpar is worth trying with anxious patients who have a history of abusing alcohol or benzodiazepines. Because alcohol is something adults have access to, these clients may drink but the alcohol does not interact negatively with the buspirone. Finally, Stahl (2000) wrote that buspirone/BuSpar may help older clients with anxiety because it is well tolerated and does not seem to have significant pharmacokinetic drug interactions.

The Case of Meredith

Meredith, a 38-year-old married defense attorney, has suffered from extreme anxiety for most of her life. She has a very strong aversion to psychotherapy and believes there should be a pill to cure her worries. Over the years, she has expressed a dislike for the benzodiazepines (she tried several) because they often induced drowsiness and fatigue. She also tried an SSRI, which made her more agitated after two weeks.

At her next appointment, her primary care physician suggested buspirone/BuSpar, a drug that for some reason Meredith had not known about. She began a course of buspirone/BuSpar 15 mg b.i.d. for her anxiety. After about six weeks Meredith noted a decrease in her daily levels of anxiety and reactions to stress. She also felt herself gain some perspective on the professional and personal issues that she often avoided. She recognized that the buspirone/BuSpar did not impair her level of functioning at work, and in fact she found she was more effective now that her anxiety had diminished. She also appreciated that the side-effect profile of buspirone/BuSpar was better than that of the benzodiazepines.

Meredith took the buspirone/BuSpar for over 18 months and then recognized a need for psychotherapy to address conflicts and issues not resolved by the medication, exercise, or stress reduction techniques that she incorporated into her life. In the treatment, Meredith focused on her sense of isolation and unhappiness in her marriage, her surfacing sexual feelings toward women, and the pain from her childhood because her family moved 10 times to different cities. Once in therapy, after seven months Meredith stopped taking the buspirone/BuSpar. Meredith is one of many who discovered buspirone/BuSpar as an effective anxiolytic.

Review Questions

- How are nonbenzodiazepines similar to and dissimilar from benzodiazepines?
- Why is buspirone a good medication for people recovering from drug or alcohol use problems?

SECTION FIVE: NEWER APPROACHES TO ANXIOLYTIC MEDICATIONS

Learning Objectives

- Be able to discuss two new approaches to anxiolytic medications.
- Know the *DSM-5* changes to Anxiety Disorders.

In the first edition of this book, we discussed propranolol/Inderal (a beta-blocker) and clonidine/Catapres (a hypertension medication) as potential anxiolytics. Since then there have been no studies

showing strong statistical significance for those agents in treating anxiety. Interestingly, as many states are decriminalizing marijuana, cannabis, some of the psychoactive elements in cannabis are being explored for anxiolytic properties. Cannabidiol (CBD) is one of 60 active cannabinoids found in cannabis sativa. In animal models, it produces significant anxiolytic properties (Almeida et al., 2013; ElBatsh, Assareh, Marsden, & Kendall, 2012). It has also been found to be useful in reducing anxiety in healthy volunteers suggesting that future trials with people who suffer from Anxiety Disorders are warranted (de Mello Schier et al., 2012). As the United States rethinks its drug laws and drug schedules, it may be that decriminalization brings to the market effective and affordable anxiolytics either through decriminalizing cannabis or designing medications from the active elements of cannabis. In addition to cannabis compounds, we will discuss kava and melatonin as anxiolytics in the chapter on herbaceuticals.

Other newer approaches to anxiolytics include focusing on the corticotropin releasing factor type 1 (CRF1) receptor. The peptide CRF plays an important role in the proper functioning of the stress response system through its action on CRF1 receptors. The hypothesis here is that in anxiety disorders in people with early life trauma, the trauma may have affected the CRF1 receptors via epigenetics. In these cases, it seems in animal models that blocking the CRF1 receptor brings about anxiolysis (Kehne, 2007). Another agent, Etifoxine/Stresam, has been around since the 1960s and seems to exert an anxiolytic effect as a translocator protein that enhances neurosteroidogenesis and as a weak direct GABAa receptor enhancer. The drug, which is also used for axonal regeneration, has been shown to block panic in rodents (Nothdurfter et al., 2011) and shows promise for treating PTSD (Pinna, 2014).

We would be neglectful if we did not add that psychotherapy has been shown to be very effective in the treatment of *DSM-5* Anxiety Disorders (remember these no longer include OCD or PTSD). In a recent meta-analysis, Cuijpers et al. (2013) found that there was no statistical difference between the efficacy of psychotherapy and pharmacotherapy for 27 studies focusing on Anxiety Disorders. This included studies where anxiety was being treated with antidepressant medication and studies where the anxiety was being treated with anxiolytic medications. Even when medication is combined with psychotherapy we tell clients that the medication provides a "chemical window of opportunity" during which it may be easier for the client to begin therapy but which is not necessary to carry on with for years.

The Case of Starr

Starr, a local 18-year-old high school track and field star living in Colorado, began to get very nervous during track season and this worsened before each track meet. Her symptoms were increased heart rate, sweaty palms and feet, and palpitations. As a result of these symptoms, she experienced a loss of concentration and confidence. She discussed this mounting problem with her coach, who suggested she talk to her family physician. The physician prescribed a low dose of buspirone/BuSpar. Starr reported that the medication made her feel tired and sometimes even more nervous. At about this time, Starr experimented with eating cookies with cannabis in them. As a result, she experienced an anxiolytic effect that she said made her feel "normal" again. She continued to use cannabis (eating it in baked goods) on the weekend and as her track team did not have a drug testing requirement her use was never detected. She claims that the anxiolytic effects lasted well into the week. Although Colorado decriminalized cannabis for recreational use she is still underage for legal use of the substance and is hiding this from her parents who think she is still taking buspirone. In Starr's case how would you weight the risks and benefits of what she is doing?

Review Questions

- How might cannabinoids be used to develop anxiolytic medications?
- How would you describe the changes to the Anxiety Disorders in *DSM-5*?

SECTION SIX: SSRI TREATMENT OF ANXIETY

Learning Objectives

- Have a general idea of what the anxiolytic mechanism is for SSRI antidepressants when they reduce anxiety.
- Understand that clients will have a heterogeneous response to SSRIs and it is hard to predict client to client who will benefit from them.

Clinicians have long known that antidepressants also reduce anxiety in clients taking them. Recall from Chapter Five that anxiety and depression are often comorbid; in fact, several opponents of categorical psychiatry feel anxiety and depression may form two ends of a symptom continuum. Researchers as early as Klein (1967) have noted the impact of antidepressants on symptoms of anxiety. Although most antidepressants seem to have some value in treating anxiety (Rickels & Rynn, 2002), some of the more chemically atypical agents such as bupropion do not, and actually may exacerbate anxiety. Clinicians must also allow for the possibility of an unpredicted, idiosyncratic response. Because, as we have pointed out, depression and anxiety are probably overdetermined disorders, it is not possible to state with certainty what the impact of taking any particular medication will be.

Serotonin appears to be implicated in anxiety either through the serotonin transporter (SERT) or the 5-HT1a receptor. The serotonin transporter-linked polymorphic region has two variations; one short and one long (Lee et al., 2005). People with the short form who experience stressful life events are more likely to develop psychological symptoms (Celada, Bortolozzi, & Artigas, 2013). In studies where mice are bred without 5-HT1a receptors, these mice show more susceptibility to anxiety in anxiogenic situations and because all neurotransmitter systems in the brain influence one another, knocking out 5-HT1a receptors in these mice also seems to alter GABA functioning (Celada et al., 2013).

The Case of Katrina

Katrina, a 57-year-old widow who worked as a secretary for a local grocery distributor, developed immobilizing anxiety symptoms about four years after her husband's death. In fact, over time she was diagnosed with Generalized Anxiety Disorder, Panic Disorder with Agoraphobia, and Persistent Depressive Disorder (previously Dysthymia in *DSM-IV*). Katrina staunchly opposed taking any form of medication, even aspirin or vitamins, but she did believe in talk therapy. She said, "I have heard many people on television and radio speak to the benefits that they received from psychotherapy." In fact, after her husband's death Katrina was helped a great deal by a female therapist at the local mental health center. The therapy was supportive and insight-oriented and lasted six months on a weekly basis, with two follow-up sessions.

Katrina had sought help from a cognitive-behavioral male therapist, a feminist therapist, a support group for people suffering with anxiety and phobias, a hypnotherapist, and now a psycho-analytically oriented psychotherapist. None of the approaches appeared helpful in reducing Katrina's symptoms. Four of the five therapists recommended she have a psychiatric evaluation. Katrina refused all recommendations.

In her work with the dynamic therapist, Katrina gradually discovered aspects of her resistance to any changes and great distrust in both modern medicine and medications. Her therapist diligently explored these issues with her and began to teach her about more recent psychopharmacologic developments related to anxiety disorders. Katrina became slightly more open to discuss the possibility of a psychiatric assessment, and she expressed interest in the SSRIs. Eventually Katrina saw a psychiatrist who prescribed paroxetine/Paxil, and she reluctantly agreed to it. After eight weeks, Katrina noticed a lessening of her fears and anxiety. Her panic all but disappeared. She did have several life issues that she continued to address with her therapist, but the SSRI treatment greatly reduced her symptoms of anxiety.

In Katrina's case, by addressing her intrapsychic issues her therapist was able to maximize therapeutic impact by combining a medical model intervention with an intrapsychic intervention. Katrina improved, and 16 months later titrated off the paroxetine/Paxil. We summarize the efficacy of antidepressants later, while discussing pharmacologic interventions by disorder.

The Case of Nicole

Nicole, a 35-year-old single woman, sought, from her psychiatrist, relief for a long-standing depression with features of anxiety. At the time of referral, Nicole was experiencing great difficulty sleeping, constant worry, mild panic, and a constant depressive affect (mood). Her physician prescribed paroxetine/Paxil at 10 mg and told her to increase to 20 mg at the end of the first week. Nicole noticed during the first week that she was more agitated and slept even less. Because her doctor had not warned her about these possible side effects, she increased the dosage at the end of the week to 20 mg. By the second day after the increase, Nicole was experiencing total panic and terror. At times she could not breathe, and in her hypervigilant state she could barely speak to her neighbor, who wisely called the EMT service. Nicole was taken to the emergency room at the local hospital, where she was prescribed a mild tranquilizer. The attending physician called her psychiatrist, and they agreed that Nicole was experiencing an SSRI-induced panic attack and she was taken off the paroxetine/Paxil. When Nicole recovered from her panic attack, her psychiatrist prescribed alprazolam/Xanax p.r.n. and encouraged her to seek therapy. He also indicated that if she still felt depressed in about two weeks, he would try a different class of antidepressant.

The Case of Rhonda

Rhonda was a 38-year-old divorced mother who had been in weekly therapy about a year. Near the end of the first year of her work, Rhonda became very depressed and requested a psychiatric consult. The psychiatrist recommended sertraline/Zoloft, a new SSRI that had just received FDA approval. Rhonda began the sertraline/Zoloft at 100 mg and soon was taking 200 mg per day. She reported feeling better but noticed she was losing large amounts of her beautiful hair daily, which she linked directly to the sertraline/Zoloft. Her therapist recommended she talk to the psychiatrist, who checked the side effects and found nothing about hair loss. However, she decreased the sertraline/Zoloft for Rhonda to 100 mg daily and the hair loss ceased.

I (Rak) also noticed this hair loss in two other female clients who took sertraline/Zoloft at 200 mg. I reported this to a middle manager at Pfizer, who indicated he would look into the situation, but I never received a further response. Sertraline/Zoloft now is seldom prescribed at 200 mg per day.

Review Questions

- What is the therapeutic mechanism of action of SSRI antidepressants when they work for anxiety?
- What would you tell a client who was starting an SSRI medication regimen hoping to alleviate anxiety?

SECTION SEVEN: ANXIOLYTIC THERAPY BY DIAGNOSIS

Learning Objective

- Know the general treatment approaches for each diagnosis.

As stated earlier, in this section we summarize recommended therapies for anxiety symptoms by diagnosis. We summarize the pharmacologic interventions and also touch on the psychological interventions. As we have stated from the beginning, an integrative view of the topic demands that these interventions be held in mind so that the reader does not unwittingly become mesmerized by the word magic of pharmacologic interventions. We cover GAD, Panic Disorder, Agoraphobia, and Social Anxiety Disorder and Specific Phobia. Even though PTSD is no longer considered an Anxiety Disorder proper (it has its own category in *DSM-5*), we will touch on anxiolytic treatment of that disorder.

Generalized Anxiety Disorder

GAD is considered the basic anxiety disorder, because it is characterized by intense, unfocused anxiety. *DSM* criteria for this classification require excessive anxiety and apprehensive expectation more often than not for at least six months before the diagnosis is made. Adults must manifest three of the symptoms in the symptom list; children, only one. In children this used to be called Overanxious Disorder of Childhood and has a high comorbidity with ADHD and Major Depressive Disorder as well as other anxiety disorders. The focus of the intense anxiety varies developmentally. Adults tend to worry about minor daily life events, whereas children tend to worry about athletic, academic, or social competence. It is crucial that clinicians explore the worry of children and adults for other emotions such as sadness, loss, rage, and other symptoms that reflect the aspects of "worry." People with GAD are vigilant regarding potential threats in the environment but do not have particular images of threats. These people actually show less physiological responsiveness (heart rate, blood pressure, respiration) to anxiety-provoking stimuli than do people with other anxiety disorders. For this reason people with this disorder have been called "autonomic restrictors." This may be explained as follows.

Recall that the autonomic nervous system regulates involuntary sympathetic and parasympathetic functions. Autonomic restriction has been linked to intense thought processes or worry that never develops to specific, consistent images of potential problems. The images would elicit more negative emotions. Their style keeps such autonomic restrictors from feeling these potentially negative emotions but also from working through their anxiety in therapy (Barlow & Durand, 2002).

Pharmacological Treatments for GAD

GAD is considered a challenging disorder to treat. Although benzodiazepines have been a staple of treatment until recently, they do not alleviate all symptoms and are significantly correlated with increased costs due to things like falls and accidents while under the influence of the drugs (particularly in elderly clients) (Berger, Edelsberg, Treglia, Alvir, & Oster, 2012). Also, benzodiazepines carry the risk of tolerance and dependence whereas drugs like SSRIs and buspirone do not and have similar efficacy (Bandelow et al., 2013; Mokhber et al., 2010). Although most benzodiazepine users do not abuse their medication, some question whether it is worth the risk to use them long-term (Baldwin, 2012). Many researchers (such as Schatzberg, Cole, & DeBattista, 2010) thus believe buspirone is the ideal medication of first choice for GAD. As noted, Bandelow and colleagues (2013) found that buspirone/BuSpar compared favorably with the benzodiazepines. Unlike benzodiazepines, buspirone/BuSpar cannot be used on a p.r.n. basis. Like the SSRI antidepressants, it seems to require daily dosing to exert its effects. Buspirone/BuSpar may also take two to four weeks for the full therapeutic benefit to be achieved. Recent research on the SNRI antidepressants (e.g., Effexor/venlafaxine; Prestiq/desvenlafaxine) are as useful for GAD as SSRIs and buspirone/BuSpar. One persisting problem is that many clients discontinue treatment with SSRIs and SNRIs because of the side-effect profile and many state a preference for benzodiazepines (Table 6.6). There are a great number of unmet needs in the population of people suffering GAD and hopefully some of the newer anxiolytics in development will provide relief with fewer side effects (Chollet, Saragoussi, Clay, & Francois, 2013).

Psychological Treatments for GAD

Regardless of the pharmacotherapy used when treating GAD, it is important to combine medication with some form of counseling or psychotherapy. The long-term nature of the condition and the lack of long-term efficacy studies both support supplementing medication with a psychosocial intervention.

TABLE 6.6 Psychotropic Medications That Combine With SSRIs to Treat OCD

SSRI and Buspirone
SSRI and Trazodone
SSRI and Lithium
SSRI and Benzodiazepine
SSRI and Zolpidem
SSRI and typical antipsychotic
SSRI and atypical antipsychotic

© Cengage Learning®

In reviewing the treatment literature, Bandelow et al. (2013) found that variations of cognitive-behavioral therapy (CBT) consistently show superiority over no treatment at all. These authors also note that the dropout rates in psychosocial treatment trials have been low and that the combination of CBT with progressive relaxation and/or exposure seems to have the best possibility of long-lasting change.

This recommendation is not intended to rule out other types of therapy such as psychodynamic therapy but, as is often the case, there are more studies of CBT and behavior therapy, partly because they are easier to study with operationalized variables. Psychodynamic therapy for GAD aims to help clients gain awareness of unconscious conflicts and underlying anxiety-provoking drives, recognize the environmental cues that activate anxiety, and understand the origins of anxiety in early life experience. Three questions typically underlie this treatment:

1. What inner drive is the client afraid of?
2. What consequences of overt behavioral expression of the drive does the client fear?
3. What psychological and behavioral measures does the client take to control the drive?

In seeking to answer these three questions, the clinician also confronts various perplexing symptoms expressed by the client, and defense mechanisms that initially hinder the therapy. Clients considered good candidates for insight-oriented therapy are those willing to engage in (and capable of) introspection and to reflect on that introspection, those who can tolerate the expression of painful psychological material, and those who can form meaningful relationships. It is important that these clients be motivated to aim for psychological change and growth as opposed to just symptom relief.

Panic Disorder

As noted earlier, in *DSM-5* and *ICD-10* (and the forthcoming ICD-11) Panic Disorder is uncoupled from Agoraphobia. Panic Disorder is typically treated in two phases. The first is aimed at reducing the frequency and/or intensity of the panic attacks. This phase is frequently accomplished pharmacologically. The second phase involves administering the psychosocial treatment in the hope of decreasing the dysfunctional responses that become panic attacks (American Psychiatric Association, 2000a). Interestingly, numerous drugs that affect different parts of the central nervous system all seem effective in reducing panic attacks (Speigel, Wiegel, Baker, & Greene, 2000). For the first phase of treatment, high-potency benzodiazepines are very effective, work quickly, and reduce anticipatory anxiety. Over 60 trials on benzodiazepines have been made on subjects with Panic Disorder, and the data suggest that these clients continue to improve up to six months, at which point gains stabilize. These medications can be prescribed p.r.n., so clients need only take the dose when they feel in imminent danger of a panic attack. Obviously, the more frequently clients use any benzodiazepine, the more likely the problem of tolerance and dependence.

Numerous trials have been conducted to assess the efficacy of antidepressants for the treatment of Panic Disorder. Summarizing literature across 15 years, Perry et al. (2006) noted that approximately 67% of subjects could be said to respond to treatment with tricyclic antidepressants and MAO inhibitors. "Response" was defined as anywhere from an 80% reduction in panic attacks to complete remission. SSRI medications generally showed a 60% response rate, where response was defined as a decrease in panic severity. Several SSRI compounds have on-label FDA approval for treatment of Panic Disorder, including sertraline/Zoloft and paroxetine/Paxil.

Several psychosocial interventions are highly successful for the second phase of Panic Disorder treatment, and from an integrative perspective we would be remiss if we omitted mention of these. Traditionally, treatment centered on gradual exposure to feared situations (in cases where agoraphobia was a component) and anxiety-coping mechanisms such as relaxation. A recent study estimated costs associated with the treatment of Panic Disorder. Costs included the cost of the treatment as well as indirect costs like lost productivity. Cognitive behavior therapy had lower overall costs associated with it than cognitive therapy plus SSRIs and SSRIs alone (van Apeldoorn et al., 2014). With the changes in how we approach health care in the United States especially, studies like this are important to sort out what is going to do the most good and provide the best value.

Social Anxiety Disorder and Specific Phobias

Because *DSM-5* has just this year (at time of this writing) uncoupled Agoraphobia from Panic Disorder, we have no treatment guidelines proper for Agoraphobia. For our purposes, think of it as similar to the approaches we will discuss for treating Social Anxiety Disorder and Specific Phobias. Although Social Anxiety Disorder (previously Social Phobia in *DSM-IV*) and Specific Phobias may vary in the focus of the fear, they share several similarities that allow us to group them together in this section. They both seem to be an outgrowth of an evolutionary mechanism that prepared humans to flee dangerous situations, and they are both problematic in that the flight response is out of proportion to the actual danger posed by the situation. In the past few decades, we have seen a rise in studies on the physiological underpinnings of these disorders including genes, neurotransmitters, the hypothalamic-pituitary-adrenal (HPA) axis, and epigenetic triggers in the environment (Dalrymple, 2012; Gimenez et al., 2014; Lueken et al., 2013). It should also be noted that some (Dalrymple, 2012) wonder if Avoidant Personality Disorder is not really the same disorder or perhaps two disorders on the same spectrum. Again, these are all disorders for which several effective psychological interventions are available and we will touch on those briefly.

Social Anxiety Disorder

Having a Social Anxiety Disorder (SAD) is being extremely and painfully shy. Just as it can be hard to differentiate SAD from Avoidant Personality Disorder, it can be hard to differentiate SAD from shyness as well. It manifests as a marked or persistent fear of one or more social or performance situations in which the person is exposed to unfamiliar people or possible scrutiny. The main fear is that the person fears acting in a way that will be humiliating or embarrassing to him- or herself. Although social anxiety disorder treatments are newer, group therapy involving role-play and rehearsal of the feared situation both seem effective (Turk, Heimberg, & Hope, 2001). As with specific phobias, exposure to the anxiety-provoking situation is an important part of the treatment. Also as with specific phobias cognitive behavioral treatments are very efficacious in treating SAD (Schreiber, Heimlich, Schweitzer, & Stangier, 2013; Willutzki, Teismann, & Schulte, 2012). There have also been studies supporting a newer variation of cognitive therapy called mindfulness-cognitive behavior therapy in treating anxiety disorders (Kim et al., 2013).

Given that psychological treatments are so effective, what is the rationale for prescribing medications? Again, the answer is that often the medications can give clients a window of opportunity (of relief from symptoms) that then allows them to confront their issues in counseling and make the necessary changes. This is particularly important for clients who are so limited by their symptoms that they cannot fulfill important obligations. Research studies support that pharmacotherapy is effective in reducing the severity of symptoms in the short term but cognitive therapies are more effective reducing symptoms and changing avoidance behaviors in the long term (Dalrymple, 2012). SAD in particular has received a great deal

of attention over the past five years from the makers of SSRI medications. Several SSRI medications have received FDA approval for treating SAD, including Paxil/paroxetine and Zoloft/sertraline. SNRI agents like Effexor/venlafaxine are also used to treat SAD. Two-thirds also respond to MAO inhibitors and the tricyclic clomipramine/Anafranil but, as noted in Chapter Five, the SSRI side effects are less difficult to manage than those from MAO inhibitors or TCAs.

Review Question

- What are the first-line choices of medication for Generalized Anxiety Disorder, Panic Disorder, Social Anxiety Disorder and Specific Phobia?

SECTION EIGHT: FOCUS ON PSYCHOLOGICAL, CULTURAL, AND SOCIAL ISSUES

Learning Objectives

- Think about the extent to which culture and the pace of Western societies contributes to anxiety.
- Consider how popular media could be used more effectively to educate lay people about what counseling and psychotherapy can offer.

PSYCHOLOGICAL ISSUES

Anxiety Disorders: Myth or Reality

The debate about the nature and source of anxiety continues. Is anxiety a product of an overwhelming state of tension (Barlow & Durand, 2002), a sign of psychological conflict (Freud, 1925), or both (Gabbard, 1994)? If we examine anxiety from a psychological perspective it is possible to arrive at one point of agreement: Clinicians who treat clients suffering from anxiety disorders understand that these clients have cognitive, affective, and interpersonal struggles that are entwined in their anxiety symptoms. No medication is going to address all of these struggles, which is where psychotherapy enters the picture. In every case we reviewed and shared here, counseling played a crucial role in the client's recovery. When talking with clients, we find that psychological issues range from anxiety resulting from situational stress to severe PTSD. Each disorder potentially encompasses underlying issues and conflicts that cannot be ameliorated by medication alone.

I (Rak, the second author of this book) have trained to become a psychoanalyst. This training involved four to five days a week treatment focused on psychological conflicts and is designed to prepare one to be a psychodynamic therapist. (A psychoanalyst provides four- to five-day-a-week treatment focused on the psychological conflicts of the patient who usually lies on a couch. Intensive psychotherapy is one- or two-day-a-week counseling that is eclectic in nature, and psychodynamic psychotherapy is counseling or therapy that is guided by psychoanalytic principles, but is not an analysis.) My view of profound anxiety resonates with that of some clinicians in the field. I believe serious anxiety can be understood only in the context of the transference in intensive psychotherapy where counselor and client search beyond the symptoms for underlying beliefs, feelings, and attitudes, conscious or unconscious. These conflicts and wishes repeatedly trigger the client's anxiety and must be integrated into the client's concept of self before any long-lasting relief can be accomplished. Taking a broader perspective, Barber and Luborsky (1991) have argued that specific anxiety disorders required varied treatments with different clients. Psychodynamic psychotherapy may be the treatment of choice for those clients who are psychology minded and willing to invest the time to explore their anxiety. Clients who want more direction from their mental health clinician may do better with a cognitive behavioral approach. Other clients whose anxiety is directly tied to a felt need to make difficult but necessary choices (such as whether to keep a safe but boring job or risk an exciting but less secure job) will likely benefit from an existential approach to

therapy. As we have discussed throughout the chapter, anxiolytics have a range of effectiveness with symptoms of anxiety disorders, but they may or may not be the total solution for the client's problem. Understanding the intrapsychic elements of each client's anxiety guides us in selecting an appropriate counseling intervention to complement whatever medication regimen they may be on.

Gabbard (1994) concluded that the treatment of anxiety disorders must begin with careful and thorough psychodynamic evaluation. In making this evaluation the therapist should be aware that the symptoms may only be the proverbial "tip of the iceberg" for the client. The mental health professional needs to assess the nature of the client's underlying fears, capacity to tolerate treatment that explores those fears, worry that the anxiety is destroying the self, and the client's relationship with important others or lack thereof. After an assessment and evaluation, the professional considers the range of treatments for anxiety, including brief therapies, cognitive-behavioral therapy, existential and humanistic therapies, psychodynamic theory, psychoanalysis, and long-term expressive-supportive psychotherapy. In cases such as those presented in this chapter, the professional must consider which approach may be most helpful to each client.

More recently a unified protocol for the transdiagnostic psychodynamic treatment of anxiety disorders was developed that draws from empirically supported treatment principles. These principles are: (1) socializing the client for therapy, (2) motivating the client and setting goals, (3) establishing the helping alliance (relationship), (4) identifying a core conflict thought to underlie the anxiety, (5) focusing on the warding-off, wish/affect, (6) modifying internalized object relations, (7) understanding and modifying defenses and avoidance, (8) modifying sense of self, and (9) ending therapy and setting up relapse prevention (Leichsenring & Slazer, 2013). In addition, short-term psychodynamic therapies have been shown to be effective for anxiety disorders (Bressi, Procellana, Marinaccio, Nocito, & Magri, 2010).

We believe the complex issues that arise in clients contribute to the complexity and mystery of anxiety disorders. Some clients maintain their high levels of anxiety in order to live out their lives in a compromised fashion. In one example provided earlier, I (Ingersoll) worked with a client who chose not to pursue the exciting job opportunities and stay in the safe but boring job. Although his anxiety decreased significantly after making his choice, he was then beset by bouts of depression. From an existential perspective the client had traded freedom for comfort and this was signaled by the depression. He re-entered treatment five years later when another opportunity to take a more exciting but less secure job presented itself and his anxiety reappeared. Some clients can find relief only from supportive counseling, whereas others require compulsive behaviors to distract them from their suffering. This strategy of seeking relief through distraction is one of the prominent motivations driving the consumer culture in the United States. From an existential perspective, the consumer culture provides distractions from the anxiety that comes when one is aware of the freedom one has and the consequences of trading it for security. For the client with the job dilemma, his current (but boring) job paid well and he was able to afford expensive pleasures (like vacations), but the relief these pleasures provided was temporary. It is most beneficial to clients not to oversell medications as a definitive treatment, but to help them understand that anxiety is an important sign of issues to explore in counseling or psychotherapy.

Cultural Issues

The pressures of American culture in general are enormous external contributors to anxiety especially in the post-9/11 era. The continued struggle for civil rights for all Americans, psychological responses to war, the horror of the terrorist attacks, the corruption of many working the stock market, an increasing mistrust of government, the increased turmoil and violence of our youth, and the dismantling and or transformation of traditional values all trigger anxiety reactions. Our culture is infused with paradigms of violence, revenge, conquest,

and dominance. The influence of culture is a powerful variable in understanding the rise of anxiety disorders. The impact of these external stressors varies with the psychological makeup of each client.

The American tendency, particularly in the consumer culture and mass media, to glorify violence continues to make major contributions to stress and anxiety in Americans, although evolutionary dynamics related to reproduction can always account for a certain percentage of violence (fighting for the best mate to reproduce with) (Wright, 1994). Violence is also reinforced by unrealistic portrayals in almost all mass media (Bushman & Anderson, 2001). The question remaining is the extent to which this contributes to anxiety, but it is certainly a useful working hypothesis in that being the target of or viewing aggression increases anxiety.

Tseng (2001) further elaborated on the external cultural pressures of anxiety by exploring its cross-cultural dimensions. He addressed the issues of how different cultures reveal their emotions. Some do so with gestures and facial expressions, others with words, still others through the body. Some cultures have highly elaborate cultural ways of expressing emotions through "somato organ language," incorporating into the language words or terms that represent somatic pain without a complete awareness of its psychological origins for affective expressions. For instance, *fa pi qi* ("lost spleen spirit," meaning losing one's temper) and *gan fuo da* ("elevated liver fire," meaning emotionally irritated) in Chinese are equivalent to organ language expressions used in English, such as "butterflies in stomach" or "a pain in the neck" (p. 292).

Tseng further elaborated that it is difficult for patients to present a clear picture of their distress if they are from a culture where the condition is viewed as a holistic experience rather than as a series of specific symptoms from the descriptive psychiatry perspective. Tseng further discussed specific culture-related syndromes such as Dhat syndrome in India (fear that excessive semen loss will result in illness) and Malignant Anxiety syndrome in Africa (intense feelings of fear and anger from extreme cultural disruption that lead to homicidal feelings). From the cultural perspective, it is clear that anxiety disorders are subject to a variety of cultural influences and the cultural "language of expression" of the client. Therapists need to be alert to these both subtle and overt manifestations of anxiety from clients. Most therapists in practice today, especially in urban settings, encounter increased numbers of clients from diverse cultural backgrounds.

Social Issues

From the perspective of third-party payers (managed care), the most appropriate treatment for a client (counseling) may be cost-effective but is not always valued in Western culture. In the United States, pharmaceutical companies have two lobbyists for every member of senate and congress. This is an enormous amount of lobbying power that drives legislators to favor giving money via Medicaid and Medicare to pharmaceutical interventions rather than talk therapy interventions. Think of it this way: when was the last time you saw a commercial for counseling? This further deepens the dilemma we have noted so often throughout the book: that psychotropic drugs alleviate many symptoms of anxiety disorders, even though we do not fully understand the pharmacokinetics and the pharmacodynamics of the drugs, yet they do not necessarily lead to deep and maintained gains for all clients. The pressures from managed care to treat most, if not all, anxiety disorders with psychotropics and brief models of counseling are enormous. It is crucial that we become and remain alert to clients whom these strategies do not help.

As detailed in other chapters, the role and influence of the pharmaceutical companies cannot be overlooked in treating anxiety disorders. The surge in the uses of SSRIs for anxiety conditions indicates the drive of these companies to influence the psychiatric treatment market with an arsenal of psychotropics. This occurs in the context of growing confusion, as discussed in earlier chapters, about distinctions between anxiety and depressive disorders and about their comorbidity.

Review Questions

- To what extent do you think the stress of daily life contributes to Anxiety Disorders?
- What would a commercial for counseling and psychotherapy look like?

SUMMARY

In this chapter, we have provided an overview of both the psychotropics and the therapeutic interventions used with anxiety disorders. In one sense you, the reader, may feel optimistic about both interventions. We caution that many therapists are surprised to discover, after what they feel were successful courses of psychotherapy, that their clients have developed new or altered symptoms and that their suffering has increased.

Medications to treat anxiety are among the most prescribed psychotropic medications in Western societies. Anxiolytic medications have evolved a great deal from the barbiturates and similar central nervous system depressants to the point where an array of medications may be used to treat client anxiety depending on the diagnosis. Although researchers have made strides in the pharmacologic treatment of anxiety, we believe that therapists must approach this work with wisdom and humility. For all we know about the psychotropic medications that can be used for anxiety disorders, we still encounter the powerful and insidious nature of human anxiety that has psychological, cultural, and social dynamics. We are learning that beneath the anxiety lie some of the fundamental struggles of human existence, struggles that cannot be altered easily, if at all.

CHAPTER SEVEN

Antipsychotic Medications
The Evolution of Treatment

Many readers may begin this chapter with some familiarity with antipsychotic medications. Others may think antipsychotic medications or the research related to them has not affected their lives. These latter readers may be wrong. Have you ever taken a prescription antihistamine such as Seldane or Allegra? Perhaps got over motion sickness with a compound that included promethazine? If so, your life has been affected by research into antipsychotics. As with so many other areas of research in psychotropic medication, antipsychotics and theories about their use have been developed through combined scientific effort, clinical research, market-driven agendas, and serendipity. Let's look at some history to introduce this topic. The primary source for the following is Healy (2002).

THE CURRENT IMPACT OF ANTIPSYCHOTICS

In a video designed for psychiatrists (Novartis Pharmaceuticals, 1998), a young man suffering from treatment-resistant schizophrenia is shown in an inpatient setting. Although his psychotic symptoms are temporarily under control, he is so incapacitated by medication side effects that he can barely walk across a small room. His movements are jerky contractions of muscle groups that he can hardly control. Anyone who has treated clients taking conventional antipsychotic medications knows that this young man is living a worst-case scenario in which the treatment is worse than the disorder

being treated. The video progresses, showing the young man at monthly intervals as he is slowly weaned off the medications causing the side effects, and gradually titrated onto a new medication (clozapine). With each passing month, we see that the young man's psychotic symptoms remain under control but that he is gradually regaining control of his body. In the final video frame, we see the same young man enjoying a game of basketball and apparently having no problems with movement or symptoms of psychosis.

This was one of the first videos promoting what we describe later as an atypical antipsychotic, and at the time of their development most of us believed that clozapine and drugs modeled after its molecular structure launched another revolution in psychopharmacology. It was hoped that (as was hoped in the SSRI revolution in antidepressants) the new antipsychotics would change the way psychotic disorders are treated as well as the quality of life that patients can expect during treatment. As we will see, although newer agents do work better for some but not all people with schizophrenia, the newer agents have problematic side effects similar in impact (if different in quality) as the older agents. Also, the claims that newer medications worked better than the older ones now seem to be untrue (Jones et al., 2006; Lieberman et al., 2005).

This chapter is divided into seven sections. The first is an overview of schizophrenia and the spectrum of symptoms being treated. The second focuses on theories of neuroleptic antipsychotic action. Section Three is an overview of the side effects of first generation, neuroleptic medications. Section Four is an introduction to the first atypical antipsychotic, clozapine/Clozaril. Section Five covers the rest of the drugs modeled on clozapine called serotonin-dopamine antagonists. Section Six looks at newer compounds and theories of how to create more effective antipsychotics. The final section looks at psychological, cultural, and social issues relevant to antipsychotic medications.

SECTION ONE: SCHIZOPHRENIA

Learning Objectives

- Have a sense of the complexity of theories of etiology for schizophrenia.
- Be able to discuss why the name "schizophrenia" is not terribly useful.
- Understand positive symptoms, primary negative symptoms and secondary negative symptoms.

Schizophrenia "... definitely involves genetic factors the precise genes and gene-environment interactions are yet to be clarified" (Keshavan, Tandon, & Nasrallah, 2013, p. 4). As Stober et al. (2009) concluded, "the phenotypic complexity, together with the multifarious nature of the 'group' of 'schizophrenic psychoses' limits our ability to form a simple and logical biologically based hypothesis of the disease group" (p. 129). Schizophrenia shares many heritable factors with Bipolar I disorder, suggesting there may be an underlying genetic basis for both disorders that runs on a continuum. At the more severe end of the continuum, the person is afflicted with schizophrenia; at the less severe end (if it is fair to use that phrase in regard to any of these disorders), the person is afflicted with Bipolar I Disorder (McIntosh et al., 2006). Ultimately, though, schizophrenia is a disorder with a heterogeneous presentation involving multiple genes that may each have relatively small effects. Etiological factors also include differences in brain structures (Hartberg et al., 2011), white matter or the glial cells in the brain (Frances, 2013), and neurochemical variables

(although nothing as simple as dopamine imbalance as was believed in the mid to late 20th century). Prevalence among adults is thought to be between 1 and 1.5% of the adult population (American Psychiatric Association, 2013). Keshavan (2013) has advocated eliminating the name "Schizophrenia" because it conveys an inaccurate characterization of the symptoms, has acquired a negative connotation (like "lunacy"), and belies what we are learning neurobiologically about the disorder. Keshavan et al. (2013) have suggested an acronym "CONCORD," which stands for "youth onset conative, cognitive and reality distortion" (p. 1). As Keshavan notes, we do not take lightly renaming a disorder but the label of "schizophrenia" seems to be obsolete.

One of the most distressing aspects of schizophrenia is that it seems to be correlated with premature death. Even more disturbing is that we still have to discern if this is related to the disorder, the medications people with the disorder take, or both. Joukamaa and colleagues (2006) did a 17-year follow up of 99 people with schizophrenia. Of the 99, 39 died in that 17 years. Adjusted for age and sex and other diseases, the risk for premature death was significantly higher than expected. The deaths also increased as the number of neuroleptics taken increased. Even though we have agents to treat the symptoms of schizophrenia, as noted above, they do not really differ much from one another in general effectiveness and what is needed is that we understand the mechanisms underlying the illness and its progression. Until we can accomplish this, we will remain stuck in symptom management (Kane & Correll, 2010).

The Spectrum of Symptoms in Schizophrenia

In *DSM-5* (APA, 2013), the category Schizophrenia and Other Psychotic Disorders of *DSM-IV* has been changed to Schizophrenia Spectrum and Other Psychotic Disorders. Many aspects of the *DSM-5* were designed to reflect the International Classification of Mental and Behavioural Disorders (ICD-10) (WHO, 1992), which includes Schizotypal

Personality Disorder under the Schizophrenia heading. So in *DSM-5,* the spectrum of disorders also contains a spectrum of symptoms. The spectrum of symptoms in schizophrenia includes both positive and negative symptoms. This concept derives from the work of the 19th-century neurologist John Hughlings Jackson. **Positive symptoms** of schizophrenia are things the client experiences but likely should *not* be experiencing, such as **hallucinations**, **illusions**, **delusions**, and **paranoia**. Clients with positive symptoms usually lack insight into the sense outsiders have that these experiences are not real or normal and frequently cannot distinguish between them and the consensual reality shared by most others.

Negative symptoms of schizophrenia are deficits in the client's functioning expressed as things like **anhedonia** (lack of pleasure in life), isolation, withdrawal, flat or restricted affect, and reduced motivation. These negative symptoms severely affect quality of life for afflicted clients and can be exacerbated by certain antipsychotic medications clients are given to control the positive symptoms. In addition to the positive and negative symptoms, clients suffering from schizophrenia experience conceptual disorganization, which used to be called "**thought disorder**." This disorganization can range from concrete thinking to severe **loose associations** and **word salad**. These symptoms may also severely reduce clients' quality of life (Thaker & Tamminga, 2001). From an integrative perspective, all these symptoms need to be addressed. Although pharmacological interventions are the first line of treatment for schizophrenia, it is also important to include psychosocial and educational components (American Psychiatric Association, 2000a).

Gelman (1999) divides the history of medicating psychotic disorders into four periods. The first period encompasses the 1950s and 1960s and began with the appearance of chlorpromazine (Thorazine). In this period, the mechanisms of action for chlorpromazine were not known, and although many people believed this drug would usher in an age of deinstitutionalization, others felt it would likely just make hospital wards more manageable.

The second period begins in the early 1960s with the emphasis (begun in the Kennedy administration) of community care versus hospital care. At this time, the National Institute of Mental Health was labeling antipsychotics "**antischizophrenic**." At this time, psychological explanations for mental disorders were dropped in favor of medical model theories. Some writers at the time (Swazy, 1974) even posited that chlorpromazine was a "**magic bullet**" for schizophrenia (which it never was). This second period ends in the 1980s with the disappearance of such overly optimistic views. By the 1970s, clinicians accepted that neuroleptics could produce "alarming side effects, non-profound benefits in most cases, and no benefit at all in many" (Gelman, 1999, p. 7).

The third period, encompassing the 1980s and early 1990s, found many clinicians still clinging to the vague medical model notion of a chemical imbalance as causing schizophrenia despite the theory being increasingly falsified. Although researchers and clinicians began to understand schizophrenia as a complex, overdetermined disorder, many psychiatrists continued to follow the chemical imbalance theory (old habits die hard and it is easier to feign certainty than to live in ambiguity). Research during this period birthed the atypical antipsychotics, and for many psychiatrists these drugs seemed to continue to support the chemical imbalance theory, although they operate very differently from the neuroleptics that actually spawned the theory. Neuroleptics block dopamine-2 (D2) receptors whereas the atypicals block mostly serotonin receptors and some D2 receptors but not as many as neuroleptics. That these drugs that massively block serotonin receptors work as well as neuroleptics that block D2 receptors calls into question how schizophrenia could possibly be just a dopamine imbalance.

The fourth and current period began in the mid-1990s and continues to the present. This period is marked by new imaging technology that allows neurologists and psychopharmacologists to more closely examine the brain and the effects of medications on the brain. During this period, researchers will likely continue to construct newer theories to account for the action of antipsychotic medications.

Review Questions

- What are some of the variables currently considered as important to the etiology of schizophrenia?
- Why is the label "schizophrenia" inaccurate and what could replace it?
- Describe positive symptoms, primary negative symptoms, and secondary negative symptoms.

SECTION TWO: THEORIES OF NEUROLEPTIC ACTION FROM THE MEDICAL MODEL PERSPECTIVE

Learning Objectives

- Understand the dopamine hypothesis of schizophrenia and how it has been falsified.
- Be able to describe the primary dopamine tracts in the brain and how neuroleptic medications are thought to work.
- Know the four classes of extrapyramidal side effects (EPS).
- Know two classes of medications regularly used to treat EPS.

In this section, we outline the mechanism of action in typical antipsychotics (neuroleptics), detail their common side effects, and discuss how to deal with side effects. It is interesting that neuroleptics, and chlorpromazine/Thorazine in particular, were widely used before their mechanisms of action were isolated. As you are now aware, this is not unusual in the history of psychopharmacology, and the neuroleptics were being used on a global scale before their mechanisms of action were identified.

The Dopamine Hypothesis of Schizophrenia

The **dopamine hypothesis of schizophrenia** (the first "chemical imbalance" theory for the disorder) actually was formulated in the 1960s but had no impact on the field of psychiatry until the 1970s. The hypothesis proposed that schizophrenia was caused by an undefined problem in dopamine transmission. The hypothesis grew out of the realization that chlorpromazine/Thorazine and haloperidol/Haldol both seemed to interrupt dopamine transmission and decrease the symptoms of schizophrenia. Equally, abuse of amphetamine drugs that stimulate dopamine can cause symptoms indistinguishable from schizophrenia in some but not all people. As you may recall from Chapter Five, this is similar to the **amine hypothesis of depression**. It posits a simple (too simple) cause-and-effect relationship from observations of medical trials. As in other cases, though, the reality is far more complex, and emotional defense of the simple dopamine hypothesis today carries the same authority as emotional proclamations espoused by the Flat Earth Society.

So how was the dopamine hypothesis developed, and what relevance has it for mental health clinicians? Since the early administration of chlorpromazine/Thorazine, researchers had noted that the drug caused symptoms similar to those in Parkinson's disease (so named for James Parkinson, who outlined the symptoms in 1812). Carlsson and Lindqvist (1963) proposed the first variation on the dopamine hypothesis, but remember that at the time people knew little about neurotransmitters and nothing at all about neurotransmitter receptors. Arvid Carlsson discovered dopamine in the central nervous system, where, researchers learned, dopamine was also a precursor to norepinephrine. Studies with reserpine/Serpalan demonstrated that it depleted norepinephrine and serotonin from the brain, but when these neurotransmitters were replaced they did not counter the effects of the reserpine/Serpalan. Carlsson and his colleagues, hot off their discovery that dopamine was also present in the brain, assumed that dopamine too was depleted by reserpine and discovered that giving research animals a precursor for dopamine (levodopa/Carbidopa) did in fact reverse the effects of reserpine/Serpalan. Thus was born the first variation of the dopamine hypothesis—that psychoses were somehow related to deficiencies in dopamine.

The first response to this theory was that it did not make sense, because chlorpromazine/Thorazine did not empty the presynaptic neuron of dopamine (recall that researchers had not yet learned about receptors). Carlsson and Lindqvist (1963) demonstrated that chlorpromazine/Thorazine and haloperidol/Haldol acted on the postsynaptic neurons. Only after Solomon Snyder and Candace Pert confirmed the presence of receptors could researchers make the conceptual leap linking the effects of chlorpromazine/Thorazine to dopamine receptors. Snyder, Banerjee, Yamanura, and Greenberg (1974) also demonstrated that there were many dopamine receptors, and subsequent research showed that antipsychotic drugs had a particular affinity for binding at the dopamine-2 (D2) receptor. This paved the way for the inordinate focus on receptors in today's pharmacologic research. Researchers concluded that neuroleptic drugs such as chlorpromazine/Thorazine and haloperidol/Haldol blocked the D2 receptors, preventing dopamine from binding at those receptors and exerting an effect. Thus, decreasing dopamine activity in this manner lessened symptoms of schizophrenia in many patients. When researchers assumed that people suffering from Parkinson's disease were suffering from decreased dopamine activity, this hypothesis further explained why people taking neuroleptics might suffer Parkinsonian side effects. Although the drug they were taking, not Parkinson's disease, had disrupted their dopamine transmission, the result was the same.

This variation of the dopamine hypothesis was supported by observations of amphetamine users as well. Researchers had long known that heavy amphetamine users could develop symptoms similar to those seen in schizophrenia. Because amphetamines were later shown to increase dopamine in the synaptic cleft, it made sense that if problems in dopamine transmission could cause schizophrenia, drugs that artificially increased dopamine levels might cause symptoms similar to those of schizophrenia, just as decreased levels of dopamine would cause symptoms similar to those of Parkinson's disease.

To summarize: It is now clear that neuroleptics (also called *typical antipsychotics*) bind to a subfamily of dopamine receptors called the D2 receptors. Here the drugs act as **antagonists**, meaning they block the receptor but exert no effect. They merely block dopamine molecules from binding. The dopamine molecules would exert an effect if they *could* bind, but they are prevented from doing so as long as the person is taking a neuroleptic medication. The dopamine hypothesis was a mainstay for understanding drug treatment for schizophrenia until the 1990s.

The following two cases illustrate both (1) the use of neuroleptics to treat disorders in the spectrum of schizophrenia and (2) the reliance on the dopamine hypothesis as the cornerstone for treating schizophrenia until the early 1990s. This approach met with both success and failure, showing that the dopamine hypothesis was too simplistic. Despite warnings from researchers such as Solomon Snyder and Arvid Carlsson that the hypothesis was merely a correlation and should not be mistaken for a cause-and-effect relationship, by the 1970s the dopamine hypothesis of schizophrenia was quite popular. It is still espoused by some clinicians with great certainty today and that is an error because we also know that agents that block serotonin receptors and glutamate receptors can decrease psychotic symptoms in some but not all people. The serotonin hypothesis was developed by observing that drugs with strong serotonergic agonism like lysergic acid diethylamide (LSD) can cause psychotic-like hallucinations in some but not all users (and these are actually usually visual unlike most psychotic hallucinations) and (as noted above) newer antipsychotics massively block serotonin and decrease psychotic symptoms in some but not all people. Finally, the glutamate hypothesis is that excessive release of excitatory neurotransmitters like glutamate and acetylcholine causes deterioration in the frontal cortex that causes the symptoms of schizophrenia. As Advokat, Comaty, and Julien (2014) conclude "… none of these models completely explains nor exactly mimics the phenotypic presentation of behaviors associated with schizophrenia" (p. 340).

THE CASE OF COLIN

Colin, a 27-year-old father of four, began to notice that he experienced strange thoughts, maybe voices, during his workday. His wife noticed that he was more agitated and tense at home, even impatient with the children. In his work as a media specialist at a major university, Colin had a range of responsibilities linked to a very tight schedule. His schedule had become all but impossible with the layoff of his assistant and he was under the most pressure he had ever been under in his career. His immediate supervisor noticed his growing disorganization at work and a gradual deterioration of his performance. Colin insisted he was receiving messages that preoccupied his mind and distracted him from his daily routine. He became frightened and paranoid, and said people were out to destroy him. He stopped sleeping and eating, and believed his food was poisoned. Finally his wife called the emergency room and was advised to bring Colin in as soon as possible. He resisted her efforts, but finally agreed to go when his best friend insisted he should to demonstrate to the world that he was not insane.

Colin was hospitalized for 18 days and prescribed 24 mg of a typical antipsychotic called thiothixene/ Navane. Colin also participated in group and art therapy during his hospitalization. On release, Colin continued the thiothixene/Navane (reduced to 12 mg a day) and began individual and couples therapy at a mental health center. Colin continued both therapies for several years, stopping the thiothixene/Navane after nine months. Ten years after his hospitalization, Colin remains relatively stable both at work and at home, leading an active and productive life. Colin was never hospitalized again, nor did he decompensate to such a state that he needed to go back on thiothixene/Navane or into the hospital. This episode occurred in the early 1980s, and the diagnosis at the time was Brief Reactive Psychosis (what *DSM-5* would label Brief Psychotic Disorder).

Colin's case also illustrates several of the perspectives we have discussed in this book. He suffered from a brief but serious cognitive impairment that included hearing voices, losing some contact with reality, and becoming paranoid. From the medical model perspective, Colin had psychotic symptoms and was hospitalized for them. The neuroleptic, thiothixene/ Navane, was very helpful, and Colin never developed

any serious side effects. It is important to note that six months after his recovery, Colin found a different position with more promotion potential and less stress. As usual though, the medical model perspective provides only part of the story. From the psychological perspective, Colin experienced enormous pressure to earn more money for his growing family at the same time he learned of his parents' divorce. He also learned there was little promotion potential for him at work, and he began to sense a growing stress with his wife. Culturally, Colin, as a second-generation Irishman to the United States, was ashamed of the dramatic nature of his psychological disorder and his need to take a psychotropic medication. The influence of his family's rigid interpretation of Catholic dogma made Colin ashamed to share this experience with others. In addition, Colin felt a covert stigmatization at work from his immediate supervisor, who was Japanese and who failed to grasp the seriousness of Colin's illness and to be empathic toward him during his recovery. His supervisor also had a work ethic that seemed to view an enormous workload as a source of pride rather than the burden Colin felt it was.

Therapy was invaluable to Colin as he focused on some personal issues that bothered him and also worked on many of the difficulties in his marriage. Throughout the therapy, Colin became alert to the signs that indicated that he could become ill again and, as of this writing, he has had no further serious problems.

THE CASE OF ETHEL

For many years, Ethel suffered from what *DSM-IV* called Undifferentiated Schizophrenia accompanied with many negative symptoms. Ethel's psychiatrist had prescribed 600 mg of chlorpromazine/Thorazine daily. Because Ethel was single and lived alone, it was very difficult for her case manager to assess how compliant she was with her medication, including her benztropine/Cogentin (taken to treat side effects from her chlorpromazine/Thorazine). Over a period of two years, Ethel had to be hospitalized six times, for periods ranging from eight days to four weeks, because she was unable to function or care for herself. Eventually, the pattern became clear: Ethel would stop taking her chlorpromazine/ Thorazine and gradually retreat into a nonfunctioning catatonic state. During her last hospitalization, the treatment team recommended haloperidol/ Haldol by injection on a monthly basis to assist her with compliance. This strategy altered Ethel's response to her illness. Although it remained essential for her to take her benztropine/Cogentin orally, getting an injection once a month at the mental health center ended her cycle of hospitalizations, seemed to ease her negative symptoms, and allowed her to participate in group activities sponsored by the center.

Neuroleptic therapy by injection was a strategy implemented for noncompliant patients before the advent of the atypical antipsychotics. This intervention was only partially successful, because many clients remained resistant to treatment with all neuroleptics and/or suffered such serious side effects that neuroleptic treatment became a burden.

Side Effects of Neuroleptic Medication

Perhaps one of the greatest influences for the development of newer antipsychotic medications was the side effects of the neuroleptic medications. Table 7.1 lists the most common neuroleptic drugs still in use today. Note that all these drugs are associated in different degrees with the difficult side effects we describe next.

To fully understand the side effects of neuroleptic antipsychotic medications, we must look at four

TABLE 7.1 Examples of Neuroleptic (Typical) Antipsychotics

Generic Name	Class or Subclass	Brand Name	Daily Oral Dose
Chlorpromazine	Phenothiazine (aliphatic)	Thorazine	150–1000 mg[a]
Promazine	Phenothiazine (aliphatic)	Sparine	25–1000 mg
Triflupromazine	Phenothiazine (aliphatic)	Vesprin	20–50 mg
Fluphenazine	Phenothiazine (piperazine)	Prolixin	2–20 mg
Perphenazine	Phenothiazine (piperazine)	Trilafon	8–40 mg
Trifluoperazine	Phenothiazine (piperazine)	Stelazine	5–30 mg
Mesoridazine	Phenothiazine (piperidine)	Serentil	75–300 mg
Thioridazine	Phenothiazine (piperidine)	Mellaril	100–800 mg
Chlorprothixene	Thioxanthene	Taractan	30–600 mg
Thiothixene	Thioxanthene	Navane	6–50 mg
Haloperidol	Butyrophenone	Haldol	2–40 mg
Molindone	Dihydroindolone	Moban	20–225 mg
Loxapine	Dibenzoxazepine	Loxitane	30–150 mg
Pimozide	Diphenylbutylpiperidine	Orap	2–12 mg

© Cengage Learning®

[a]Schatzberg, Cole, and DeBattista (1997) have summarized research suggesting that little benefit is gained from chlorpromazine by exceeding a dose 400 mg a day.

TABLE 7.2 Four Primary Dopamine Pathways in the Brain

Name	*Location*
Mesolimbic pathway	Projects from the ventral tegmental area of the brain to the limbic system. Plays a role in emotional behavior.
Mesocortical pathway	Projects from the ventral tegmental area of the brain all the way to the cerebral cortex. Plays a role in cognition.
Nigrostriatal pathway	Projects from the substantia nigra of the brain stem to the basal ganglia and is part of the extrapyramidal nervous system.
Tuberoinfundibular pathway	Projects from the hypothalamus to the pituitary and governs prolactin release.

© Cengage Learning®

primary dopamine pathways in the brain that are affected by these medications. Table 7.2 summarizes these pathways, and then we discuss each.

The Four Primary Dopamine Pathways in the Brain

The Mesolimbic Pathway

Without dispute, the mesolimbic pathway is most clearly associated with the positive symptoms of schizophrenia. Stahl (2013) has noted that the auditory hallucinations, delusions, and even thought disorder symptoms of schizophrenia have been correlated with this pathway. Stahl has suggested that perhaps the dopamine hypothesis of schizophrenia should be renamed the "mesolimbic dopamine hypothesis of positive psychotic symptoms" (p. 374), because that more accurately describes the correlation between neuroleptic medications acting at this brain site and decreased symptoms. Obviously one problem in medicating clients with schizophrenia is that the effects of the medications (at least to date) cannot be isolated to this one dopamine pathway.

The Mesocortical Pathway

The mesocortical pathway is related to cognition, but its role (if any) in the symptoms of schizophrenia is undetermined. It does appear that the blockade of the dopamine-2 receptors in this pathway by neuroleptic medications causes an emotional blunting (sometimes referred to as **flat affect**) and cognitive problems that look like thought disorder. This has sometimes been called **neuroleptic-induced deficit syndrome** (Stahl, 2013). Neuroleptic-induced deficit syndrome is particularly problematic, because it mirrors the negative symptoms of schizophrenia that we discussed at the beginning of this chapter. Part of the ongoing debate is whether neuroleptic medications acting on this pathway actually exacerbate the negative symptoms of schizophrenia and in turn degrade the client's quality of life. Further, if clients have pronounced negative symptoms before receiving neuroleptic medication, such medications may make the symptoms worse.

The Nigrostriatal Dopamine Pathway

The nigrostriatal dopamine pathway as part of the extrapyramidal nervous system governs motor movements. Any deficiency of dopamine in this pathway causes a movement disorder. Parkinson's disease is caused by a deficiency of dopamine in this pathway, in turn caused by degeneration of dopamine neurons in the pathway. What we describe later as extrapyramidal symptoms are the **Parkinsonian side effects** that result when neuroleptic medications block dopamine receptors in this pathway and cause movement disorders. One of the more serious disorders is **tardive dyskinesia**, or late-appearing abnormal movement. Although the effects of neuroleptics on this pathway and thus movement confirmed initial hypotheses about the role played by dopamine in their mechanism of action, such effects have also confirmed fears that for some clients the treatment may be as difficult to live with as the symptoms.

The Tuberoinfundibular or Hypothalamic Pathway

Ironically, the physically shortest dopamine tract we will discuss has the longest name. The tuberoinfundibular pathway (also called the hypothalamic pathway) is much shorter than the previous three and, as noted in Table 7.2, controls the prolactin levels that normally rise in breast-feeding women. The firing of dopamine neurons in this pathway inhibits the release of prolactin, precluding lactation. When a woman is pregnant, part of the hormonal changes she experiences include inhibition of these neurons. This inhibition increases prolactin release so the woman can lactate to feed her child after birth. Herein lie more problematic side effects from neuroleptic medications. When the medications artificially inhibit the dopamine neurons in this pathway by blocking DA receptors, the result is an unintended increase of prolactin and symptoms such as galactorrhea (breast secretion) and amenorrhea (cessation of menses) in females as well as development of female secondary sex characteristics in males. Clients of both genders may also experience sexual dysfunction.

Given this overview of important pathways affected by neuroleptic medications, you can surmise the basic problem. As we noted, the only antipsychotic actions from these medications result from their blockage of D2 receptors in the mesolimbic pathway. The blocking of D2 receptors in the remaining three pathways result in undesirable side effects. In addition, neuroleptics are "dirty" drugs, meaning that they not only block dopamine receptors but also may block histamine, acetylcholine, and adrenergic receptors. These properties also result in undesirable side effects. Having introduced the different ways in which side effects can occur from neuroleptic medication, let's now look more closely at the primary side effects of these medications. Please note that this discussion of the topic is not exhaustive and does not include

rare side effects. These descriptions should give clinicians a sense of what clients may expect and what to listen for as clients describe effects they are experiencing.

Allergic Reactions to Neuroleptics

Allergic reactions to neuroleptics occur in approximately 7% of patients and usually manifest between two weeks and two months of treatment. The primary symptom is a rash on the face, neck, upper chest, or extremities. The rash (local or general) results in red pimples accompanied by a burning or stinging sensation. These are usually treated with **antihistamines** or, in more severe cases, steroids (Malhotra, Litman, & Pickar, 1993).

Anticholinergic Effects of Neuroleptics

As the name implies, anticholinergic effects of neuroleptics result from the neuroleptic medication blocking acetylcholine receptors in both the peripheral and the central nervous systems. The secondary results are called **autonomic side effects** because of their impact on the autonomic nervous system. The primary CNS side effect related to anticholinergic action is **delirium**. The peripheral effects of anticholinergic action are described later. Note that all these side effects may be exacerbated if the client is also taking an anticholinergic agent with the neuroleptic. We explain the rationale for using these agents later, when we address extrapyramidal symptoms.

Blurred Vision

The anticholinergic action of neuroleptics can paralyze the ciliary muscle in the pupil of the eye, causing difficulty in focusing on objects within a close field of vision. Sometimes prescribers lower the dosage temporarily or recommend reading glasses to provide relief (Perry, Alexander, & Liskow, 2006). We have found that although not all clients experience this (or any other side effect), those who do often prefer to have the doctor change their medication (and honestly who can blame them?).

Dry Mouth

Dry mouth can be particularly bothersome for clients, depending on the strength of the effect. Both the antihistaminic and anticholinergic effects of neuroleptics cause dry mouth. Many clients can obtain relief with sugarless gum or candy, but many clients find it necessary to carry a drinking bottle with them at all times. Our clients often preferred sweetened, caffeinated soft drinks, which, combined with other poor dietary habits, exacerbated the weight gain associated with the antihistaminic effects of neuroleptics.

Constipation

Constipation can be seriously aggravated by neuroleptic medication, although it may resolve as the client adjusts to the medication. Routine use of laxatives is to be discouraged (Perry et al., 2006). Malhotra and colleagues (1993) noted that in severe cases, constipation can progress into fatal intestinal dilation or paralytic ileus. Paralytic ileus can result in death through intestinal obstruction. Although this is rare, clients need regular checkups with regard to intestinal functioning.

Urinary Retention

Urinary retention may be noticed two to four weeks from beginning the neuroleptic regimen. According to Perry and colleagues (2006), blocking the acetylcholine neurons affects the detrusor muscle that governs the flow of urine. Although the effect is dose related, acute urinary retention is a sign for the prescribing professional to consider another medication as it can lead to kidney problems and bladder or urinary tract infections.

Withdrawal Reactions

Although neuroleptic medications are not drugs of abuse per se, regular and long-term use can induce tolerance, which can lead to withdrawal reactions if medications are discontinued abruptly. The symptoms usually begin two or three days after discontinuation and include headache, nausea, vomiting, diarrhea, and insomnia. Any client who has taken a neuroleptic for at least one month should have the medication tapered off if it is to be discontinued. Perry et al. (2006) recommend at least a one-week period (inpatient) or a two-week period (outpatient) where the dosage is titrated down before the drug is discontinued. Although it is more associated with the atypical antipsychotics, hypersalivation can also occur in people taking neuroleptics. Essali and colleagues (2013) have noted that this is an understudied phenomenon and although they believe anticholinergic drugs may be helpful, more research is necessary.

Cardiovascular Side Effects from Neuroleptics

As with some of the antidepressants we discussed in Chapter Five, neuroleptics can cause orthostatic hypotension, which is due to the antiadrenergic effects of these drugs. This effect inhibits the normal constriction of blood vessels associated with postural change, resulting in the lightheadedness and dizziness characteristic of orthostatic hypotension (Malhotra et al., 1993). This side effect usually begins within the first few hours or days of treatment and is more pronounced when the neuroleptic has been administered **parenterally** (by injection). In most cases, clients can easily manage this by standing up slowly and by elevating their feet when lying down. In cases where clients have complained about this effect, lowering the medication dose has also been effective as long as the therapeutic effects are not diminished to the point that symptoms begin to interfere with the client's life again. Clients on neuroleptics may also experience electrocardiogram changes, which are of debatable clinical significance. Although case reports exist of lethal cardiovascular events in people taking neuroleptics, they have not been linked to the neuroleptic medication per se.

Dermatological Side Effects from Neuroleptics

Perhaps the most common dermatologic side effect is photosensitivity. This sensitivity to sunlight occurs in approximately 3% of clients taking neuroleptic medications. Most cases are related to chlorpromazine/Thorazine, but all clients on neuroleptics should limit their exposure to the sun and should use sunscreen and protective clothing. Approximately 1% of clients on neuroleptics develop a bluish pigmentation in their skin. This rare effect depends on the neuroleptic used, dosage, and extent of exposure to sunlight. These disorders are thought to be much less frequent today because use of neuroleptics has decreased and lower doses are used (Perry et al., 2006).

Endocrinological Side Effects of Neuroleptic Medications

Neuroleptics can cause hormonal side effects partly because of their impact on dopamine transmission in the tuberoinfundibular pathway, described earlier. As mentioned, galactorrhea and amenorrhea can occur in females. It is important to note that breast enlargement and engorgement can occur in both males and females (Sullivan & Lukoff, 1990). Elevated prolactin levels may subside within two to three days of discontinuing treatment of oral antipsychotics, but in some cases this may take weeks or months (Perry et al., 2006). In addition, clients may experience polydipsia (excessive thirst and water drinking) or a deficiency of sodium in the blood (hyponatremia).

Weight Gain

Studies done in the 1970s correlated weight gain with neuroleptic medications. The average gain was approximately 13 pounds. Weight gain is tied to the antihistaminic properties of the neuroleptics, as is drowsiness and sedation (Advokat et al., 2014), but it can be exacerbated by poor choices like sugary drinks to ease side effects like dry mouth. Perry et al. (2006) caution that although weight gain may be a property of neuroleptic medications, it may also be due to a combination of factors such as the medication, a sedentary lifestyle, and poor diet habits. Although these authors encourage clinicians to monitor patients' weight, they remind us that under no circumstances should clients use amphetamine-based appetite suppressants, because of the connection between dopamine stimulation and exacerbated symptoms.

Extrapyramidal Symptoms Caused by Neuroleptic Medication

As you may recall from our discussion of the nigrostriatal dopamine pathway in the brain, neuroleptic medications block the dopamine-2 receptors in this pathway and cause movement disorders. These EPSs, can range from mild to severe, and may have early or late onset. For most clients, these symptoms are problematic and are one reason that many psychiatrists believe newer, atypical antipsychotics should be the first line of treatment.

Early-Onset Extrapyramidal Symptoms

Estimates of early-onset EPSs fluctuate wildly, ranging between 2 and 95% of clients taking neuroleptics (Lavin & Rifkin, 1992). **Dystonias** or **dystonic reactions** occur in 2 to 10% of clients on neuroleptic medications. The onset is sudden (1 to 3 days after neuroleptic medication is taken) and consists of involuntary contractions of possibly any striated muscle group. The most common dystonic reactions are in the muscles of the head and face, producing tics, facial grimacing, or spasms. The reactions are possible with all neuroleptics but are less likely with the piperazine phenothiazines (e.g., fluphenazine/Prolixin) (see Table 7.1). Although these side effects often cease without treatment, they can be easily treated with Benadryl or benztropine/Cogentin, an anticholinergic agent. The etiology of dystonic reactions is not known.

The term *akathisia* refers to a subjective experience of motor restlessness, a condition that is much more difficult to treat than dystonic reactions. In our clinical work with clients, the psychological experience of this particular side effect can be profound. Clients report feeling that they cannot sit still, and they tap their foot/feet, pace back and forth, shake their hands, or rock back and forth when standing. Observed behaviorally, they are always in constant motion. The incidence of akathisia in studies ranges from 21 to 75% (Perry et al., 2006). The majority of clients who develop akathisia experience symptoms within about two months. Schatzberg et al. (1997) note that sometimes akathisia has been misdiagnosed as psychotic agitation. Obviously, this misdiagnosis may lead doctors to increase the dosage of the very compound causing the problem.

One sign from which to discern the difference between psychotic agitation and akathisia is the degree of psychological contact the client can make. It is important that someone who has a therapeutic alliance with the client talk to him or her about the symptoms. Most clients suffering from akathisia can, to some extent, describe the symptoms and differentiate them from psychotic symptoms they have experienced in the past. Schatzberg and colleagues note that asking the client whether the restlessness is "a muscle feeling or a head feeling" (p. 145) often helps differentiate akathisia (the muscle feeling) from anxiety that may accompany agitation (the head feeling). These authors consider that to assume akathisia over agitation is to err on the side of caution. Doctors may treat akathisia with a benzodiazepine, an anti-Parkinsonian agent such as benztropine/Cogentin, or even a beta-blocker such as propranolol/Inderal. Although some clients may not even be aware of their akathisia, the symptoms greatly distress others. Furthermore, sometimes agents used to treat akathisia exacerbate the sedation the client experiences, making such treatment problematic.

Parkinsonism is a set of side effects that manifest as muscular rigidity, slowed movement, tremors (usually in the hands), or **bradykinesia** (fatigue when performing repetitive motion). The tremors may occur at rest or while in motion and may include the mouth, chin, and lips. Clients with Parkinsonism appear depressed, but it is important to differentiate this from actual depression. The incidence ranges in studies from 2 to 56% of clients taking neuroleptics. Again it depends on the neuroleptic used, the dosage, and the individual's response to it. Parkinsonism is typically treated with anticholinergic agents (such as benztropine/Cogentin). There is debate as to whether or not all neuroleptics should be given with an anti-Parkinsonian agent (Stanilla & Simpson, 1995). Advocates claim that doing so precludes the appearance of many extrapyramidal symptoms, and opponents claim the neuroleptics are toxic enough without adding a second agent if not needed.

Late-Onset Extrapyramidal Symptoms

Two identified late-onset EPSs are similar to the early-onset symptoms and differ only in the time it takes them to manifest. Frequently these are called tardive syndromes, meaning delayed-onset, abnormal, and involuntary movement disorders (Fernandez & Friedman, 2003). Bear in mind that the word *tardive* means "late appearing"; thus, tardive dystonia and tardive akathisia are the same as dystonic reactions and akathisia as described earlier, but with a much later onset (sometimes after a patient has taken the neuroleptic for years). Although there is no developed literature regarding these two late-onset EPSs, there is a great deal of literature on tardive dyskinesia.

Tardive dyskinesia is a late-appearing abnormal movement of the mouth, lips, and tongue that may be accompanied by involuntary twitching and jerking of muscles (choreic movement). The primary differential diagnoses include Huntington's chorea and other disorders that affect the basal ganglia (Casey, 1993). The most common symptoms are sucking and smacking lip movements, lateral movements of the jaw, and puffing of cheeks with tongue-thrusting motions (Perry et al., 2006). Tardive dyskinesia affects on average 15 to 20% of clients on neuroleptics, although gender (7:1 male-to-female ratio), age, diagnosis, dosage, and duration of neuroleptic regimen all seem to play a role. Perry and colleagues (2006) noted, tardive dyskinesia is seen in approximately 5–10% of patients being treated with neuroleptics who are over 40 years of age but can also occur in up to 80% of elderly patients. In general, people with schizophrenia (likely due to the drugs they are taking) have a 31 times higher chance of developing tardive dyskinesia than those in the general population (Merrill, Lyon, & Matiaco, 2013).

There are several theories of etiology for tardive dyskinesia, including hypersensitivity to dopamine, imbalances between the dopamine and acetylcholine systems, GABA dysfunction, and excitotoxicity. Most recently, a theory has been proposed that oxidative stress and resulting structural abnormalities are the key factors in people who develop tardive dyskinesia (Kulkarni & Naidu, 2003). At present, there is no one accepted theory.

Tardive dyskinesia is unpredictable. Although a six-month regimen of neuroleptics is generally considered safe, some patients develop tardive dyskinesia after only a few weeks of taking neuroleptics. When clients show signs of tardive dyskinesia and the neuroleptic is discontinued, often the symptoms vanish within weeks to months. Tardive dyskinesia appears irreversible in some cases, whereas in others it may only remit years after the neuroleptic is discontinued. Schatzberg et al. (1997) noted that about 25% of their clients developed dyskinesia when the neuroleptic was tapered off or stopped. Dyskinesia develops in some individuals who have never been exposed to neuroleptics (Merril et al., 2013). Schatzberg and colleagues (1997) state there is no single effective or standard treatment for tardive dyskinesia and clinicians should consider the risks and benefits of extended treatment with neuroleptics in patients likely to be kept on the medication more than a few months.

Schatzberg and colleagues (1997) conclude that "this issue must be discussed with the patient and his or her family unless there are defensible clinical reasons for not doing so" (p.151). From our clinical experience, the only reasons for not discussing this with clients and/or family members is if a client's symptoms preclude making psychological contact and the family members are clearly judged to be incapable of acting, or unwilling to act, in the client's best interest. Although most of the newer atypical antipsychotics are not associated with tardive dyskinesia, there is still a risk with some like risperidone/Risperdal. It appears that the incidence of tardive dyskinesia in the newer antipsychotics is substantially lower than in the neuroleptics (Dolder & Jeste, 2003; Friedman, 2003; Lykouras, Agelopoulos, & Tzavellas, 2002).

Neuroleptic Malignant Syndrome

Although rare, neuroleptic malignant syndrome (NMS) is a potentially life-threatening complication of neuroleptic medications. Although rates of occurrence are low, they should be noted. Approximately 1% of all psychiatric admissions may have this response to standard neuroleptic medications. Hyperthermia, severe extrapyramidal symptoms, and autonomic disturbances characterize NMS. Caroff and Mann (1993) have noted that the onset may occur within an hour to two months after the first dose of the neuroleptic. In most cases, the clients show signs within a week. Once NMS begins, it progresses rapidly over a one- to three-day period. If the medication is discontinued in time, most cases resolve within a month. Fatalities from NMS are rare, because use of neuroleptics has decreased and the syndrome is detected early.

Agents to Treat Extrapyramidal Side Effects

Anti-Parkinsonian agents are used for treating early-onset extrapyramidal symptoms. Recall that these side effects result from neuroleptic-induced blockade of dopamine receptors in the nigrostriatal pathway that cause decreased dopamine transmission. Table 7.3 lists drugs commonly used to treat EPSs. More recently, experimental studies have been conducted to examine calcium channel blockers (e.g., diltiazem/Cardizem, nifedipine/Procardia, nimodipine/Nimotop, and verapamil/Veralan) as agents to treat EPSs but more research is needed (Essali, Deirawan, Soares-Weiser, Adams, 2011).

Looking at Table 7.3, readers may sense the paradox of all the agents listed. As for the dopaminergic agent (amantadine), you may ask, "If neuroleptics are decreasing dopamine transmission, won't the addition of a dopamine agonist worsen symptoms?" Similarly, you may look at all the anticholinergic agents and wonder, "If neuroleptics cause anticholinergic symptoms, won't adding an anticholinergic agent worsen these side effects?" Both are good questions. To understand why any of these agents may be given to a client taking neuroleptic medication for psychotic symptoms, it is first important to understand something we discussed in Chapter Two, the delicate balance of neurotransmission and the ripple effect of how impact on one neurotransmitter system eventually influences others.

Recall that although most neurons produce only one type of neurotransmitter, most neurons have receptors for multiple neurotransmitters. When we clinicians interfere with neurotransmission by introducing an agent such as a neuroleptic, we set in motion a ripple effect that can upset the function

TABLE 7.3 Drugs Commonly Used to Treat Extrapyramidal Side Effects

Generic Name	Brand Name	Type of Drug	Daily Dosage Range
Amantadine	Symmetrel	Dopaminergic	100–300 mg
Benztropine	Cogentin	Anticholinergic	2–6 mg
Biperiden	Akineton	Anticholinergic	2–8 mg
Diphenhydramine	Benadryl	Anticholinergic	50–300 mg
Ethopropazine	Parsidol	Anticholinergic	100–400 mg
Procyclidine	Kemadrin	Anticholinergic	10–20 mg
Trihexyphenidyl	Elixir	Anticholinergic	4–15 mg

© Cengage Learning®

and balance of many other systems. One of these is the cholinergic system. It seems the neurons that make acetylcholine depend on dopamine transmission. If we interfere with dopamine transmission, we disrupt acetylcholine transmission as well. Thus, one theory about extrapyramidal symptoms is that they result from disruption in balance between dopamine neurons and acetylcholine neurons. Therefore, two ways to restore balance logically present themselves. The first is to decrease the acetylcholine transmission so it "evenly matches" the dopamine transmission. That is done with anticholinergic agents. The second solution is to boost dopamine transmission so it more evenly matches acetylcholine transmission. The obvious challenge here is not to increase it in an area or in a way that exacerbates the psychotic symptoms that were the problem in the first place.

Both solutions to addressing EPSs have their problems. Although amantadine/Symmetrel does in fact diminish dystonia, akathisia, and Parkinsonism more effectively than placebo, it also causes orthostatic hypotension, skin rashes, and GI disturbance and can exacerbate psychotic symptoms or induce agitation. Similarly, anticholinergic agents effectively treat dystonia, akathisia, and Parkinsonism, but can cause allergic reactions (rash or dermatitis), increase heart rate, exacerbate all anticholinergic side effects listed earlier for neuroleptics, cause urinary retention,

impair memory, and may induce confusion and/or delirium. Although helpful with EPSs, clearly neither type of agent is a panacea, and prescribing professionals must carefully balance the intended therapeutic effects with the emergence or exacerbation of side effects.

Table 7.4 describes the rational prescribing practice recommended by Perry et al. (2006).

The following two cases address some of the complex side effect issues linked to neuroleptics

TABLE 7.4 Rational Prescribing Practice for Treating Extrapyramidal Symptoms

First, try lowering the dose of the neuroleptic or switch the client to an atypical antipsychotic.

Generally speaking, anticholinergics should not be routinely added as prophylactics when a client is prescribed neuroleptic medication.

Every three months reassess a client who is prescribed medication for EPSs, because not all clients need long-term treatment with these agents.

If a client does not respond to one agent, try another, because responses differ person to person.

There is no support for combining anticholinergic agents.

© Cengage Learning®

and potential dependency issues related to some anticholinergics.

THE CASE OF TEANA

Teana, a 37-year-old divorced biracial mother of three, suffered from Schizoaffective Disorder and polysubstance dependence. Most recently, her presenting symptoms seemed more like the positive symptoms of schizophrenia than those of a manic profile. The psychiatrist was acutely aware of Teana's polysubstance dependence. Both Teana and her case manager vouched for the fact that Teana was attending Narcotics Anonymous (NA) and was not currently using any drugs of abuse. The psychiatrist reluctantly prescribed fluphenazine/Prolixin 20 mg daily, accompanied by the anticholinergic benztropine/Cogentin 2 mg daily.

About a month later, Teana scheduled an appointment with the psychiatrist, indicating that it was an emergency. Both the psychiatrist and case manager were puzzled, because she had enough medication for 90 days. In the waiting room, another case manager overheard Teana talking about what a "sweet" high she got from that "cognitive stuff" and that she was totally out and needed more. The case manager alerted the psychiatrist, who took Teana off the benztropine/Cogentin and substituted a dopaminergic, amantadine/Symmetrel. Teana was upset and acted out both in the physician's office and in the waiting room, and she went back to using for a time. Eventually, she returned to her drug treatment and accepted the amantadine/Symmetrel in place of the benztropine/Cogentin.

THE CASE OF MAURICE

Maurice, a 39-year-old, single, auto assembly-line worker, became acutely psychotic at work. He spoke in a "language" that could not be understood, and he appeared delusional and paranoid. He was hospitalized for seven weeks and released on 30 mg of trifluoperazine/Stelazine daily. Maurice could not return to work, and three months after being released from the hospital he was evicted from his apartment. He had been homeless and on the streets for over four months when he was accepted by a Christian house of hospitality, which offered to house him and monitor his medication. Over time, Maurice changed from the positive symptoms of Schizophrenia to an array of negative symptoms. He became withdrawn, isolated, and detached, with slurred speech and impaired movement. The monk who was in charge of the house noticed that he seemed fatigued, that his hands trembled constantly, and that his movements were rigid and very slow. He called the mental health center to alert them to these changes in Maurice, and the psychiatrist saw him the following week. The case manager also had reported that Maurice had seemed more withdrawn lately. The psychiatrist evaluated Maurice, found he was suffering from Parkinsonism, and treated him with benztropine/Cogentin, an anticholinergic.

Maurice's symptoms improved gradually, but he never returned to any previous level of functioning. He remained in a state of isolation with minimal Parkinsonian symptoms, but with little hope of improving the quality of his life. We lost track of Maurice when he was recommended for clozapine/Thoarazine in 2000. He had already been on neuroleptics for 13 years.

Uses and Efficacy of Neuroleptic Medications

Thus far, you are likely aware that the neuroleptics we have described have several drawbacks. Despite persistent and troublesome side effects, how well do these traditional agents really work? As we noted while summarizing the history of neuroleptics, compared to no medication at all they were a breakthrough. The questions remain, though, what is the efficacy today for neuroleptics? For what disorders are clinicians likely to see them employed? Pies (2005) has emphasized that the main indication for any antipsychotic is, of course, for psychosis. He noted that although it is not necessarily inappropriate to use an antipsychotic for a nonpsychotic disorder, antipsychotics are often misused for other conditions, such as agitation.

Certainly this is where the "practice" of medicine comes in and doctors must make clinically informed judgments to the best of their ability. At the same time, mental health clinicians should be aware of the difference between common and uncommon uses for neuroleptics. Table 7.5 lists common uses of antipsychotics outlined by Pies (2005) and Stahl (2013).

And what about efficacy? As you learned in Chapter Five, many antidepressants fare no better than placebo in controlled trials, making the question of efficacy an important one to explore in great depth. All the available neuroleptic (typical) antipsychotics have conclusively been shown to be more effective than placebo in reducing the positive symptoms of schizophrenia. The positive symptoms are typically the target symptoms, because they are the most disruptive to the client and others in the client's life. However, negative symptoms do

not respond well (if at all) to neuroleptics (Kane & Marder, 1993).

The most recent large-scale studies we have are the Clinical Antipsychotic Trials of Intervention Effectiveness (CATIE) (Lieberman et al., 2005) and the Cost Utility of the Latest Antipsychotic Drugs in Schizophrenia Study (CUtLASS1) (Jones et al., 2006).

Although some clients may respond within hours to days of receiving a neuroleptic, an adequate trial should be at least four weeks, and maximum improvement in symptoms is expected to occur within the first six months of therapy. Although evidence suggests that early antipsychotic treatment in recently diagnosed clients improves long-term outcomes, over two to three years, the relapse rates of even those with a diagnosis of first-time psychosis are in the 60 to 90% range (Szymanksi, Cannon, Gallagher, Erwin, & Gur, 1996). Table 7.6 summarizes strategies outlined by Perry et al. (2006) for clients who do not respond to neuroleptics or who respond only partially.

Clearly, although they offer some relief from the symptoms of psychosis, neuroleptics carry side effects so severe that many clients are not motivated to comply with medication regimens. Interestingly though, clients drop out of treatment with the older neuroleptics at about the same rate as the newer serotonin-dopamine antagonists (Zyprexa/olanzapine; Risperdal/risperidone) (Advokat et al., 2014). The only drug that may still be better for treatment-resistant cases is Clozaril/clozapine and it is to that drug that we turn next. A final note:

TABLE 7.5 Common Uses for Neuroleptic Medications

Schizophrenia

Schizophreniform Disorder

Brief Psychotic Disorder

Schizoaffective Disorder

Major Depression with Psychotic Features

Psychosis secondary to cocaine intoxication

Manic states

Dementia related to various causes/disorders

Noncompliant client in an acute setting where fast onset of action is desired

Noncompliant client needing intramuscular formulations

Tics associated with Tourette's syndrome

Severe cases of Obsessive-Compulsive Disorder

Agitated State of PTSD

TABLE 7.6 Strategies for Clients Taking Neuroleptics Who Partially Respond or Do Not Respond

Continue the same neuroleptic at the same dose.

Increase the dose of the current neuroleptic.

Switch to a different class of neuroleptic.

Add another medication to the neuroleptic.

Switch to an atypical (second-generation) antipsychotic.

neuroleptics may have uses outside of psychiatry. Advokat et al. (2014) noted that the neuroleptic thioridazine/Mellarill can kill an antibiotic resistant bacteria called *Staphylococcus*. It does so by removing glycine from the cell wall thus weakening it and allowing the antibiotics to then move in for the kill. So who knows how many other useful functions these drugs may have even if we eventually stop using them to treat schizophrenia?

Review Questions

- What is the dopamine hypothesis of schizophrenia and how has it been falsified?
- What are the four primary dopamine tracts in the brain and how are they affected by neuroleptic medications?
- What are the four classes of EPS?
- What are two classes of medication to treat EPS?

SECTION FOUR: CLOZARIL: THE PROTOTYPE FOR ATYPICAL ANTIPSYCHOTICS

Learning Objectives

- Be able to describe what makes the atypical antipsychotics atypical.
- Give a general summary of the mechanisms of action and side effects for clozapine.
- Understand potential drug–drug interactions that may be dangerous for people taking clozapine.

There were two early attempts to develop antipsychotics that were structurally different from the neuroleptics. Molindone/Moban was a structurally unique molecule in that it resembled the neurotransmitter serotonin. Despite this similarity, its binding properties resemble neuroleptics in the affinity for dopamine receptors. Although its use is less frequently associated with tardive dyskinesia, it

seems to induce many of the same early-onset EPSs of the neuroleptics. Its efficacy is similar to that of haloperidol/Haldol, and these similarities lead researchers to group it with the neuroleptics. Loxapine/Loxitane is structurally more related to serotonergic antipsychotics (such as clozapine/Clozaril) than a neuroleptic, but it too functions more like a neuroleptic than like anything else. Loxapine/Loxitane binds to both dopamine and serotonin receptors but has many of the same side effect problems as the neuroleptics.

THE CASE OF BONNIE

Bonnie experienced her first psychotic episode when she was 17 years old. Bonnie's mother had been institutionalized off and on for 18 years, diagnosed with Schizophrenia. Her father left Bonnie and her mother when Bonnie was only 2 years old, and she had no siblings. Bonnie had been diagnosed with Schizophrenia, Disorganized subtype (under *DSM-IV* criteria. In *DSM-5* all subtypes of schizophrenia have been eliminated). She suffered from delusions, magical thinking, and bizarre behavior such as storing feces in Mason jars under her bed, believing they would turn to gold if stored long enough. Bonnie would masturbate openly with little concern for where she was and would only say, "The voices are fucking me."

Bonnie showed marked negative symptoms and conceptual disorganization. These became substantially worse when she was treated with neuroleptic medication. When Bonnie was referred to the partial hospitalization program (PHP), she was 28 years old. She had three children of her own with three different men but had lost custody because of her inability to care for them. She was not allowed visits with them in their foster home because her bizarre behavior upset them. On first coming to the PHP from an inpatient unit, Bonnie was taking 500 mg of chlorpromazine/Thorazine daily as well as 6 mg of benztropine/Cogentin. This medication produced pronounced EPSs and worsened her anhedonia and social withdrawal. Over the course of two years, the psychiatrist at the PHP switched Bonnie's medication four times (constantly adjusting dosages), trying to maximize the therapeutic benefits and minimize the side effects. The best combination seemed to be haloperidol/Haldol (20 mg daily) and benztropine/Cogentin (2 mg daily). This "best" combination, the doctor reluctantly agreed, allowed Bonnie to reside in a maximum-supervision group home and attend (but rarely participate in) PHP programming. Apparently, Bonnie was in for a life living on the fringes of society.

In 1990, we became aware of a new drug called clozapine/Clozaril and a patient management program sponsored by Novartis Pharmaceuticals. As a person suffering from treatment-resistant Schizophrenia with pronounced negative symptoms, Bonnie was an ideal candidate for the program. Further, her Social Security disability benefits covered the costs of the medication. The program was rigorous, including weekly blood draws to check Bonnie for potentially lethal side effects (described later). After several months, Bonnie was titrated off her haloperidol/Haldol and benztropine/Cogentin and titrated onto clozapine/Clozaril. Although she experienced many of clozapine's/Clozaril's side effects (weight gain, excessive salivation, GI upset), these seemed acceptable compared to what she had experienced on the neuroleptic.

Further, several months into treatment the PHP staff noticed a pronounced change in Bonnie. One day as she was coming to the PHP to have her blood drawn, a staff member greeted her, joking that she looked as if she had just gotten up. Bonnie, who had rarely responded with more than one- or two-syllable answers, turned to the staff member and said, "Yes, as you can see I am quite tired." This marked a dramatic decrease in Bonnie's negative symptoms. She began to participate in groups and to engage in conversations with other clients about day-to-day activities. Further, she became more independent in the group home and moved to a moderate-supervision setting. Perhaps the most rewarding aspect of her case was that she improved to the point that she was allowed to (and could enjoy) biannual visits with her children, who lived about an hour away. Certainly Bonnie did not fully recover from Schizophrenia, but the clozapine/Clozaril brought about a diminishment of symptoms that greatly improved her quality of life. At last check, Bonnie was still stable and tolerating the clozapine/Clozaril therapy.

A NEW ERA

As we have noted, the discovery of antipsychotic drugs in 1950 was a breakthrough in treating mental illness. Lieberman (1997) noted that the magnitude of this advance in psychiatry has been compared to the discovery of insulin for diabetes, antibiotics for infectious disease, and anticonvulsants for epilepsy. At the same time, almost a half-century's experience with these compounds has made clinicians and consumers painfully aware of their limitations. According to Essali, Haasan, Li, and Rathbone (2009), 25–33% of patients treated with neuroleptics are treatment-resistant. Even when patients respond, Lieberman (1997) noted that almost 50% of patients respond only partially to treatment. And, as you have seen, the therapeutic effects of the neuroleptics predominantly reduce the positive symptoms; neuroleptics are less beneficial for the negative symptoms and conceptual disorganization. Finally, the therapeutic effects of neuroleptics come with a great number of side effects. It is important to note; however, that paying attention to clients' subjective distress over these side effects helps doctors titrate medications and clients participate in treatment (Taira, Hashimoto, Takamatsu, & Maeda, 2006).

Lieberman drew the metaphor that after 40 years of wandering in the proverbial pharmacological wilderness (1950 to 1990), many researchers and clients thought the introduction of clozapine/Clozaril was the gateway to a "promised land." Alas, though it brought improved treatments to some clients, the horizon of the true "promised land" will continue to recede from sight until the etiology of schizophrenia is understood.

Although clozapine/Clozaril was actually synthesized in 1959, it took 30 years before it was released for use in the United States. What makes clozapine/Clozapine atypical? First, the majority of its binding action takes place at serotonin sites rather than dopamine receptors. Second, it alleviates psychotic symptoms while causing significantly fewer extrapyramidal side effects. Third, it is a more effective antipsychotic agent than conventional neuroleptics. Finally, clozapine/Clozaril has an impact on both the negative and the positive symptoms of schizophrenia. Melzer (1993) noted that clozapine/Clozaril is very effective in treating a set of symptoms we have been referring to as *conceptual disorganization* (Lencz, Smith, Auther, Correll, & Cornblatt, 2003). Haloperidol/Haldol has typically been the neuroleptic baseline against which all other antipsychotic drugs are tested. In numerous studies, clozapine/Clozaril was more effective than haloperidol/Haldol (Wahlbeck, Cheine, Essali, & Adams, 1999). More recently, the CATIE research indicated that clozapine/Clozaril is still better than other serotonin-dopamine antagonists after failure on a first agent (Lieberman et al., 2005).

Placebo Versus Active Control Trials

Before exploring the atypical antipsychotic medications, we want to briefly note an important difference in the way newer antipsychotic medications are tested. In the introduction to Part Two and in Chapter Five, we covered the problem of placebo response, particularly with regard to antidepressant medications. In tests of newer medications designed to help people suffering from psychotic symptoms, an ethical problem arises with placebo-controlled trials. First, placebo responses from people suffering psychotic disorders have historically been very small in number, which raises the ethical concern of testing new medications against placebo. If a person is suffering from psychotic symptoms, it simply is not ethical to withhold treatment from the person for the purposes of having the person in a placebo control group. Therefore, new antipsychotics are frequently tested against the older neuroleptic medications. Such *active control trials* (Fleischhacker et al., 2003) are more designed to test the medication's side effect profile than to test efficacy against placebo. For the most part, the newer antipsychotics (with the exception of clozapine/Clozaril) work

just as well as haloperidol/Haldol but have a more favorable side effect profile.

Mechanisms of Action

How does clozapine/Clozaril work? Whereas we noted the mechanism of action in neuroleptics focused on the blocking of dopamine receptors, clozapine/Clozaril is one of the most complicated drugs on the market. Researchers have found it has noteworthy interactions with at least nine neurotransmitter receptors. Six of the nine receptors are dopamine or serotonin receptors. Researchers currently do not know which of these receptors (or which combination of receptors) accounts or account for the antipsychotic effects. Table 7.7 details the mechanisms of action of clozapine.

Reviewing Table 7.7, perhaps the most striking thing you note is that the primary mechanism of action is strong serotonin antagonism and weak dopamine antagonism. Recall that all the neuroleptics worked by powerful dopamine antagonism, particularly at the D2 receptor. As far as clozapine/Clozaril goes, although the overall effects on dopamine are weak, those effects are more pronounced on the D1 receptor than the D2 receptor. Without having to understand the biochemistry involved, you can draw the significant conclusions: (1) This compound is more effective in treating schizophrenia than neuroleptics that rely solely on D2 antagonism, and (2) this result weakens any interpretation of the dopamine hypothesis of schizophrenia that ties symptoms to dopamine transmission. On the other hand, it was recently postulated that clozapine/Clozaril exerts antipsychotic action by *transiently* occupying D2 receptors as opposed to the prolonged occupation of receptors seen in neuroleptics (Seeman, 2014).

The most that can be said is that by significantly interfering with dopamine transmission, neuroleptics can attenuate the positive symptoms of schizophrenia. There have also been some more recent papers suggesting that clozapine/Clozaril acts as an antagonist at glutaminergic NMDA receptors (Schwieler, Engberg, & Erhardt, 2004). This makes sense because some current studies are looking to NMDA

TABLE 7.7 Mechanisms of Action of Clozapine

Receptor	Action	Strength of Action
Dopamine 4	Antagonist (blocks receptor, most DA antagonism here)	Weak
Dopamine 1	Antagonist (blocks receptor)	Weak
Dopamine 2	Antagonist (blocks receptor)	Weak
Dopamine 3	Antagonist (blocks receptor)	Weak
5-HT2	Antagonist (blocks receptor)	Strong
5-HT2C	Antagonist (blocks receptor)	Strong
5-HT3	Antagonist (blocks receptor)	Strong
Histamine	Antagonist (blocks receptor)	Unknown
Ach	Antagonist (blocks receptor)	Unknown
Adrenergic	Antagonist (blocks receptor)	Unknown

© Cengage Learning®

antagonists to treat both schizophrenia and Bipolar I Disorder (Javitt, 2010). Schatzberg et al. (1997) remind us that clozapine/Clozaril, although an exciting development, is not a panacea. They warn, "The drug does have problems and dangers, it does not work for everyone, and patients who are helped substantially may still be far from well" (p. 157). With those cautions in mind, we turn now to the side effects of clozapine/Clozaril.

Clozapine/Clozaril Side Effects

We cover the more common side effects of clozapine/Clozaril here. Those seeking a more elaborate discussion, including rare side effects, should see Perry et al. (2006) or Pies (2005).

Agranulocytosis

The most potentially dangerous side effect of clozapine/Clozaril is agranulocytosis. This hematologic (related to blood-performing organs) side effect causes white blood cell (WBC) count to drop dramatically in about 1.2% of treated patients. In a sense, this problem is related to the normal functioning of the immune system. In such cases, the clozapine/Clozaril molecule attaches to the

white blood cells, which the body then mistakenly interprets as foreign substances and discards. Mounting evidence suggests that people who develop agranulocytosis have a genetic predisposition to it. After clozapine has been around for more than one generation of clients to receive it, researchers will likely know more about this disposition. Approximately half of the clients quit taking clozapine/Clozaril because of this hematological side effect (Davis, Fuller, Strauss, Konicki, & Jaskiw, 2013).

The first reports of agranulocytosis came from Finland in 1975, where 13 trial subjects had the reaction and 8 died from resulting secondary infection. Of the 73 agranulocytosis cases reported in the United States, 84% occurred in the first 3 months of treatment, 12% between 3 and 6 months, and the remaining 4% after 6 months. So the longer clients tolerate the drug, the less likely they are to develop agranulocytosis (Pisciotta, 1992). Clients must be monitored closely, though, and the manufacturer (Novartis Pharmaceuticals) mandates a weekly white blood cell count for the first six weeks. If all goes well, the monitoring is every four weeks. This mandate is based on the hope that the white

TABLE 7.8 Common Side Effects of Clozapine

Type	*Side Effect*	*Proposed Cause*
Hematologic	Agranulocytosis	Potentially lethal drop in white blood cell count related to drug binding to white blood cells and immune system response
Autonomic	Constipation Hypersalivation Nausea/vomiting Syncope	Likely caused by anticholinergic and antiadrenergic properties
Cardiovascular	Hypertension Hypotension ECG changes	Possibly caused by antiadrenergic properties
Metabolic	Weight gain	Possibly caused by antihistaminic and antiserotonergic properties
Neurologic	Delirium Seizures	Rarer effect caused by anticholinergic properties Mechanism not known
Psychiatric	OC symptoms	Possibly caused by antiserotonergic properties
Sexual dysfunction	Anorgasmia Impotence Priapism Decreased libido	Possibly caused by antiadrenergic or anticholinergic properties
Other CNS effects	Problems with temperature regulation	Mechanism not known

© Cengage Learning®

blood cell decrease is gradual and that therefore advance warning is possible. All patients must be cleared through a national registry (the Clozaril Patient Management System, at http://www.cloza-pineregistry.com/faq.aspx.), and the doctor and pharmacy are responsible for making blood counts as long as the patient is on the medication. Most patients stay on between 200 and 350 mg per day. Despite these precautions, 12 fatalities had occurred by 1994, with 5 of these people dying despite drug discontinuation. A baseline white blood cell count must be obtained before the first dose is given, and the cell count must be 3500/mm or higher. If the WBC falls below 3000, clozapine/Clozaril should be discontinued and never given again. The client should also be admitted to a hospital for observation. Table 7.8 lists the side effects of clozapine/Clozaril, drawn from Perry et al. (2006).

A final note, more recently (Shuman, Trgoboff, Demler, & Opler, 2014) several studies have been reviewed that point to certain drug classes, in combination with clozapine/Clozaril, increase the chance of hematological adverse side effects. Autonomic agents like asthma medications, anti-infective agents like antiviral medications or antibiotics, proton-pump inhibitors that decrease gastric acid and other drugs for the gastrointestinal system are all correlated with an increase in hematological side effects.

Although nonmedical mental health professionals do not prescribe medications, it is important that they know of these potential adverse effects so they can advocate for the client if necessary. Clozapine/Clozaril is still the least prescribed atypical antipsychotic because of all the blood monitoring that is necessary.

Autonomic Side Effects of Clozapine

Autonomic side effects result from the antiadrenergic and anticholinergic actions of clozapine/Clozaril. These include constipation, hypersalivation, nausea/vomiting, and syncope (fainting or passing out). For some clients, the constipation may be severe. Dosage reduction, increased exercise, and increased fluid intake may alleviate the problem. Hypersalivation is a still unexplained side effect that a significant percentage of clients experience (Hodge & Jespersen, 2008; Perry et al., 2006). This typically manifests as excessive drooling at night but may include gagging. Although this decreases over the first two to three months, it will likely persist at some level. Clinicians have treated this with anticholinergic medications and some patients have sought out Chinese herbal medicines but there is no consensus on how to treat this (Essali et al., 2013). Other clinicians try to help clients adjust by sleeping with a towel on their pillow. This latter solution was in fact preferred in the case of Bonnie, given earlier. Although Bonnie was bothered by the salivation, she did not want to take any additional medications—and who could blame her?

Nausea and vomiting may occur after weeks or months of treatment, because there are large numbers of serotonin receptors in the gut that the drug affects, but the exact etiology is still unclear. Taking the medicine with food may help some clients. Syncope is a transient loss of muscle tone that may be localized or more general leading to unconsciousness. It appears dosage related, and reducing dosage may solve the problem.

Cardiovascular Side Effects

Cardiovascular side effects may range from hypertension to hypotension and tachycardia. Hypotension is more often reported (11 to 13% of clients) than hypertension (4% of clients). Although dosage reduction may alleviate both symptoms, tolerance to the hypotensive side effects usually develops within a month (Perry et al., 2006). As for tachycardia, the client may experience an increase in heart rate of 20 to 25 beats per minute. Onset is usually within a week of starting clozapine/Clozaril, and although the symptom may decrease, it rarely abates completely. Although other atypical antipsychotics can cause QTc interval problems, clozapine does not seem to be among them (Grande, Pons, Baeza, Torras, & Bernardo, 2011). The QTc interval is the measure of the time between the start of the "Q" wave and the end of the "T" wave in the heart's electrical cycle (the "c" stands for "correction"). This represents electrical depolarization and repolarization of the ventricles. A lengthened QTc interval is a marker for torsades de pointes (ventricular tachycardia) that can cause sudden death. We will say more about this below in discussing other atypicals.

Metabolic

The most problematic metabolic side effect is weight gain, with clients gaining between 9 and 25 pounds on average. This is problematic to both patients and doctors as the weight gain can then lead to the onset of type II diabetes (Hodge & Jespersen, 2008). Males gain more weight than females and the weight gain seems to happen in three stages suggesting different underlying neural mechanisms (Pai, Deng, Vella, Castle, & Huang, 2012). The first stage is an initial period from baseline to 3 months, the second a steady increase between 3 and 18 months and the third a plateau after this point (Pai et al., 2012). The side effect is thought to be due to antihistaminic and antiserotonergic mechanisms of action in clozapine. In a retrospective analysis of weight gain across several different atypical antipsychotics, Wirshing et al. (1999) concluded that weight gain associated with clozapine/Clozaril tended to be most persistent. In the case described earlier, Bonnie gained a total of 30 pounds over two years of clozapine/Clozaril treatment. She was close to her ideal weight at the start of treatment, and this side effect troubled her. She did not want to discontinue the medication, although.

Neurological Side Effects

Of the neurological side effects in Table 7.8, the one of greatest concern is seizures. Grand mal seizures can occur in patients on high dosages. The maximum dosage is 900 mg a day. Approximately 5% of clients receiving between 600 and 900 mg suffer from seizures, about 3% of those receiving dosages between 300 and 600 mg develop seizures, and some 1% of those receiving up to 300 mg develop seizures (Perry et al., 2006). If seizures occur, discontinue clozapine/Clozaril until the patient has a normal neurological exam. If the neurological exam is normal, clozapine/Clozaril can be reintroduced at 50% the original dose. Sometimes anticonvulsant medication can be used with clozapine to preclude further seizures.

Extrapyramidal Side Effects

As noted, clozapine/Clozaril is associated with a low incidence of severe EPSs. Approximately 3% of clients experience muscular rigidity or tremor, and approximately 6% develop akathisia. There have been no reports of dystonias or late-onset EPSs.

In general, Damkier, Lublin and Taylor (2011) wrote that optimizing clozapine/Clozaril treatment, in addition to watching for the adverse events described here, requires the following:

- Working together with the patient and the family to monitor therapeutic and side effects
- Keeping plasma levels above 350–420 ng/mL in a period of at least 12 weeks to gauge responsiveness
- Augmenting clozapine/Clozaril with Lamictal/lamotrigene, ECT, or another antipsychotic if the response is partial
- Diminishing side effects by reducing the dose when possible
- If reducing the dosage relieves side effects but interferes with main effects try adding another antipsychotic medication

Review Questions

- Given that clozapine/Clozaril is the first "atypical antipsychotic," what is it that makes it "atypical" compared to neuroleptics?
- What are the primary mechanisms of action and side effects of clozapine/Clozaril?
- Which side effect is potentially lethal and how is it monitored?
- What are potential drug–drug interactions that may be dangerous for people taking clozapine/Clozaril?

SECTION FIVE: THE SEROTONIN/ DOPAMINE ANTAGONISTS

Learning Objectives

- Understand what the differences are between the different SDAs. Are they unique or are they "me too" drugs?
- Know what the common side effects are across the SDAs.
- Understand the problem with QTc intervals and why Serlect/sertindole was taken off the market.

Despite its side effects, clozapine/Clozaril shifted the momentum of antipsychotic research. Starting with the introduction of chlorpromazine/Thorazine in 1952 and the dopamine hypothesis of schizophrenia, there was little research on how to treat clients who did not respond to neuroleptic medication (Lopez-Munoz, Alamo, Rubio, & Cuenca, 2004). The creation and introduction of clozapine ushered in a new research direction in antipsychotics. Whereas researchers up to this point had focused on antihistamines and dopamine antagonists, clozapine/Clozaril raised a new possibility, which was that some combination of serotonin balanced against dopamine antagonism would have an antipsychotic effect. Further, this approach held much more promise for impacting both positive and negative symptoms. Serotonin dopamine antagonists (SDAs) have been developed in the hopes of maximizing therapeutic benefits. Since clozapine's/Clozaril's U.S. release in 1989, several drugs have been developed that to differing degrees are intended to balance serotonin against dopamine antagonism. SDAs are atypical antipsychotics patterned after clozapine/Clozaril.

Another way to view this mechanism is by looking at relative percentages of antagonism of various receptors (Stahl, 2013). With therapeutic doses of neuroleptic agents, 70 to 90% of D2 receptors are blocked with little (if any) blockage of serotonin receptors. With therapeutic doses of clozapine, only 30 to 60% of D2 receptors are blocked, whereas 85 to 90% of serotonin receptors are blocked. SDAs fall midway on the range, with 30 to 50% of D2 receptors blocked and 60% of 5-HT receptors blocked. As noted above, it is still assumed that some D2 blockage is necessary to get an antipsychotic effect but it can be transitory blocking rather than longer term blocking.

The primary goal for side effects has been to eradicate the risk of agranulocytosis. Many new atypical medications have been developed that are "clozapine/Clozaril-like" without causing agranulocytosis. Note that although these agents appear generally just as effective as neuroleptics, they are not as effective as clozapine/Clozaril. Although many clients prefer the side effect profiles of the newer drugs, others seem to prefer the neuroleptics (Jones et al., 2006; Lieberman et al., 2005). Table 7.9 lists the SDA antipsychotics.

The Specter of Side Effects

Before exploring the individual SDA compounds, we want to emphasize that the primary problems driving this research were the lack of EPSs in clozapine/Clozaril and the presence of agranulocytosis in clozapine/Clozaril. The underlying theme of these forces was legal liability. With this liability in mind, apparently the most problematic side effect with the SDAs is related to a cardiac process called the *QTc interval*. The QTc interval is the length of time the heart's natural pacemaker (the sinuatrial node) ventricles need to electrically discharge and repolarize. The sinuatrial node is impulse-generating tissue and

TABLE 7.9 Atypical (Second Generation) Antipsychotics

Generic Name	Brand Name	Date Released
Risperidone	Risperdal	1994
Risperidone Consta	Risperdal	2003
Risperidone M-Tab	Risperdal M-Tab	2003
Olanzapine	Zyprexa	1996
Olanzapine & fluoxetine	Symbyax	2006
Paliperidone	Invega	2009
Paliperidone	Invega Sustenna	2009
asenapine	Saphris	2009
Sertindole	Serlect	1997
Quetiapine	Seroquel	1998
Ziprasidone	Geodon	2001
Ziprasidone Intra Muscular	Geodon	2002
Amisulpride	Solian (in Europe)	1997
iloperidone	Fanapt	2009
Lurasidone	Latuda	2010
Aripiprazole	Abilify	2002

© 2015 Cengage Learning®

prolonging its QTc interval can cause cardiac arrhythmia, including a potentially serious condition called *torsades de pointes (TdP)* and sudden death. The antihistamine Terfenadine/Seldane had a similar effect and was therefore taken off the market. This effect also caused drug regulation authorities in the United Kingdom and United States to pull the SDA sertindole (sertindole/Serlect) off the market between 1999 and 2001. After postmarket analyses it was relaunched in Europe in 2005, a move the FDA strongly disagreed with (Pae, 2013).

Healy (2002) notes that many other antipsychotics, including neuroleptics, have this side effect, which came to light when Paul Leber of the FDA had experts testify on both sides of the argument. Presently the drugs with the most profound effects on QTc interval are contraindicated in patients with cardiac conditions, but as with all newer drugs, only time will tell how significant this potential side effect is. It is also important to understand that other drugs may contribute to QTc prolongation and that these medications are contraindicated with sertindole (Table 7.10). The side effect is also present to a lesser degree in neuroleptics, antidepressants, stimulants, and anxiolytics (Advokat et al., 2014). Mental health clinicians should check with prescribing professionals for more information about drug–drug interactions related to QTc prolongation. An overview of QTc can be found at http://www.sads.org/, a website devoted to sudden arrhythmia death syndromes.

In addition to the problems with QTc prolongation, atypical antipsychotics are now clearly linked to an increased risk for type 2 diabetes and other metabolic problems (Lebovitz, 2003). People taking certain atypical antipsychotics (clozapine/Clozaril, olanzapine/Zyprexa, and quetiapine/Seroquel but not risperidone/Risperdal) are almost 15% more likely to develop adult-onset (type 2) diabetes than those taking neuroleptics (Newcomer, 2005). The American Diabetes Association and the America Psychiatric Association have recommended clients on these medications have blood drawn and tested for insulin resistance every 6–12 months. Liberty, Todder, Umansky, and Harman-Boehm (2004); Lindenmayer and Patel (1999); and Goldstein et al. (1999) noted that the use of atypical agents is associated with increased risk of diabetes and diabetic **ketoacidosis** in adults. Koller, Cross, and Schneider (2004) have reported the same problem in pediatric populations. Liberty et al. (2004) and Lebovitz (2003) recommend screening patients for risks associated with the disorder prior to putting them on an atypical antipsychotic regimen, and then monitoring them closely. In September 2003, the FDA requested that manufacturers of atypical antipsychotics update their product information labeling to contain additional information about diabetes and hypoglycemia.

TABLE 7.10 Common Side Effects Associated With Sertindole

Type	Description	Percentage of Patients
Autonomic	Dry mouth, decreased ejaculatory volume	Unknown
Cardiovascular	Prolonged QTc interval Hypotension, dizziness	Unknown Unknown
Hematologic	None noted at this point	
Hepatic	None noted at this point	
Metabolic	Weight gain of 5% body weight May be associated with increased risk of diabetes	Unknown
Endocrinologic	Minor, short-term prolactin increase	Unknown
Gastrointestinal	None noted at this point	
Neurologic	None noted at this point	
Respiratory	Rhinitis (nasal congestion)	Unknown

© Cengage Learning®

Currently researchers are trying to sort out how much increased risk users of atypical antipsychotics may have for developing diabetes or hyperglycemia and what the mechanisms of this risk may be. It is also important to sort out this risk from the increased incidence of diabetes and hyperglycemia in the general population (Brown University Psychopharmacology Update, 2003). One study comparing the risk in olanzapine/Zyprexa versus risperidone/Risperdal found that cases of patients on olanzapine/Zyprexa seem associated with significantly higher risk of medication-related diabetes (Fuller, Shermock, Secic, & Grogg, 2003). Alas, whereas researchers once believed that moving from neuroleptic antipsychotic medications to atypical antipsychotic medications resulted in fewer medical complications and higher quality of client life, that conclusion seems ill-founded (Abidi & Bhaskara, 2003).

Risperidone/Risperdal

Risperidone/Risperdal was the second atypical or second generation antipsychotic introduced in 1994. It was called a "novel" antipsychotic (Perry et al., 2006) because at low doses it does not cause EPSs but does at higher doses. This reversal arises because its dopamine antagonism is far greater than that of clozapine/Clozaril. On the positive side, it is not associated with agranulocytosis. There is a long-acting, injectable formulation of risperidone/Risperdal (Resperdal Consta) now and the oral formulation is now generic. The injectable, long-acting form of risperidone/Risperdal appears efficacious and well tolerated (Kane et al., 2003). Compared to clozapine/Clozaril, risperidone/Risperdal seems slightly less effective, although these studies also show mixed results (Perry et al., 2006). Stahl (2013) notes that risperidone/Risperdal has a far simpler pharmacologic profile than clozapine/Clozaril but still seems to decrease positive and negative symptoms.

There are some EPSs with risperidone/Risperdal, particularly at higher doses. Although risperidone/Risperdal does not block histamine or acetylcholine receptors, some weight gain is still associated with it but only about half as much as

other second generation antipsychotics like olanzapine/Zyprexa and quetiapine/Seroquel. Because the SDA side effects can vary we include tables of the side effects for each SDA. Table 7.11 summarizes the side effects associated with risperidone/Risperdal. An active metabolite of risperidone (9-hydroxy-risperidone) was synthesized and approved in 2006 as paliperidone/Invega. It is more effective than placebo and (not surprisingly) has a side effect profile similar to risperidone/Risperdal. In 2009, the FDA approved a parenteral formulation of paliperidone/Invega called Invega Sustaenna/paliperidone palmitate for the treatment of acute schizophrenia and for treatment in the maintenance phase. Risperidone/Risperdal is also approved for the maintenance phase of Bipolar I Disorder as a monotherapy or an adjunctive therapy to lithium/Lithobid or valproate/Divalproex. It is also indicated for treating irritability in individuals diagnosed with Autism.

Olanzapine/Zyprexa

Olanzapine/Zyprexa was approved in 1996. It has on-label approval to treat schizophrenia bipolar disorder with mixed or manic specifiers as well as the maintenance phase of Bipolar I Disorder.

When compared in clinical trials, olanzapine/Zyprexa performs as well as haloperidol/Haldol without EPS but with weight gain. As doses increase so does the blockade of D2 receptors. We do not yet have much data comparing olanzapine/Zyprexa with clozapine/Clozaril. Olanzapine/Zyprexa has a chemical structure similar to clozapine but is different from both clozapine/Clozaril and risperidone/Risperdal. This unique structure differs enough from both the latter compounds as to have neither agranulocytosis nor short-term EPSs associated with it. There is a very low incidence of tardive dyskinesia with long-term use. Olanzapine/Zyprexa is not as sedating as clozapine/Clozaril but is associated with weight gain. A parenteral formulation of olanzapine (Zyprexa Relprevv) was approved in 2009. There is a post-injection delirium/sedation syndrome (PDSS) so patients must be under observation for three hours after injection and have someone with them when they leave the facility

TABLE 7.11 Common Side Effects Associated With Risperidone

Type	Description	Percentage of Patients
Autonomic	None noted	
Cardiovascular	Prolonged QTc interval	Unknown
	Hypotension, dizziness	10%
Hematologic	None noted, no agranulocytosis	
Hepatic	None noted, no monitoring necessary	
Metabolic	Weight gain of 7% body weight	18%
	Increased risk of diabetes	
Endocrinologic	Increased prolactin levels	Unknown
Gastrointestinal	Nausea	18%
Neurological	Agitation/anxiety	58%
Early-onset EPS	Dose related	
Tardive dyskinesia	Dose related	
Neuroleptic malignant syndrome	2 cases noted by 1997	
Respiratory	Rhinitis (nasal congestion)	Approx. 9%
Other	Headache	16%
	Insomnia	54–58%
	Sedation	Approx. 9%

© Cengage Learning®

where they got the injection (Advokat et al., 2014). Table 7.12 outlines the common side effects for olanzapine.

Quetiapine/Seroquel

Quetiapine/Seroquel has a chemical structure similar to clozapine/Clozaril but has some atypical advantages. First, it appears to be associated with no prolactin increases nor EPSs. It is approved for use in the maintenance treatment of schizophrenia, the manic phase of bipolar disorder and can but used adjunctively in major depressive disorder and Bipolar I disorder. As with other SDAs, the goal with quetiapine/Seroquel was to have the therapeutic effects of clozapine/Clozaril without the agranulocytosis. At this point quetiapine/Seroquel is not associated with agranulocytosis. It has a half-life of about seven hours, which may necessitate dosing two to three times a day. In 2007, extended release versions of quetiapine/Seroquel were approved. Table 7.13 details the side effect profile for quetiapine/Seroquel. It should be noted that Advokat et al. (2014) commented that quetiapine/Seroquel has been used inappropriately to promote sleep in settings like prisons and we have seen this in many foster care homes. This drug also can disrupt the QTc interval so should only be used under the closest supervision. Others have criticized quetiapine/Seroquel as a largely "me too" drug (Prescrier International, 2011) because in

TABLE 7.12 Common Side Effects Associated With Olanzapine

Type	Description	Percentage of Patients
Autonomic	Constipation, dry mouth	Approx. 8%
Cardiovascular	Minor changes in blood pressure	Unknown
Hematologic	None noted, no agranulocytosis	
Hepatic	Minor changes in enzyme levels	Unknown
Metabolic	Weight gain Increased risk of diabetes	Unknown
Endocrinologic	Increased prolactin levels	Unknown
Neurologic	Early-onset EPS	Dose related
Tardive dyskinesia	Unknown	
Neuroleptic malignant syndrome	No cases known	
Other	Sedation	26%

© Cengage Learning®

TABLE 7.13 Common Side Effects Associated With Quetiapine

Type	Description	Percentage of Patients
Autonomic	Constipation, dry mouth	Approx. 6%
Cardiovascular	Prolonged QTc interval Dizziness Orthostatic hypotension Tachycardia	None noted Approx. 7% Approx. 6% Approx. 4%
Hematologic	None noted at this point	
Hepatic	None noted at this point	
Metabolic	Weight gain	None noted
Endocrinologic	Prolactin increase	Rare
Gastrointestinal	Dyspepsia	Approx. 4%
Neurologic	None noted at this point	
Respiratory	Rhinitis (nasal congestion)	Unknown
Other	Sedation Priapism	18% Rare

© Cengage Learning®

two large-scale meta-analyses, it has not shown therapeutic advantage over other treatments.

Ziprasidone/Geodon

Ziprasidone/Geodon is the sixth atypical antipsychotic to be released. It was initially slated for release with the brand name of Zeldox but the FDA felt there were too many new drugs with brand names that began with "z," so it was released as Geodon. Like all other SDAs, ziprasidone/Geodon blocks a combination of dopamine and serotonin receptors. Unlike the other SDAs, ziprasidone/Geodon is an agonist of a particular serotonin receptor (the 5-HT1a receptor), giving it a buspirone/BuSpar-like action. Some feel this may make the drug useful for depressive symptoms as well (Dunner, 2007). As with the other SDAs, the most common side effects of ziprasidone/Geodon are sedation, nausea, constipation and/or diarrhea, dizziness, restlessness, respiratory congestion, and some uncontrollable movements such as tremor and shuffling. As with several other drugs in this category, clients need to be monitored for prolongation of QTc interval (Rivas-Vasquez, 2001). Ziprasidone/Geodon seems to induce less weight gain than olanzapine/Zyprexa but also does not seem as efficacious (Grooten et al., 2009). Ziprasidone/Geodon is also available in parenteral formulations beginning in 2003. Ziprasidone/Geodon is also associated with QTc interval prolongation. The following case demonstrates the effective use of ziprasidone/Geodon after a long and complex history with neuroleptics and their side effects.

THE CASE OF MELANIE

Melanie, a 16-year-old high school sophomore, was referred to a psychiatrist because she developed psychotic symptoms. She was very disorganized and suffered from visual, olfactory, and auditory hallucinations. She was first put on 25 mg of chlorpromazine/Thorazine, and she experienced an array of side effects, including severe postural hypotension. Melanie was taken off the chlorpromazine/Thorazine, and thiridazine/Mellaril at 25 mg was attempted, with

the same result. Even with benztropine/Cogentin, Melanie developed severe postural hypotension. This prevented her from working and going to school, because she was very lightheaded and fainted frequently. Therefore her psychiatrist switched her to first trifluoperazine/Stelazine and then haliperodol/Haldol, and with both Melanie developed akathisia with restlessness and pacing. She felt as if she was "crawling out of her skin." These side effects persisted even with trihexiphenidyl/Artane to combat this movement disorder.

After many trials she and her psychiatrist found she could tolerate perphenazine/Trilofon at 4 to 8 mg and up to her eventual stabilizing dose of 16 mg. Melanie stayed on the perphenazine/Trilafon for many years, with very good results. Her psychiatrist noted that during this time her organization improved. Although her course fluctuated, she was able to graduate from college, marry, and have a child while on the perphenazine/Trilafon; the child was born healthy. She became an effective K-6 teacher and mothered her child well. Later, she developed a severe tardive dystonia that affected her neck and back muscles, and she suffered incapacitating back spasms that hot baths or massages could not assuage. Gradually, she was taken off the only neuroleptic that helped her, perphenzine/Trilafon, which she had taken for 17 years.

After careful consideration and evaluation, her psychiatrist now put Melanie on quetiapine/Seroquel 400 mg, but she experienced a very serious relapse. This was her first psychotic break in over a decade, so for the time Melanie was put back on perphenzine/Trilafon and the dystonia (which never fully went away) worsened. Her psychiatrist also tried the SDAs risperidone/Risperdal and olanzapine/Zyprexa but both were too sedating. Then in June 2001 Melanie began a course of treatment with ziprasidone/Geodon, with great success. Her tardive dystonia is improving and although she cannot risk going off the medication to have another baby, Melanie is learning to cope with this limited sense of choice. Melanie had no drowsiness on ziprasidone/Geodon. Finally, she told her psychiatrist that her feelings were back and she was learning how to love.

This case reflects the efforts of a diligent and determined psychiatrist and a courageous patient. They addressed each medication and side effect dilemma as it arose and sought to provide options from among both the neuroleptic and the serotonin-dopamine antipsychotics. Issues from several perspectives were certainly addressed during the course of treatment. The most significant factor was that the quality of Melanie's life improved.

Review Questions

- What are the main differences between the different SDAs?
- What are the common side effects of the non-clozapine/Clozaril SDAs?
- What is QTc prolongation and why was sertindole/Serlect taken off the market?

SECTION SIX: NEWER AGENTS

Learning Objectives

- Understand how the newer agents compare to the atypical antipsychotics.
- Be able to critically examine adjunctive therapies like adding aripiprazole/Abilify to antidepressants.

Amisulpride/Solian

At the time of this writing, amisulpride/Solian is available in Europe and Australia. It is classified an atypical antipsychotic but is not an SDA. It is a specific antagonist for D2 and D3 receptors. At between 400 and 800 mg a day, amisulpride/Solian appears effective in treating schizophrenia but dosing has been a poor predictor of response with the drug (Bowskill, Patel, Handley, & Flanagan, 2012). Amisulpride/Solian is unique in that it has high specificity for blocking D2 and D3 receptors in the limbic system but not in other areas such as the basal ganglia. At low doses it blocks autoreceptors, but at high doses it shows postsynaptic antagonism. This increases DA action in the limbic

system at low doses and decreases DA action at high doses. The combination seems to result in low EPSs. In low doses, it also seems to alleviate depression and dysthymia but would not be subject to the same types of abuse as other dopaminergic compounds (such as amphetamines) (Danion, Rein, Fleurot, & the Amisulpride Study Group, 1999; McKeage & Plosker, 2004). In controlled studies, amisulpride has been associated with the following side effects: insomnia, anxiety, and agitation (5 to 10% of clients); sedation, constipation, nausea, vomiting, and dry mouth (2% of patients); and weight gain, acute dystonia, tardive dyskinesia, hypotension, and QTc prolongation. Amisulpride/Solian has also been associated with increased prolactin release. Researchers have recently concluded that amisulpride/Solian is equal in efficacy to risperidone/Risperdal and may surpass it in subsequent studies (Sechter et al., 2002). Researchers have tried treating fibromyalgia with amisulpride/Solian but it was poorly tolerated by study participants (Rico-Villademoros et al., 2012). As with any new drug, only time will tell whether this drug is contributing anything new or improved.

Lurasidone/Latuda

Lurasidone/Latuda was approved to treat schizophrenia in 2009 and bipolar depression in 2013 (Belmaker, 2014; Loebel et al., 2014). Lurasidone/Latuda is an antagonist of 5-HT2a, 5-HT7, 5-HT1a and D2 receptors (Awad et al., 2014). In many trials it is superior to placebo and as effective as olanzapine/Zyprexa. In other studies patients switched from their current antipsychotic to lurasidone showed improvements in self-reported health status (Awad et al., 2014). Side effects include some EPSs (Parkinsonism and akathisia), sedation, agitation and some nausea. It does not appear to affect QTc intervals.

Iloperidone/Fanapt

Iloperidone/Fanapt was approved in 2009 for the treatment of schizophrenia. It is considered a second-generation atypical antipsychotic whose primary mechanism of action is 5-HT2a and D2 antagonism (Weiden, 2012). It has greater binding capacity at the 5-HT2a receptor than the D2 receptor. It can cause mild QTc disruption and weight gain although it seems to produce lower EPS than haloperidol/Haldol or risperidone/Risperdal (Dargani & Malhotra, 2014). In a "switch study" conducted by Weiden et al. (2014), there were no significant differences in efficacy or safety/tolerability between iloperidone/Fanapt, risperidone/Risperdal, olanzapine/Zyprexa, and aripiprazole/Abilify (Rado & Janicak, 2014). Arif and Mitchell (2014) also noted that iloperidone/Fanapt lacks a clear benefit over other drugs for schizophrenia. Although early trials produced only modest results, later trials that used slower initial dosing found iloperidone/Fanapt to be equal to other non-clozapine/Clozaril antipsychotics (Rado & Janicak, 2014).

Asenapine/Saphris

Asenapine/Saphris was approved for the treatment of schizophrenia and manic or mixed specifiers for Bipolar I Disorder in 2009. It also was approved in 2010 as an adjunct to lithium or valproate for Bipolar I Disorder. It comes in a unique formulation of dissolving tabs that require no eating or drinking for 10 minutes after putting the tab in the mouth. The mechanism of action involves more receptors than most antipsychotics (other than clozapine/Clozaril). Advokat et al. (2014) note that it is chemically similar to the antidepressant mirtazapine/Remeron. It binds antagonistically to D1, D2, D3, D4, and D5 receptors, 5-HT2a, 5-HT2c, 5-HT1a, alpha-1 and H1 (histamine) receptors. According to Cortese, Bressan, Castle, and Mosolov (2013) asenapine/Saphris is effective in treating the positive symptoms of schizophrenia in acute situations and has **prophylactic** value. The most common side effects include dizziness, akathisia, and sedation. It is associated with weight gain but better than olanzapine/Zyprexa in this area (Kemp et al., 2014). In two 3-week trials, asenapine/Saphris was reported to lead to improvements in self-reported health-related quality of life (Michalak, Guiraud-Diawara, & Sapin, 2014). It should be noted that other studies from countries outside the United States are emerging in the literature suggesting that while all atypical antipsychotics may decrease psychotic symptoms, they may be

correlated with a decreased quality of life due to adverse effects that limit mobility as well as socioeconomic factors (de Araujo et al., 2014).

Aripiprazole/Abilify

Aripiprazole/Abilify is an antipsychotic that may open up yet another approach to treating the symptoms of schizophrenia. It has FDA approval for treating schizophrenia, the maintenance phase of Bipolar I Disorder, as an adjunctive treatment for depression, and for irritability associated with Autism Spectrum Disorders. It is sometimes said to be the first third-generation antipsychotic (neuroleptics being the first generation and atypicals being the second). It was approved in 2002 and presents us with yet another set of mechanisms of action. It appears to be a potent partial agonist of D2 receptors, a partial agonist of 5-HT1a receptors, and an antagonist of 5-HT2a receptors (Dhillon, 2012). These studies indicate that it is better than haloperidol/Haldol at treating positive and negative symptoms as well as having fewer side effects. Bristol-Myers Squibb filed a regulatory application with the FDA, and the drug was approved in November 2002 (Barclay, 2002). Aripiprazole/Abilify is available in oral and parenteral formulations. In 2007, the FDA approved aripiprazole as an "add-on" drug for depression (Rosen, 2007).

Stahl (quoted in Manisses Corporation, 2002) stated that aripiprazole/Abilify belongs to a class of drugs called *dopamine system stabilizers* although we would contend that until the dopamine system has conclusively proven to be "unstable" in patients with schizophrenia or Bipolar I Disorder, the phrase dopamine system stabilizer may be more marketing than clinical reality. Aripiprazole/Abilify seems to have a decent side effect profile, and does not seem to cause QTc prolongation but can cause weight gain, tardive dyskinesia, neuroleptic malignant syndrome and hyperglycemia (prescribing information at http://www.drugs.com/pro/abilify.html). In 2007, aripiprazole was approved as an adjunctive treatment for depression in adults if the antidepressant did not seem to be working. This was based on two studies that lasted six weeks with 743 patients whose depression had not lifted despite the fact they were taking an antidepressant (Hellerstein et al., 2008; Nelson et al., 2010).

This particular use of aripiprazole/Abilify seems odd to us. First of all to use a powerful, expensive antipsychotic drug with possibly serious side effects for nonpsychotic depression does not make sense in a risk–benefit analysis. Why not increase the antidepressant dose, add another antidepressant or change antidepressants altogether (Reidbord, 2009)? This points to pharmacoeconomic gains more than therapeutic gains. Antipsychotic drugs are increasingly being used for mild mood disorders and insomnia. We should be rightfully alarmed that prescriptions for antipsychotics increased from 28 million in 2001 to 54 million in 2008. Also, the use of these drugs for off-label indications doubled between 1995 and 2008. It is probably no coincidence that money pharmaceutical companies spent advertising antipsychotics increased from $1.3 billion in 2007 to $2.24 billion in 2010 (Friedman, 2012). From an integrative perspective this adjunctive practice seems highly questionable.

Review Questions

- How do newer agents like aripiprazole compare to the atypical antipsychotics like olanzapine?
- What are some problems in the risk–benefit analysis of adjunctive therapies like adding aripiprazole/Abilify to antidepressants.

SECTION SEVEN: FOCUS ON OTHER PERSPECTIVES

Learning Objectives

- Practice empathizing with the experience of people suffering from schizophrenia.
- Understand how stigma interferes with medication adherence.
- Be able to discuss how advocacy is even more important based on what we know about pharmacoeconomics.

PSYCHOLOGICAL CONSIDERATIONS

What is it like to experience psychotic symptoms? One of our clients told us that to suffer from schizophrenia was to suffer from interminable boredom. This client knew what it felt like to be intellectually and interpersonally engaged and knew what her symptoms were robbing her of. Her treatment with olanzapine/Zyprexa was an important part of her recovery, and her psychotherapy was another crucial component. Another client spoke of his experience in terms of stark terror. He was plagued by voices he felt sure were demonic in origin, and he was convinced his very soul would not survive his ordeal. For this client, a series of seven antipsychotic medications were tried, with only minimal success. Counseling with an ego-strengthening focus helped this client retain some quality of life. We note these narratives because we have encountered clinicians who thought people with psychotic disorders could not benefit from counseling or psychotherapy. Quite to the contrary, such clients are unlikely to improve much if only treated with medication.

Sayre (2000) examined clients' perceptions of their symptoms. Their perceptions fell into five distinct themes, summarized in Table 7.14.

Regardless of the extent to which one agrees with the ultimate truth of each conclusion, each theme obviously opens a gateway for counseling and

TABLE 7.14 How Clients Understand Their Symptoms, by Theme

Theme	My symptoms are ...
Disease	... the result of a brain disease
Psychology	... related to my personality and behaviors
Crisis	... the result of a trauma or crisis
Ordination	... a sign of significance or special power
Punishment	... a punishment for past behavior

© Cengage Learning®

psychotherapy. When a client with psychotic symptoms can make psychological contact, it is crucial that a trained therapist begin establishing a relationship with the person so that when able to use it, that person has access to therapy that will help him or her through the psychological realm. The type of therapy employed will vary with the developmental level of the client. Many clients with psychotic disorders are struggling with establishing adequate ego functioning, and counseling them should focus on ego-strengthening techniques. Some clients who have adequate ego functioning may be struggling with transpersonal development. These clients are likely a minority, but they do exist, and several clinicians have offered guidelines for working with them (Grof, 1998, 2000; Lukoff, Lu, & Turner, 1996).

In addition Seeman and Seeman (2012) reviewed publications in three databases between 2001 and 2012 looking for studies about clients' attitudes toward taking medication. They found about 60 studies relevant to their goal of understanding these attitudes. Themes extracted from these papers fell into three main themes. The first was control by medication and of medication where many felt under the control of the medication and wanted more control over their medication regimen. The second theme was a sense of dependence on the medication and prescriber. This was often a negative attitude as they felt it restricted their lives. Finally, the third theme was stigma from using antipsychotic medication. Nonmedical mental health therapists need to listen for such theme as they relate to adherence.

Lauriello, Lenroot, and Bustillo (2003) provided an overview of some of the counseling approaches that have shown success with clients suffering from schizophrenia. Although the studies reviewed did not favor psychodynamic approaches, they found that personal therapy, cognitive behavioral therapy, social skills training, and family therapy all had some support in the literature. In addition to vocational and job coaching, these treatments are an important part of an overall treatment plan and have been shown to decrease the number of hospitalizations that clients experience (Bichsell, 2001; Fenton & McGlashon, 1997)

In the spirit of an integrative approach, it is also important to note that clients who have significant improvements on atypical antipsychotics may also suffer psychological sequelae. Weiden, Aquila, and Standard (1996) point to clients experiencing "awakenings" phenomena, in which their improvement allows them to be more in touch with their losses and psychological pain. Weiden et al. (1996) concluded that the long-term psychological issues many clients must deal with include changes in self-image, sexuality, and intimacy concerns. That such researchers are addressing these issues alongside medication management is encouraging and leads us to our discussion of counseling and psychotherapy with clients who are suffering from schizophrenia.

Dealing With Ambivalence About Taking Medication

Clinicians encounter many clients who are ambivalent about taking medication that is going to cause them severe side effects. Even though the newer medications hold promise for allowing clients to regain a great deal of functioning, there is no getting around the side effects of weight gain, potentially fatal blood disorders, the risk of diabetes, and annoying side effects such as hypersalivation. The most important thing (as in any form of counseling or psychotherapy) is the quality of the therapeutic alliance. Counselors who have a good relationship with the client and client's family (or caregivers) know the client's personality, the client's values, and the client's degree of insight and the extent to which symptoms are impairing their ability to function.

Although not a unitary concept, insight assessment is possible and to a large extent depends on the qualities of the therapeutic alliance just listed. Insight includes awareness of the illness, relabeling of symptoms and treatment compliance (Chan et al., 2014; Konstantakopoulos et al., 2014) and is highly correlated with cognitive functioning (Ouzir, Azorin, Adida, Boussaoud, & Battas, 2012). We are also learning that although only a minority of people with schizophrenia act out violently, the more insight the client has the more easily clinicians can predict (and head off) violent outbursts (Ekinci & Ekinci, 2013). David and Kemp (1997) summarized five psychological barriers to insight. The first two are psychopathology and cognitive deficits. Both interfere with the abstract reasoning processes that are necessary to have a sense of how others are experiencing you. If these deficits are a result of symptoms and medication reduces the symptoms, then after the deficits have been addressed clinicians can work with the client. The third and fourth barriers to insight are ego defense mechanisms and aspects of personality. Assuming the client can make psychological contact, these can be handled within the context of the therapeutic relationship. The last barrier to insight is culturally and socially determined attitudes, which may be intricately woven together with ego defenses and aspects of personality. Ideally, an integrative assessment will take these social and cultural attitudes into account. When consciously acknowledged by the clinician, they can be worked with in the counseling relationship.

Issues from the Cultural Perspective

The Culture of Stigma

Perhaps the most prominent issue from the cultural perspective is stigma (Seeman & Seeman, 2012). The idea of suffering from a mental/emotional disorder still carries the belief, shared by many, that the afflicted person is somehow "defective," not equal to others in the eyes of society, and, in some cases, even being justly punished by whatever god there may be. Although the United States and other countries have made strides in addressing this through education, advocacy, and community action, stigma still persists (Corrigan et al., 2000; Penn & Corrigan, 2002; Schreiber & Hartrick, 2002). In our brief historical outline of the antipsychotics, you saw how when the first neuroleptics were leading to deinstitutionalization of recovering clients, towns lobbied hospitals with petitions to keep the recovering people behind hospital walls (Healy, 2002).

In some societies a stigma is equally associated with the use of psychotropic medications. Jorm (2000) detailed a study in which many people expressed negative beliefs about medication for mental health disorders, although they favored medication for physical disorders. As we have argued in this book, a healthy skepticism about what medications can and cannot provide is important; however, negative beliefs about medication can also develop into negative beliefs about people who choose to take such medications. This is where mental health clinicians can intervene with advocacy and education. It should be noted that a recent study also commented on stigmatization of individuals receiving psychotherapy. The perspectives of mental health consumers reflected in the study is that they are portrayed particularly negatively in the media. The researcher in this case felt that this stigma may prevent people from seeking help in the first place (Ben-Porath, 2002).

The issue of stigma is particularly pronounced in severe disorders such as schizophrenia. Positive and negative symptoms of schizophrenia severely decrease clients' quality of life by decreasing their social interactions or the receptivity of others to interacting with them. Add the severe extrapyramidal side effects associated with neuroleptic medications, and the problem is unnecessarily compounded. We say "unnecessarily" because more and more clinicians are advocating the atypical antipsychotics as a first line of treatment. It is important for mental health clinicians to participate in this advocacy. Assuming a client is willing to take a medication to deal with the life-disrupting symptoms of schizophrenia, that client deserves every opportunity to be given the most effective agent with the fewest side effects. At this point, clozapine/Clozaril is still reserved for treatment-refractory clients, because of the risk of agranulocytosis. However, the SDAs (olanzapine/Zyprexa in particular) may be excellent first-line medical treatments for schizophrenia (Psychlink, 1998). As most clinicians are aware, the lives of many people with schizophrenia have been so disrupted by their symptoms that they frequently lack financial resources such as health insurance. Many of these clients receive Medicaid or Social Security disability. Therefore, those responsible for paying for treatment may balk at the cost. Advocacy must be directed to these payers, which takes us next to the social issues.

Social Issues

Pharmacoeconomics

Perhaps the most important obstacle to the widespread adoption of atypical antipsychotics is cost. Pharmacoeconomics is an area of which mental health clinicians need to be aware (van Luijn, 2012). Ernst et al. (2000) found that physicians often do not know the cost of generic and brand name medications. Even when they do know the cost of generic versus brand name, some studies show it does not affect prescribing habits (Polinski et al., 2008) especially when prescribers have negative views of the generics (Shrank et al., 2011). Bearing in mind that over a 12-year period a new drug may cost $400 million to $500 million to bring to market, the costs of newer agents are going to be substantially more than older ones. Brand-label atypical antipsychotics cost approximately eight times what similar generic drugs cost. In 2014 in the United States, a 30-day supply of olanzapine costs approximately $392 and a 30-day supply of generic olanzapine/Zyprexa is $12. A 30-day supply of clozapine is approximately $300 whereas generic clozapine/Clozaril is $34. There are always questions though about the equivalence of generic compounds (Lam, Ereshefsky, Toney, & Gonzales, 2001).

In the United States, the decisions about what drugs to use for Medicaid patients are made by state formulary boards, pharmacy committees, or state medical directors and pharmacy directors. In a 1998 video symposium (Psychlink, 1998), pharmacologist Larry Ereshefsky and psychiatrists Bill Glazer and Jay Fawver reviewed a protocol for lobbying state officials, which can be useful to mental health professionals. Depending on the regulatory agency and personnel involved, clinicians cannot assume that audiences for advocacy know about the symptoms of schizophrenia and so are advised to consider the following steps when advocating for atypical antipsychotics to be routinely available to indigent clients. This protocol can also be helpful in educating the public about the long-term benefits of allowing clients access to the atypical antipsychotics. One of the problems we run into is that high-cost medications are frequently targets of cost-containment.

Although only 1.1% of the population is thought to suffer from schizophrenia, 30% of those patients are on Medicaid. Since they were first introduced in the 1990s atypical antipsychotics have become the first line of treatment and accounted for 15% of all Medicaid spending in 2005. Since then Medicaid programs and Medicare Part D prescription programs require prior approval or some other restriction for at least one antipsychotic (Seabury et al., 2014). Because of the vulnerable nature of these patients disruption of medication routine can have adverse consequences. Seabury et al. (2014) estimated that restrictive formulary policies in 24 states studied resulted in a 2% point increase in the prison population due to more mentally ill people being arrested. This increased the nationwide prison population by 9920 prisoners and $362 in costs.

When advocating for formulary fairness, make sure the parties involved (whether a formulary board or the lay public) understand the positive and negative symptoms of schizophrenia. Next, explain the mechanism of D2 blockade and the severe side effects associated with it. A discussion of compliance is important, because many clients go off neuroleptic medications to avoid the severe side effects. Clinicians should then discuss how the newer atypical antipsychotics are more complex drugs than the neuroleptics, with multiple mechanisms of action. These more complex molecules are associated with better outcomes. It is also important to emphasize that each atypical is structurally different from the others, to preclude the assumption that one atypical is just as good as any other. Much like antibiotics, some clients respond to one atypical and not to another, so it is important that prescribing professionals have access to all of them.

Efficacy and Compliance

As we have documented here, the atypical antipsychotics appear to have at least equal efficacy on the overall symptoms and seem better tolerated than neuroleptics. Although the initial excitement over the atypicals was somewhat euphoric, more recent studies note that it may be time to tone down that excitement (Volavka et al., 2002). Still, clozapine/Clozaril and the SDAs seem to have better side effect profiles than do the neuroleptics and are at least as good as the neuroleptics at addressing the symptoms of schizophrenia. Although clinicians hoped as recently as 1998 that the atypicals would clearly improve quality of life and decrease suicidality, these hopes have yet to be consistently confirmed (Sernyak, Desai, Stolar, & Rosenheck, 2001). As far as compliance goes, clients do seem more likely to continue taking clozapine/Clozaril as opposed to haloperidol/Haldol, because clozapine/Clozaril offers greater symptom relief and reduced side effects (Rosenheck et al., 2000).

Whom Do We Trust?

A final note is called for as we end this long journey through the world of antipsychotic medications. Readers are likely aware that many issues remain unresolved about just how good the newer, atypical antipsychotics are. One variable that continues to play a role from an integrative perspective is the economic power of pharmaceutical companies. It is interesting that many of the initial studies that were optimistic about the revolution atypicals could bring about were funded by pharmaceutical companies and were short-term studies. One of the latest studies that suggests the initial response to the atypicals was too enthusiastic was sponsored by the National Institute of Mental Health, with only moderate funding from the pharmaceutical industry. We hope that through such independent, large-scale, long-term studies, the truth will be easier to pursue. Healy (2002) documented how Eli Lilly Pharmaceuticals recruited well-known figures from psychiatry beginning in the 1970s to conduct research and write papers. He connected this effort to meta-analyses on drug efficacy that have been written entirely by people on the pharmaceutical company payroll. One example is the meta-analysis on fluoxetine/Prozac that appeared in the *British Medical Journal* (Beasley et al., 1991), supposedly refuting the connection between fluoxetine/Prozac (a Lilly product) and suicide. It stated, "Until then, papers written solely by company personnel would never have been published in a leading journal like the *British Medical Journal*. This article cracked the dam that had separated the academic and commercial universities" (p. 263). That crack in the dam has unleashed a flood and we ask, where is that flood leading us?

More recently many pharmaceutical companies are paying increasingly expensive fines for things like unlawful marketing practices. In the first edition of this book, the largest criminal fraud settlement was when the Warner Lambert division of Parke Davis Pharmaceuticals paid $479 million for criminal fraud in promoting the off-label use of gabapentin/Neurotin for adolescents diagnosed with Bipolar I Disorder. In 2013 Johnson & Johnson agreed to pay $2 billion for unlawful marketing of risperidone/Risperdal and paliperidone/Invega. Johnson & Johnson's Janssen unit settled claims that marketed risperidone for children and the elderly without approval and that it paid kickbacks to physicians and to Omnicare Inc., the largest pharmacy for nursing homes (Bloomberg News, 2013). In addition Abbott Laboratories paid $1.5 billion to resolve criminal and civil investigations of the off-label use of valproic acid/Depakote (United States Department of Justice, 2012). Lawsuits such as these are actually leading some pharmaceutical companies to close their neuroscience divisions (Greenberg, 2013).

Review Questions

- What do you think makes it hard to empathize with the experience of people suffering from schizophrenia?

- How does stigma around schizophrenia interfere with medication adherence?

- Based on what you know about Pharmacoeconomics, what are some important advocacy issues for clients?

SUMMARY

Antipsychotics play a vital role in the treatment of severe mental and emotional disorders such as schizophrenia. Although there are many theories of how antipsychotics work, the jury is still out on what these medications tell us about the nature of schizophrenia and its etiology. Until recently, antipsychotic medications were basically all neuroleptic and worked through dopamine antagonism. The creation of clozapine/Clozaril and now the SDAs has opened a new avenue of treatment for schizophrenia and provided more options to clients with the disease. No drug can be taken without a cost and the newer antipsychotics are still associated with side effects. For the newer medications such as clozapine and the SDAs, there is a new concern about these medications inducing diabetes and other metabolic problems. Newer compounds such as aripiprazole will likely help us continue developing theories about the nature of schizophrenia. Although medication is a first line of treatment for schizophrenia, mental health clinicians must remain advocates of psychosocial interventions to improve the quality of life for people with schizophrenia. In addition, mental health professionals must remain mindful of the pharmacoeconomics of the newer, more expensive antipsychotics and advocate for indigent clients to have access to these drugs.

CHAPTER EIGHT

Mood Stabilizers

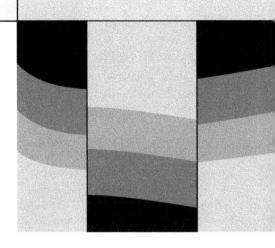

Bipolar I Disorder (BPI) is an incapacitating, severe mental illness that affects approximately 1% of the population (APA, 2013). It usually has its onset in adulthood and early onset is age 13. Despite this, there has been an epidemic of misdiagnosing children who act out as having Bipolar I Disorder. In an effort to stem the tide of misdiagnoses, the American Psychiatric Association (APA) included an untested, new diagnosis in *DSM-5*. It is called Disruptive Mood Dysregulation Disorder and deals with acting out, aggressive behavior, and tantrums that are developmentally abnormal as defined by the criteria. The consensus now is that for a child to be diagnosed with Bipolar I Disorder she or he must show evidence of sustained, inappropriate euphoria and grandiosity. We discuss this further in Chapter Nine but the context of mood stabilizers is changing radically and we hope, in this chapter, to not just introduce you to the medications that are grouped under the mood stabilizer category, but also help you understand the rapidly changing context of diagnosing and treating Bipolar I Disorder.

This chapter is divided into eight sections. The first explores the curious history of the phrase mood stabilizer and discusses what an effective mood stabilizer should do. The second section covers an overview of Bipolar I Disorder and its symptoms. Section Three provides some history on how some of the medications in use were discovered and developed. Section Four focuses on lithium, the first drug used specifically for Bipolar I Disorder or what used to be called Manic-Depressive Illness. Section Five discusses anticonvulsants used to treat Bipolar

I Disorder. Section Six covers newer treatments like lamotrigine/Lamictal. Section Seven takes us back to the atypical antipsychotics and details their use in Bipolar I Disorder. Finally Section Eight discusses cultural and social issues related to mood stabilizers.

SECTION ONE: MOOD MISNOMERS

Learning Objectives

- Understand the history of the phrase "mood stabilization."
- Be able to state what makes a drug a good mood stabilizer.

The very phrase "mood stabilization" is curious. Webster's New Universal Unabridged Dictionary (1989) notes that a stabilizer makes or holds things stable. That is simple enough, but the very nature of mood in us human beings is rarely stable. In fact, our range of affect and the manner in which we express it may be one of the hallmarks of being (or becoming) human. Clinically speaking, "normal" mood is referred to as a state of "**euthymia**." This word, however, has two slightly different meanings. The more clinical meaning of euthymia is a state that is neither manic nor depressed. Simple enough—perhaps too simple where human beings are concerned. A more important meaning of "euthymia" is rooted in the etymology of the word (almost never referred to by mental health clinicians). The original Greek meaning of *euthymia* is being "tranquil or joyous." *Eu-* is a Greek prefix meaning "good or well," and *thymus* refers to "mind." Unfortunately, clinicians typically restrict the word *euthymic* to the shallower, clinical meaning, of "neither manic nor depressed." Perhaps we would better serve clients if we aimed for the original meaning. Imagine what mental health delivery would be like if joy and tranquility were viewed as desirable goals for clients! As philosopher Alan Watts (1973) noted, mental health clinicians seem to be suspicious of things such as joy and prefer that consensual reality be defined as the frame of mind one has going to work on Monday morning. Be that as it may, mood stabilization is the practice of introducing pharmacologic agents that keep clients' moods within parameters clinically described as "normal" or "euthymic." The psychotropic agents used to do this are called **mood stabilizers**.

The phrase "mood stabilizer" was first used in 1985 by Guy Chouinard who suggested that combining estrogen and progesterone may create a mood stabilizer (Healy, 2008). The phrase *mood stabilizer* did not come into use until the mid-1990s and it was not a phrase scientifically gleaned from years of painstaking research on how certain drugs affected patients. No, it was pressed into use by Abbott Laboratories marketing their newly patented Depakote/valproic acid (Healy, 2013). Depakote was approved for the manic phase of Bipolar I Disorder in 1995 but, as Healy (2013) points out, this is not surprising because any sedating drug will produce a change in people suffering from mania. At the time there were relatively few manic patients and many sedatives on the market. Abbott's license did not allow them to claim Depakote would stop mood swings or act as a prophylactic. They dealt with this by emphasizing the ambiguous phrase "mood stabilization" in their marketing of Depakote. It was ambiguous enough to be the perfect marketing term. Even psychiatry began using it and admitting that as a field, psychiatry did not really know what it meant (Sobo, 1999). There were no peer-reviewed papers on "mood stabilizers" in 1990 and over 100 in 2000 (Healy, 2013).

Regrettably, as you will see, these so-called mood-stabilizing agents rarely bring clients the deeper experience of euthymia, described by the ancient Greeks as tranquil or joyous. In this society, suspicion of joy is perhaps reflected in the severe restriction of access to those drugs that actually seem to induce joy. More often, clients taking mood stabilizers report feeling constricted mood, something even less than the normal fluctuations of mood. Clinically, such clients are described as being neither manic nor depressed, but many tell us this is not a pleasant state. What does it mean to feel *neither* manic nor depressed? Describing a state by what it is *not* [called the *via negativa* or *apophatic* (without images) in the spiritual logic of St. Thomas of Aquinas] usually fails to give a clear picture of what the state really *is*. We suspect that the clinical meaning of euthymia is perhaps more word magic retreated to by exhausted clinicians who simply want to say, "The client is neither manic nor depressed." So we are somewhat back where we started.

In an effort to operationalize for readers the mysterious phrase "mood stabilizer," we use the parameters set by clinical logic and draw on the work of Schou (1997) and Keck (Interactive Medical Networks, 2001). Schou noted that a mood stabilizer should have far-reaching effects. Ideally, it should show efficacy for relieving manic episodes and depressive episodes, and as a prophylactic treatment, for preventing any further severe mood symptoms. Keck agreed, noting that mood stabilizers should (1) show efficacy in an acute manic phase, (2) show such efficacy in one stage of Bipolar illness without exacerbating another stage, and (3) show some efficacy for mood, psychotic, and cognitive symptoms. Keck also added that mood stabilizers should show some efficacy as a prophylactic (Interactive Medical Networks, 2001). The key to these definitions is that an ideal mood stabilizer does more than simply calm a person suffering from mania. That calming could easily be accomplished with one of the benzodiazepines described in Chapter Six or one of the neuroleptics described in Chapter Seven; however, the neuroleptic would have little impact on the depressive symptoms or as a prophylactic.

Clinically, the words used to describe mood disorders are important for understanding mood stabilizers. We all need to understand the terms bequeathed to us from *DSM-IV* to describe mood symptoms that may require mood stabilization. Although *DSM-5* has changed "Mood Disorders" to two separate categories

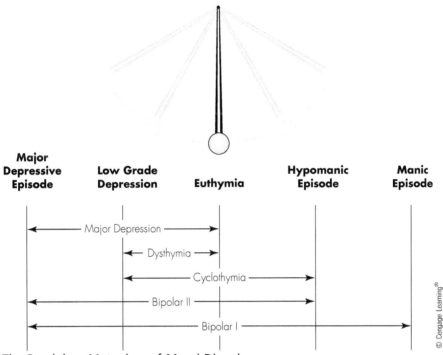

FIGURE 8.1 The Pendulum Metaphor of Mood Disorders

(Depressive and Bipolar Disorder), this exercise is still useful. Figure 8.1 offers the metaphor of a pendulum to illustrate these concepts.

As you can see in Figure 8.1, euthymia is at the pendulum's center, implying a "centered" state, meaning normal. In the figure, elevated mood is shown as movement to the right of euthymia and depressed mood is shown as movement toward the left of euthymia. Mood elevated above normal is not described as pathology in *DSM* even when it reaches hypomanic levels. Hypomanic episodes were new in *DSM-IV* (American Psychiatric Association, 1994), have been retained in *DSM-5* (APA, 2013) and remain difficult to diagnose. The primary difficulties lie in confirming the symptoms and in the fact that hypomanic symptoms eventually shade into manic symptoms. No "hard and fast" line separates them. Hypomanic episodes are described in terms exactly similar to manic episodes, except they are of shorter duration and less severe. As the pendulum of mood moves further to right toward elevated mood, the

next descriptor is "manic episode." This is mood so elevated that it is "sufficiently severe to cause marked impairment in social or occupational functioning or to necessitate hospitalization to prevent harm to self or others" (American Psychiatric Association, 2013, p. 124). In the direction of depressed mood, there is a low-grade depression spectrum referred to in *DSM* first as Persistent Depressive Disorder (previously Dysthymia in *DSM-IV*) and finally Major Depression, described in Chapter Five. Figure 8.1 includes arrows, spanning the range of a client's mood, that correspond to *DSM* criteria for particular disorders. Mood stabilization comes into play in Cyclothymia (fluctuations between hypomania and persistent depressive disorder), Bipolar II Disorder (fluctuations between major depression and hypomania), and Bipolar I Disorder (fluctuations between major depression and mania).

We are primarily concerned in this chapter with medications used to treat Bipolar I Disorder, colloquially known as "manic-depressive illness."

Although so-called mood stabilizers are used to treat Schizoaffective Disorder, Bipolar II Disorder, Borderline Personality Disorder, and Cyclothymia, these uses are not yet systematic, the literature is inconsistent, and mood stabilization focuses on manic symptoms (Delgado & Gelenberg, 2001). We cover lithium and several anticonvulsant medications, some of which have demonstrated efficacy for treating Bipolar I Disorder and others that are still under study. We also discuss atypical antipsychotic medications, as well as a new, hybrid medication combining olanzapine/Zyprexa with fluoxetine/Prozac (brand name Symbyax). Because there are so many brand names and formulations of lithium (e.g., Lithobid, Eskalith, Lithonate), we will depart from our generic/Brand name presentation in this case and simply refer to it as "lithium." We will do the same when discussing valproic acid and use the term *Valproate*.

Note that the literature on medications for Bipolar I Disorder often use "mood stabilizer" as synonymous with "antimanic." We use the phrase "mood stabilizer." It is also important to note that the so-called mood-stabilizing medications described in this chapter are increasingly being used in an attempt to control aggressive behavior, particularly in children and adolescents (Viesselman, 1999). We discuss this use as well as the fact that little research supports this practice in the next chapter.

Review Questions

- What is your reaction to the origin of the phrase "mood stabilizer?"
- What qualities make a drug a good mood stabilizer?

SECTION TWO: BIPOLAR I DISORDER

Learning Objectives

- Be able to understand the challenges in identifying the etiology and proper treatment of Bipolar I Disorder.
- Know the spectrum of symptoms as well as the challenge of the specifiers "mixed episode" and "rapid cycling."

As noted, Bipolar I Disorder is predominantly characterized by symptoms that meet the criteria for major depression and symptoms that meet the criteria for mania. The estimated **lifetime prevalence** fluctuates between 0.4 and 1.6% of the adult population (Kessler et al., 1994). In *DSM-5,* there are new categories replacing what were Mood Disorders in *DSM-IV.* One such category is Bipolar and Related Disorders that includes Bipolar I, Bipolar II, and Cyclothymia.

Prevalence estimates are very difficult to come by, and some practices used to justify them are questionable. In Ohio in 2003, a psychiatrist on a cable-access news program stated that the incidence of Bipolar I Disorder is significantly higher than currently believed. To support this assertion, he cited some survey research (Hirschfeld et al., 2003). He did not say that the survey in question was extrapolating diagnoses from a 10-item questionnaire (which is not clinically ethical), that the 10-item questionnaire had only fair validity, and that 10 of the 11 authors received substantial financial support from pharmaceutical companies. This was hardly a good citation of a supposedly objective, scientific study. Our point is that most viewers may not have even bothered to look up the study to which the speaker was referring and might believe him simply because he was a psychiatrist.

Estimates have sometimes been made for how many people are thought to suffer from Bipolar I, II, and Cyclothymia. These estimates are about 4% of the population (Advokat, Comaty, & Julien, 2014) but that is not an appropriate practice. In preparation for the release of the *DSM-5,* some advocated that all these disorders should be placed on a continuum called Bipolar Spectrum Disorder (Akiskal & Banazzi, 2006; Ghaemi, Ko, & Goodwin, 2002; Paris, 2009). In *DSM-5,* Bipolar and Related Disorders were given their own category but it is NOT a spectrum. The concern with the spectrum idea was the possibility that clients who showed symptoms of irritation or inattention (especially children and adolescents) would get misdiagnosed under the bipolar spectrum umbrella with Bipolar I Disorder (Baroni, Lunsford, Luckenbaugh, Toubin, & Leibenluft, 2009; Paris, 2009).

And it should be added that the *DSM-IV* Task Force rejected the idea of childhood Bipolar Disorder because there was not enough evidence (Frances, 2013). Although some researchers (Alloy et al., 2012; Walsh, Royal, Bronw, Barrantes-Vidal, & Kwapil, 2012) have explored what they call a "soft" Bipolar Spectrum, currently Bipolar I, Bipolar II, and Cyclothymia should be conceived of as discrete disorders rather than thinking of Cyclothymia or Bipolar II as leading to Bipolar I or diagnosing subthreshold symptoms.

The mean age of onset for Bipolar I Disorder is 18 (Weissman, Bruce, Leaf, Florio, & Holzer, 1991). The American Psychiatric Association (2013) describes Bipolar I Disorder as a long-term illness with a variable course. The association estimates that 90% of clients who suffer a single manic episode repeat the experience. The majority of manic episodes (60 to 70%) occur immediately before or after an episode of major depression (American Psychiatric Association, 2013). Most patients seek treatment for depression and may be misdiagnosed with unipolar depression for years (Angst et al., 2011). There are several specifiers for the disorder (that used to be subtypes in *DSM-IV*), mixed episode and rapid cycling being the most difficult to treat. Mixed episode is when the person has both symptoms of depression and mania. Rapid cycling is when the person has four or more episodes (manic or depressive) in a 12-month period. In addition, 60% of people suffering from Bipolar I Disorder have comorbid substance use issues and substance use is correlated with a greater risk of switching from depressive symptoms to manic symptoms (Ostacher et al., 2010).

Scientists do not know what causes Bipolar I Disorder. This is surely dismaying to the clients who suffer its symptoms, but the truth is, the well-intentioned theorists who share a strong medical model perspective tend to theorize exclusively from this perspective. Although a great deal of attention has been placed on heritability, this focus has not provided clues as to the etiology of Bipolar I Disorder other than giving people the luxury of speculating that it *may* be genetic. From

an integrative perspective, this hypothesis is not terribly useful. It might be just as useful to say that the disorder "appears karmic." Some promising developments are occurring in molecular psychiatry, but more work needs to be done before a coherent theory can be articulated (Manji, Moore, Rajkowska, & Chen, 2000). Despite the ignorance about etiology, as with Schizophrenia, the spectrum of symptom presentation in Bipolar I Disorder requires comment.

Symptoms in Bipolar I Disorder

Bipolar I Disorder is unique in that symptoms manifest heterogeneously, which influences treatment (Pacchiarotti et al., 2013). About half of all clients suffering from Bipolar I Disorder have psychotic symptoms and these clients respond less well to some treatments, lithium in particular (Bowden, 1998). Most clients suffering from Bipolar I Disorder return to adequate functioning between episodes (approximately 80%); however, many require continued pharmacologic interventions to avoid future episodes. As with Schizophrenia, clients with Bipolar I Disorder are at a greater risk for suicide: the completion rate is 10 times that of the general population (Advokat et al., 2014).

Researchers estimate that 35 to 50% of clients who do stay on medication are likely to suffer relapse despite medication compliance (Advokat et al., 2014). Many clinicians assume that patients stabilized will continue on the medication indefinitely. There is some evidence in favor of slowly titrated withdrawal in patients who have made therapeutically based life changes and seem able to manage their illness. We say more about this later when we explore the disorder from various perspectives.

Review Questions

- Why is treating Bipolar I Disorder so difficult?
- What specifiers are harder yet to treat effectively and why do you think that is?

SECTION THREE: SOME HISTORY ON MOOD STABILIZERS

Learning Objectives

- Be able to describe some of the accidental events that went into the discovery of lithium.

In the 19th century, a popular theory called *uric acid diathesis* was a dominant concept in medicine used to explain the etiology of disorders as diverse as manic-depressive illness and cardiac problems (Healy, 2002). As Barlow and Durand (2002) have noted, "diathesis" means vulnerability (as in the diathesis–stress model of psychopathology), in this case, vulnerability to the effects of the uric acid on one's system. Uric acid is a breakdown product of urea, which is a compound, found in urine as a result of protein metabolism.

In the 19th century, as today, theories followed the technologies available to test them. The ability to peer inside neurons is followed by theories of mental disorders that hypothesize intraneuronal (and interneuronal) causes, as you saw in our Chapter Five discussion of depression (remember the molecular/cellular theory of depression?). In the 19th century, chemical analysis was the newest technology of that time, so researchers used it to investigate substances eliminated from the body and then proposed theories about disorders, based on the analysis. Although the uric acid diathesis theories are now recognized as no more accurate than the chemical imbalance theories of depression, they did provide a starting point for research that led to lithium being used for Bipolar I Disorder.

Uric acid was also found to be a major constituent in kidney stones and gout. Gout is a painful inflammation of the joints, caused by uric acid in salt form settling in joints. In the 19th century, gout was also linked to disturbances in mood (although these surely could have been side effects of the unpleasant experience of having gout). In 1817, a new element called *lithium* had been discovered. Lithium is a light, positively charged metal ion that has been used therapeutically in a number of ways for almost 200 years. Researchers realized that lithium dissolved kidney stones, so perhaps it would be useful for other disorders related to uric acid. From a period spanning 1840 to 1870, Alexander Ure and Alfred Garrod began experimenting with lithium as a treatment for disorders believed related to uric acid (Lenox & Manji, 1998).

As Healy (2002) documents, the effects of lithium on **urates** gave rise to an industry in lithium-laced products. Although many readers may know that Coca-Cola at one time had coca leaf extract as one of its ingredients, you may be surprised to know that 7-Up came on the market as a lithium-containing beverage. Spring waters containing lithium were carried by spas and were supposed to induce a sense of well-being, and lithium was even used as a salt substitute for patients with heart problems. As early as 1870, the Danish neurologist Carl Lange (co-creator of the James-Lange theory of emotions) found that lithium had therapeutic effects in clients with manic-depressive illness. In the United States, William Hammond gave lithium to patients with mood disorders and also reported positive results (Healy, 2002). One problem with lithium, however, is that in large enough doses it can be toxic, and there were some fatalities from these enthusiastic additive uses of the substance. This, coupled with the decline of the uric acid diathesis hypothesis of illness, contributed to the FDA removing lithium from the market in 1949. Ironically, this same year a little-known psychiatrist from Australia was about to put lithium "back on the map."

Developments Down Under

John Cade was a psychiatrist and state hospital superintendent in Australia in the mid 20th century. Under the influence of the uric acid diathesis theory, Cade hypothesized that a toxin that entered the brain caused mania. He further asserted that this toxin could be detected in urine. He proposed injecting uric acid from manic patients into guinea pigs, thinking that if the hypothetical toxin were active, it would induce manic activity in the guinea pigs. Alas, uric acid is highly toxic and the first guinea pigs died. He then decided to dissolve the acid by mixing it with a metal to form a soluble salt. After failing with a number of metals, he found lithium ideal for his mixture. He then injected the dissolved mixture of uric acid and lithium into the guinea pigs, and they responded not with mania but lethargy. Cade thought the lethargy was a calming effect and eventually tried injecting just lithium into the guinea pigs. It had the same effect (in actuality, the lithium did not calm the guinea pigs, it just made them sick). At any rate, although this was not at all what he had expected to find, Cade (1949) concluded that lithium might have some effects on mood (calming what he called "psychotic excitement"), and he proposed to test it in humans, including himself (Snyder, 1996). Although Cade had some success using lithium in manic patients, several of his patients died from its toxicity (Healy, 2002).

Although some give Cade all the credit for discovering lithium (Snyder, 1996), others (Healy, 2002) cite the important contributions of Morgens Schou, a Danish researcher. Schou (1978) did the first randomized, controlled trials that demonstrated the efficacy of lithium. Although Cade had some success, it was anecdotal and not based on standard trials. Schou's research confirmed the usefulness of the compound and led to standards for safe dosage levels. Note that there is still no theoretical basis for lithium's use. As Snyder (1996) concludes, "One of the fascinations of the discovery process is that we often find the right answer by looking in the wrong place" (p. 119).

As noted, lithium was taken off the market in 1949 (the same year it appeared to have efficacy for manic-depressive illness) and was not reapproved by the FDA for psychiatric use until 1970. Some think part of the reason for this time lag was that because lithium is a naturally occurring element, no pharmaceutical company could get a patent on it, thus limiting its profitability. The toxicity of lithium was surely another reason for the caution in approval. The early deaths related to lithium were all caused by lithium-induced cardiac problems. Researchers now think these cases were all cases of lithium toxicity,

but when monitored and given in appropriate doses, the cardiac side effects of lithium are typically minor (Tilkian, Schroeder, Kao, & Hultgren, 1976). As we outline later, lithium therapy must be closely monitored, because the therapeutic dose is very close to the toxic dose. The only FDA-approved use of lithium is for mood stabilization.

Review Question

- What are some of the accidental discoveries that went into figuring out lithium could be used to treat Bipolar I Disorder?

SECTION FOUR: LITHIUM: THE PROTOTYPICAL MOOD STABILIZER

Learning Objectives

- Be able to give an overview of at least four mechanisms of action of lithium and why we think they may help in Bipolar I Disorder.
- Be able to describe the categories of side effects from lithium.
- Know the profile of who is a good candidate for lithium.

As noted, lithium is a naturally occurring, positively charged alkali metal ion. Johan August Arfvedson in Stockholm, Sweden, discovered it in 1817. Its name derives from the Greek *lithos,* meaning "stone" because Arfvedson discovered it in a mineral source. It can be mixed with magnesium and aluminum to form metal alloys, is used in some glasses and batteries, and of course has use in psychopharmacology. It has been assumed that lithium has good efficacy in treating acute mania as well as being a prophylactic for both manic and depressive episodes (American Psychiatric Association, 2000a) and was the drug of first choice for Bipolar I Disorder. The problem is that in "real life," many patients stop taking it because of its difficult side effect profile. Right now, anticonvulsants and atypical antipsychotics are more often the first drugs prescribed because clients do not want to be bothered with side effects and the blood testing necessary when taking lithium. Many still feel that lithium has the best efficacy in studies compared to other drugs and that it enhances the effects of antidepressants (Grof & Muller-Oerlinghausen, 2009). As usual, though, there are disagreements in the literature and the differences between what works in short-term studies versus what is necessary managing a chronic disorder are different things (Post, 2010). The evidence for lithium to treat bipolar depression is weaker than for its effectiveness in bipolar mania. Lithium does seem (when clients adhere to prescription) to have strong efficacy in maintenance of euthymia and prevention of relapse (Malhi, Tanious, Das, Coulston, & Berk, 2013).

Throughout the mid to late 20th century we had consistent support for the idea that long-term lithium therapy correlated with decreased suicide rates in clients suffering from Bipolar I Disorder (Goodwin & Ghaemi, 1999). Lithium may also have neuroprotective properties, which would mean that Bipolar I Disorder is progressive and/or degenerative and lithium protects neurons from the progression of the disorder. As with most hypotheses, more work needs to be done to confirm this one (Manji et al., 2000). Lithium is least effective in clients suffering from mixed episodes or rapid cycling of mood symptoms (Bowden, 1995). Lithium is typically available in capsules, tablets, slow-release tablets, and as lithium citrate syrup (Keck & McElroy, 2002). Common lithium formulations are listed in Table 8.1.

Peak plasma levels for lithium are reached by about three hours but lithium is not fat soluble and does not cross the blood–brain barrier easily. Because of this, the therapeutic dose can be close to the toxic dose which as you can imagine is problematic. Clients show an initial response within one week to one month of beginning lithium therapy. Because of this time lag and because clients suffering from manic symptoms may endanger themselves or others, additional medications may be used, including typical antipsychotics and

TABLE 8.1 Examples of Lithium Formulations

Generic	*Brand Names*	*Formulation*
Lithium citrate	Cibalith-S	Syrup
Lithium carbonate	Eskalith	Capsule
	Eskalith-CR	Scored tablet
	Lithobid	Tablet
	Lithotabs	Tablet
	Lithane	Gelatin capsule

© Cengage Learning®

benzodiazepines (Advokat et al., 2014). Once a client starts to show a response to lithium, symptoms usually diminish quickly. If lithium is discontinued abruptly during the manic phase of the illness, relapse may occur rapidly (Perry, Alexander, & Liskow, 2006). Lithium is not metabolized and is excreted unchanged by the kidneys which puts a strain on them. Thus, long-term lithium users should be screened regularly for markers indicating kidney damage (Rybakowski et al., 2012).

As with all mental disorders, we do not know what causes Bipolar I Disorder. This makes finding an effective intervention challenging and severe mental disorders like BPI seem to be rooted in the brain, which makes things even more complicated as we are just beginning to realize how little we know about the brain. In placebo-controlled studies, approximately 60 to 80% of clients suffering from mania show some level of response to lithium over placebo. Some researchers (Grof & Alda, 2001; Grof, Alda, Grof, Fox, & Cameron, 1993) challenge this estimate and believe that the response rate is closer to 50%. Chen, Mehta, Aparasu, Patel, and Ochoa-Perez (2014) concluded that monotherapy with atypical antipsychotics was more effective and safer than monotherapy with mood stabilizers for adolescents. Because in many cases people are treated with multiple medications, it is harder to specify response rates to one. Grof (2006) has summarized research into a profile of patients who are good lithium responders. So, we might ask, what are the "symptoms" of a good lithium response? According to Grof, they include:

- Complete remission between episodes
- Depressive symptoms are more vegetative in nature (similar to what we said about depression in Chapter 5)
- The person does not meet criteria for rapid cycling or mixed episode specifiers
- No significant psychiatric comorbidity (but remember in some studies up to 60% of people with BPI meet criteria for substance use disorders)
- Episodic course in another family member

Another way to look at this is that combination therapy has become standard practice but even there it depends on the presentation of symptoms. For example, lithium seems most effective for enhancing the effects of antidepressants for refractory patients. Anticonvulsants plus lithium seem to provide better protection against relapse than just lithium (Leng et al., 2008). On the other hand, combination therapies that we seemed to think had efficacy in the first edition of this book, turned out not to. The most common practice was adding antidepressants to mood stabilizers, which Sachs et al. (2007) concluded did not improve response. Lithium treatment cannot occur until clients have several lab tests done, including checking sodium, calcium, and phosphorous levels, and an electrocardiogram, urinalysis, thyroid battery, and complete blood cell count.

Because the average duration of a manic episode is three months, plasma levels of lithium effective for the client should be maintained for three to six months afterward. If lithium is to be discontinued, Perry et al. (2006) recommend that the daily dosage be tapered by 25% each day over a period of four weeks. About half of patients stabilized successfully on lithium and then switched to placebo relapse within six months. There are stories of patients relapsing in a few days, but these are not from controlled studies and are rare.

Unlike antidepressants, there are more often significant statistical differences between lithium and placebo groups in participants with Bipolar I Disorder. Clearly something is happening, but what? To address

that question, we begin by discussing the mechanisms of action of lithium.

Mechanisms of Action

The pharmacology of lithium is incredibly complex and a matter of ongoing speculation. Lithium affects different parts of the brain differently at different times when different doses are used. Lithium's effects extend to multiple neurotransmitters and second-messenger systems.

As all researchers point out, we are still uncertain of the key factors in lithium's effectiveness. Table 8.2 outlines the mechanisms of action we know lithium exerts. Note that part of the complexity of lithium is due to the fact that it can affect the brain differently in different regions (e.g., increasing neurotransmitter release in some areas and decreasing release of the same neurotransmitter in other areas). These mechanisms are summarized from Malhi et al. (2013); Perry et al. (2006); and Schatzberg, Cole, and DeBattista (1997).

The best-studied effects of lithium are on serotonin, and these effects also demonstrate the complexity of lithium's pharmacodynamics. After short-term use (one to two weeks), lithium appears to increase serotonin synthesis by increasing tryptophan reuptake in synapses. After two to three weeks, it appears to enhance release of 5-HT from neurons in the parietal cortex and the hippocampus. Long-term taking of lithium seems to cause downregulation in 5-HT1 and 5-HT2 receptors. Again, how these effects may relate to mood is currently unknown.

Lithium's effects on norepinephrine (NE) are equally curious. Lithium appears to increase the rate of norepinephrine synthesis in some parts of the brain. It decreases excretion of norepinephrine metabolites in manic patients but increases excretion of norepinephrine metabolites in depressed patients. Lithium appears to block postsynaptic DA receptors, which seems to partly explain the controlling effects on mania and psychosis. There appears to be evidence that lithium affects the **G-proteins** in second-messenger systems. Apparently it inhibits some enzymes, in particular second-messenger systems, which in turn is believed to bring about some of the therapeutic effects.

TABLE 8.2 Mechanisms of Action of Lithium

Neurotransmitter System	Effects
Serotonin	Increase in tryptophan (precursor) uptake after short- and long-term treatment. General increases in serotonin levels. Increased release of serotonin in the hippocampus, hypothalamus, and parietal cortex. Serotonin receptor decreases in hippocampus. Long-term administration causes downregulation of 5-HT1 and 5-HT2 receptors.
Dopamine	Long-term administration diminishes neostriatal dopamine activity. May block the effects of highly sensitive DA receptors, thus decreasing the behaviors associated with DA stimulation.
Norepinephrine	Increases rate of synthesis of NE in some parts of the brain but decreases the synthesis in other parts. Decreases the excretion of NE metabolites in manic patients and increases the excretion of NE metabolites in depressed patients.
Second-messenger systems	Lithium appears to reduce the activity of second-messenger systems in undetermined ways.
Ionic effects	Lithium, being a positively charged metal ion, may have stabilizing effects on neurons in the CNS.
Inhibiting Intracellular Enzymes	Inhibition of glycogen synthase kinase-3 (GSK-3) increases Beta-catenin that stimulates axon growth and cell survival.
Neuroprotection	Antioxidant properties may protect brain from oxidative stress.

© 2015 Cengage Learning®

We know that in BPI, there are gray matter deficits, meaning, that compared to unaffected individuals and those who had brain scans after lithium treatment, people suffering from BPI seem to have reduced volume in the subgenual and anterior cingulate cortex as well as the prefrontal cortex. Some of these reductions are hypothesized to be the result of excitotoxicity caused by glutamate-induced stress. In patients (some but not all of course) who have responded to lithium treatment, these gray matter reductions decrease or vanish in subsequent brain scans positing a neuroprotective mechanism in lithium (Malhi et al., 2013).

If even after reviewing our brief description of lithium's mechanisms of action you are confused, you are not alone. Scientists do have molecular clues as to lithium's pharmacodynamics, but these clues do not help explain how it alters mood. From an integrative perspective, this is likely because mood cannot be explained in terms of brain chemistry alone. In fairness though, researchers have likely only seen the proverbial "tip of the iceberg" in terms of lithium's mechanisms of action, and continued research will likely yield a deeper understanding of its effects on brain chemistry.

Theories of Lithium Action

The short answer to the question "How does lithium work?" is "We don't know." Because researchers do not really know what causes Bipolar I Disorder, it is hard to draw definitive conclusions as to how lithium corrects the disorder in people who respond to it as a treatment. Next, we briefly outline some medical model theories that have implications for psychosocial interventions as well.

Lithium and Neurotransmission
The Amine Theory Revisited

In Chapter Five, we discussed the amine theory of depression, which in essence proposed that people whose nervous systems did not produce enough amines (specifically norepinephrine) become depressed. From here, it was a simple leap to propose that some people's nervous systems produce amines erratically, sometimes producing too many, and at other times producing too few. When the nervous system of such afflicted people produces too many amines, the result is manic mood. When the person's nervous system produces too few amines, the result is depression. This appeared to have limited support in that lithium is correlated with decreased norepinephrine metabolites in manic patients and increased NE metabolites in depressed patients. These data led researchers to conclude that lithium helped the body achieve some innate homeostasis (dare we say, "chemical imbalance?") that had been lacking. Obviously, in light of how complex lithium's effects are, this chemical imbalance theory also turns out to be as oversimplistic and inadequate as is the chemical imbalance theory of depression.

Lithium's Ionic Impact on Neurotransmitter systems

That lithium is a positively charged metal ion may account for lithium's effects on the nervous system. As Preston, O'Neal, and Talaga (2002) note, "Since neurotransmitter production, release, and reuptake rely on various ions (sodium, calcium, potassium, and magnesium), lithium's ionic properties may affect neurotransmission-mediated depression and mania" (p. 187). This hypothesis is certainly plausible. As you saw in Chapter Two, all neurons have ion channels that allow the passage of positively or negatively charged particles into the cell. We noted that an influx of positively charged ions (such as sodium) tends to excite cells and an influx of negatively charged ions (such as chloride) tends to inhibit or hyperpolarize cells. We will now cover hypothesized mechanisms of action for lithium using an algebra equation metaphor. Both the etiology of BPI and the actions of lithium involve multiple (maybe dozens) variables that could be said to resemble an algebra equation with many unknown variables. Each of these hypothesized mechanisms may play a part of the action of lithium

and all may not be necessary to bring symptom relief in BPI. Until we know more about the etiology of BPI though, we don't know which equation variables we can dispense with.

Dopamine

Dopamine (DA) is an excitatory neurotransmitter that many researchers believe is an important variable in the equation in the symptoms of BPI and lithium's action. During mania, DA metabolites are increased in some but not all patients which may point to an increase in actual DA (Cousin, Butts, & Young, 2010). If DA transmission is elevated during mania then it may prompt a balancing (homeostatic) mechanism that could then cause depression. Animal models of lithium action show extracellular DA to decrease after the introduction of lithium. The postsynaptic actions of DA are mediated by G-protein receptors, which then stimulate second messenger systems like adenyl cyclase (AC) and cyclic adenosine monophosphate (cAMP). Research suggests that lithium also alters the function of these units in ways that may be neuroprotective.

Glutamate and NMDA Receptors

Glutamate (Glu) like DA is an excitatory neurotransmitter. Michael, Erfurth, Ohrmann (2003) first hypothesized that glutamate was elevated in manic episodes. N-methyl-D-aspartate (NMDA) receptors, among other things, control many aspects of memory and plasticity. They also open ion channels that can increase sodium and calcium, positively charged ions that would increase cell firing. With chronic lithium administration, lithium binds to NMDA receptors and this causes downregulation of the NMDA receptors and enhanced Glu reuptake (Malhi et al., 2013).

GABA

GABA is an inhibitory neurotransmitter that plays crucial roles in modulating Glu and DA. Here again, we see the complexity of trying to understand the relationship between neurotransmitter families. Patients with BPI are thought to have diminished GABA transmission that then leads to increases in excitatory transmission via DA and Glu. This leads to excitotoxicity that in turn causes cell loss and perhaps accounts for the decreased brain structure volume in patients with BPI. Lithium increases the level of GABA in the plasma and spinal fluid of people and so supposedly it also increases it in the central nervous system.

Lithium's Effect on Second-Messenger Systems

In the late 1980s and early 1990s, researchers proposed that intraneuronal effects caused lithium's therapeutic effects. They specified second-messenger systems as a primary site where lithium exerted a powerful influence. In this theory, the lithium acts to modulate these systems, in some cases slowing them down and in others speeding them up (Avissar & Schreiber, 1989; Malhi et al., 2013; Weber, Saklad, & Kastenholz, 1992). Recall from Chapter Two that second-messenger systems may play a role in neuronal excitation and subsequent firing. In this theory, the slowing of the second-messenger systems may decrease cell firing and (theoretically) decrease manic symptoms. It now appears these may be only one of many effects that ultimately translate into therapeutic gains. Some of the second-messenger systems are responsible for the production of brain-derived neurotrophic factor (BDNF) that (recall from Chapter Five) acts as a brain cell nutrient repairing cells and stimulating neurogenesis. Lithium seems to enhance the production of BDNF in parts of the brain.

Lithium and Circadian Rhythms

As early as 1990, researchers have sought to explore the connection between Bipolar I Disorder and sleep–wake cycles that are part of our circadian rhythms (biologic cycles within the course of a day) (Goodwin & Jamison, 1990). This theory reflects the psychosocial intervention of optimizing sleep and setting regular patterns of sleep and wakefulness with clients suffering from Bipolar I Disorder. The circadian rhythm hypothesis of lithium's action derives from the fact that lithium slows the circadian rhythm in species ranging from plants to human beings (Lenox & Manji, 1998). Although studies with humans are hampered by several ethical limits that do not constrain animal models, it appears that lithium significantly slows and lengthens the circadian cycle. More recently, McCarthy et al. (2013) tied BPI disorder to those genes tied to the circadian cycle. Their research conclusions suggest that lithium enhanced the resynchronization of circadian rhythms and that may be one therapeutic mechanism in the equation of symptom relief.

Side Effects of Lithium

Approximately three-fourths of clients on lithium experience side effects (American Psychiatric Association, 2000b). The side effects are a primary reason for clients to stop taking the drug (Atack, 2000; Advokat et al., 2014). One problem is that the therapeutic dosage is often close to the toxic dosage, so the drug requires regular blood monitoring in clients. The side effects of lithium are summarized in Table 8.3 and then described more fully in the text. The types and degrees of side effects clients will suffer are difficult to estimate. The literature on side effects has always given broad ranges of the percentage of patients complaining of adverse effects (35 to 93% according to Lenox and Manji, 1998)—so broad as to be not much help. Price and Heninger (1994) noted that the side effects increase as the serum levels of the drug increase. It is important to note that clients will have different numbers and degrees of side effects, and that lithium's difficult side effect profile is a main reason that continued research on different mood stabilizers is important. When the percentage is generally known, we have also listed in parentheses the proportion of clients thought to suffer from a given side effect. Data for Table 8.3 are drawn from Lenox and Manji (1998); Perry et al. (2006); and Schatzberg et al. (1997).

CNS Side Effects of Lithium

The cognitive side effects of lithium may be the most troubling for clients but remain the least studied (Jamison & Akiskal, 1983; Lenox & Manji, 1998; Shaw, 1986). From the psychological perspective, clients say lithium decreases creativity

TABLE 8.3 Side Effects of Lithium

Type of Effect	Description
CNS effects	Contradictory evidence of deleterious cognitive effects on concentration, memory, and creativity Seizures can occur as a result of lithium toxicity
Neuromuscular	Tremors at rest or although moving (4%–65%) Muscle weakness (40% in short-term treatment)
Gastrointestinal	Chronic nausea, diarrhea, occasional blood in stool
Endocrine	Weight gain (11%–64%), Hypothyroidism (approx. 4%), Goiter (approx. 6%), Elevated thyroid-stimulating hormone (30%)
Renal	Polyuria/polydipsia (20%)
Dermatologic	Acne and rashes, Aggravation of psoriasis, Alopecia
Hematologic	Increase in white blood cells (75%–100%)
Teratogenic	Increased risk of Epstein's anomaly, a congenital heart defect characterized by displacement of the tricuspid valve
Sexual	Decreased libido in males and females, erectile dysfunction in males

© Cengage Learning®

and concentration and increases forgetfulness. Schatzberg et al. (1997) have noted that forgetfulness is one of the most common reasons given by clients who stop taking lithium. The few existing studies have produced conflicting data. Judd, Squire, Butters, Salmon, and Paller (1987) reported slowed rate of central information processing with short-term use of lithium. Some of these effects seem to diminish with long-term use, suggesting there is some accommodation to the effects. More research on this problem is warranted, and clinicians should monitor cognitive functioning in clients receiving lithium. Cognitive impairment can also be a sign of lithium toxicity.

Neuromuscular Side Effects of Lithium

The most reported neuromuscular side effect of lithium is tremor. The tremor can occur while the client is at rest or moving. The incidence of tremor (like most estimates of side effects) is quite broad (4 to 65%) but the symptom is directly correlated with the client's lithium level. Emotional stress and stimulants such as caffeine can worsen the tremor. Although the tremor is reversible with discontinuation of the medication, it may also be controlled by lowering the lithium dosage or by administering a beta-blocking agent (such as that described in Chapter Six). Although the source of lithium-induced tremor is uncertain, it is not related to the extrapyramidal side effects caused by neuroleptics described in Chapter Seven. Several studies have shown that medications used for EPS are ineffective with lithium-induced tremor. General muscle weakness is also a common neuromuscular side effect of lithium and is reported in about 70% of clients within the first two weeks of taking lithium. Again, this side effect is dose related and appears to resolve on its own after the first two or three weeks of lithium use.

Gastrointestinal Side Effects of Lithium

Gastrointestinal (GI) side effects can range from mild to severe, with milder effects that include bloating and slight abdominal pain and severe effects that include nausea and vomiting. It is important for clinicians to monitor these side effects closely, because they are also signs of lithium toxicity. Perry et al. (2006) noted that GI side effects frequently subside on their own and can be diminished if the medication is taken with food. Sometimes, the daily required dosage can be divided into more numerous, smaller portions. Although there are currently sustained-release formulations of lithium, studies indicate no real benefits in terms of side effect profile.

Endocrine Side Effects of Lithium

The most problematic endocrine-related side effect of lithium is weight gain. It has been clearly tied to lithium use and is another of the more common reasons that people stop taking lithium (Peselow, Dunner, Fieve, & Lautin, 1980). Weight gain is variable, ranging from about 7 to 60 pounds. Clients who are overweight to begin with seem to gain more weight while taking lithium. Also, the better the therapeutic response to lithium, the more weight the person typically gains (Perry et al., 2006). Although the reasons for the weight gain are not entirely clear, lithium does exert an insulin-like effect in lowering blood glucose levels and inducing hypoglycemia. This hypoglycemia then promotes eating and weight gain. Dietary regulation and exercise require close monitoring by a physician, because both can disrupt levels of lithium in the client's system. Lithium treatment may also disrupt thyroid functioning, most commonly through an increase in thyroid-stimulating hormone.

Renal Side Effects of Lithium

The most common renal side effects of lithium administration are **polydipsia** (chronic, excessive thirst) and **polyuria** (excessive urination). These effects occur in about 20% of clients on lithium. The polyuria is caused by lithium reducing the kidneys' ability to concentrate urine. Although these effects may wear off on their own, lowering the dosage or discontinuing the drug can relieve them. A more problematic (albeit rarer) side effect from lithium is inflammation of the renal tubules, blood vessels, and surrounding tissue (called *interstitial nephritis*). Although rare, it can cause renal scarring and destruction. Patients exposed to multiple

periods of lithium toxicity are at greater risk for this disorder. These side effects have led to the recommendation that clients on lithium have kidney function checked every 6 to 12 months (Schatzberg et al., 1997).

Dermatologic Side Effects of Lithium

The dermatologic side effects of lithium include various rashes and outbreaks on the skin, aggravation of existing dermatologic conditions, and hair loss (alopecia). Cases of rashes, acne, or other outbreaks on the skin may resolve by themselves. Lowering the dosage frequently relieves them. Few studies have been done on hair loss and lithium treatment. Although more rare than other dermatologic problems, it seems associated with disrupted thyroid function. On discontinuation of the drug, hair loss stops and hair typically regrows. The mechanisms of action of these dermatologic side effects are at present unknown.

Sexual Side Effects of Lithium

Only a few studies have looked at incidence of sexual dysfunction related to lithium use. These and anecdotal clinical evidence suggest that lithium does interfere with sexual functioning. Note that hypersexuality is sometimes associated with mania, and for such clients, returning to baseline levels of sexuality may seem like impairment but that is only relative to the hypersexual state they experienced in manic episodes (Rojansky, Wang, & Halbreich, 1992). Under double-blind conditions, lithium has been reported to cause decreased libido as well as erectile failure (Vinarova, Uhlir, Stika, & Vinar, 1972).

Lithium Toxicity

As noted, the therapeutic dosage of lithium is frequently close to the toxic dosage. Prescribing professionals cannot know the correct dose in advance, because each person eliminates lithium at different rates. In addition, lithium is one of the few psychotropic medications that is not highly fat soluble. As a result, it has a more difficult time crossing the blood–brain barrier and requires higher concentrations in the blood to reach adequate concentrations in the central nervous system (Lickey & Gordon, 1991). Clients must have regular blood tests to ensure that their levels are within safe parameters.

The balance of lithium in a person's bloodstream is delicate. Many things can affect it, including physical and emotional stressors that alter sodium levels. For example, changes in diet and exercise can easily lower sodium levels, which in turn alter the plasma levels of lithium to the point where the person could suffer lithium toxicity. In some documented cases, medical illnesses seemed to tip the balance and bring about toxicity (Decina, Schlegel, & Fieve, 1987). Because the kidneys excrete lithium almost intact, any impairment of kidney functioning (such as mild dehydration, reduced salt intake, or dieting) can result in lithium toxicity.

The toxicity is of a type described as "excitotoxicity" (West, 1996). This means the brain's excitatory neurotransmitter systems become overstimulated and produce excess calcium (a positively charged ion) and free radicals and break down cell defenses. West and Melzer (1979) studied clients under severe psychological stress and found these clients were at higher risk for developing lithium toxicity. These authors were concerned that the ego disintegration typical of severe mental and emotional disorders actually functioned as a risk factor for lithium toxicity; ironically, it was ego disintegration that partially made people candidates for lithium. Also note that clients with a history of brain injury may have increased vulnerability to lithium toxicity (Moskowitz & Altshuler, 1991).

Lithium toxicity primarily affects the brain. The symptoms include confusion, slurred speech, loss of balance, tremor, GI upset, and possibly coma and death. Although some of these symptoms are side effects that are most likely to occur at the beginning of therapy, if they emerge in a client who has been on lithium for some time, the drug should be discontinued and immediate medical attention should be sought (Lickey & Gordon, 1991). There is no antidote to lithium poisoning, and the condition is usually treated by halting the drug administration and giving the client sodium-containing fluids. If the toxicity is serious enough,

TABLE 8.4 Signs of Lithium Toxicity

Nausea

Drowsiness

Confusion

Dizziness

Mental dullness

Slurred speech

Muscle twitches

Irregular heartbeat

Blurred vision

© Cengage Learning®

other medical interventions may be necessary (Paragas, 1984). Julien (2001) notes that complete recovery from lithium toxicity can take weeks to months, depending on the severity of the case. Table 8.4 summarizes the signs of lithium toxicity.

Some authors (Sheean, 1991; West, 1996) feel that the dangers of lithium toxicity are minimized in the literature. Sheean (1991) estimated that 10% of lithium toxicity survivors suffer some permanent neurologic damage. Aronson and Reynolds (1992) recommend that clients have their blood checked as close as possible to 12 hours after the last dose. At this time, the drug absorption is complete and allows for the most consistent reading. Dennison, Clarkson, O'Mullane, and Cassidy (2011) noted that lithium toxicity occurred at the rate of about 6 cases per 100,000 clients in their sample from Cork County, Ireland. In many of those cases, the toxicity seemed to be the result of lithium interacting with other medications so polypharmacy must be closely monitored in patients taking lithium. Mental health clinicians often have to help clients organize schedules to make sure these tests are done consistently. Although lithium toxicity is a problematic side effect, the chances of developing it can be greatly reduced through conservative dosing strategies, care in combining lithium with other medications, regular blood monitoring, and educating clients and significant others about the core symptoms (Delva & Hawken, 2001).

Lithium and Aggression

An important footnote to lithium in the history of psychopharmacology is the work of Michael Sheard. He has conducted several studies exploring the effects of lithium on aggressive behavior (Sheard, 1971; Sheard, 1975; Sheard & Marini, 1978; Sheard, Marini, Bridges, & Wagner, 1976).

Sheard began his work on rodents, assuming that because serotonin was implicated in aggression and because lithium affected serotonin transmission, it might affect levels of aggression in rodents. These initial studies seemed to indicate that lithium did decrease aggression, so he then treated prison inmates with lithium in a placebo-controlled study. Although lithium had no impact on nonviolent behaviors such as lying and stealing, it appeared to fully suppress serious assault in the inmates, as guards observed and documented. Sheard's conclusion was that only impulsive aggression was affected. More importantly, on discontinuation of lithium, the aggression returned. Sheard's work laid the basis for many different populations being treated with lithium for aggression. As we discuss in Chapter Nine, children and adolescents are among those who receive lithium and other mood stabilizers for aggressive behavior and diagnoses like Conduct Disorder (Malone, Luebbert, Pena-Ariet, Biesecker, & Delaney, 1994)

Although lithium therapy is still an effective treatment for the symptoms of Bipolar Disorder (Baldessarini, Tondo, Hennen, & Viguera, 2002), that alone does not mean clients comply with lithium treatment. In addition, not all clients have a therapeutic response to lithium and need alternatives. After presenting some cases of clients taking lithium, we discuss those alternative treatments.

Lithium Cases

The following cases illustrate several different ways in which lithium has been used in mental health treatment.

The Case of William

Near the end of summer William, a 27-year-old, single construction worker, began to act very oddly and irrationally. He missed work or was often late. Coworkers noticed that he seemed "hyper" and silly, because he would toss tools, speak rapidly, and lose his train of thought. Friends recognized that William, an avid sports fan, was becoming obsessed with the owner of the local professional football team. William would talk at great lengths about his long conversations with this man and the inside advice he gave William just before each season. At present, he said the two of them were in intense discussions about strategies for the preseason games. One evening William's girlfriend, Sharon, called two of his best friends, a psychologist and attorney, to alert them of William's increasing bizarre behavior. She said he had invested most of his savings in what she believed was a scam to save dying children in Africa, was not sleeping, and had extreme mood swings she had never seen before. This evening she was afraid, because when he stormed out of her house, he told her he was going to walk on the center rail of the major highway at sunrise and he believed only the traffic driving west would be able to see him. He also believed this was the only way he could communicate with the sports owner about a disagreement they had had about a rookie on the team. She indicated she had never seen him like this, and she said she felt that William had slept little in recent weeks.

Eventually his two friends found William at the local YMCA, where he was being escorted out by police for creating a scene and using profanity with the manager. His friends spoke to the police, who released William to them. Over the next several hours, William talked with his friends about many grandiose plans, his paranoid fears, his worries that there wasn't enough time in a day, and his growing, spiteful hatred of the football team owner. Gradually, after long and circuitous arguments, William's two friends convinced him he needed medical help and took him to the emergency room of a local hospital. William was admitted and put on lithium carbonate, 450 mg, three times a day, until he stabilized and was discharged. At the three- and six-month follow-up, William remained stable and his blood levels remained in the therapeutic range. Now, 10 years later, William has had only one, minor manic episode, which did not demand hospitalization. He no longer takes the lithium and leads a relatively normal life. He is now married, with three children, and continues to work in construction.

The Case of Lincoln

Lincoln is a 38-year-old trade laborer who has suffered from Bipolar I Disorder for 19 years. He has had to be restrained or arrested for 31 of his 32 hospitalizations. Lithium, supportive counseling, and case management have failed to manage his disorder. It is important to mention that the lithium worked well enough to stabilize Lincoln so that he could be discharged from the hospital, but even when taken as prescribed, it could not keep him from decompensating into a psychotic and manic state. In these states, Lincoln becomes menacing and violent. During his manic episodes, no one can talk to or reason with Lincoln, and he seems to become more agitated and grandiose when safety personnel or mental health staff attempt to reason with him, resulting in hospitalization and restraint.

On discharge, Lincoln could return to work for short periods of time, but eventually he would again begin to decompensate into a manic state. His psychiatrist recommended both case management and a counselor. Lincoln began a 10-year counseling regimen with the same counselor. The work was problematic and very difficult. It emerged that Lincoln was the oldest of seven children and that his domineering father was an alcoholic. As a child, Lincoln had sustained several beatings from his father, and yet as an adult he intermittently worked for him. The counselor could not predict when Lincoln would become manic and often found out about the episodes only after Lincoln was hospitalized. It appeared there was no way to break the cycle of Lincoln's hospitalizations, and he refused any other medications beside lithium and diazepam/Valium for his

agitation. His severe Bipolar I Disorder with psychotic features and extreme manic states seemed impossible to control or manage.

During the 10th year of treatment, Lincoln recognized for the first time that he could self-admit to the hospital without the struggle of being either forcibly taken in or probated. This was a major breakthrough, and he externalized this decision by blaming the episode on his counselor when he spoke with the hospital staff. His counselor accepted this twist of events and worked with Lincoln to help him understand how this hospitalization was different from all the rest. Lincoln was never hospitalized again, except for the time he volunteered to participate in the Depakote/valproic acid studies at a local research hospital. During the study, Lincoln unfortunately got the placebo, and his mania went off the charts. He had to be put in isolation and administered both lithium and valproic acid/Depakote. This was also quite a learning experience for him.

When he returned to therapy, still on lithium and valproic acid/Depakote, Lincoln began to explore his family-of-origin issues, his current depressive feelings and enormous fear of them, and his desire to have a relationship with a woman. The combination of drugs seemed to stabilize Lincoln, and the counseling deepened his understanding of himself and his illness. He eventually married and managed to establish his own business, but he remains on his medication, is alert for side effects, and tries to cope with the anxiety and hyper states in his life.

Lincoln suffered tremendously from his Bipolar I illness, yet he managed to find the resilience to survive the numerous hospitalizations and connect with a counselor who maintained a tolerant, empathic, and focused relationship with him until he could begin to manage his illness in a more proactive way. In therapy, he explored intrapsychic issues and cultural examination of the impact of his Eastern European heritage. It is a miracle that Lincoln survived his illness and chaotic life. Both the combined drug therapy and the counseling facilitated Lincoln's improvement.

The Case of Kelly

Kelly is a 39-year-old, married, African American art teacher with no children. Over the holiday break, her husband noticed increased signs of agitation in Kelly, along with insomnia and heightened irritability. He also noticed that her daily activity increased dramatically and he could not keep up with everything she was trying to accomplish.

Kelly's state became so exaggerated that other family members became quite worried. Kelly would call members of her family at all hours of the night and try to enlist them in her ongoing activities. Finally, her husband had the good judgment to take Kelly to her family physician. She assessed Kelly briefly and referred her to a psychiatrist, whom she called immediately to alert her about Kelly's manic state. The psychiatrist evaluated Kelly the next day and recommended that she begin a course of lithium. She began on 450 mg daily and gradually increased to 1350 mg. The psychiatrist spoke with Kelly and her husband about lithium toxicity. Kelly returned to work and took the lithium as prescribed. She also had her blood levels checked regularly over the next several months. She never had a case manager or therapist.

In the seventh month, Kelly's husband began to notice a change in her skin, indicated by acne and rashes, one of the known side effects of lithium. Both he and Kelly noticed her continued drowsiness, frequent nausea, and mild dizziness. Kelly also complained of forgetfulness and mental dullness as she tried to remember her lessons for class. Most recently, she complained of blurred vision. She contacted her family physician, who immediately consulted with the psychiatrist who recognized the signs of lithium toxicity. He saw Kelly immediately, diagnosed toxicity from the signs, discontinued the lithium, and began sodium fluids. Even after this intervention, it took Kelly eight weeks to recover from the symptoms of lithium toxicity. She did not try another mood-stabilizing agent and tried to manage her rather moderate mood symptoms with diet, exercise, and meditation.

Review Questions

- What are four therapeutic effects of lithium and why do we think they help BPI disorder?
- What are the categories of side effects from lithium?
- What kind of client seems a good candidate for lithium?

SECTION FIVE: ANTICONVULSANTS AS MOOD STABILIZERS

Learning Objectives

- Understand the mechanisms of action that may be useful in using anticonvulsants to treat BPI.
- Understand the categories of side effects from anticonvulsants.

Anticonvulsant medications are used in treating Bipolar Disorder and appear to have some efficacy as antimanic agents. Researchers initially hypothesized that manic episodes resemble seizures in the sense that they "kindle," or "catch fire," just as fires "kindle" and then if enough kindling is present, the fire (manic episode) grows. For clients with seizure disorders, each episode seems to increase the probability of later episodes or to act as "kindling" for these later episodes. This was tied to reports about manic episodes, in that many clients who suffer from a manic episode are more likely to suffer from subsequent episodes. Thus, earlier episodes are said to somehow "kindle" the brain for other episodes. This theoretical similarity has been used as a justification for treating mania with anticonvulsants and birthed a line of research in which drugs that are approved as anticonvulsants seem to find their way into trials for treating Bipolar I Disorder. Since the first edition of this book, the support for the kindling theory has been inconsistent at best (Bender & Alloy, 2011). Some researchers have gone so far as to relabel the anticonvulsants "neuromodulators" when they are used to treat BPI

(Advokat et al., 2014). Our position is to discard the kindling theory and to *not* add more labels to existing compounds. The search for the etiology and drug mechanisms to treat BPI are confusing enough without muddying the waters with unnecessary terms. As with schizophrenia, the most important thing with Bipolar I Disorder is research that will uncover the etiology, not more drugs and labels for existing drugs. The following anticonvulsant medications are used in treating Bipolar Disorder and mania.

Carbamazepine/Tegretol

Researchers developed carbamazepine/Tegretol in the late 1950s as an anticonvulsant medication with efficacy in treating epilepsy. Pharmaceutical companies introduced it to the European market in 1960. In the early 1960s, physicians believed carbamazepine/Tegretol had beneficial psychotropic effects in people taking it for epilepsy, and in the 1970s, Japanese researchers documented its effectiveness in manic-depressive illness (Keck & McElroy, 1998). This latter research was confirmed in the late 20th century in a double-blind, crossover trial (Ballenger & Post, 1980). The FDA approved carbamazepine/Tegretol in 1974 as an antiepileptic drug for adults, in 1978 as an antiepileptic for children over 6 years of age, and finally in 1987 as an antiepileptic without age restriction. Carbamazepine/Tegretol comes in several liquid formulations (solutions, syrups) as well as slow-release and chewable formulations.

Mechanisms of Action in Carbamazepine/Tegretol

Table 8.5 summarizes the mechanisms of action for carbamazepine/Tegretol.

As you can see from Table 8.5, carbamazepine/Tegretol has many proposed mechanisms of action; however, researchers do not know which ones, or which combinations, account for carbamazepine/Tegretol's efficacy in clients suffering from Bipolar I Disorder (Keck & McElroy, 2002). Keck and McElroy (1998) and Mitchell and Malhi (2002) have proposed two basic mechanisms in

TABLE 8.5 Proposed Mechanisms of Action for Carbamazepine/Tegretol

Reduce neuronal firing through inhibition of sodium channels

Increased potassium conductance

Decreased glutamate release

Increase in adenosine receptors

Also alters neurotransmission mediated by NE, 5-HT, DA, GABA, Substance P, and aspartate

© Cengage Learning®

carbamazepine/Tegretol that may influence the symptoms of Bipolar Disorder. The first is effects on ion channels to reduce the firing of neurons, and the second is effects on presynaptic and postsynaptic neurotransmission.

Ion Channel Effects of Carbamazepine/ Tegretol

Recall from Chapter Two that each neuron has ion channels that allow the influx of either positively charged or negatively charged ions. The influx of positively charged ions increases the likelihood of a cell firing, and the influx of negatively charged ions decreases the likelihood of the cell firing. Carbamazepine/Tegretol seems to reduce neuronal firing by binding to and deactivating sodium ion channels. Sodium is a positively charged ion, and when its ion channel is deactivated it cannot enter the neuron and exert its excitatory effects. Some studies in the late 20th century supported the notion that carbamazepine/Tegretol increases potassium conductance, which is strange because potassium is positively charged and that would seem to increase cell excitation (Post, Weiss, & Chuang, 1992). More recent research more often supports the idea that carbamazepine/Tegretol ultimately decreases potassium conductance because it decreases calcium entry, which is necessary for activating potassium channels (Thomas & Petrou, 2013).

These mechanisms occur shortly after a person takes the drug and account for carbamazepine/Tegretol's anticonvulsant properties. These mechanisms do not explain why it is an effective mood stabilizer, however, the mood-stabilizing effects usually do not appear for 10 to 14 days (Perry et al., 2006).

Carbamazepine/Tegretol's Effects on Neurotransmission

Carbamazepine/Tegretol has numerous effects on neurotransmission. It decreases glutamate release (recall from Chapter Two that glutamate is an excitatory neurotransmitter) and affects norepinephrine, dopamine, and adenosine. Adenosine was not covered in Chapter Two but is what is called a *neuromodulator,* which is similar to a neurotransmitter except that its actions are not limited to the synaptic cleft. Carbamazepine/Tegretol causes an increase in adenosine receptors, which overall, would have an inhibitory effect on the nervous system. As noted, knowledge of these mechanisms has not helped explain why carbamazepine/Tegretol has efficacy for manic-depressive symptoms.

Efficacy of Carbamazepine/Tegretol in Bipolar Disorder

Although the scant literature supports the efficacy of carbamazepine/Tegretol for manic-depressive symptoms, the drug does not appear as effective as once thought (Dardennes, Even, Bange, & Heim,

1995; Kleindienst & Greil, 2002). For patients who have never had a mood stabilizer, lithium outperforms carbamazepine/Tegretol (Hartong, Moleman, Hoogduin, Broekman, & Nolan, 2003). Although other researchers challenge this view, carbamazepine/Tegretol is listed as a second-line treatment for mania. Like lithium, response to carbamazepine/Tegretol is correlated to the dosage and many nonresponders have been on inadequate doses of the drug. Studies have also supported carbamazepine/Tegretol as a maintenance therapy for manic-depressive illness (Kishimoto, Ogura, Hazama, & Inoue, 1983). Many researchers believe that trials with appropriate methodologies and adequate samples would find carbamazepine/Tegretol equal to lithium in efficacy (Mitchell & Malhi, 2002).

Side Effects of Carbamazepine/Tegretol

Table 8.6 summarizes the more common side effects associated with carbamazepine/Tegretol, according to Perry et al. (2006) and Schatzberg et al. (1997).

Dermatologic Side Effects of Carbamazepine/Tegretol

Within two weeks to five months of beginning carbamazepine/Tegretol, approximately 7% of users

TABLE 8.6 Common Side Effects Associated With Carbamazepine/Tegretol

Type	Description
Dermatologic	Rash that may foreshadow WBC problems
Endocrine	Hyponatremia (dangerous drop in sodium levels), Water intoxication
Gastrointestinal	Nausea, vomiting
Hematological	Leukopenia (elevated WBC count), Agranulocytosis (rare), Aplastic anemia (rare)
Hepatic	Elevated liver enzymes (20%)
Neurologic	Sedation/ataxia, dizziness, Dystonic reactions
Psychiatric	Delirium, hallucinations, Minimal cognitive impairment
Teratogenic	Associated with craniofacial defects and spina bifida

show general dermatologic problems such as rash or acne. Some data connect these dermatologic side effects to a more serious side effect of bone marrow suppression, particularly in children (Silverstein, Boxer, & Johnson, 1983). Another possible side effect is Stevens–Johnson syndrome, a rash involving the skin and mucous membranes. The lesions can include conjunctivitis as well as oral and genital lesions. Severe forms of the syndrome can include hepatitis and pneumonia and can be fatal. Once detected, this syndrome resolves when medication is discontinued. Recently, hypersensitivity to carbamazepine/Tegretrol has been linked to a family of genes referred to as *human leukocyte antigen (HLA)* (Tangamornsuksan, Chaiyakunapruk, Somkrua, Lohitnavy, & Tassaneeyakul, 2013). One particular allele of this family (HLA-B*1502) is correlated with Stevens–Johnson syndrome response to carbamazepine/Tegretol. This is one of those findings that moves the era of pharmacogenetics closer as now researchers recommend screening for this allele prior to treating a patient with carbamazepine/Tegretol (Amstutz et al., 2013).

Endocrine Side Effects of Carbamazepine/Tegretol

Carbamazepine/Tegretol can cause sodium depletion (hyponatremia) as well as water intoxication (defined as too much water in the body). Although this occurs in only 5% of clients, hyponatremia can be fatal if not corrected. The symptoms of sodium depletion include headache, nausea, puffiness about the face, muscle weakness, and disorientation. Frequently lithium is combined with carbamazepine/Tegretol, and sodium depletion (as noted earlier) can in turn cause lithium toxicity.

Gastrointestinal Side Effects of Carbamazepine/Tegretol

The most commonly experienced GI side effects of carbamazepine/Tegretol are vomiting and nausea. If people experience these side effects, their dosage can be reduced to resolve the side effect. Frequently, clients experience this while the prescribing professional is titrating the dose upward. In that case, the prescribing professional usually slows the titration.

Hematologic Side Effects of Carbamazepine/Tegretol

Elevated white blood cell counts (leukopenia) are experienced in approximately 12% of adults and 7% of children taking carbamazepine/Tegretol. Symptoms include fever, sore throat, and ulcers in the mouth. Although the blood count should be monitored for problems, most blood counts return to baseline without intervention (Sedky & Lippmann, 2006). Patients with low counts should be monitored every two weeks for the first three months of medication treatment. If the count falls below a certain point (3000 per millimeter), the drug should be discontinued. This same problem exists with oxcarbazepine/Trileptal, which is a metabolite of carbamazepine/Tegretol (Milia et al., 2008). More problematic are agranulocytosis (drop in white blood cell counts) and aplastic anemia (failure of the bone marrow to produce white and red blood cells).

Hepatic Side Effects of Carbamazepine/Tegretol

The most common side effect related to the liver is an elevated level of liver enzymes that govern metabolism. This side effect occurs in about 20% of clients on carbamazepine/Tegretol and is generally thought benign. There are rare occurrences of liver toxicity, the majority of which occur in the first four weeks of treatment. Symptoms include fever, jaundice, rash, anorexia, and/or nausea. If liver toxicity occurs, the medication should be discontinued.

Neurologic Side Effects of Carbamazepine/Tegretol

Two of the most common side effects of taking carbamazepine in general are sedation and dizziness. These typically occur within the first few weeks of therapy. Some children on carbamazepine/Tegretol experience dystonic reactions in the first two to three weeks of treatment. This response is possibly due to dopamine antagonism. If carbamazepine/Tegretol is combined with lithium, about 12% of clients taking the combination risk neurotoxicity.

Symptoms include confusion, disorientation, slurred speech, and problems with coordination.

Psychiatric Side Effects of Carbamazepine/Tegretol

No estimates exist on how many people experience psychiatric complications from carbamazepine/Tegretol, but the typical symptoms include delirium and hallucinations, insomnia, irritability, and mood lability. If these occur, the medication should be discontinued. There are also reports of some minimal cognitive impairment from carbamazepine/Tegretol; however, this impairment is not as great as is reported with lithium.

Teratogenic Side Effects of Carbamazepine/Tegretol

The use of carbamazepine/Tegretol in pregnant women has been associated with craniofacial defects, spina bifida (underdeveloped neural tube), underdeveloped fingernails, and developmental delays. Although some studies dispute these figures, there is not enough evidence to support safe use during pregnancy. Researchers recommend pregnant women avoid carbamazepine/Tegretol and valproic acid/Depakote (Werler et al., 2011).

OXCARBAZEPINE/TRILEPTAL

Oxcarbazepine/Trileptal can be thought of as a safer version of carbamazepine/Tegretol that may actually replace it in clinical practice (Advokat et al., 2014). It is carbamazepine/Tegretol with an oxygen molecule attached to one of its rings, which allows for an easier metabolism. It seems to have similar efficacy and side effects in treating BPI in adults but is not different from placebo in children and adolescents (Wagner et al., 2006).

THE CASE OF MOLLY

Molly is a 24-year-old single woman who has suffered from Bipolar I Disorder for over a year. She has had a great deal of difficulty on lithium, and her attending physician recognized that carbamazepine/Tegretol had just received FDA approval for use with Bipolar I Disorder in adults. He titrated Molly off the lithium and began a course of treatment on the carbamazepine/Tegretol. Over time, Molly noticed that her intermittent manic symptoms lessened while she was taking Tegretol, and she agreed to begin therapy to focus on issues surrounding her sexual orientation and great issues of anxiety and concern about "coming out" as a lesbian.

In this case, the carbamazepine/Tegretol served as an important alternative to lithium, and it stabilized Molly enough that she was able to explore other psychological issues in counseling. Another outcome of the counseling was that Molly was able to tolerate her depressive symptoms and link them to the losses she experienced in her life and to deep personal sadness. Molly remained on carbamazepine/Tegretol for six years and then successfully titrated off the psychotropic with minimal adverse effects. Molly's case is a good illustration of how psychotropic medication provides a window of opportunity for clients to explore intrapsychic issues.

THE CASE OF ROGER

Roger, a 32-year-old single male has suffered from a variety of mood and psychotic disorders over the past decade. Sometimes his chronic manic symptoms would intensify and Roger would become psychotic and have to be hospitalized. During these hospitalizations, Roger was given various diagnoses: He was variously diagnosed with Schizophrenia, Schizoaffective Disorder, Cyclothymia, and Bipolar I Disorder. He was treated with several medications, including lithium, perphenazine/Trilafon, loxapine/Loxitane, haloperidol/Haldol, and thiothixene/Navane. None of these medications seemed very helpful to Roger, and his case remained a mystery to his psychiatrist.

Recently, Roger was prescribed carbamazepine/Tegretol for his symptoms, and after three months he began to report some relief from his chronic manic symptoms. After six months on the drug, however, Roger began to experience continuous auditory and tactile hallucinations. He had never experienced either of these symptoms before, although the variety of his symptoms was extensive. After a careful assessment, his attending psychiatrist recognized that there was a very strong possibility that Roger was experiencing psychiatric side effects of the carbamazepine/Tegretol. The psychiatrist discontinued the medication, and after about five days the hallucinations disappeared.

Given the complexity and range of Roger's symptoms and diagnoses, it is remarkable that his psychiatrist was able to link his hallucinations to an adverse reaction to the carbamazepine/Tegretol rather than to new psychotic symptoms. This case is a good illustration of the importance of good medical care, particularly where multiple medications are involved.

VALPROIC ACID

Valproic acid is another anticonvulsant that is used as a mood stabilizer. There are several formulations of valproic acid with different names, including Divalproex, Depakene, Depacon, and Depakote. We use *valproate* because that is the most general term in use. Valproate was first synthesized as a sodium salt by George Carraz in 1962. Its initial use was as a solvent, and its anticonvulsant properties were not discovered until 1963. This discovery (like many in psychopharmacology) was made by accident: In France, researchers were mixing valproate (as a solvent) with other compounds thought to have anticonvulsant properties. The researchers soon discovered that the other compounds worked only when mixed with valproate and that only the valproate had anticonvulsant properties. It was tested and introduced as an anticonvulsant in Europe in 1967. Abbott Laboratories obtained a license for it as an anticonvulsant in 1983. In 1987 and again in 1991 Abbott was granted a patent and a new method to produce semisodium valproate, which differed from the original valproate by only one sodium ion. Abbott claimed it had a better gastrointestinal side effect profile. In 1995, Abbott won FDA approval for using valproate to treat acute manic episodes.

TABLE 8.7 Proposed Mechanisms of Action for Valproate

Inhibits sodium and calcium channels
Slows metabolism of GABA
Increases release of GABA
Inhibits reuptake of GABA
Unspecified effects on gene expression

© 2015 Cengage Learning®

Mechanism of Action

Table 8.7 summarizes proposed mechanisms of action for valproate.

Valproic acid differs chemically from all other anticonvulsants and psychotropic compounds. Like carbamazepine/Tegretol and lithium, it has many mechanisms of action. Scientists do not know why it acts effectively as an anticonvulsant or as a mood stabilizer. One theory, summarized by Keck and McElroy (1998), is that valproate slows down metabolism of GABA by attaching to the enzyme that breaks down GABA (GABA transaminase). Second, it increases GABA by inhibiting its reuptake. Third, valproate may inhibit sodium channels hyperpolarizing neurons. Finally, valproate may affect gene expression in ways that are therapeutically beneficial but not yet understood (Oguchi-Katayama et al., 2013). Recall from Chapter Two that GABA serves an inhibitory function in the nervous system, so any agent that increases its presence would increase inhibition of the nervous system.

Efficacy of Valproate in Bipolar I Disorder and Aggression

Current data suggest that valproate is as effective as lithium in treating acute mania and may be more effective than lithium in mixed-state or rapid-cycling subtypes of Bipolar I (Bowden et al., 1994; Freeman, Clothier, Pazzaglia, Lessem, & Swann, 1992; Mitchell & Malhi, 2002). Schatzberg et al. (1997) have noted that open trials indicate that valproate is also effective as a prophylactic. The antimanic effects of valproate begin within 7 to 14 days of a patient beginning the medication. It is currently being used in both children and adults (Wagner et al., 2002).

Some support exists for the notion that valproate is better tolerated than lithium. French researchers Lambert and Venaud (1992) noted in their study that valproate decreased aggression in animal models, may increase cognitive functions in humans (as opposed to the impairment of cognitive function associated with lithium), and may provide "awakening" effects on personality. An example would be a client whose emotional flattening and avolition improve after being put on valproate. Perry et al. (2006) make the point that in comparing valproate to lithium, it is important to separate the participants in various studies into those who have taken lithium and responded, those who have taken it and not responded, and those who have never taken it. This would give us more accurate information on how valproate compares to lithium, but many researchers do not give the participants' lithium history. It appears that valproate is also useful in reducing aggression and irritability in people suffering from personality disorders. Like lithium, it also seems useful in treating reactive/affective/defensive/impulsive (RADI) aggression (Padhy et al., 2011).

Side Effects of Valproate

Table 8.8 outlines the most common side effects of valproate. Note that the percentage of clients who suffer from a given side effect varies, as does the reported percentage of side effects, depending on which source you consult.

Cardiovascular Side Effects of Valproate
Edema is a condition characterized by swelling of body parts, particularly the limbs. Pitting edema is when pressure applied to the swelled area leaves a pit for some time after the pressure is released. This is caused by excess fluid under the skin and in the tissue outside the blood vessels. The condition is caused by excess salt in the system, and the valproate in some manner seems to disrupt the balance of salt in the system. Although this side effect is relatively

TABLE 8.8 Common Side Effects Associated With Valproate

Type	Description
Cardiovascular	Pitting edema
Dermatologic	Transient alopecia
Endocrinologic	Weight gain
Gastrointestinal	Anorexia Nausea, indigestion, Vomiting, Transient diarrhea
Hematologic	Neutropenia (low count of a particular white blood cell) Thrombocytopenia (low platelet count)
Hepatic	Increase in hepatic enzymes, Hepatotoxicity
Neurologic	Sedation, Fatigue, Confusion, Headache
Teratogenic	Neural tube defects, Craniofacial defects

© Cengage Learning®

rare, clients should know how to recognize it and report it to the doctor if it occurs.

Dermatologic Side Effects of Valproate
The transient alopecia (hair loss) that is a side effect of valproate is similar to that seen with lithium. The hair tends to regrow when the drug is discontinued and may regrow even if the drug is continued. Obviously, most clients find this distressing enough to discontinue medication.

Endocrinologic Side Effects of Valproate
Weight gain and increased appetite are common side effects of valproate. Perry et al. (2006) note that although dietary counseling may be recommended, caloric restriction may not solve the problem. Although it is hard to determine which clients suffer from this side effect and how much they gain, all clients should have baseline weight measured before beginning valproate therapy.

Gastrointestinal Side Effects of Valproate

This category of side effects of valproate has the broadest range. It is the second most common set of side effects attributed to valproate. Although many clients suffer from gastrointestinal side effects, researchers really do not understand the mechanisms of action. Both Perry et al. (2006) and Schatzberg et al. (1997) have emphasized that often these side effects can be alleviated by changing the formulation of valproate used. In addition, an over-the-counter histamine blocker such as Pepcid can also provide relief.

Hematologic Side Effects of Valproate

Platelet dysfunction (thrombocytopenia) can be a problem for clients on valproate. The symptoms include easy bruising or bleeding. Platelet levels can be checked, and if the counts are low, the prescribing professional can lower the dose or try a different medication. Another problem in this category is neutropenia, which is a low count of a particular type of white blood cell. Again, if this occurs, the drug dosage can be decreased or the medication discontinued.

Hepatic Side Effects of Valproate

The most common hepatic side effect from valproate is elevated levels of liver enzymes. This side effect, which seems benign, occurs in almost half the participants taking valproate in some studies. A more serious although rare problem is hepatotoxicity. This may be fatal and can be detected through tests of liver functioning. Symptoms of hepatotoxicity include lethargy, vomiting, anorexia, and weakness.

Neurologic Side Effects of Valproate

Sedation is the most common neurologic side effect of valproate. Less commonly, clients may experience headache, fatigue, and confusion. Small studies have also reported onset of hand tremor within one month of beginning treatment.

Teratogenic Side Effects of Valproate

Like carbamazepine/Tegretol, valproate is associated with increased risk of neural tube defects and craniofacial defects in infants of mothers taking valproate.

As can be seen from the side effect descriptions of lithium, carbamazepine/Tegretol, and valproate, there are some very unpleasant side effects associated with all these drugs. Although they all show efficacy to some extent in treating the symptoms of Bipolar I Disorder, many clients will not take them because of the side effect profiles. In addition, the truth is that scientists still do not understand why any of these medications are effective against the symptoms of Bipolar I and aggression. For these and many other reasons, the search continues for better mood stabilizers.

THE CASE OF JOSÉ

José is a 15-year-old Latino student who was placed in a Severe Emotionally Disturbed (SED) classroom for his aggressive and acting-out behavior. José had beaten up several boys and one girl over the past three years, and one of the boys had to be hospitalized for head injuries. After a recent fight, one of José's teachers noticed that José became very tired, even though he was the violent and uncontrolled aggressor. He slept in the dispensary for over an hour, and when he woke up he seemed very dazed and disoriented. The teacher consulted with the school psychologist, who was aware of many studies and efforts to administer mood stabilizers to aggressive youth. The psychologist also wondered if José might be experiencing some sort of atypical seizure disorder. As a result, the intervention teams met with the mother (his parents were divorced) and recommended a psychiatric consult for José.

José was referred to a psychiatrist who had an excellent reputation for treating children and adolescents. After a careful evaluation of José that included a complete neurological evaluation, he recommended that José begin a combined psychotropic medication treatment of lithium and carbamazepine/Tegretol for his atypical seizure disorder and extremely aggressive behavior.

The intervention team included an explanation of this pharmacologic treatment in their staff meetings, and they monitored the administration of both drugs while José was at school. This therapy, along with milieu support, greatly reduced José's outbursts and his aggressive behavior. In fact, over the next 18 months he only threatened, but did not assault, one student.

THE CASE OF BEVERLY

Beverly, age 67, is a widow of 17 years who has suffered from Schizoaffective Disorder for over 17 years. Her psychiatrist had tried to manage her extreme manic episodes with both lithium and carbamazepine, with only marginal effectiveness. Over time, Beverly had several side effect problems with lithium, including tremors, weight gain, goiter problems, severe rashes, and muscle weakness. Carbamazepine/Tegretol was ineffective in managing her manic episodes, which often necessitated that Beverly be hospitalized for long periods.

Beverly was not responsive to counseling, because she lacked insight and seemed to blame all her problems on either her husband's death or bad luck. She did connect with a female case manager, who helped her with daily living and survival skills, medication management, and support with her loneliness. The case manager was very knowledgeable about psychotropic medications, and she wondered if Depakote/valproic acid might be helpful to Beverly. She not only brought her idea to the attention of the staff psychiatrist but also spoke with Beverly about the medication. Beverly began a course of treatment on Depakote/valproic acid, and her manic episodes and symptoms diminished significantly. She was hospitalized once for a brief period over the next four years, and she had minimal side effects on the Depakote.

In this case, the knowledge, experience, and diligence of the mental health professional helped the client and alerted the psychiatrist to an alternative medication. This decision addressed Beverly's extreme suffering from her manic symptoms and the side effects. When counselors are well educated about psychopharmacology, they can competently assist both the client and the attending physician.

Review Questions

- What are the mechanisms of action that may be useful in using anticonvulsants to treat BPI?
- What sorts of side effects do anticonvulsants have?

SECTION SIX: NEWER ANTICONVULSANTS AS MOOD STABILIZERS

Learning Objectives

- Understand the hypothesized therapeutic effects of using these agents on BPI disorder.
- Know what some of the more dangerous side effects are.

Ever since valproate first showed promise as a treatment for Bipolar I Disorder, the search has continued for new mood stabilizers. Most drugs approved as anticonvulsants were considered for efficacy as mood stabilizers. Newer anticonvulsants may hold promise as mood-stabilizing agents, but they must be thoroughly researched, because their structures, effects, and side effects are heterogeneous (Calabrese, Shelton, Rapport, & Kimmel, 2002). Although research has just begun on these agents, the following sections summarize what we know about them so far. Table 8.9 lists newer anticonvulsant agents being researched for efficacy in treating Bipolar I Disorder.

Lamotrigine/Lamictal

The FDA approved Lamotrigine/Lamictal as an anticonvulsant in 1994. Since that time, researchers have been studying its efficacy in treating Bipolar I Disorder, making it the most studied of the newer anticonvulsants (Yatham et al., 2002). Macdonald and Young (2002) had hoped that in terms of its efficacy, lamotrigine/Lamictal would be promising but the study

TABLE 8.9 Newer Anticonvulsants Being Investigated for Efficacy in Treating Bipolar I Disorder

Generic Name	Brand Name
Oxcarbazepine	Trileptal
Lamotrigine	Lamictal
Topiramate	Topamax
Gabapentin	Neurontin

© Cengage Learning®

TABLE 8.10 Side Effects of Lamotrigine/Lamictal

Side Effect	Percentage Reporting
Dizziness	38%
Headache	29
Double vision	28
Unsteadiness	22
Nausea	19
Blurred vision	16
Sleepiness	14
Rash	10
Vomiting	10

© Cengage Learning®

results since then have been disappointing and inconsistent. Lamotrigine/Lamictal has shown some initial efficacy in preventing relapse in BPI but is not useful for acute mania or depression (Advokat et al., 2014).

Mechanism of Action of Lamotrigine/Lamictal

Although lamotrigine/Lamictal is still under study, research to date has identified several mechanisms of action. The drug seems to stabilize neuronal membranes by blocking sodium, calcium, and potassium ion channels. Lamotrigine/Lamictal also inhibits release of glutamate in the hippocampus. Recall from Chapter Two that glutamate is an excitatory neurotransmitter. Thus, inhibiting glutamate would generally tend to inhibit the neurons in those areas of the brain. This may result in an overall decrease in excitability in the brain that accounts at least for its anticonvulsive properties.

Side Effects of Lamotrigine/Lamictal

Table 8.10 summarizes the side effects so far known from taking lamotrigine/Lamictal. Unlike the other side effect tables in this chapter, these are not listed by category, on which more research is needed.

Probably the most serious side effect in Table 8.10 is the rash, which could be related to Stevens–Johnson syndrome, an immune-complex-mediated hypersensitivity disorder where the epidermis separates from the dermis and that may be fatal (which we discussed above in the section on carbamazepine/Tegretol). Children and adolescents are more susceptible to

this so lamotrigine is not indicated for anyone under the age of 16 (Kazeem et al., 2009). Clients taking lamotrigine/Lamictal who notice a rash should contact their doctor immediately. In addition to these, some psychiatric side effects have been reported, including depression, confusion, irritability, and mania (Asghar, 2002; Ferrier, 1998).

Preliminary Conclusions About Lamotrigine/ Lamictal for Bipolar I Disorder

Although there have been some positive reports on lamotrigine/Lamictal, its use in treating Bipolar Disorder may lie in using it as an adjunct to complement other agents such as lithium. Lamotrigine/Lamictal seems to have the most impact on unipolar depression, typically being significantly more effective than placebo. It is also useful for preventing future depressive episodes. Although it has not yet shown efficacy in treating acute mania, it may be a useful complement for unipolar depression (Calabrese et al., 1999). As Hurley (2002) noted, lamotrigine/Lamictal costs two to four times as much as lithium and when this is considered along with lamotrigine/Lamictal's adverse effects and efficacy, it does not seem like a strong contender as a mood stabilizer.

Topiramate/Topamax

Topiramate/Topamax is a new anticonvulsant that has shown some promise in open trials for treating Bipolar I Disorder. Although initial studies seemed to indicate that weight loss was a side effect (Marcotte, 1998), recent analyses indicate that any lost weight is regained after 12 to 18 months of therapy (Gordon & Price, 1999). At this point, it appears that topiramate/Topamax may serve as a useful adjunct to more traditional mood stabilizers in treatment-resistant cases (Chengappa, Gershon, & Levine, 2001; Letmaier, Schreinzer, Wolf, & Kasper, 2001). Topiramate/Topamax alone is no better than placebo for the treatment of mania (Kushner, Khan, Lane, & Olson, 2006).

Gabapentin/Neurontin

Gabapentin/Neurontin was introduced to the United States in 1993 as an anticonvulsant. In addition, it has been used off label for a variety of disorders, including BPI Disorder, impulsive behaviors, anxiety disorders, substance use disorders, and chronic pain. Some of these uses have proven quite problematic, and we return to this issue later. Gabapentin/Neurontin is designed to mimic the effects of GABA in the central nervous system (and is hence referred to as a GABA analog). Although initial trials proved promising (Stanton, Keck, & McElroy, 1997), later controlled studies and meta-analyses have found gabapentin/Neurontin no more effective than placebo (Frye et al., 2000; Maidment, 2001; Pande, Crockatt, Janney, Worth, & Tsaroucha, 2000). Gabapentin may yet show efficacy for agitation in psychiatric patients (Megna, Devitt, Sauro, & Mantosh, 2001), but thus far it has not sufficiently demonstrated antimanic properties. At the time of this writing, a great deal of controversy surrounds gabapentin/Neurontin and criminal fraud in its off-label uses that we explain shortly.

One of the more promising groups of agents are the newer antipsychotics covered in Chapter Seven. We now review the use of these in treating Bipolar I Disorder and finish the section by giving overviews

of newer agents that may yet rise to prominence as useful compounds.

Review Questions

- What are some of the mechanisms of action for lamotrigine and topiramate?
- What are some potentially dangerous side effects of these drugs?

SECTION SEVEN: ATYPICAL ANTIPSYCHOTICS AS MOOD STABILIZERS

Learning Objectives

- Understand what the hypothesized mechanisms of action are for using atypical antipsychotics for BPI.
- Know the side effects and how they relate to the side effects of lithium and anticonvulsants.

Throughout the book, we have written about the lack of accuracy in the *DSM* categories and in the psychotropic drug categories. For example, we noted that drugs categorized as antidepressants seem to have efficacy for a variety of disorders. So are they really "antidepressants" proper? The same problem crops up when we consider the use of atypical antipsychotics for Bipolar I Disorder. Olanzapine/Zyprexa was approved in 2000 for treating Bipolar I Disorder. Although the dosing is somewhat higher for Bipolar I Disorder than for Schizophrenia, current evidence suggests that olanzapine/Zyprexa may also be useful in the long-term treatment of Bipolar I Disorder and is at least as effective as lithium (Berk, Ichim, & Brook, 1999). In a large, randomized, clinical trial, Tohen et al. (2002) concluded that olanzapine/Zyprexa was more effective than valproate in treating acute mania over a three-week period. More recently, Derry (2007) examined five trials of treating BPI with atypical antipsychotics and found they were better than placebo. Derry felt the antipsychotics had efficacy in treating both phases of the disorder, but more recent research by Singh, Chen and Canuso (2012) contradicts this and implies they only have efficacy for the manic stage. They did produce weight gain. The other consistent finding seems to be that even when symptoms are in remission, patients on atypical antipsychotics for BPI have significantly poorer quality of life ratings than those in the control group. Yen et al. (2008) believed that adverse effects from the medications was a big part of this.

Current research is also looking at risperidone's/Risperdal's role in treating mania. Because these medications must be used at higher doses than those used for treating schizophrenia, there is an increased risk of tardive dyskinesia. It also seems that atypical antipsychotics, although showing promise for treating mania, may induce depression in some clients with BPI Disorder (Yatham, 2002). The most attractive feature of the atypical antipsychotics is the possibility that they would be better tolerated in terms of side effects than any of the mood stabilizers discussed so far. Although not associated with side effects such as hair loss, they are associated with weight gain, sedation, and the increased risk of diabetes (in some cases) that may be equally problematic for some clients (McIntyre, 2002).

One of the newer uses of atypical antipsychotics is as complements for another mood stabilizer (Kafantaris, Coletti, Dicker, Padula, & Kane, 2001). Delbello, Schwiers, Rosenberg, and Strakowski (2002) outlined a course of treatment for adolescents diagnosed with Bipolar I Disorder, complementing valproate with quetiapine/Seroquel. The study found that the combination therapy was more effective than valproate alone. Likewise, Weizman and Weizman (2001) concluded that the atypicals had promise both alone and when used in addition to other mood stabilizers, although these authors point readers to the debate on whether or not the atypical antipsychotics have significant advantages in terms of side effects.

Review Questions

- What are the hypothesized mechanisms of action for using atypical antipsychotics to treat BPI?
- How do you think the side effect profiles compare between atypicals, anticonvulsants, and lithium?

GENERAL CONCLUSIONS ON MOOD STABILIZERS

Although we have yet to explore mood stabilizers through the other perspectives of the integrative model, we can draw some conclusions from the medical model summary of these drugs covered thus far. First, as we noted at the beginning of the chapter, the very notion of mood stabilization is as illusive as the etiology of Bipolar I Disorder. All the medications discussed in this chapter were originally developed to treat other conditions, and their effects on mood states were accidentally discovered. Researchers really need to understand the etiology of Bipolar I Disorder and the action mechanisms of the effective drugs before they can move forward to designing drugs and other treatments specifically to treat Bipolar I Disorder. The inclusion of the phrase "and other treatments" implies that causes of Bipolar I Disorder may in fact not be limited to biological ones. From an integrative perspective, looking at psychological and even spiritual aspects of the disorder may help therapists radically redirect treatment efforts. Finally, it is becoming clear that the most difficult aspect of mood stabilization is the prophylactic one. Mitchell and Malhi (2002) noted that one large problem with researching this area is that clients eligible for the trials usually suffer from less severe forms of the disorder. This makes the clinical trial easier to carry out but decreases the generalizability in the field.

SECTION SEVEN: ISSUES FROM OTHER PERSPECTIVES

In this section, we explore some of the many issues surrounding mood stabilizers that frequently are not covered in psychopharmacology books. From an integrative perspective, there are numerous non-pharmacologic issues that, if engaged, could have profound implications for treatment.

Psychological Issues
Bipolar Illness and Creativity

Several of our students have asked whether there is a significant connection between Bipolar I Disorder and creativity. Jamison (1989) conducted a study with an admittedly small number of participants that supported the notion that clients who identified themselves as artists seemed to have a higher incidence of manic-depressive illness. Jamison (1993a, 1993b) revisits this study with several other case studies that seem to support the hypothesis. At the time she noted that medical model theorists resist this connection; however, much current work supports it as accepted now by the medical community (Ricciardiello & Fonaro, 2013). In a family study with 300,000 people, Kyaga et al. (2011) found that people with BPI and healthy siblings of people with BPI and Schizophrenia were over-represented in the creative professions. One difficult question is how treatments may stifle creativity, raising the question as to whether the treatment is worse than the disorder. The case of Robert illustrates this situation.

The Case of Robert

Robert worked as a visual artist, suffered severe mood swings, and met the criteria for Bipolar I Disorder. When he was depressed, he described himself as being in a liminal state between life and death. In this liminal state, he claimed to "peer across the narrow vale" that separated the living and the dead. In peering across that valley, Robert felt overwhelmed by the immensity of both the horrors and beauty of being alive; he became acutely aware of the needless cruelty that human beings inflict on one another. His conclusion was that most people were suicidal and expressed their suicidality outwardly in cruel actions. In such periods, he frequently contemplated suicide, and the only thing that stopped him was a profound

conviction that suicide did not bring about the cessation of consciousness that, in these states, Robert so desperately desired. As a practicing Wiccan, Robert believed souls would continue to deal with the same problems in the afterlife that they faced in this life, so suicide would not be "an easy out." Robert's practice of Wicca also led him to see his own alienation from mainstream society as an illness of the society more than his illness. To cope, Robert drank and abused opioids until he could create a buffer of numbness between himself and the terrors and pain of the world.

When Robert was in a manic mood, his creative output was indeed amazing. He was able to capture on canvas the rapture he could feel in contemplating the beauty of life as well as the desolation that so frequently overtook him. He could often work for days and even weeks on little or no sleep. Robert's manic episodes usually ended in a more restrictive setting as he would take his paintings out to museums and offer them to personnel there for display. His insistence and manner usually resulted in law enforcement officers being called and transporting Robert to an inpatient facility. Although certainly disruptive, Robert never threatened or hurt anyone.

After his third manic episode, Robert was stabilized and agreed to try lithium therapy. He suffered from forgetfulness, weight gain, sexual dysfunction, and hand tremors. Although the forgetfulness and hand tremor interfered with his painting, he said it was his total *lack* of mood that he found unacceptable. He said in essence that the medication took away all feeling and passion from his mind. He said it reminded him of the "zombie powder" used in voodoo ceremonies in the B-grade horror movies he watched. In addition, Robert found the regular blood testing uncomfortable and disruptive to his life. He discontinued lithium under his doctor's care after three months. The doctor then tried treating Robert with divalproex, with similar results.

Robert eventually stopped all medical treatments for his condition and chose instead to return to his previous lifestyle. Family members twice tried to have him involuntarily committed but were unsuccessful. Robert stated that if his condition were going to kill him at least he would be able to function as an artist until death. While on medication, he was not an inconvenience to society, he said, but neither was he fully alive. In his last therapy session, Robert said he did not expect his therapist or most people to understand, because most people hated life and hated to see anyone truly living the mystery of it. When told by family that his lifestyle was a risk to his well-being, he was fond of quoting the saying, "The candle that burns twice as bright burns half as long."

Again, from an integrative perspective there is much to reflect on in Robert's story. Do people have a right to live as they wish even if that lifestyle may cause them impairment and distress and possibly shorten their life? Is Robert really any different from other people who engage in unhealthy behaviors (such as smoking, fighting, creating unnecessary anger and stress for themselves and others)? Certainly it would be ideal if a medication existed that his doctor could have used to treat Robert without the severe side effects on his creativity, but this has never been an ideal world.

Robert's story also brings in the spiritual aspects of life. Although many adherents to positivism and the medical model perspective abhor the mere mention of the word, if spirituality reflects a person's ultimate concerns in life then Robert's spirituality was an important component of his story. From an integrative perspective, clients' spirituality is as important as the medications they are taking and the cultural/social context in which they find themselves.

Compliance with Mood Stabilization Therapy

Cases such as Robert's raise the issue of compliance with mood stabilizer therapy. One of our clients said to us, "I don't like taking lithium, but I seem to always get in trouble when I don't take it." This client—let's call him Jack, for convenience—was suffering some fairly severe side effects from lithium in the early 1990s but had failed to respond to carbamazepine/Tegretol. Weight gain and forgetfulness particularly bothered Jack. In addition, Jack, like Robert, deeply disliked having blood drawn and found the regular blood testing very difficult to comply with. On one occasion he went on a drinking binge, almost winding up in the emergency room. He recovered from that but became deeply depressed over his situation. Twice the doctor had titrated Jack off lithium, and twice he relapsed within 18 months. The relapses were crushing blows to his sense of self-efficacy, and he began to refer to himself as a "chemical cripple."

Compliance can be a difficult challenge for clients who are taking lithium. Studies on compliance show that about half the clients who begin lithium therapy stop taking the drug against medical advice. This also holds true for other mood stabilizers such as carbamazepine/Tegretol and valproate. Predictors regarding who is likely to be noncompliant include clients with histories of noncompliance, clients with denial regarding the severity of their illness, and the length of time the client has been on the mood stabilizer (the longer, the less compliant) (Scott & Pope, 2002). Most clients stop taking the medication because of the side effects, and it is not hard to understand why (Silverstone & Romans, 1996). As we see later, numerous medications may be as effective as lithium in treating Bipolar I Disorder, and mental health clinicians need to be prepared to advocate for their clients should lithium be unacceptable to the client. Although some clients can manage their symptoms without medication, many may require long-term or even lifelong pharmacologic intervention. For these people, the dangers of going off medication include not only relapse but also a significantly increased risk for suicide (Baldessarini, Tondo, & Hennen, 1999).

We have also found from the psychological perspective that clients tend to miss the "high" associated with manic states. There is no simple solution to this other than to establish a good therapeutic alliance with the client and, early in the relationship, to construct a history of the client's symptoms, making sure you discuss the symptoms that were most troubling for the client. When the client misses the manic states, it is important to balance what may be an idealization of these past states with the reality of the problems they caused the client. This dialogue must take place within a trusting relationship. Family therapy and support can also help clients face difficult existential issues. The bottom line, though, is that it is not the mental health clinician's job to "talk the client into" staying on medications. If the client cannot come to this decision autonomously, then clinicians need to explore alternatives to lithium therapy.

SECTION EIGHT: ISSUES FROM THE CULTURAL AND SOCIAL PERSPECTIVES

It is not rocket science to notice some oddities about aggression in U.S. society in general. The author Kurt Vonnegut (1991) has pondered aggression in the United States and what it means that we live in a time when killing is a leading entertainment form. Although many scholarly works support this description (Shifrin, 1998), we recommend instead that readers check their local cable listings. Other estimates indicate that many categories of violent crime have increased between the 1980s and 1990s, and this may continue into this 21st century (Goldstein & Conoley, 1998). The linguist and activist Noam Chomsky (2002) has noted that U.S. society has a history of violent imperialist policies requiring that citizens be distracted to other things (such as forms of violent entertainment). When you pair this aspect of U.S. society with the rates of psychotropic medication use, you may begin to wonder if perhaps everyone needs something to "take the edge off."

In Chapter Nine, we discuss the controversy that surrounds diagnosing younger and younger children with Bipolar I Disorder. At this point, though, we want to examine from an integrative perspective the connection between the violent nature of U.S. society and the use of "mood-stabilizing" medications. We have already noted that more and more mood stabilizers are being prescribed off label to treat children who engage in aggressive/violent behaviors, but we question if this is really treating the cause of the behaviors. The American Academy of Pediatrics (Shifrin, 1998) has summarized the literature that has concluded that viewing violence on television does influence the aggressive behaviors of children. Nevertheless, few studies look at how much violence children are exposed to who are also being treated with mood stabilizers for violent medication.

From an integrative perspective, we would do well to examine any correlation between viewing such violence on television or in video games and being on mood-stabilizing medication. Further, as we document in Chapter Nine, resources are decreasingly available for psychosocial interventions with children who have suffered or witnessed violence. Psychosocial interventions help children make meaning out of these horrible experiences, and the meaning they make has everything to do with how well they function after the event (Garbarino, 1998).

Although in U.S. society we discourage and punish some forms of aggression, others are blatantly rewarded. A good example is marketing strategies. Marketers frequently use martial vocabulary speaking of "conquering" a market, "exploiting" a competitor's weakness, or "destroying" the competition. The culture of marketing takes on special meaning in the pharmaceutical industry and, as we noted earlier, requires special monitoring.

The lawsuit discussed below, regarding the anticonvulsant gabapentin (Neurontin), illustrates some of the problems of aggressive marketing.

The Gabapentin Controversy: Corruption in Corporate Culture

As we noted earlier, studies from the medical model have not supported gabapentin as having efficacy in treating Bipolar I Disorder. Yet the drug continues to be prescribed off label. One such prescription became the center of this mess. This story was reported on National Public Radio on January 16, 2003 (Prakash, 2003). Although drug companies must follow rules in promoting medications to physicians, there are also ways around these rules. The case in question deals with a 16-year-old who committed suicide while under the care of his doctor, ostensibly for Bipolar I Disorder. The doctor was treating the teenager with gabapentin/Neurontin, although the young man said it was not helping.

The patient's statements make sense in light of a review of the literature that does not support gabapentin as having efficacy for Bipolar I Disorder.

What has come to light and became the center of a criminal fraud lawsuit is that the drug's manufacturer (Warner-Lambert, a subdivision of Parke-Davis) was accused of illegally marketing the drug for unapproved uses. The basic strategy was that the company encouraged the off-label use of gabapentin/Neurontin by directing money at influential doctors, who then wrote favorable reports for medical journals about gabapentin's efficacy in Bipolar I Disorder. By also talking about such findings at meetings of professional organizations, drug companies create "buzz" about the possible uses and increase the probability of increased off-label experimentation by others in the field. The "loophole" is that a company cannot market a drug for off-label uses but can "educate" doctors about those uses.

Parke-Davis contracted with a company called Medical Education Systems in Philadelphia, paying MES $160,000 to develop 12 scientific papers to "support epilepsy education." In actuality, three of these papers were on gabapentin/Neurontin and Bipolar I Disorder. The documents indicate that Parke-Davis made sure the articles printed what it wanted included, preapproved the authors and topics, and even chose the journals to which they would be submitted. According to the NPR story, some of the papers may have been entirely written by MES ghost-writers. The NPR reporter interviewed a former editor-in-chief of the *New England Journal of Medicine,* who stated that this arrangement is not unusual and that pharmaceutical companies often hire medical education companies to write such papers and then pay prominent physicians to basically sign the paper.

In another story, Prakash (2002) documented that Warner-Lambert/Parke-Davis planned the strategy to promote gabapentin for unapproved uses and that a company committee formulated the strategy. This strategy was enacted after the company determined in 1995 that clinical trials would be too expensive and take too long. The fear was that by the time the clinical trials were completed, the patent on gabapentin would have expired, and competitors would flood the market with generic formulations of the compound. The lawsuit involving Parke-Davis's Warner-Lambert division (recently acquired by Pfizer) maintained that this strategy was illegal. In addition, Warner-Lambert withheld one study from publication that concluded gabapentin was less effective than placebo for treating Bipolar I Disorder. The question arises, to what extent did the illegal strategy contribute to the physician prescribing gabapentin for the young man who committed suicide?

We are aware that we are writing this at a time when corporate scandal has been prominent in the headlines, first with the Enron scandal and then the WorldCom story. We feel the gabapentin story describes an extension of the immoral practices that seem to be such a large part of the U.S. corporate culture. Any integrative view of psychopharmacology must take this corporate culture into account when considering the impact of pharmaceuticals on the person. Any mental health clinician operating in the United States must consider these perspectives when treating clients taking psychotropic medication. Ideally, clinicians can get the client's agreement to monitor prescriptions for off-label uses of medications and when necessary, advocate for the client. As noted, the pharmaceutical company Pfizer acquired the Warner-Lambert division of Parke-Davis and was held responsible for the subdivision's activities between 1996 and 2000.

Pfizer pleaded guilty to criminal fraud and agreed to pay $240 million in criminal fines (the second-largest ever in health care fraud) and an additional $152 million in civil fines to be shared among state and federal Medicare agencies (Journal News.com, 2004). Perhaps the most difficult thing to comprehend is that this fine was a fraction of the money made through the off-label uses of gabapentin. *Time* magazine (2004) estimated that gabapentin/Neurontin made Pfizer $2.7 billion in 2003 and that 90% of that figure was from off-label uses. This would mean that almost $2.25 billion was made in off-label uses, making the $430 million in fines a proverbial "drop in the bucket."

Ingersoll, Bauer, and Burns (2004) have explored the role of advocacy in light of possible corruption in the corporate culture of the pharmaceutical industry. These authors recommend the following steps. First, mental health clinicians must know how to read and evaluate research. In an ideal world this would be enough, but in the real world clinicians must also work to understand how papers come to be published and whether the trial was conducted by a neutral party or a vested interest (including the pharmaceutical company itself). Clinicians need to know how well psychological treatments work and advocate with their professional organizations to focus on this material in professional journals and conferences. In addition, clinicians need to know the limits of diagnostic categories and that they are not descriptions of diseases capable of a single allopathic treatment but rather clusters of symptoms occurring together that can help guide treatment. Finally, mental health clinicians should consider advocating for regulatory oversight of pharmaceutical marketing to preclude dishonest or misdirected marketing efforts.

The Role of the Law in Pharmaceutical Company Regulation

Certainly, the gabapentin/Neurontin suicide described in the last section has components that should be addressed from the social perspective. First and foremost are the laws that allow companies to use loopholes such as the ones described. All too often there is an assumption that if something is not against the law, there is no problem. This of course ignores the rich history of unjust laws in our, as well as other, societies as well as discriminant enactment and adjudication. What protection does the individual citizen have when competing with vested power interests such as pharmaceutical companies that have the power to speak directly to elected representatives who supposedly represent us all? Here oversight—supervision—becomes an issue. Although many say that government oversight of corporations is already too great in this country, this is hard to believe when you look at scandals such as those involving Enron, World-Com, and now Pfizer. If anything, these scandals point to the need for further oversight and for internal checks and balances on the government regulatory agencies and courts, as well as legislation, and on media and advertising.

The Social Costs of Bipolar Disorder

Another social issue that needs to be considered concerns the social costs of Bipolar Disorder as well as the costs of treatment. An interesting study by Wyatt, Henter, and Jamison (2001) looked at the social costs of the disorder and then tried to estimate the amount society saved by using lithium. Reporting that the estimated social cost of manic-depressive illness in 1991 was roughly $45 billion, these authors noted that by comparing the actual social costs and the projected costs had lithium never been introduced, they could estimate how much money was saved. Recall that the FDA did not approve lithium for manic-depressive illness until 1970, so estimated social costs from that year in 1991 dollars may be considered an estimate of typical social costs prior to lithium's approval.

These authors concluded that in terms of direct social costs, lithium appeared to save approximately $8 billion a year, or a total of over $170 billion. These direct costs included inpatient and outpatient care and research dollars. In addition, the authors sought indexes of indirect costs and estimated that introducing lithium saved society approximately $155 billion. Indirect social costs included factors such as lost productivity of wage earners, homemakers, and caregivers as well as the unhappiness and waste of those people who languished in institutions or of those who, without lithium, may have committed suicide. Although many complex variables cannot be represented adequately in such studies, it is safe to assume that although not a perfect treatment, lithium has worked well enough for enough individuals to effect substantial savings in the social costs of treating manic-depressive disorders. The unaddressed issues in large-scale "guesstimates" about "costs to society" include general questions about the relative health of the society and the pointed question: If the society were healthier, would the need for intrusive interventions such as lithium treatment remain the same?

CONCLUSION

We hope this chapter on mood stabilizers has at least increased the complexity with which readers think about the issue. In many ways, the topic is like the mythic Hydra, with each problem representing a head. Once one head is cut off, several more arise in its place. Probably, until scientists can more clearly outline the etiology of manic-depressive illness, clinicians will continue to approach treatment in a "hit-or-miss" fashion. Although newer research on the human genome may accelerate the quest for the "perfect" medication, research must also continue examining the most effective psychosocial treatments for clients who take medications as well as for those who choose not to.

SUMMARY

Bipolar I Disorder is a serious and, in many ways, mysterious mental/emotional disorder. Although there are medications that help people suffering from the disorder, researchers are still unclear as to how the disorder develops and how to discern which medications will work best for individual clients. Although the drugs to treat Bipolar I Disorder are referred to as *mood stabilizers,* this is an inexact term. The oldest mood stabilizer is lithium, although researchers are not clear exactly how it exerts its therapeutic effects. Although lithium is still in use, not all clients respond well to it and many must try other medications. Alternatives to lithium include carbamazepine/Tegretol and valproic acid. Both of these compounds have proven efficacy for treating Bipolar I Disorder. There are several new drugs that the jury is still out on including oxcarbazepine, lamotrigine/Lamictal, and topiramate/Topamax. As with antidepressants, pharmaceutical companies must be closely monitored in the claims they make for mood stabilizers, as the gabapentin/Neurontin controversy illustrates. Because so little is known about the etiology of Bipolar I Disorder, it is important to take an integrative view of efficacy claims made by pharmaceutical companies.

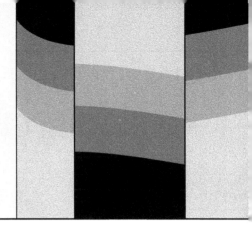

PART THREE

Newer Issues

This part of the book explores new ground in psycho-pharmacology on five important topics: the use of psychotropics with children, herbaceuticals, addiction medicine, drug-assisted psychotherapy and the use of psychotropics in the elderly. There is nothing new about prescribing psychotropic medications to children; however, in the last decade there has been an exponential increase in this practice. One of the biggest problems with this practice is that very few psychotropic medications are FDA approved for use in children, and the younger the child is developmentally, the more that child's nervous system differs from an adult's. In addition, we are seeing annual decreases in the amount of funding set up to support mental health services for children. From an integrative perspective this is a disaster, because many mental and emotional problems children experience are treated very effectively to psychosocial interventions. If no resources are provided for these interventions, then more and more children are referred for medication therapy alone despite an absence of evidence to support such referrals. Finally, an integrative view of this issue requires people to examine this culture's view of children. If work and achievement are given higher priority than family, where does that leave children?

Much has been written on herbaceuticals, but the topic is really just becoming accessible to English-speaking audiences, because the majority of the research has been conducted in European countries and published in journals written in European languages. Herbaceuticals are somewhat controversial in general in the United States, because technically they can be sold as "supplements" and do not require FDA oversight. As such, there is no guarantee on dosage, potency, or quality of formulation. Without FDA oversight, it is unlikely that herbaceuticals will be prescribed for mental or emotional disorders. We also cover the controversial marijuana plant in the herbaceuticals chapter. Although this book does not cover the pharmacology of drugs of abuse, a substantial case has been made for marijuana having medicinal uses, and we review that literature.

The other new ground we cover in this edition is Logan Lamprecht's chapter on drugs used to assist recovery from addition, Ingmar Gorman's chapter on using drugs like MDMA to assist psychotherapy and the final chapter on psychotropic medication use in elderly clients.

CHAPTER NINE

Medicating Children

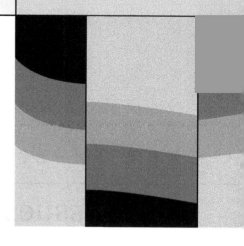

This chapter is divided into seven sections. Section One is an overview that discusses current trends in medicating children, problems the trends cause, and directions for the future. It also discusses developmental issues. Section Two focuses on stimulant medication and the diagnosis of attention deficit hyperactivity disorder (ADHD). Section Three focuses on research on combined interventions and particularly the Multimodal Treatment Study (MTA study) of Children with ADHD. Section Four focuses on children taking mood stabilizers. Section Five focuses on antipsychotics and children. Sections Six and Seven focus on anxiolytics and antidepressants in children, respectively.

SECTION ONE: PERSPECTIVES, DILEMMAS, AND FUTURE PARADIGMS

Learning Objectives

- Understand the problematic increase in psychotropic medications for children despite a dearth of evidence of the effectiveness of these drugs.
- Have a general understanding of the impact of the FDA Modernization Act and the Best Pharmaceuticals Act for Children.
- Be able to state the "developmental unknowns" associated with giving kids psychotropic medications.

Thus far, we have explored the medical model and psychological, cultural, and social perspectives as they relate to psychopharmacology. In this chapter, we

demonstrate that using psychotropic medications with children and adolescents raises particular problems and concerns from several perspectives. As discussed in Chapter Three, we frequently see explanations and justifications from the medical model perspective used to reduce childhood disorders to chemical and genetic problems, excluding crucial consideration of environmental traumas, developmental foreclosures, or life stressors.

We explore child and adolescent psychopharmacology primarily from the medical model perspective but complement this approach with information from the other perspectives (psychological, cultural, and social). We set the stage by exploring the current status of the treatment of children and adolescents with mental and emotional disorders. This chapter is structured differently from the others in this book. We begin by discussing the context from the social and cultural perspectives and the problems with prescribing psychotropic medications to children. Then we cover an introduction to stimulants used to treat symptoms of ADHD. Finally, we give the status of their current use since the last edition of the book if that is possible.

THE COMPLEX STATE OF THERAPY

Dr. Frank O'Dell, Professor Emeritus of Counseling in the College of Education and Human Services at Cleveland State University, has argued in all his lectures on counseling children and adolescents that the United States is an "anti-kid" society (Personal Communication, 2001). By that he means fewer and fewer therapists and psychiatrists choose to treat or continue to work with children in counseling. To support his argument, O'Dell points out that resources for children, including the number of hospital beds in mental health wards for children, have been shrinking. He believes the rules of managed care companies, dwindling personnel resources, and increasing difficulty in working with parents or guardians and their struggling children all contribute to the current trend. This has been a problem for at least 45 years. The American Academy of Child & Adolescent Psychiatry (AACAP) (2001) summarized the following facts, which support O'Dell's assertion, indicating little has changed:

- There is a dearth of child psychiatrists. Satcher (2001) stated further that many barriers remain that prevent children, teenagers, and their parents from seeking help from the small number of specially trained professionals who are available and that places a burden on pediatricians, family physicians, and other gatekeepers to identify children for referral and treatment decisions (U.S. Department of Health and Human Services, 2001).
- The AACAP's report projected that between 1995 and 2020, the need for child and adolescent psychiatrists will increase by 120%, whereas the need for general psychiatry is projected to increase at 22% for the adult population.
- McCarty, Russo, and Rossman (2011) demonstrated that only 13% of youth with suicidal behaviors and ideation receive mental health services.
- In November 2010, the Coalition for Juvenile Justice estimated that up to 75% of teenagers in the juvenile justice system nationwide have a diagnosable mental disorder, and these numbers continue.
- One in 10 children suffers from mental illnesses severe enough to impair development. Fewer than 1 in 5 children get treatment for mental illness.

The U.S. Department of Health and Human Services (2001) concluded that burgeoning numbers of children are suffering needlessly because their emotional, behavioral, and developmental needs are not being met by the institutions and systems created to care for them. As the number of children and adolescents needing psychological treatment rises and the number of service providers falls, the primary treatment modality becomes psychotropic medications rather than therapy. Imagine if you were a parent of one of these children.

Debner (2001a) reported that in a one-year period, 350 children needing hospitalization were turned away from hospitals in the Boston area. This phenomenon is occurring in most major U.S. cities and is exacerbated by hospitals holding onto children who are ready to be discharged, because there is no suitable placement for them. In another article, Debner (2001b) noted that the chief pediatricians from the five major academic health centers in Massachusetts indicated there is a serious crisis in psychiatric services for youth in the state. The doctors said they and their staffs could not find appropriate therapy and other mental health services for mentally ill children. As a result, many such children deteriorate to the point of crisis. Thomas and Holzer (2006) reported that America suffers from a serious long-term shortage of child psychiatrists that is taking a toll on young people, their parents, and their doctors. It is further recognized that the demand for psychotropic drugs is intense in spite of dangerous side effects.

The *Washington Post* (2002) published an article about a woman who desperately needed a psychiatric evaluation for her teenage daughter and who left 36 phone messages for various psychiatrists. She received only four replies. All the replies were from practitioners who refused to take the case because they did not treat adolescents. The article further detailed how, more and more, in-network providers (clinicians) prefer not to take patients covered by managed care plans, because reimbursements are so low and restrictions so numerous. The article also highlighted the disparity and arguments between the treating professionals and spokespeople from managed care companies. It is more than fair to say that desperate parents and anguished children are caught in the political policy dilemma over the cost and reimbursement of mental health treatment for children and adolescents.

Since the first edition of this book, there has been a movement to train more primary care physicians in pediatric mental health services to try to address the shortage of pediatric mental health professionals. Aupont et al. (2013) describe a model called Targeted Child Psychiatric Services designed for primary care physicians as well as child psychiatrists. This was associated with improved access to the child psychiatric services that exist, helped identify optimal care settings for patients and helped pediatricians be more likely to accept a patient back after that patient had been under psychiatric care.

Another problematic topic is who dispenses medications in schools. Most states have a policy on this and many states have a Nurse Delegated Medication Administration program (Ryan, Katsiyannis, Losinski, Reid, & Ellis, 2014). Most standardized curricula include trainings of approximately 30 hours with 8-hour updates every two years or so. These are by and large directed by professional nurses (Spector & Doherty, 2007). Nationwide lists of states and their programs can be found at http://www.nasbe.org/healthy_schools/hs/bytopics.php?topicid=4110&catExpand=acdnbtm_catD and http://www.healthin schools.org/health-in-schools/health-services/school-health-services/school-health-issues/medication-management/state-policies-on-administration-of-medication-in-schools.aspx.

THE EXPLOSION OF PSYCHOTROPIC MEDICATION PRESCRIPTIONS FOR CHILDREN AND ADOLESCENTS

With diminishing psychological supports for children and adolescents, using psychotropic medications with them has become the treatment of choice, even though the majority of medications used with them lack FDA "on-label" approval for them (Werry, 1999). Researchers currently estimate that between 7.5 and 14 million children in the United States experience significant mental health problems (Riddle, Kastelic, & Frosch, 2001; Wozniak, Biederman, Spencer, & Wilens, 1997). These statistics vary a little from Satcher (2001),

cited earlier; clearly, millions of children in this country require mental health services. Children are increasingly prescribed psychotropic medications as part of their treatment; in many cases, the medications replace the therapy (Jensen et al., 1999; Phelps, Brown, & Power, 2002). Given the explosion in the use of psychotropic medication with children, it is important also to note that this population has been *excluded* from clinical trials of these drugs. Hence, decisions about juvenile medication obviously rest more on extrapolation of adult data to children and adolescents than on direct research and evaluation of the safety and efficacy of psychotropic medication with children (Riddle et al., 2001; Vitiello & Jensen, 1997).

Coyle (2000) indicated that 80% of all medications prescribed to children and adolescents in the United States have not been studied for the safety and benefit of these populations. As of 2011, The National Institutes of Health indicated that methylphenidate, lithium, all atypical antipsychotics, lorazepam, and amitriptyline were still on the highest priority list of needs in Pediatric Therapeutics of drugs to be studied in pediatric populations.

Even though there is a black box warning related to the risk of increased suicidality in children and adolescents prescribed SSRIs and SNRIs, the use of these psychotropic agents has increased with children and adolescents (Markowitz & Cuellar, 2007). The trend in treating children and adolescents with off-label psychotropic medications, mostly in lieu of counseling and psychotherapy, has triggered concern both in the general public and the mental health community. Coyle (2000), Furman (1993), and Zito (Zito et al., 2000, 2003) argue that there is little or no evidence to support psychotropic drug use with very young children and conclude that such treatment could have harmful psychological, developmental, and physical effects. In a multinational study, American youths were three times more likely to be on an antidepressant medication than their peers in Denmark, Germany, and the Netherlands (Zito et al., 2006). In 2010, the pharmaceutical companies research protocols were really challenged when uncovered pharmaceutical studies on many highly utilized psychotropics were found to be no more efficacious than the placebo. In fact, the second author has personal communications with several psychiatrists in their fourth or fifth decade of practice who question the overall effectiveness of psychopharmacology with patients, especially children (Ramirez, Personal Communication, 2014).

In another multinational study, Zito et al. (2008) found that the annual prevalence of youth taking psychotropic medication was threefold greater in the United States than in the Netherlands and Germany. The atypical antipsychotics represented 5% of antipsychotic use in Germany but 66% in the United States. Interestingly, though, anxiolytics were twice as common in Dutch youth than as in U.S. or German youth.

With proper research, mental health professionals may be able to head off disasters such as aspirin precipitating Reye's syndrome or valproate leading to sudden death in infants (Riddle et al., 2001). Given the lack of knowledge about the long-term and adverse effects of psychotropic medication on children, it is crucial that mental health clinicians be alert to the impact of these drugs on children and advocate for youth when the evidence that such drugs would be helpful is questionable (Ingersoll, Bauer, & Burns, 2004). At this point, we would like to introduce a case that highlights many of the treatment and medication dilemmas children and adolescents encounter.

THE CASE OF PHILLIP

Phillip is a 7-year-old first-grader from a single-parent home. His mother is on public assistance, and he is the oldest of four boys. Although some of the details of his developmental history are sparse, Phillip began to exhibit impulse control problems at the age of 2 years and 4 months, shortly after his father moved out of the house. He was hyper-vigilant, easily distractible, aggressive with his younger sibling, and frequently irritable. Initially, his mother believed he was going through a stage of rebelliousness, but after several months she became concerned about his behavior and mentioned this to the pediatrician. After a brief examination, the pediatrician indicated that Phillip was likely suffering from ADHD and recommended against medication unless his behavior got too out of control at home. However, she felt he would need a course of methylphenidate/Ritalin, a prescription stimulant, once he began preschool. Phillip's mother accepted this recommendation and planned to have him evaluated when he began preschool. Phillip's behavior improved slightly over the next several months, without therapy or psychotropic medication.

When he began preschool, it took only a few days before all his active symptoms returned. After observing him for several weeks, the teacher recommended to Phillip's mother that he see a physician to be assessed for a stimulant medication. After the evaluation, the physician prescribed 10 mg of methylphenidate/Ritalin daily for Phillip. Methylphenidate/Ritlain is one of the most common stimulants used for symptoms of ADHD in children. It is intended to reduce inattentiveness, distractibility, impulsivity, and motor hyperactivity, with a goal of improved academic productivity. Phillip's symptoms slightly improved over the next eight weeks, but his aggressive behavior toward other children increased. Phillip's mother noticed more unpredictable behavior at home, as well as sleeplessness and restlessness followed by long periods of lethargy. She took him back to his physician, who referred them to a psychiatrist. The psychiatrist, after a three-session assessment, diagnosed Bipolar I (BPI) Disorder, took him off the methylphenidate/Ritalin, and prescribed 50 mg of carbamazepine/Tegretol daily and 0.01 mg of clonazepam/Klonopin. The carbamazepine/Tegretol was used to reduce his manic symptoms. This antiseizure medication has over time been found very effective with Bipolar Disorder (Phelps et al., 2002).

The clonazepam/Klonopin was used to address Phillip's anxious and agitated symptoms. This antianxiety medication often relaxes children and reduces anxiety without inducing sleep.

Many of Phillip's symptoms diminished, but his mother noticed both a sluggishness and apathy in him that were new. Over the course of the next year, Phillip's teacher addressed several of his learning and cognitive processing problems. Up to this point, the focus of Phillip's treatment had been psychopharmacologic. No psychosocial interventions were given to Phillip, as is often the case (Phelps et al., 2002). No one seemed to have any awareness or discussion about the optimal level of medication for Phillip, and there was no referral for a psychosocial assessment. As his symptoms worsened, he was evaluated by a psychiatrist schooled in prescribing adult psychotropic medications off label to children. Finally, Phillip's mother took him to see a therapist, who focused on Phillip's attachment issues, his phobic anxiety triggered by sudden loss or the anticipation of sudden loss, and his physiologic symptoms, which the therapist considered powerful side effects of the pharmacologic therapy.

Analysis of Phillip's Case

Analyzing the case, Phillip was treated by pharmacology in the medical model method and rational thinking centered on pharmacology dominated the case. The combination of methylphenidate/Ritalin and carbamazepine/Tegretol on Phillip's system was supposed to reduce some of his externalizing symptoms in the constellation of ADHD or Bipolar I disorders, but the psychological aspects of his personality were ignored. Not until much later in the course of his illness did Phillip get some assistance in those domains. Culturally, Phillip's mother had little power in society and was torn between accepting the opinion of the medical experts, and watching the negative impact the medications were having on her son. As mental health professionals, we need to understand the medical psychiatry's rapid efforts to address most disorders of childhood and adolescents with psychotropic medication. Far too often, medicating professionals view talk therapy and other psychosocial interventions as ineffective and second rate. Because medical professionals hold more power in our society than mental health professionals, their medical opinions are frequently given more weight. Today, psychiatrists burdened by enormous caseloads are open to what is known as split-treatment, a joint effort by the mental health professional and psychiatrist to plan and integrate treatment and be vigilant for client manipulation.

We must integrate care into a larger model of treatment that addresses each of the four perspectives equally and where mental health professionals' opinions on mental health treatment are given more weight. In addition, the power of pharmaceutical companies must be monitored. Bodenheimer (2000) has documented numerous cases where companies prevented important research findings from being published because they were not favorable regarding the compounds being tested. To what extent may such situations affect clients like Phillip? This will be discussed later in the chapter.

Remember, Phillip was in the 4 to 7 age range when he began treatment. Coyle (2000) comments that there is "no empirical evidence to support psychotropic drug treatment in very young children and that such treatment could have deleterious effects on the developing brain" (p. 1060). Furman (1993) posited that psychiatrists in the United States are recklessly "out of control" in prescribing methylphenidate/Ritalin and other stimulants for children, in contrast to the extreme caution that physicians in almost all European countries use in recommending this treatment approach. With the increasing trend to medicate a younger and younger population (Zito et al., 2000), mental health professionals not only need to understand the impact and therapeutic effectiveness of these medications, but also their limitations and potential for harming children.

THE MEDICATION OF CHILDREN AND THE FEDERAL LAWS

As we have noted in previous chapters, the laws of the land hold great influence over cultural and social paradigms. To a large extent, laws are the result of a dynamic interaction of forces that influence other areas such as socioeconomic status and the fiscal systems of a society. Socioeconomic status and fiscal systems shape laws in very powerful ways, and people with financial resources are able to buy influence with lawmakers. This is nothing new, but bears stating in this chapter. Although recent legislation has been introduced to address

TABLE 9.1 Major Emphases of Recent Legislation on Pediatric Pharmacology

Law/Rule	Summary
FDA Modernization Act (Public Law Number 105-115, 1997)	Recognizes rights of children as patients Sets specific standards for research of pediatric drugs Encourages pediatric labeling
Best Pharmaceuticals for Children Act (Public Law Number 107-109, 2002)	Voluntary pediatric studies of currently marketed drugs Created list of all pediatric drugs needing documentation Requires timely labeling of pediatric drugs Establishes a mandate to include children of all cultures in studies Voluntary studies of new drugs
Pediatric Rule Bill of 2002[a]	Required timely pediatric studies and adequate labeling

[a]Child & Family Services Improvement Act: Language on how the use of medications is to be monitored.

© Cengage Learning®

the many problems of prescribing psychotropic medications for children, most such laws require only voluntary testing of psychotropic drugs, diminishing any real impact. In this section, we summarize recent laws and comment on them, beginning with a summary in Table 9.1.

FDA Modernization Act

Buck (2000) traced the unfolding need for greater specific labeling of drugs used with patients less than 18 years of age. The burgeoning use of almost all drugs approved for children by the FDA compelled pediatric health care providers to use these drugs off label without a clear knowledge of dosing, administration, or adverse-effect information. In 1992, the FDA took steps to improve both pediatric labeling and research, which resulted in support for building a network of pharmacologic research by the National Institutes of Health (NIH). These efforts began to address the problem, and passage of the FDA Modernization Act (1997) for the first time set specific requirements to tighten regulations relating to pediatric pharmacology. This law encouraged pediatric labeling on drugs used widely with children and adolescents where the lack of labeling might lead to serious misuse. However, the FDA website (2013) warns that users of methylphenidate/Ritalin may have an erection lasting many hours. This from an agency that still cannot

conduct pediatric studies that evaluate the full impact of the drug on that population.

This law goes a long way toward recognizing the rights of children as patients, protecting their health, and assisting pediatric providers with essential information. Unfortunately, the law did not go far enough. Many practitioners and lawmakers felt the need for a comprehensive law to mandate pharmacologic research, monitor it, and further protect children.

The Best Pharmaceuticals for Children Act

On January 4, 2002, President George W. Bush signed Public Law Number 107-109, the Best Pharmaceuticals for Children Act (Dodd, 2001), with the anticipation that it would address many of the dilemmas and controversies surrounding the eruption in use of pharmaceuticals for children. This law aims to initiate critical studies with pharmaceuticals already prescribed to a population for whom there exists little research, and it tightens the monitoring and development of new drugs released for children and adolescents. The law seeks to integrate viewpoints on medicating children with the medical, cultural, and social perspectives. Unfortunately, its most powerful provisions regarding the conduct of pharmaceutical companies are voluntary.

The Best Pharmaceuticals for Children Act (BPCA) has 19 sections that can be viewed at http://www.fda.gov/RegulatoryInformation/Legislation/FederalFoodDrugandCosmeticActFDCAct

/SignificantAmendmentstotheFDCAct/ucm148011
.htm). This law encourages voluntary pediatric studies of already marketed drugs, the so-called off-label
psychotropic drugs in widespread use with children,
and it creates a research fund for studying these
drugs (see http://blogs.fda.gov/fdavoice/index.php
/tag/best-pharmaceuticals-for-children-act-bpca/).
Both efforts are critical to understanding the effectiveness and efficacy of psychotropic medications for
children and adolescents. Further, the law establishes
an ongoing program for the pediatric study of drugs,
including a list of all drugs for which documentation is
needed. This aspect of the law is monitored by the
commissioner of the FDA and the director of the
National Institutes of Health, who have the power
to make written requests to pharmaceutical companies
for pediatric studies. The law requires timely labeling
changes for pediatric drugs under study.

As of this edition, the status of most pharmaceuticals
for children and adolescents remains similar to what it
was in 2006. There was the black-box effort with
SSRIs and SNRIs, but they are prescribed at rates
higher than in 2006 (Cummings & Fristad, 2007)
and most other psychotropics are used with children
and adolescents to quiet anxiety, agitation, and rage.

However, the pharmaceutical companies continue
to challenge the Pediatric Rule on all fronts and now
it is 2014 and most important drugs for children have
not been studied with a pediatric group. So goes the
Pediatric Rule. On October 17, 2002, the U.S. District Court for the District of Columbia ruled that the
FDA did not have the authority to issue the Pediatric
Rule and has barred the FDA from enforcing it. The
Pediatric Rule would have required timely pediatric
studies and adequate labeling of all human drugs.

Child and Family Services Improvement Act

The Child and Family Services Improvement Act of
2011 (Public Law 112-34) includes new language
that addresses the social-emotional and mental health
of children who have been traumatized by maltreatment. State Child and Family Services Plans now
have to include details about how emotional trauma
associated with maltreatment and removal is
addressed. They also have to describe how the use
of psychotropic medications is monitored.

A WORD ON CROSS-CULTURAL PERSPECTIVES

Tseng (2003) proposed many variables and differences in prescribing psychotropic medications to
children and adolescents from various cultures. He
stressed that one must consider not only the physician's attitudes about treating people from different
cultures, but also the patients' perspectives on how
they feel about psychotropic medications. Thus, the
giving and receiving of medications has many
implications. This factor is greatly enhanced for
children and adolescents, because the physician
must not only communicate with the parents
about the diagnosis and the psychotropic medications (neither of which may make sense in the parents' worldview) but must also weigh carefully the
cultural issues that the family brings to treatment.

Tseng (2003) also addresses the enculturation
issues of children. His research has described how
not every culture emphasizes the fast-paced and
often accelerated approach to growing up that char-
acterizes the United States. **Enculturation** is
defined as a process through which an individual,
starting in early childhood, acquires a cultural system through the environment, particularly from
parents, school, and so on. Some cultures, such as
many Asian cultures, have a laid-back attitude
toward babies and toddlers that is more indulgent.
Yet later, they show a dramatic shift for these children, who, when they arrive at latency, the developmental period between the ages of 6 and 11 or
12, experience enormous pressure to be diligent
and to achieve. Thus, as clinicians treat children
and adolescents from all cultures, they need to
reconsider cross-cultural adjustment and revise the
psychosocial stages of Erikson (1968), which
depended on developmental understandings in a
particular culture.

With the upsurge in the use of psychotropic medications, it is impossible to monitor the expected and
unexpected adverse effects. Given the expanding
knowledge of the varying developmental trajectories
of children from other cultures, mental health practitioners and psychiatrists need to exercise further
caution when prescribing psychotropic medications

for these children. Lin and Poland (1995) described in detail the remarkably large interindividual variability in drug responses and side effect profiles. This can be partially accounted for in differences of ethnicity and/or culture apart from physiological pace. Some cultures are very suspicious of medication and may delay the decision for more than a year.

Lin and Poland (1995) have made significant contributions to the understanding of **cultural psychiatry** and to the fact that genetic factors associated with individual and ethnic backgrounds contribute greatly to responses to medication in children, adolescents, and adults. Kirmayer and Ban (2013) note that cultural differences in self and personhood are equally important. All researchers we reviewed point to variations within the same ethnic group and variations among ethnic groups. This further complicates the integrative dilemma, which is how to view psychopharmacology and cases from the four perspectives outlined in Chapter One as well as consider important developmental lines and levels. Mental health professionals recognize that researchers have much to learn about psychopharmacology with children and adolescents, as shown by the research cited in this chapter. We need to integrate our growing understanding of cultural psychiatry with our limited understanding of how psychotropic medications work in children. The Best Pharmaceutical Act for Children (2002) provided for including in studies children from various racial and ethnic backgrounds. The law calls for studying the impact of medications on children of different cultures.

PSYCHOLOGICAL PERSPECTIVES OF CHILDREN AND ADOLESCENTS

Medicating children and adolescents for all types of psychological disorders is a solution that only reflects partial truth. The overt behaviors and symptom profile for which they receive medication may only mask the deeper psychological wounds of loss, trauma, abuse, sibling rivalry, neglect, sexual abuse, or gender conflict. Furman (2000) has indicated that if mental health professionals carefully examined the overuse of stimulants with children, they would discover a variety of conflicts and problems fueling the hyperactive behavior. These issues could include cruelty in the home, harsh toilet training, neglect, sexual abuse, delay in language development, and more.

Young children cannot address their inner conflicts without the help of a caring therapist and the modality of play therapy, yet far too often they are diagnosed with Bipolar I or ADHD and medicated in an attempt to quickly suppress their active symptoms. There should be far more effort to get the child to a therapist to uncover the underlying cause(s) of the child's anguish, but this requires resources that, at the time of this writing, lawmakers are not giving a high priority.

The American Academy of Pediatrics (2011) for ADHD makes clear that parent and teacher assessments at home and school, respectively, along with clinical review and examination by pediatrician or psychiatrist, often omit psychological assessment of the child by a mental health professional to rule out abuse, neglect, loss, sleeplessness, or other potential causes of hyperactivity or mania. In this protocol (the AAP guidance), the psychology and clinical history of the child are treated as unimportant. Many authors unfortunately support rapid assessment of ADHD children to speed up treatment with stimulant medication.

OPPOSITION TO THE CURRENT TREND OF MEDICATING

Opponents to exclusive medication treatment for ADHD, Bipolar I, and other conditions have pointed out significant regional variations in the amount of psychotropic medications prescribed to children and wide variations in regional diagnostic criteria for ADHD and other conditions (Safer, Zito, & Fine, 1996; Wolraich, Hannah, Pinnock, Baumgaertel, & Brown, 1996). These variances have legislators and mental health advocates from various regions of the country clamoring for more judicious use of psychotropic medications with children, with more careful attention to the range of adverse effects from them, and a more formalized protocol for diagnosing ADHD, Bipolar I, and other conditions. This protocol should go well beyond the traditional oral report from teacher to parent about a child's externalizing behavior. Opponents of psychotropic medication use in children call for a more specific and guided differential diagnosis of these disorders because the symptoms commonly overlap with Oppositional Defiant Disorder, Conduct Disorder, Major Depressive Disorder, various anxiety disorders, and many developmental disorders (American Academy of Child and Adolescent Psychiatry, 2007; August, Realmuto, MacDonald, Nugent, & Crosby, 1996). Many researchers and practitioners still feel that ADHD in particular is a myth and that the explosion in use of the diagnosis renders differential diagnosis impotent (Armstrong, 1997; Furman, 2000). Furman (2000) concluded,

> I have tried to trace the thinking that followed the discovery of the vastly different approaches in the United States and Europe to the management of the active or overactive child.... This thinking led to the conclusion that ADHD is not a specific disorder or pathological entity but rather a collection of symptoms that could be manifested by a child in distress, a child in conflict within himself and/or with his environment. It has no more specificity than that, and likewise methylphenidate has no specificity in producing its effects.... Suppressing these symptoms by "subduing" the child with medication hides from all the source of the child's troubles, precludes his being able to obtain mastery of his troubles through understanding, and subjects him to a false label of brain pathology. (p. 141)

Furman, now deceased, indicated that his conclusions were not new but simply ignored.

AN OVERVIEW OF PEDIATRIC AND ADOLESCENT PSYCHOPHARMACOLOGY

By the time this text has been published, only a handful of psychotropic medications will have been approved as on label for the preschool age group. Examples include methylphenidate/Ritalin, amphetamine/Adderall, haloperidol/Haldol, and chlorpromazine/Thorazine (Zito et al., 2003). Methylphenidate/Ritalin is now under great scrutiny (Zaicek, 2009). For preschool-age children, it is aggressive behavior that generally triggers a referral for treatment (Bassarath, 2003). A few more psychotropic medications have been approved for use in older children and adolescents (Kluger, 2003), but those (such as the antidepressant fluoxetine) are hotly debated because of suicidal risk. Table 9.2 lists as many medications as we were able to find with on-label approval for children.

We have mentioned the national dilemma that more children and adolescents demand psychological services each year, yet there are fewer service providers. Concurrent with this expanding problem is the dramatic increase in the use of psychotropic medications off label for a variety of mental and emotional conditions and disorders. Although this is problematic in and of itself, the focus on psychological and interpersonal factors in treating children and adolescents has dangerously diminished. Whereas it used to be common practice for child psychiatrists to choose in each case from among drug therapy—primary drug therapy and secondary counseling, or primary counseling and secondary drug therapy (Kraft, 1968)—today these choices are rarely discussed routinely.

Also note that *DSM* criteria are primarily normed on adults and are more difficult to apply with children. House (1999) has indicated that over half of the time, children who meet the criteria for one mental or emotional disorder meet criteria for other disorders as well. This multiple nature of children's problems frequently results in a polypharmacy approach and requires careful decisions by the physician and/or treating team (Brown & Sammons, 2002). How carefully those decisions are made varies from setting to setting and clinician to clinician and are more random today (Leslie, 2011).

Researchers do know that the preschool years are one of the key developmental periods for maturation of the brain dopamine system, which is targeted by stimulants (Coyle, 2000). The FDA approved package insert on methylphenidate/Ritalin warns against

TABLE 9.2 Drugs with FDA On-Label Approved Uses in Children

Generic Name	Brand Name	Dosage	Ages
ADHD Medications			
Methylphenidate	Ritalin	10–60 mg	6 and older
Immediate Release (IR)	Methylin	20–60 mg	6 and older
Methylphenidate	Ritalin SR		
Sustained or Extended	Metadate SR		
Release (SR/ER)	Concerta		
Methylphenidate			
Transdermal	Daytrana	10 mg/9 hours	6 and older
Dextroamphetamine	Focalin	5–40 mg	6 and older
Dextroamphetamine			
Extended Release	Focalin XR	10–40 mg	6 and older
Lisdexamfetamine	Vyvanse	30–70 mg	6 and older
Amphetamine/Dextroamphetamine	Adderall	5–40 mg	3 and older
Atomoxetine	Strattera	.5 to 1.4 mg	6 and older
Guanfacine	Intuniv	1–4 mg	6 and older
Clonidine	Kapvay	.1 to .4 mg	6 and older
Antipsychotics/Mood Stabilizers			
Aripiprazole	Abilify	2–30 mg	For BPI 10 and older
		2–15 mg	Irritability/Autism 6 and older
		2–30	Schizophrenia 13 and older
Risperidone	Risperdal	.25–3 mg	Autism 5 and older
		.5–6 mg	BP Mania 10–17
		.5–6 mg	Schizophrenia 13–17
Olanzapine	Zyprexa	2.5–20 mg	BPI/Schizophrenia 13 and Older
Paliperidone	Invega	2.5–20 mg	BPI/Schizophrenia 12–17

(continued)

TABLE 9.2 Drugs with FDA On-Label Approved Uses in Children (continued)

Generic Name	Brand Name	Dosage	Ages
Quetiapine	Seroquel	50–600 mg	BPI 10 and older
		50–800 mg	Schizophrenia 13 and older
Lithium	Eskalith	900–2400 mg	BPI 12 and older
	Lithobid	900–1800	?
Neuroleptics			
Chlorpromazine	Thorazine	.5–200 mg	Psychosis 6 and older
Haliperodol	Haldol	.5 to .15 mg	Tourette's 3–12
Pimozide	Orap	.05–2 mg	Tourette 12 and older
Antidepressants			
Escitalopram	Lexepro	10–20	12 and older
Fluoxetine	Prozac	10–20	for depression 8–18
		10–60	for OCD 7–17
Fluvoxamine	Luvox	25–200 mg	for OCD 8–17
Sertraline	Zoloft	25–200	for OCD 6–17
Amitripyline	Elavil	25–100	for depression 12 and older
Clomipramine	Anafranil	25–100	for OCD 10 and older
Imipramine	Tofranil	30–100 mg	depression 12 and older
		25–75 mg	eneuresis 6 and older
Protriptyline	Vivactil	15–20 mg	depression 12 and older

its use with children under age 6. Given all the unknowns, many scholars and physicians are concerned about the quality and care and the current explosion of prescribing practices with preschoolers. Mental health professionals do not have enough clear evidence about how preschoolers respond to psychotropic medications, and researchers are very uncertain about the impact of such medications on the development of preschoolers. Let's examine some of the major developmental issues.

Developmental Issues

For many of you, this section on human growth and development in children and adolescents is a review. Most texts on development emphasize cognitive, language, moral, and psychosocial developmental paths. We briefly consider these lines of development and include others that are potentially affected by the ingestion of psychotropic medication. Understanding development is further complicated by the construct of **developmental lines**—the simultaneous occurrence of several aspects of human growth and development.

Developmental Lines

Although there are dozens of lines of human development, this multiplicity is still not a focus for mental health professionals outside of developmental studies. What should be common knowledge for mental health professionals is still peripheral to their training. For example, the Council for the Accreditation of Counseling and Related Educational Programs (CACREP) requires only one human development course for a master's degree in school or clinical mental health counseling. There may be dozens of lines of human development. These include physical development, cognitive development, emotional development, sexual development, moral development, spiritual development, kinesthetic development, socioemotional development, gender identity, and role-taking ability. These are just a few of the lines of development to which every person has access, and, for the most part, everyone proceeds through them unevenly.

The sheer number of developmental lines and the fact that most people proceed unevenly through them raise enormous, unaddressed issues for psychopharmacology. We noted earlier that scientists know very little about how brains develop and that many researchers are concerned that psychotropic medications could profoundly damage the brains of children and adolescents when taken long term. Glen Elliott, director of the Langley Porter Psychiatric Institute Children's Center of the University of California at San Francisco, noted that the current use of psychotropic medications on children "has outstripped our knowledge base . . . we are experimenting on these kids without tracking the results" (Kluger, 2003, p. 51). For example, even when an adolescent truly appears to suffer from Bipolar I Disorder, the sequelae of mood stabilizer side effects such as weight gain and perhaps hair loss are likely to be more devastating for

a person of that age than for an adult—but there is no research on such psychological issues.

Perhaps the greatest problem of studying child and adolescent psychopharmacology from the four integrative perspectives is that whenever the issue of medicating children comes up, the only perspective represented is that of the medical model. A good example is a *Time* magazine cover story, by Kluger (2003) that basically explores only the medical model perspective, with only minor attention to psychological, cultural, and social issues. The same article presents a diagram showing what parts of the brain are believed to be correlated with different mental or emotional disorders. At no point in the article does the author state that these areas are hypothesized to be *correlated with* symptoms and there is no evidence that they *cause* symptoms. This remains true as of the second edition of this book.

As we have noted throughout the book, many symptoms that are psychogenic in origin register in the brain, but this does not mean the symptoms were *caused* by the brain. This bias toward the medical model perspective leads laypeople to assume that mental/emotional disorders, whether in children or adults, are strictly medical disorders. This assumption is not currently supported by the evidence we have been covering in this book. A full-scale multimodal approach to mental and emotional disorders in children and adolescents considers medication and possible brain pathology as only one part of the story in a very complex interaction of tentative causes and interventions.

Developmental Pharmacology

Developmental psychopharmacology is a newer area of research that studies brain development focused on brain plasticity (the brain's ability to shape itself to environmental or chemical input) and sensitive periods (during which experience can alter neural representation before hardwiring occurs) (Carrey, Mendella, MacMaster, & Kutcher, 2002). Pediatric psychopharmacology is an equally young enterprise with the first published reports dated in 1937 but by the 1980s the United States had become the world leader in medicating children (Riddle, Walkup, & Vitiello, 2008).

Although these disciplines are examining development strictly from the medical model perspective, its overarching question is, "What happens in the complex process of neural development when an infusion of psychotropic medications is introduced to address particular environmental stressors during periods of accelerated brain development?" Compared to adults, children and adolescents respond to psychotropic medications in different and distinctive ways that have implications for efficacy and safety (Vitiello & Jensen, 1995). The rate at which prescriptions of psychotropic medications have grown for children despite the dearth of research to support their efficacy raises the question "are we doing too much or too little?"

Epstein (2001) posited that active brain growth spurts occur stagewise in correlation with Piagetian types of development. Thus, a child who is making the transition from the sensory motor stage to Piaget's preoperational stage is in a very active brain growth stage (from age 2 to 4 years). Epstein cites Boothroyd (1997), who noted that lexical knowledge and syntactic knowledge grow rapidly until age 4. At about 6 (from age 6 to 8), the next rapid brain growth period parallels Piaget's concrete reasoning stage, where a child begins to think logically about experienced inputs, the concrete operational stage. Epstein discussed the next brain growth period as slow (from age 12 to 14 years), a time of practicing and consolidating new networks in preparation for the next rapid brain growth stage (between ages 14 and 16 years). Psychotropics often are administered to preschoolers in the rapid growth period between ages 2 and 4 years, and to early-latency children between the ages of 6 and 8 years. Mental health professionals do not know enough about the impact of both on-label and off-label psychotropics in these rapid brain growth periods to be administering them to children and adolescents. Bramble (2003) concluded that given the changing nature of pediatric pharmacology and developmental pharmacology, this society needs a rapid expansion of pediatric research and academic inquiry into the impact of psychotropics

on children's development. The second author in an extensive review of developmental pharmacology articles found only those supported fully by pharmaceutical companies or ones that cost between $29.50 and $40.00. Almost all recommended the use of a psychotropic as a first-line intervention. Interestingly, the pharmaceutical companies signed documents stating that they had no "conflict of interest." In addition, the medications being used are only partially successful 40–50% of the time (Rapoport, 2013).

Another problem with pediatric psychopharmacology is **polypharmacy**: the use of more than one psychotropic simultaneously, a usage that interacts with children's metabolism in a variety of unpredictable ways (Brown & Sammons, 2002). Clinicians who observe children and adolescents under the influence of polypharmacy are often startled not only by the dramatic change in the clients' affective and behavioral state but also by the array of side effects they experience. Tonya, a very aggressive 12-year-old, was placed on olanzapine/Zyprexa (an atypical antipsychotic), sertraline/Zoloft (an SSRI antidepressant), lorazepam/Ativan (an anxiolytic), and valproate/Divalproex (a mood stabilizer). This combination of medications was ostensibly for what appeared to the attending psychiatrist as Bipolar I with severe agitation and aggression in the manic phase. Tonya's symptoms diminished, but her teacher noticed new ones: slurred speech, mild tics, and a constant staring off without responding when addressed. Now, rather than disrupting the class, she slept through it. Although from the perspective of the teacher and other students this was an improvement, was Tonya being helped, or was she merely medicated into submission when she might have been more fundamentally helped with assessment and therapy from a wider interpersonal perspective?

Other developmental considerations include adverse cardiovascular effects. We have many reports of sudden deaths of children and adolescents treated with psychotropic medications, including methylphenidate/Ritalin, TCAs, SSRIs, bupropion/Wellbutrin, lithium, and most neuroleptic medications. Gutgesell et al. (1999) detailed the cardiovascular and electrophysiologic effects of commonly used psychotropic medication, which can be deadly. Although the precise causes of the deaths have not been documented, severe heart spasms (cardiac arrhythmias) and delayed repolarization of the heart rhythm (delayed QTc interval) make the heart muscle vulnerable to possibly lethal changes (such as ventricular tachycardia). These tragedies call on mental health professionals to be vigilant and cautious when prescribing psychotropic medication. With many high-risk medications, cardiovascular monitoring is particularly important. In fact, Wagner and Fershtman (1993) recommended ECG monitoring at baseline and during drug therapy for children and adolescents who are on the medications associated with cardiovascular side effects. Brown and Sammons (2002) argued that the use of most psychotropic medication exceeds data available for efficacy, effectiveness, and safety.

Many concerns also remain related to the physiological impact on children who take psychotropic medication. One is the controversy about the impact of stimulant treatment on brain growth in children (Bell, Alexander, Schwartzman, & Yu, 1982). Researchers have recently learned that methylphenidate and other stimulants decrease blood flow to selected parts of the brain, specifically the cortex area that controls conscious movement (Zeiner, 1995). In a recent study (Castellanos et al., 2002), the research team concluded that developmental trajectories for all brain structures, except caudal, remain parallel for children and adolescents in ADHD patients and controls. This suggested that genetic and early environmental influences on brain development in ADHD are fixed, nonprogressive, and unrelated to stimulant treatment.

However, initial brain scans of patients with ADHD showed significantly smaller brain volumes in all regions than what appeared in the brain scans of the controls. In general, because of brain plasticity (the brain's ability to shape itself), it is possible for children to be highly susceptible to a negative impact on their brain development during one period of development and less so in another period of development (Carrey et al., 2002). Does

treatment with psychotropic medications constitute a negative impact? These authors further concluded that researchers are only beginning to understand the long-term effect of psychotropic medication on neuron cell factors and their overall impact on brain development. All these developmental concerns or issues involve potential adverse effects for children and adolescents taking psychotropic medication.

At this point, we cover the different categories of medications used on children and adolescents. We begin the next section with a more thorough treatment of stimulant medications.

Review Questions

- What are some of the main problems with the increase in psychotropic medication prescriptions for children?
- What was the impact of the FDA Modernization Act and the Best Pharmaceuticals Act for Children? Name at least three changes these acts initiated.
- What are the "developmental unknowns" that make prescribing psychotropic medications for children problematic?

SECTION TWO: STIMULANT MEDICATION

Learning Objectives

- Understand the mechanism of action and side effects of stimulant medications.
- Be able to discuss the type of symptoms stimulants seem most helpful for.

Even though stimulants are currently the best-studied psychotropic medication used on children, many issues regarding their use are still unresolved. Because stimulants are prescribed almost exclusively for children, we have included information on them in this chapter. Before discussing some of the controversial issues, let's examine some background and general information on these widely prescribed medications.

Some History

The first known stimulant in the West was cocaine. It was isolated in 1859 by a German chemist named Albert Niemann and was given to Bavarian soldiers to decrease fatigue. In 1884 Karl Koller perfected its use as an analgesic during eye surgery. His assistant, a young neurologist named Sigmund Freud, was off visiting his fiancé at the time and so missed out on credit for that discovery. Freud had been personally experimenting with cocaine and wrote the paper "Uber Coca" ("On Cocaine") prior to realizing its addictive qualities (Freud & Carter, 2011). Many people in South American societies still regularly chew coca leaves with little ill effect, because unprocessed leaves are far less dependence inducing than is refined cocaine powder (Siegel, 1989). Efforts to synthesize amphetamine began in 1887, when physicians believed it useful for treating asthma. This belief emerged from the use of an herbaceutical called *ma huang* in Chinese medicine. *Ma huang* is discussed more thoroughly in Chapter Ten on herbaceuticals, but for now understand that it is the ingredient ephedra that is central to the story of amphetamines. This ingredient produces the bronchial dilation that relieves the wheezing of asthma.

In the 1920s, a Chinese pharmacologist working for Eli Lilly (K. K. Chen) was working to isolate and synthesize ephedra from ma huang. He succeeded in synthesizing a compound so structurally similar to ephedra that it was named *ephedrine*. Although this could be taken orally, the goal for asthma treatment was a compound that could be inhaled. Gordon Alles succeeded in developing another variation of the molecule that could be delivered in an inhaler. Called Benzedrine, this variation was successful in treating asthma. Aside from treating asthma, it also seemed to induce euphoria. People soon realized they could open the inhaler and ingest the contents for what became known as "the amphetamine rush." This also became a popular pastime on college campuses during exams. Amphetamines were experimented with to

manage a number of disorders, and one of their early uses was treating children for what was described as "overactivity."

Werry has asserted that research in psychopharmacology for children began with publication of Bradley's (1937) paper on how amphetamine seems to calm overactive children and help children with learning disabilities. The only other noteworthy investigations of the same period were studies on the effects of antihistamines on children (Connors, 1972). These works are thought to be the only primary contributions to child psychopharmacology until very recently (Werry, 1999).

Bradley's work reemerged in the 1960s after psychiatry began moving away from a psychodynamic model toward the biological model dominant today. Psychiatrists at that time were not well trained in the statistical methods that were becoming the norm in evaluating medications. They turned to psychologists for assistance. The psychologists emphasized the need to look at medication effects on learning and academic performance (Werry, 1999). Such research has, until very recently, remained focused primarily on stimulant medication.

Research in pediatric psychopharmacology received an unintentional boost in the 1960s with the creation of a diagnosis called Minimal Brain Dysfunction (MBD). MBD was one of the several precursors to the current ADHD diagnosis. MBD was treated with stimulant medications such as methylphenidate. Although later discarded because it was too vague, the MBD diagnosis did much to lead to the development of a norm for a methodology with which to evaluate the effects of drugs, and particularly stimulants, on children.

In World War II, German, British, American, and Japanese soldiers all used amphetamines, a practice still common in the U.S. Air Force to help pilots keep alert on bombing missions (Knickerbocker, 2002). After World War II, the Japanese had such huge surpluses of amphetamines that they marketed them to civilians. These drugs were advertised for the elimination of drowsiness and repletion of spirit. Researchers estimate that by 1948, 5% of the Japanese population between the ages of 15 and 25 was dependent on amphetamines.

After World War II, it became evident that amphetamines have appetite suppressant qualities, and chemists tried to tease these out from the reinforcing properties that were connected to abuse. However, most of these initial efforts (such as methylphenidate/Ritalin) failed, and then the drugs were simply marketed as amphetamines.

The amphetamine molecule is a simple and highly malleable molecule that acts as the chemical template for over 50 pharmacologically active substances (Grilly, 1994). Amphetamine is basically made of two compounds (isomers) labeled "L" and "D" amphetamine. D-Amphetamine is more potent and was marketed as Dexedrine. A minor modification in this molecule yields methamphetamine marketed as Methedrine. Other variations of the amphetamine molecule can produce MAO inhibitors. Modifying amphetamine to dimethoxy-methylamphetamine (DOM) produces a psychedelic compound similar to mescaline, and further modification produces the empathogen methylene-dioxymethamphetamine (MDMA, street name "ecstasy"). The latter was a promising psychotherapeutic compound until criminalized (Eisner, 1994). The therapeutic effects revolved around chemically induced states of empathy, euphoria, and well-being that facilitated insights that were then to be integrated into clients' normal awareness (Stevens, 2009).

Table 9.3 outlines stimulant medications used to treat ADHD in children.

Mechanisms of Action in Amphetamines

Amphetamines exert almost all their effects by causing the release of norepinephrine and dopamine from the synaptic vesicles into the synaptic cleft. There are different mechanisms for amphetamines to act as dopamine agonists and the number of mechanisms used depends on the type of amphetamine. There are two isomers of amphetamine, "L" and "D." The "L" isomer amphetamine mechanisms of action include:

- Pure reuptake inhibitor for DA
- No presynaptic activity
- Enhances NMDA receptor response
- Weak block monoamineoxidase
- 80% metabolized
- The classic L-isomer amphetamine is methylphenidate/Ritalin

The D-isomer amphetamine mechanisms of action are similar to those of cocaine and include:

- Reuptake inhibition of DA (inhibit DAT)
- Drug taken into terminal by DAT & depletes vesicles (causes DA transporter to act in reverse) thus releasing DA from the presynaptic neuron
- Enhances NMDA receptor response
- Weak block of monoamineoxidase (MAO)
- Releasing NE from presynaptic neuron

Amphetamine/Dexedrine is the classic D-isomer amphetamine but is less prescribed than Adderall. Mixed amphetamine salts/Adderall includes D-amphetamine.

TABLE 9.3 Stimulant Drugs Used to Treat ADHD in Children

Generic Name	Brand Name	Type of Drug	Daily Dose
Amphetamine and D-amphetamine compound	Adderall	Stimulant	5–40 mg
D-Amphetamine	Focalin	Stimulant	5–40 mg
Methylphenidate	Ritalin	Stimulant	5–60 mg
Lisdexamfetamine	Vyvanse	Stimulant	30–70
Atomoxetine[a]	Strattera	NE reuptake inhibitor	0.5–1.2 mg

© Cengage Learning®

[a]Atomoxetine is not a stimulant but an SNRI (see Chapter Five).

In a study comparing methylphenidate to cocaine, Volkow et al. (1995) noted that although the mechanisms of action and effects are similar, methylphenidate clears more slowly from the brain, which, they hypothesize, makes it less dependence inducing. Readers are encouraged to think critically about this result, because when a similar mechanism of slow clearance is invoked to defend cannabis (marijuana) as low in dependence-inducing qualities, it is often rejected (De Fonseca, Carrera, Navarro, Koob, & Weiss, 1997). Either the mechanisms discussed decrease the probability of dependence or they do not. Pharmaceutical and political agendas should be separated from this debate so that people can objectively examine the issues. In previous chapters, we have listed the adverse effects of psychotropics being discussed. With ADHD, these effects are interwoven into the complex presentation of the stimulants. We ask you to consider why in the continent of Europe (an area of the world that has about the same population as the United States), stimulant medications are used with children for only about 5 to 8% of the treatment population so treated in the United States. Now let us examine the *DSM-5*.

ADHD Diagnosis and Assessment

According to the *DSM-5,* the diagnostic criteria for attention–deficit/hyperactivity disorder are

A. Either (1) or (2):
  (1) six or more of the following symptoms of inattention have persisted for at least five months to a degree that is maladaptive and inconsistent with developmental level:

  Inattention
  (a) often fails to give close attention to details or makes careless mistakes in schoolwork, work, or other activities
  (b) often has difficulty sustaining attention in tasks or play activities
  (c) often does not seem to listen when spoken to directly
  (d) often does not follow through on instructions and fails to finish schoolwork, chores, or duties in the workplace (not due to oppositional behavior or failure to understand instructions)
  (e) often has difficulty organizing tasks and activities
  (f) often avoids, dislikes, or is reluctant to engage in tasks that require sustained mental effort (such as schoolwork or homework)
  (g) often loses things necessary for tasks or activities (e.g., toys, school assignments, pencils, books, or tools)
  (h) is often easily distracted by extraneous stimuli
  (i) is often forgetful in daily activities
  (2) Hyperactivity: Six (or more) of the following symptoms of hyperactivity impulsivity persisted for at least six months to a degree that is maladaptive and inconsistent with developmental level:

  Hyperactivity
  (a) often fidgets with hands or feet or squirms in seat
  (b) often leaves seat in classroom or in other situations in which remaining seated is expected
  (c) often runs about or climbs excessively in situations in which it is inappropriate (in adolescents or adults, may be limited to subjective feelings of restlessness)
  (d) often has difficulty playing or engaging in leisure activities quietly
  (e) is often "on the go" or often acts as if "driven by a motor"
  (f) often talks excessively

  Impulsivity
  (g) often blurts out answers before questions have been completed
  (h) often has difficulty awaiting turn
  (i) often interrupts or intrudes on others (e.g., butts into conversations or games)

B. Several hyperactive-impulsive or inattentive symptoms that caused impairment are present before age 12 years.

C. Several inattentive or hyperactive–impulsive symptoms are present in two or more settings.

D. There must be clear evidence of clinically significant impairment in social, or occupational functioning.

E. The symptoms do not occur exclusively during the course of a Pervasive Developmental Disorder, Schizophrenia, or other Psychotic Disorder and are not better accounted for by another mental disorder (e.g., Mood Disorder, Anxiety Disorder, Dissociative Disorder, or a Personality Disorder). (APA, 2013, pp. 59–60)

Source: Diagnostic and statistical manual of mental disorders, 5th ed., (Washington, DC: American Psychiatric Association, 2013).

Both the "Consensus Statement" of the National Institutes of Health (1998) and the "Clinical Practice Guidelines" of the American Academy of Pediatrics (AAP) (2011) recommend careful diagnosis of ADHD and then an appropriate and judicious use of stimulants in combination with other psychosocial treatments to address the symptoms. Epstein et al. (2010) also emphasize that children treated with stimulant medication show improvement in ratings by parents and teachers but not in their level of functioning as measured by grades. Thus they note that mental health services in addition to medication are important.

In terms of assessment most protocols recommend a neurologic exam, a consultation with a psychiatrist or psychologist who specializes in ADHD, behavioral observation reports from parents, grandparents, teachers, and other school personnel. Olfson, Gameroff, Marcus, and Jensen (2003), analyzing national data, reported the increased rates of treatment from 0.9 per 100 children in 1987 to 3.4 per 100 children in 1997. They posited that this increase along with fewer treatments (counseling) per child was attributed to a broader awareness of the diagnosis by special educators, growth of managed behavioral health care, and increased public acceptance of psychotropic medications. But we ask, has the mushrooming of the ADHD diagnosis in children led to improved assessment and treatment?

The answer is mixed. Although some teachers, school administrators, and pediatricians rapidly diagnose ADHD in children, the NIH (1998), the National Institute of Mental Health (NIMH) (1996, 2000), and the AAP (2001) all have developed diagnostic guidelines for ADHD for years. More recently, The American Academy of Child & Adolescent Psychiatry (AACAP) (2007) released a practical, evidence-based practice parameter. In 2011 the same group released a practice guideline with expanded treatment of how to make the diagnosis and how to add psychosocial interventions to treatment (AACAP, 2011). The initial guideline was again updated in 2012. In all cases, these expert societies recommend a careful evaluation by a trained psychiatrist or psychologist in conjunction with teachers, mental health professionals, and family members. They recommend an evaluation period that is not rushed, so the team can rule out other conditions that might be confused with ADHD, and which includes observation and rating scales.

In a 10-year review of rating scales assessing ADHD, Collett, Ohan, and Myers (2003) concluded that *DSM IV*-based rating scales can reliably, validly, and efficiently measure ADHD symptoms in youth. In this comprehensive review, the authors evaluated the validity and sensitivity of subscales on several rating scales to assess the symptoms of ADHD. The greater use of narrowband rating scales in the assessment of ADHD can supplement and complement clinical interviews and behavioral observations in the evaluation of ADHD in children and adolescents. It is now evident that reliable and valid ADHD rating scales can augment the accuracy and specificity of diagnosis.

In a comprehensive response to the Multimodal Treatment Study (Owens et al., 2003), the authors sought to answer the layered question, "What do we treat in ADHD?" and "Who treats it?" based on the needs of the child and her or his circumstances (Paul, 1967, p. 111). Their findings were remarkable. The children least likely to respond well to a combined treatment of stimulants and milieu therapy were those with depressed parents or caregivers and severe ADHD. Owens et al. (2003) examined several outcome predictors, using nine baseline child and family characteristics. None were predictive, but the two issues discussed earlier along with a lower IQ of the identified child correlated with an outcome less-than-favorable with the combined treatment.

ADHD Efficacy, Effectiveness, and Conundrum

ADHD has been classified as one of the externalization disorders, along with Conduct Disorder and Oppositional Defiant Disorder. As opposed to the other two, stimulant medication has been the treatment of choice for ADHD for about 25 years in the United States (Phelps et al., 2002). In fact, stimulants for ADHD are the most widely researched and used medications in child psychiatry. Evidence indicates significant increase in the use of stimulants for both preschoolers and children despite the fact that the FDA approval is only for children ages 6 and older (Brown & Sammons, 2002; Riddle et al., 2001; Zito et al., 2000, 2003). The data include empirical evidence on safety, efficacy, and adverse effects.

Research demonstrates the beneficial effects of stimulants on symptoms linked with ADHD. These effects include diminished inattention, impulsivity, overactivity (Bennett, Brown, Carver, & Anderson, 1999), improved classroom attention and academic efficiency (DuPaul & Rappaport, 1993), and improved mother–child relationships (Barkley, Karlsson, Strzelecki, & Murphy, 1984). However, with all the benefits cited for the use of stimulants with ADHD, available literature to date has not supported or demonstrated that stimulants enhance school achievement (Phelps et al., 2002). Short-term efficacy studies supported the impact of stimulants on the target symptoms. From this literature, clinicians can conclude that using stimulants with children appropriately diagnosed with ADHD diminish the child's inattention, impulsivity, and hyperactivity, but do not necessarily improve his or her academic achievement. It is very possible that the child will adapt better to the demands of the classroom environment and become less externally driven. However, it would also be interesting to research whether or not stimulants improve performance in children who are not diagnosed with ADHD.

Proponents of stimulant treatment for ADHD are more convinced than ever that the disorder is passed on through heredity via the *DRD4* receptor gene and that, as twin studies have suggested, up to 80% of the variance in the trait of hyperactivity/impulsivity is now considered to be based on genetics (Barkley, 1998). Peter Jaska (1998), president of the Attention Deficit Disorder Association (ADDA), is a staunch advocate of stimulant treatment for ADHD and argues that "we cannot and will not turn back decades of scientific research on the biological basis of ADHD, medical research, educational progress, and federal disability legislation, because some people selling books claim that ADHD is a 'myth' " (p. 1). Both Jaska and Barkley are experts on the biological bases for ADHD derived from the medical model perspective and the resulting medication for treatment, but they seldom address intrapsychic, cultural, or social perspectives of ADHD.

Review Questions

- What are the mechanisms of action and side effects of stimulant medications?
- What types of symptoms are stimulants most useful for?

SECTION THREE: ADHD AND COMBINED INTERVENTIONS

Learning Objectives

- Understand the differences between the initial, two-year, and eight-year follow up of the MTA study group.
- Be able to describe conditions that may be comorbid with ADHD and why this may also be a misdiagnosis.

Interventions with ADHD usually begin with assessing the child or adolescent for oral stimulant medication, because most studies have indicated short-term behavioral improvement related to the symptoms of the disorder when stimulants are used (American Academy of Pediatrics, 2001; Barkley, DuPaul, & Connor, 1999; Phelps et al., 2002). Methylphenidate/Ritalin accounts for 90% of the prescriptions for ADHD (Advokat, Comaty, & Julien, 2014). In the late 1990s studies demonstrated that Adderall (amphetamine/dextroamphetamine) is equally efficacious but methylphenidate/Ritalin is still the leader in medications used to treat ADHD.

As noted, most consensus statements on ADHD treatment recommend psychosocial interventions that assist the family as well as the person diagnosed with ADHD. These approaches include psychotherapy, cognitive-behavioral therapy, behavioral therapy, social skills training, impulse control therapy, parenting skills training, support groups, and family therapy. Each of these approaches alone or in conjunction with stimulant medication can help ameliorate some of the symptoms of ADHD and/or address some of the underlying factors affecting the person with the disorder. The American Academy of Pediatrics (2001) first treatment guideline specifically recommended behavioral therapy as the best adjunct intervention with stimulants to establish targeted outcomes and manage the child's behavior both in the classroom and at home. They also stated that if one stimulant does not work at the highest feasible dose, the physician should recommend another. Clinicians learning about pharmacology may find it helpful to remember that stimulants generally provide only relief of symptoms, thus requiring other treatment modalities and follow-up. In a follow-up to that Bader and Adesman (2010) recommended a list of complementary and alternative treatments for ADHD. Although the American Academy of Pediatrics did not recommend these specifically they did note that essential fatty acid supplementation is well tolerated and modestly effective.

Results of the Multimodal Treatment Study for Children with ADHD (MTA Cooperative Group, 1999) demonstrated initially that stimulant treatment was slightly more effective than behavioral therapy alone, and equally effective to therapy and medication combined. It should be noted that parents preferred the behavioral therapy conditions to the stimulants-alone treatment. As with all treatment approaches for ADHD, the MTA study is not without its critics, who argue for a better match of patient with a treatment strategy tailored and selected for the individual's needs (Green & Albon, 2001). When the selected management (interventions) for a child with ADHD has not met targeted outcomes, clinicians must evaluate the original diagnosis, adjust treatments and medications, and evaluate for coexisting conditions.

Another critic of the MTA study (Leo, 2002) noted that the fanfare surrounding publication of the study "was nothing short of extraordinary" (p. 53). Leo pointed out that *ABC News* reported that results indicated drug therapy was much better than counseling for ADHD. Leo contends that the MTA study was heavily biased toward medication treatment. He claims the study's authors all had a history of strongly favoring medication, bringing their objectivity into question. He also points out that the MTA study had four groups: one received medication, one received behavior therapy, one received both, and a fourth group received no treatments from the MTA researchers but instead received standard treatment in the community. The most "robust" changes were reported in ratings by teachers and parents of children in the study. The problem with this, according to Leo, is that the investigators preselected a group of parents who believe it is acceptable to medicate children; in fact, in all cases the parents contacted the investigators to enroll children in the study. This fact, according to Leo, points to a bias in the sample.

Edwards (2002) addressed the important follow-up outcomes of studies and interventions in the wake of the report from the MTA Cooperative Group study (1999). He recommended that a specific family-based intervention be used in a mental health setting in conjunction with pharmacologic treatment. He specifically cited Parent Management Training (PMT) as an approach that through cognitive-behavioral coaching helps parents manage their child's difficulties. Whatever the method, more physicians, researchers, and clinicians are recommending family interventions with children and adolescents diagnosed with

ADHD. The research in treatment outcomes of ADHD is complicated, and we encourage you to evaluate many strategies and interventions for your clinical work, especially those that include family/ parent strategies.

The MTA study was followed up at two years and at eight years. Here is a summary of the findings. At two years, cessation of drug treatment was correlated with significant clinical decline. Continued drug therapy was correlated with moderate decline and initiation of stimulant therapy for those in control group was correlated with significant improvement (MTA Cooperative Group, 2004). So at this point again the cornerstone of treatment seemed to be with the medication. At the eight-year follow up, 33% of the subjects were still on medication (and 83% of them were on stimulants). Improvement was maintained but the group had not "normalized" meaning there were still significant achievement gaps between them and so-called "normal" controls. Thirty percent still met the *DSM-IV* criteria for ADHD (though one suspects more would meet criteria under *DSM-5* because you only need five criteria met rather than six). Overall, medicated children did better in math and reading. There was still a significant test score gap between children in the study and the control group. Also, interestingly, approximately 30% showed signs of antisocial behavior and 25% showed signs of Oppositional Defiant Disorder (Barnard-Brak & Brak, 2011; Sheffler et al., 2009). This is interesting because many specialists felt that the antisocial behavior often comorbid with ADHD was because the ADHD was untreated. It seems that there may be something else to the antisocial behavior because it seemed to persist in so many people despite their long-term treatment for ADHD.

We spoke with one interventionist who provides a learning/coaching service to children with ADHD (Joyce Kubik, Personal Communication, April 2003). Kubik not only conducts specific skill-building training/coaching for ADHD children but also conducts support groups for parents. She also gives workshops for teacher in-service programs. Her overall message is that children with ADHD are capable of developing specific learning strategies that will lead to improved academic learning and success. She outlines these specific skills in her book *S.C.O.P.E.: Student Centered Outcome Plan and Evaluation* (Kubik, 2002). The central theme of her work is to help parents and teachers find ways to help students with attention difficulties. The American Academy of Child & Adolescent Psychiatry (2001) stated,

> Research also should include the role of school and community-based professionals, as well as primary care clinicians, in delivering treatment services. Little is known about how short or long-term effectiveness varies as a function of the school and community-based professional involvement. . . . They should consider child and family outcomes and cost-effectiveness of care. Linking outcomes to service parameters is an important step in encouraging practice in system change. (p. 10)

In this summary statement, you can recognize aspects of the multimodal model that forms the basis of this book in analyzing and evaluating interventions with children and adolescents diagnosed with ADHD. It calls for more comprehensive research on the multiple factors that contribute to ADHD in children and adolescents and initiates the process to improve research on outcomes with this disorder.

ADHD and Comorbidity

The American Academy of Pediatrics (2001) also stressed that evaluation for ADHD should include an assessment for coexisting or comorbid conditions. The literature on ADHD identifies several psychological and developmental disorders that coexist in children with ADHD (Biederman, Mick, Faraone, & Burback, 2001; Phelps et al., 2002; Spencer, Biederman, & Wilens, 2002). These disorders included conduct and oppositional defiant disorders, mood disorders, anxiety and depressive disorders, mental retardation, learning disabilities, tics, substance abuse, and medical conditions. Researchers have estimated that among children with ADHD, the prevalence rate of

Oppositional Defiant Disorder is up to 35%, Conduct Disorder up to 26%, anxiety disorders up to almost 26%, and depression up to 18% (AAP, 2001). It is more difficult to estimate comorbidity rates of Bipolar Disorder, substance abuse, and tics. Most authors who discuss comorbidity and ADHD tend to discuss the issue from a pharmacologic perspective (Levy & Hay, 2001; Solanto, Arnsten, & Castellanos, 2001). This is a burgeoning and complex conundrum in the treatment of ADHD. We encourage you to be alert to the great variability in children and adolescents diagnosed with ADHD and to assess for other conditions or factors.

Susan L. Andersen (2005) studied stimulants and the developing brain. She found that the effects of stimulant drugs during different stages have unique short-term, acute effects that also influence their long-term effects. Chronic, pre-pubertal exposure alters the expected developmental trajectory of brain structure and function and results in a different topography in adulthood. She also discovered that the timing of exposure (childhood vs. adolescence), the age of examination after drug exposure (immediately or delayed into adulthood), and sex influenced observable effects. Hopefully this can provide new treatment options for ADHD.

Mental health clinicians should be able to recognize the evidence recommending cautious use of stimulants with children and adolescents diagnosed with ADHD, and should remain alert to the potential for overdiagnosis or misdiagnosis of the disorder and the extensive range of comorbid/coexisting conditions. Phelps et al. (2002) summarized issues surrounding comorbidity of ADHD, ODD, and CD related to the evidence that when two or more of these disorders occur together, the prognosis is more guarded. They also addressed the hypothesis that ADHD occurs first in the child and the symptoms of impulsivity and inattention interact with the psychosocial issues of family turmoil, parental problems, and abuse factors to trigger ODD and/or CD. Clinicians need to be alert to the range of symptoms of several disorders when assessing and evaluating symptoms of impulsiveness and hyperactivity. These conditions could emanate from psychological family and environmental factors. Although the debate continues about the effectiveness of stimulant medication with ADHD, Greenhill (1998) and NIH (1998) concluded that stimulants used for ADHD children and adolescents

1. Produce moderate to marked short-term improvement in motor restlessness, on-task behavior, compliance, and academic performance.
2. In studies of six months or longer, children fail to maintain academic improvement or improve social problem-solving skills (Greenhill, 1998, p. 53).

Atomoxetine, a Nonstimulant

Recently, atomoxetine/Strattera, a nonstimulant and a selective norepinephrine reuptake inhibitor (SNRI) has demonstrated some promising results in reducing ADHD symptoms (Brown University, 2002). It was approved for use in children ages 6 and older in 2003 and for maintenance treatment of ADHD in children and adolescents in 2008. Atomoxetine/Strattera is metabolized primarily through the CYP2D6 enzymatic pathways. It demonstrates an adverse event percentage of between 3.5 and 7% (poor metabolizers) in clinical trials. These adverse events include gastrointestinal problems, irritability, insomnia, aggression, and dizziness. As a nonpsychostimulant, atomoxetine/Straterra has potential as an alternative to the stimulants now used with ADHD. As with any new medication, only time and continued research will tell if atomoxetine will improve on the side effect profile of stimulant medications.

In a very sad and disappointing statement, the status of the treatment of ADHD has not changed in seven years since the first edition of this text.

- Children, adolescents, and adults are being diagnosed at accelerated rates.
- The first and second course of treatment is pharmaceuticals.
- Efforts by the FDA, legislation like the Best Pharmaceuticals for Children Act have been marginalized.
- Limited assistance for the poor, Medicaid, wards of the county or state, orphans and other children,

and adolescents with restricted access to quality medical care.

- A belief still that life is better through pharma—just watch TV since the Health Care Act passed in 2009.
- Society's intolerance for anxious, agitated, and aggressive children.
- Large metropolitan school systems' inability to understand the impact of bullying on students with disabilities.

So with little progress, more children take the drugs and some experience improvement whereas many others graduate to more potent pharmaceuticals.

Review Questions

- What were the differences between the initial findings of the MTA study and the two-year and eight-year follow up?
- What does the eight-year follow-up tell us about antisocial behavior and ADHD treatment?
- What conditions may be comorbid with ADHD and why may these be a case of misdiagnosis?

SECTION FOUR: MOOD STABILIZERS AND BIPOLAR I DISORDER IN CHILDREN

Learning Objectives

- Be able to think critically about the problems of putting children and adolescents on medications tested on adults.
- Be able to articulate alternatives to so-called mood stabilizing medications for children.

The *DSM-5* (American Psychiatric Association, 2013) provides the following diagnostic criteria for Bipolar Disorder, Single Manic Episode:

A. Presence of only one Manic Episode and no past Major Depressive Episodes.

Note: Recurrence is defined as either a change in polarity from depression or an interval of at least two months without manic symptoms.

B. The Manic Episode is not better accounted for by Schizoaffective Disorder and is not superimposed on Schizophrenia, Schizophreniform Disorder, Delusional Disorder, or Psychotic Disorder Not Otherwise Specified.

Criteria for Manic Episode

A. A distinct period of abnormality and persistently elevated, expansive, or irritable mood, lasting at least one week (or any duration if hospitalization is necessary).

B. During the period of mood disturbance, three (or more) of the following symptoms have persisted (four if the mood is only irritable) and have been present to a significant degree:

(1) inflated self-esteem or grandiosity
(2) decreased need for sleep (e.g., feels rested after only three hours of sleep)
(3) more talkative than usual or pressure to keep talking
(4) flight of ideas or subjective experience that thoughts are racing
(5) distractibility (i.e., attention too easily drawn to unimportant or irrelevant external stimuli)
(6) increase in goal-directed activity (either socially, at work, or school, or sexually) or psychomotor agitation
(7) excessive involvement in pleasurable activities that have a high potential for painful consequences (e.g., engaging in unrestrained buying sprees, sexual indiscretions, or foolish business investments).

C. The symptoms do not meet criteria for a Mixed Episode.

D. The mood disturbance is sufficiently severe to cause marked impairment in occupational functioning or in usual social activities or relationships with others, or to necessitate hospitalization to prevent harm to self or others, or there are psychotic features.

E. The symptoms are not due to the direct physiological effects of a substance (e.g., a drug of abuse, a medication, or other treatment) or a general medical condition (e.g., hyperthyroidism).

Source: Diagnostic and statistical manual of mental disorders (5th ed., Text Revision, pp. 123–125). Washington, DC: American Psychiatric Association, 2013.

We have seen in the past decade an increasing interest and shift in focus from Conduct Disorder (CD) and Oppositional Defiant Disorder (ODD) to Bipolar I Disorder in children and adolescents (Kusumaker, Lazier, MacMaster, & Santor, 2002; Milkowitz et al., 2014). We illustrated this in the case of Phillip at the beginning of this chapter. Although in our Chapter Eight discussion of mood stabilizers we focused on Bipolar I Disorder, in this chapter we use the more general BPI, because that is the construct common to the literature on children and adolescents. Many diagnostic scholars tell us the prevalence of BPI is growing, especially in preadolescent children, with almost no gender differences (Bland, 1997; Hirschfeld et al., 2003; Zarate & Tohen, 1996). The case for increased incidence is still undecided.

In the *Diagnostic and Statistical Manual of Mental Disorder*, 5th Edition (*DSM-5*; American Psychiatric Association [APA], 2013), BPI is the basis of a new category, *Bipolar and Related Disorders*. BPI is the centerpiece of this section, which also includes Bipolar II Disorder, Cyclothymic Disorder, Bipolar Disorders related to substance use or medical conditions, and other specified and unspecified Bipolar and Related Disorders. In order to stem the tide of BPI misdiagnoses in children, Disruptive Mood Dysregulation Disorder was introduced to the *DSM-5* section on Depressive Disorders. The jury is still out on whether this will reduce the false diagnosis of BPI in children (Margulies, Weintraub, Basile, Grover, & Carlson, 2012) or, for that matter, how we should treat Disruptive Mood Dysregulation (Jairam, Prabhuswamy, & Dullur, 2012).

There is considerable controversy regarding the appropriateness of a BPI diagnosis in children. Questions regarding the appropriateness of such a diagnosis are founded on the idea that criteria for BPI may overlap with criteria for developmental issues; other disorders usually diagnosed during infancy, childhood, or adolescence (e.g., what the *DSM-5* calls Neurodevelopmental Disorders); and

other problems known to affect people of all ages (e.g., depressive, anxiety, substance use, and impulse-control disorders) (Chang, 2008). Further, there are currently no pediatric diagnostic guidelines for BPI in children, and it is inappropriate to use the *DSM* criteria for BPI because they were normed on adults (Kowatch et al., 2005; Sahling, 2009).

One of the most problematic issues is assuming that any type of irritability or acting out is somehow related to the invalid notion of a "bipolar spectrum." Differentiating between irritability (very common in children and adolescents) and symptoms of BPI is an ethical imperative for clinicians, particularly those working in foster care or with other children and adolescents who have no one to advocate for them (Banaschewski, 2009; Sahling, 2009). Although published studies using functional brain-scanning technologies to investigate early-onset BPI are few, some show brain anomalies similar to those that correlate with adult BPI (Frazier et al., 2005). Only longitudinal studies will answer the question regarding how predictive such anomalies are for the development of BPI because brain scans can only suggest endophenotypes that are related to vulnerability to a disorder (Jackson, 2006).

The problems with the exponential increase in diagnosing pediatric bipolar disorder are many. In many children, rapid mood swings can be normal. The treatment guidelines (Kowatch et al., 2005) admit that "no one can say for sure what these children will look like when they grow up" (p. 214). This is a disturbing statement because BPI, properly diagnosed, is thought to be a chronic disorder. The authors of the treatment guidelines admit that the DSM symptoms for adult mania are problematic when used for children, but then they recommend continuing to use them. Overall, the treatment guidelines fail to draw distinctions between normal children and those really afflicted with BPI (Sahling, 2009).

Currently, the *DSM-5* diagnostic criteria for Bipolar Disorder are used for children and adolescents without any major modifications and the features providing the best distinction between ODD,

CD, ADHD, and BPI are the presence of a flight of ideas, grandiosity, and the episodic nature of the grandiosity (Carlson, 1996; Kusumaker et al., 2002). As we summarize the literature on BPI in children and adolescents, we learn that it is difficult to diagnose, more clinicians are recognizing its prevalence at an earlier age of onset, three tentative developmental theories are linked to it (McMahon & DePaulo, 1996), and more clinicians are using antimanic medications to treat BPI in both children and adolescents.

Soutullo et al. (2005) concluded that there is an overdiagnosis of Bipolar Disorder in the United States when compared to several countries like Spain, Turkey, India, Brazil, Switzerland, Denmark, and Finland. This difference may be attributed to a relative lack of data, differences in diagnostic criteria, different levels of recognition of child and adolescent psychiatry as a true specialty in Europe, clinician bias against Bipolar Disorder, an overdiagnosis in the United States, and/or a true higher prevalence of BD in the United States. It sounds like the same case with ADHD.

Viesselman (1999) addressed the general symptoms of BPI as expansive mood, inflated self-esteem, decreased need to sleep, talkativeness, flight of ideas, distractibility, psychomotor agitation, and excessive involvement with pleasurable activities. Phelps et al. (2002) addressed the fact that BPI youth often are incorrectly diagnosed as having Schizophrenia; thus, BPIs are difficult to discern in children and adolescents because many present with an agitated depressed mood rather than mania (Weller, Weller, & Fristad, 1995). Lewinsohn, Klein, and Seeley (1995) stated that pediatric clients with BPI present with more psychomotor agitation, elevated mood, increased verbalizations, inflated self-esteem, distractibility, and a decreased need for sleep. Duffy (2010) detailed with great specificity the potential genetic markers for children who might be vulnerable to inherit Bipolar I.

The treatment of choice for BPI in children and adolescents is the mood stabilizers covered in Chapter Eight. These drugs include lithium/Eskalith, Lithobid, valproate/Depakote/Depakene/Divalproex), carbamazepine/Tegretol, oxcarbazepine/

Trileptal, and olanzapine/Zyprexa. Many scholars already cited in this chapter argue against indiscriminate use of these medications with pediatric populations without further study and argue for more complete awareness of the dynamics affecting the child.

Riddle et al. (2001) discussed the finding that the older antiepileptic drugs had been well researched as mood stabilizers in adults but not in pediatric populations. Campbell, Kafantaris, and Cueva (1995) have studied lithium/Eskalith, carbamazepine/Tegretol, and valproate/Divalproex used for children with nonspecific aggression and found lithium/Eskalith was superior to placebo and to the other antiepileptic drugs in reducing aggression. One very important note: Eberle (1998) found that one type of adverse event of using valproate with girls is that of polycystic ovarian disease, which can have profound consequences for females.

In the early 21st century, children and teens are 40 times more likely to be diagnosed with Bipolar Disorder than they were in the late 20th century (Miller & Barnett, 2008). As noted above there is evidence that this is due to diagnostic inflation and not an epidemic-level increase in the disorder. Geller et al. (2012) compared lithium/Eskalith, valproic acid/Divalproex, and risperidone/Risperdal in a trial called Treatment of Early Age Mania (TEAM). The response rate for risperidone/Risperdal was significantly higher (68%) than for lithium/Eskalith (36%) or valproic acid/Divalproex (24%). Advokat et al. (2014) note that quetiapine/Seroquel and aripiprazole/Abilify are as effective as risperidone/Risperdal. As noted in the chapter on antipsychotics though, these drugs come with severe side effects like weight gain and disruption of metabolic functions that can lead to type 2 diabetes.

In our clinical work of over 40 years, we have found that the comorbid substance use disorders were a major missing piece in several cases with children and adolescents. These clients were diagnosed with ODD, CD, or BPI and seemingly did not improve with psychotherapy or psychotropic interventions. The missing link and confounding variable was their hidden polysubstance abuse or dependence, which exacerbated some symptoms and masked others. The links in the literature show how the onsets of BPD, ADHD, CD, or ODD become significant risk factors in diagnosing substance use disorders. It should be noted that any attempts to procure research papers on pediatric or child papers on the research topics of developmental pharmacology, ADHD, BP I, and pharmaceuticals related to these disorders published in 2013 or 2014 were sponsored by pharmaceutical companies and cost $39.00.

The following case may provide additional understanding of these complex variables.

THE CASE OF NICOLE

Nicole, a 14-year-old Caucasian girl currently living in a foster home, had just been referred to a Severe Emotional Disturbance (SED) unit in her school system. Nicole had a history of acting out, impulsivity, distractibility, conduct, and learning problems from a very early age. Initially, Nicole was referred to a specialist for her impulsivity and distractibility both at home and in preschool at the age of 4.

During the assessment, the clinician suspected a mood disorder but seemed to have more evidence for ADHD. He recommended a daily course of amphetamine salts/Adderall with behavior management therapy at home and school, focused on specific age-appropriate behaviors. At the time of the evaluation, he did not notice Nicole's intermittent scratching of her genital area. Over the next six months, Nicole showed little improvement in her symptoms and behaviors as a result of the amphetamine salts/Adderall and the milieu behavioral therapy. In fact, some of her behaviors worsened: she attacked other children, was cruel to animals, and was overtly curious about male and female genitals. After nine months, the psychologist consultant at the school recommended another neuropsychiatric evaluation and an outside therapist who would address some of Nicole's apparent psychological conflicts along with her behavior.

The second psychiatric evaluation yielded a change in diagnostic perspective. This time, the psychiatrist diagnosed BPI and prescribed valproic acid/Divalproex and a low dose of lorazepam/Ativan, an anxiolytic. The new therapist, a female, stopped the behavior therapy and began to treat Nicole with a combination of play therapy and insight-oriented therapy. The play produced associations to remote possibilities of earlier sexual abuse and abandonment, and the insight therapy captured her already highly critical superego (obsessive thought patterns and preoccupation with sexual act) and her deep affection for the rituals of the Catholic Church. Nicole remained on this treatment regimen for about two-and-a-half years. During treatment, she never really settled down in class or at home, but her behavior and attention were slightly more manageable. (We have all had cases where there is just enough improvement from the medication to raise expectations even if the client seems not to be making progress in many important areas of her life.) Later, Nicole developed a passion for reading 7 to 10 books a week that she got from the local library. On her trips back and forth to the library, she befriended some older boys (ages 10 to 13) who offered her street stimulants at a very low cost. Nicole welcomed the friendship and experimented with the drugs (stimulants, soapers, cocaine), but was gangraped by the boys one Saturday afternoon. Overwhelmed by this horrific sexual trauma, Nicole did not speak of it to anyone. She also immediately stopped associating with the boys. Her response to this event was alternately to withdraw into a cocoonlike isolation and to become aggressive with people.

She verbally assaulted teachers and foster parents and attacked her friends and other students. She was unreachable and totally out of control. She stopped attending her therapy sessions with the counselor, but she continued to seek street drugs.

Puzzled and frustrated, the school crisis team recommended an additional psychiatric evaluation and assessment for Nicole and possible hospitalization. This triggered a series of episodes in which she ran away, had several foster and specialized school placements, a brief stay at a juvenile detention facility, one abortion, and two attempts at drug rehabilitation for her dependence on stimulants, cocaine, and now alcohol. Somehow Nicole survived and is now in an SED classroom with a specialized social worker as an aide. She is on olanzapine/Zyprexa for psychotic mania, sertraline/Zoloft for depression and anxiety, low doses of valproic acid/Divalproex for violent and aggressive outbursts, and zolpidem/Ambien as needed for sleep. In essence, at 14, Nicole was loaded with psychotropic medications (polypharmacy). She was referred to a new female therapist, with whom she rarely spoke; when she did, she mentioned missing her former, caring play therapist, one of the most stable objects (people) in her life. Although Nicole did attend her class regularly and her behavior was quite manageable, her teachers reported very little learning progress and a total inability to interact with her classmates. Her therapist echoed much of the same descriptions, but voiced marginal hope when she and Nicole engaged in drawing or other forms of play therapy or discussed issues related to an all-loving versus all-punishing God. The concluding remarks in her individual educational plan (IEP) at school read, "No change, few academic gains, impulsive/aggressive behavior stabilized, little socialization, continues in counseling."

Examining this case from our four perspectives yields some important insights and omissions. Nicole did receive a more extensive assessment early on and participated in behavioral therapy first, which is recommended by the literature (AAP, 2001; Kusumaker et al., 2002; Phelps et al., 2002) followed by art therapy and insight therapy when the behavioral therapy failed. It is critical to note that the second therapist helped Nicole discuss psychological and cultural issues and learned about the pressure from her complicated feelings about her upbringing in the Catholic Church and her deep awareness of her self-critical feelings and thoughts.

As is so often the situation with a foster child, other social and cultural pressures intervened, such as drug abuse, negative and exploitive peer relationships, and sexual trauma. It is not clear whether Nicole ever experienced sexual or physical abuse earlier in her life. The most recent team is faced with an early adolescent girl with a long history of psychotropic and psychotherapeutic treatments whose life is further complicated and traumatized by rape and drug dependence. Given the assumption that the significant others in her life—case managers, foster parents, teachers—feel she is out of control, the attending psychiatrist then addressed her range of symptoms and conflicts with a polypharmaceutical strategy. This approach numbs and tranquilizes Nicole so she is more appropriate in her various living environments but fails to address the boiling issues, anguish, and conflicts from the other aspects of her life. Treatment for Nicole should begin by recognizing the extreme complexity of her life space and developing a treatment plan and approach to gradually help her titrate off some of her medications while addressing in counseling the complex issues of abuse, drug dependence, abandonment, and loss of self that so plague her. She will need a very extended and interpersonal treatment approach if she is to recapture hope and resiliency in her life. We also would speculate about the accuracy of her diagnosis, because of the interplay of her conflicts and varying presenting problems and lack of empathy in her counseling.

Review Questions

- What are some of the problems of putting children and adolescents on medications tested on adults?
- What alternatives do we have to so-called mood stabilizing medications for children?

SECTION FIVE: CHILDREN AND ANTIPSYCHOTIC MEDICATION

Learning Objectives

- Know the diagnoses for which typical and atypical antipsychotics are being used in children.
- Be able to discuss the problems with this practice.

Schizophrenia with adolescent onset has been noted since the earliest descriptions of the disorder. Readers will recall Emil Kraepelin's initial diagnosis of a patient as having "*dementia praecox,*" which means "youthful insanity." As Russell (2001) notes, given that the disorder has been linked with adolescents through the evolution of its diagnostic forms, one might think there would be ample treatment literature regarding these populations, but there is not. Childhood-onset schizophrenia (prior to age 12) is even rarer than adolescent onset. It is estimated that maybe 1 child in 10,000 would suffer this before the age of 12 (Remschmidt, 2002). The differential diagnosis must include substance-use disorders, depressive disorders with psychotic symptoms, and what *DSM-5* calls other neurodevelopmental disorders like Autism Spectrum Disorder (Androutsos, 2012). Even when criteria are met it is very difficult to diagnose schizophrenia in a child. The Child Psychiatry Branch at the National Institute of Mental Health (NIMH) conducted a longitudinal study of childhood onset schizophrenia. Outpatient screening accurately diagnosed 55% of the 121 cases. However, inpatient observation including medication-free observation ruled out 96 children with alternative diagnoses. Outpatient screening only accurately diagnosed 62% of this same group. The conclusion the researchers drew was that inpatient, unmedicated observation was the most accurate way to diagnose these children (Gochman, Miller, & Rapoport, 2011).

In a review of controlled studies of antipsychotic agents to treat Schizophrenia, Campbell, Rapoport, and Simpson (1999) found only one controlled study of the use of these agents with adolescents and one report on their use with children younger than age 12. Therefore, Russell (2001) notes, until more research is conducted clinicians must extrapolate from adult studies to children and adolescents, which poses many risks. Although he comments this is not cause to adopt a nihilistic attitude, it does call for clinical skepticism. Russell maintains it may be true that people with early-onset Schizophrenia have more severe forms of the disorder, but this has yet to be determined conclusively and it does not mean pharmacologic treatment will not be effective. Further, early-onset Schizophrenia seems to have more severe negative symptoms, making the atypical antipsychotics a better choice

if the children can tolerate the adverse drug effects (Botteron & Geller, 1999).

Although few data are available regarding the use of antipsychotics with childhood psychoses, in the 20th century the neuroleptic haloperidol/ Haldol was used because it tended to be less sedating (Andreasen, 2000). Because of the potential for Parkinsonian-like symptoms, this medication was often prescribed with an anti-Parkinsonian agent such as benztropine/Cogentin. Ernst et al. (1999); Phelps et al. (2002); and Riddle et al. (2001) also addressed the use of the "atypical" newer neuroleptics for children diagnosed with tics, behavioral problems in autism, psychotic illness, and nonspecific aggression. In 2004, Toren et al. (Toren, Ratner, Laor, & Weizman, 2004) did a benefit-risk assessment of atypical antipsychotics in treating schizophrenia and comorbid disorders in children. They found the atypicals seemed to work better than neuroleptics and now it seems that neuroleptics like haloperidol/ Haldol are only used if the patient does not respond to an atypical. Of the atypical, risperidone/Risperdal and olanzapine/Zyprexa seemed to improve cognitive functions and inhibit suicidal behavior. Madaan, Dvir, and Wilson (2008) noted that the FDA concluded there was enough support for using atypicals in children and approved two atypicals for childhood schizophrenia.

As we noted in Chapter Seven, evidence is mounting that atypical antipsychotics are also correlated with increased risk for diabetes and hyperglycemia and that this risk includes children and adolescents (Koller, Cross, & Schneider, 2004). Research by Correll et al. (2009) confirmed these mounting suspicions. The study concluded that use of aripiprozole, olanzapine, quetiapine, and risperidone for 12 weeks all produced weight gain, and varied in lipid and metabolic parameters. The authors called for more careful monitoring of the child's health before using an atypical. Whatever medication a clinician chooses, Russell (2001) emphasizes the need for multimodal treatment that includes psychosocial interventions such as individual and family therapy, psychoeducational counseling, and social skills training.

A more common problem is raised by Pappado-pulos et al. (2002) in a study that examines the range of off-label prescribing of atypical antipsychotics for aggression. These authors state that although in theory doctors seem to agree about optimal prescribing practices, in the "real world" there is wild disparity in the prescriptions written. Apparently, even the agreement between researchers and front-line doctors can be influenced by staff pressure, limited staff resources, managed care limits on inpatient stays, and the movement away from physical restraint.

Another problem that requires further debate and research concerns the notion that Schizophrenia is a wide spectrum of early-onset disorders manifesting in a variety of the disorder called "schizotaxia," which refers to a genetic predisposition to Schizophrenia (Meehl, 1962). Tsuang, Stone, and Faraone (2001) advocate treating Schizophrenia prophylactically. These authors maintain that the theoretically genetic predisposition toward Schizophrenia may be associated with reversible problems and may improve the child's quality of life. Despite this strong medical model perspective, they admit that psychosocial interventions may also work. They conducted a six-week trial of risperidone (prescribed at low levels) in six subjects identified as schizotaxic. They reported that five of the six reported increased cognitive abilities during the trial as well as greater enjoyment of social activities. Obviously, there is no way to determine the amount of placebo effect until a double-blind, placebo-controlled trial is done.

Great caution needs to be exercised here, as the implications are that asymptomatic children might be given antipsychotics in the hope that their diagnosis as schizotaxic is correct. The antipsychotic market currently amasses $5 billion a year, and many fear that the theory of schizotaxia is just another way of bending the parameters of diagnosis to help pharmaceutical companies profit from a new market. Currently, no diagnostic system in the world identifies adolescents in the phase *before* onset as ill, so this approach would have ramifications for the diagnosis. Ideally, the issues surrounding the politics of research and publishing described in Chapter Two, need to be more adequately addressed before any further medicating of asymptomatic

populations. As Frances (2013) noted, preventive psychiatry could only work if we know the etiology of a disorder and have a safe and effective treatment for the disorder. We have neither where schizophrenia is concerned.

In Chapter Seven, we discussed neuroleptics and their affinities for different CNS receptors, their pharmacokinetics, and pharmacodynamics. Marriage (2002) spoke to our inability to predict the response of an individual patient (child or adolescent) to a typical or atypical neuroleptic. He addressed the enormous response variation, especially with adolescent males, Asians, Native Americans, and people suffering from various forms of organicity. For children or adolescents exhibiting symptoms of psychosis, the long-term prognosis is poor (Phelps et al., 2002), and we need to learn a great deal more about the adverse side effects of both the typical and atypical medications (Riddle et al., 2001). Given the outcome of Olfson et al. (2006) National Trends Study, which indicated that children treated with second-generation medication (atypical antipsychotics) included descriptive behavior disorders (37.8%), mood disorders (31.8%), pervasive developmental disorders or mental retardation (17.3%), and psychotic disorders (14.2%), we are again reluctant to endorse atypicals as a treatment of choice for childhood psychosis.

Review Questions

- What are some of the conditions for which children are being put on antipsychotic medications?
- What are the main drawbacks to this practice?

SECTION SIX: ANTIANXIETY MEDICATIONS AND CHILDREN AND ADOLESCENTS

Learning Objective

- Understand particularly how anxiolytic medications are used with children who have school anxiety.

Despite the high prevalence of anxiety disorders in children (10 to 20%), very few controlled medication trials have been conducted. In *DSM-5*, Obsessive-Compulsive Disorder (OCD) and Post Traumatic Stress Disorder (PTSD) have been given their own categories. Children's anxiety disorders, Separation Anxiety Disorder, Selective Mutism, Specific Phobia and Generalized Anxiety. In the late 20th century, Brown and Sawyer (1998) concluded that regarding anxiolytic medication with children, "few published empirical studies support their long term efficacy for children and adolescents" (p. 83). Bernstein and Shaw (1997) noted that psychotropic medications should not be the sole intervention but should be used as an adjunct to counseling. Interventions that facilitate active mastery are important, to prevent symptoms returning after discontinuation of medication. Little has changed and almost 20 years later anxiety disorders in children are first best treated with non-pharmacological therapies like behavior therapy, cognitive-behavior therapy, and internalizing prevention programs. House (1999) noted that children's disorders can be generally grouped as externalizing (like acting out against others) and internalizing. Internalizing often results in anxiety symptoms. Young children with anxiety disorders are more likely to be depressed and to exhibit temperamental inhibition and sleep problems (Doughert et al., 2013).

The 2013 article of Rapp et al. will guide our complex study of anxiety disorders. The *DSM-5* and earlier versions have really not assisted our journey to discover effective treatments for children and adolescents suffering from anxiety disorders (AD). It is the second author's opinion that there have been too many changes in the *DSM* related to AD since 1980. Our focus needs to shift to treatment with safe and effective outcomes. Bernstein, Borschardt, and Perwien (1996) viewed these changes as placing at risk a decade of research on childhood anxiety disorders, although Phelps et al. (2002) supported elimination of some categories of childhood anxiety disorders from *DSM III-R* as a research-based simplification of the categories. Although prevalence rates vary for current anxiety disorders with children and adolescents (Botteron & Geller, 1999; Garland, 2002), incidences of Generalized Anxiety Disorders (GAD), and Separation Anxiety Disorder (SAD) are frequently thought to require both psychopharmacologic and psychotherapeutic interventions. Currently, although almost all the drugs are used off label, SSRIs such as paroxetine/Paxil, fluvoxamine/Luvox, fluoxetine/Prozac, citalopram/Celexa, and sertraline/Zoloft are prescribed for children and adolescents with anxiety disorders. Advokat et al. (2014) noted that fluoxetine/Prozac may be the best medication if medication is necessary. The current concern over safety of these medications for children and adolescents applies to their use in anxiety disorders as well as in depression. One of chronic side effect of SSRIs recognized in children is a behavioral activation (Riddle et al., 1991), like an increased agitation different from a mania. As noted earlier the Food and Drug Administration (2003) issued a Public Health Advisory stating that use of SSRIs and similar types of antidepressants with depressed children and adolescents may be linked to increased suicide rates. How this will affect use of these antidepressants for anxiety disorders remains unclear. Rapp, Dodds, Walkup, and Rynn (2013) continued to use SSRIs in their combined treatment approaches with children diagnosed with GAD, SP, and SAD. Their study gave very high marks to Cognitive-Behavioral Therapy (CBT) in conjunction with a psychopharmacological approach.

In a review of the literature on anxiolytic medications used in pediatric populations, Livingston (1995) noted mixed results with benzodiazepines and said that in cases where studies show initial results, the results fail to be significant in replications of the studies. Livingston notes that if children are going to be placed on these medications, prescribers need to "start low and go slow" (p. 248). Recall from Chapter Six, benzodiazepines such as alprazolam/Xanax and diazepam/Valium have an inhibitory impact on the CNS at the GABA receptor complex. As Advokat et al. (2014) note these drugs usually cause cognitive impairments and so are not recommended except in the case of short-term medical procedures (e.g., dental procedures).

SCHOOL ISSUES, ANXIETY, AND CHILDREN

A relevant law when addressing anxiety in children is the Individuals with Disabilities Education Act (IDEA). Services to children are provided under a number of provisions in this act, and often many *DSM* anxiety disorders can be used to qualify a child for services. The diagnostic categories of *DSM* do not automatically correspond to the eligibility categories in IDEA. The interested reader can go to http://www.ed.gov/offices/OSERS/IDEA /the_law.html for a listing of the relevant diagnoses. IDEA services focus on disability conditions that interfere with a child achieving academically or vocationally.

Anxiety disorders have been used to qualify a child for special services. A key symptom is fears associated with personal or school problems that persist over a period of time and adversely affect educational performance. Anxiety disorders are one of the most common childhood disorders and may impair a child's life even if symptoms are below the threshold for a *DSM* diagnosis. For example, some studies show "subclinical" anxiety to be highly correlated with reading difficulty (Bernstein & Shaw, 1997). Currently, studies are underway to measure the impact of bullying on anxiety (Twemlow, Fonagy, Sacco, & Brethour, 2006).

Developmental differences exist in the presentation of the anxiety disorders. For example, younger children with Separation Anxiety Disorder have far more symptoms than older children. In adolescents, somatic complaints and school refusal are more common than in younger children. Conversely, older children with GAD show more symptoms than younger ones. This is probably caused by cognitive differences, because older children have more mental tools with which to craft their worries.

Interestingly, in several studies with benzodiazepines, the medicated groups did no better than placebo controls. Two studies did yield significant differences among school refusers and children with selective mutism and social phobia. In one study, the school refusers did better than controls when given Tofranil/imipramine, a tricyclic antidepressant. The other study, on selective mutism and social phobia, showed that the experimental subjects did better than controls when given Prozac.

A related childhood disorder is Separation Anxiety Disorder. Here, the anxiety is aroused by separation from familiar people (usually parents) or leaving home. The reaction is excessive and may include fears that something will happen to the parents or to prevent reunification. Somatic complaints are also common. The distinction must be made between developmentally normal separation anxiety and this disorder. If refusal to go to school is thought to be due to Separation Anxiety Disorder, the child will go if accompanied by the parent. Although benzodiazepines and antihistamines have been used to treat this (Wozniak et al., 1997), exposure-based interventions and relaxation are likely to be more effective.

Another subthreshold condition is shyness. It is consistently correlated with adult and childhood anxiety disorders. Although common (90% of people report feeling it at some time in their lives), it can be debilitating as the person gets older. Shy men marry later and become parents later than their counterparts who are not shy. Although shy women marry and become parents at ages comparable to their counterparts who are not shy, they are less likely to attend college or work outside the home. Social phobia is a severe manifestation of shyness that afflicts about 5% of children. It delays social and emotional development. The overwhelming fear of doing or saying something embarrassing or humiliating keeps such people from eating, drinking, or writing in public or engaging in everyday conversations.

Although children generally outgrow shyness, they do not outgrow Social Phobia. Children with social phobias are usually depressed and lonely and almost always solitary. They may show extreme anxiety in situations where they feel they are being evaluated by others. The onset of Social Phobia is usually in adolescence and without treatment, the course is often chronic. There is high comorbidity with depression, other anxiety disorders, and substance abuse to self-medicate. As with other childhood anxiety disorders, the recommended treatments include rehearsal, imagery, and drug treatment with antidepressant compounds. Behavior therapy has a 70% success rate for both children and adults, with systematic desensitization and exposure being the common treatments. Although more children and adolescents are being prescribed SSRIs and SNRIs for shyness and Social Phobia, there is literature supporting the practice. Rapp et al. (2013) continued to use SSRIs as the pharmacological treatment of choice in their protocols with some success and marginal adverse effects in the pediatric population. They reported on one study that used pregabalin (Lyrica) with promising results with a pediatric population. There are too many adverse effects to pregabalin.

Review Question

- How could anxiolytics be helpful to children with school anxiety?

SECTION SEVEN: ANTIDEPRESSANTS AND CHILDREN AND ADOLESCENTS

Learning Objectives

- Understand why the black-box warning on antidepressants for children is important.
- Be able to suggest the type of monitoring necessary if a child is on an antidepressant.
- Know the "placebo problem" especially in reference to children and antidepressants.

Many reports have appeared on an increased incidence of MDD in children and adolescents. Although more studies on this have begun, there is always error in the epidemiologic methods used to gather such data, so such reports are far from conclusive (Ingersoll & Burns, 2001). As McClure, Kubiszyn, and Kaslow (2002b) noted, many approaches are used for diagnosing and treating mood disorders in children, only a few have any

empirical support. It does seem that when identified, childhood or adolescent depression is characterized by high rates of comorbidity with conduct, anxiety and attention deficit disorders, impaired social and vocational functioning, increased rates of substance abuse, eating disorders, and higher risk for completed suicide (West, 1997). Given that, it is important to consider all treatments that may be helpful when a child or adolescent does manifest symptoms of depression.

Depression (unipolar) can be very difficult to discover, discern, and diagnose in children and adolescents. In children, the symptoms manifest themselves as hyperactivity, impulsivity, and aggressiveness. Grief and loss may trigger enuresis, sleeplessness, nightmares, and extreme stubbornness, depending on the age of the child (Brown & Sammons, 2002; Riddle et al., 2001; Ryan, 2002; Viesselman, 1999). In fact, Ryan (2002) noted that depressive illnesses in children and adolescents can be protracted, recurrent, and continue into adulthood.

Newer research into the complexities of antidepressant action can help neurologists and clinicians better understand developmentally important age differences in the nervous system. Researchers are beginning to see that developing animals differ from older ones in serotonin-mediated responses. Very-early-onset stress may compromise later adaptive capacity of some of these systems (Goldman-Rakic & Brown, 1982). Juvenile depression may also differ substantially from adult depression regarding the role of noradrenergic mechanisms and thus in the responsiveness to compounds that target norepinephrine. Practitioners need to be alert to warnings such as those by Coyle (2000), who noted there is "no empirical evidence to support psychotropic drug treatment in very young children and that such treatment could have deleterious effects on the developing brain" (p. 1060).

Tricyclic Antidepressants in Children

Overall, the results have not supported data found in adult studies regarding the efficacy of tricyclic antidepressants in treating juvenile depression

(Cohen, Gerardin, Mazet, Purper-Ouakil, & Flament, 2004; Rosenberg, Holttum, & Gershon, 1994). The weight of currently available evidence suggests that TCAs as a group are indistinguishable from placebo, except in side effects (Kutcher et al., 1994; Puig-Antich et al., 1987). The highest response rate in a study is about 44%. In addition, a significant risk arises of serious cardiac problems in developing bodies. The same conclusions hold true for the TCA derivatives such as desipramine/Norpramin and nortriptyline/Trazodone. Both have been fairly well studied, and researchers have failed to show significant therapeutic differences from placebo but did show a high number of adverse side effects. In addition, both still carry the risk of cardiovascular complications.

Research has demonstrated that TCAs (and MAOIs) have not revealed greater efficacy than that for placebo, and their adverse side effect profile is extensive, including reports of sudden cardiac death (Birmaher, 1998; Brown & Sammons, 2002; Kye et al., 1996; Riddle, Geller, & Ryan, 1993; Werry, 1999). There is little support if any for the routine use of TCAs as a first line of treatment in children and adolescents. Therefore, it is disturbing that millions of prescriptions for desipramine and related compounds have been written for young people under age 18 (Goleman, 1993). Sommers-Flanagan and Sommers-Flanagan (1996) recommended that such prescriptions be reserved for special cases where other treatments have proven ineffective or intolerable and that a thorough physical (including cardiovascular exam) should be conducted before beginning the medication. TCAs should be used in children only under the following conditions:

- Full informed consent of patient and parent
- A history of lack of response to more appropriate treatments
- Full disclosure of side effect profile
- Disclosure of cardiotoxicity of these compounds
- When trials of more effective, available pharmacotherapies (SSRIs) have failed

Also, TCAs should be used with extreme caution, because the noradrenergic system (on which TCAs operate) does not fully develop until early adulthood (Goldman-Rakic & Brown, 1982). This evidence has not changed.

SSRIs in Children

As noted, the FDA (2003) has currently issued a Public Health Advisory cautioning about a possible link to the use of certain SSRI antidepressants in pediatric populations and increased suicide rates. The antidepressants in the advisory are listed in Table 9.4.

As noted, the SSRIs currently are used with children and adolescents for anxiety and depression. Fluoxetine/Prozac has received FDA approval for use in pediatric populations, and fluvoxamine/Luvox is approved for treating OCD in children (Brown & Sammons, 2002). All other SSRIs are prescribed as off label to children with depression as of this writing. Children and adolescents encounter the same adverse effects as when the SSRIs are employed with anxiety disorders. These compounds are more effective in children but not as effective as in adult samples. GlaxoSmithKline pled guilty to criminal charges for

TABLE 9.4 Antidepressants Listed in 2003 FDA Public Health Advisory

Generic Name	Brand Name
Fluoxetine	Prozac
Fluvoxamine	Luvox
Citalopram	Celexa
Escitalopram	Lexapro
Mirtazapine	Remeron
Nefazodone	Serzone
Paroxetine	Paxil
Sertraline	Zoloft
Venlafaxine	Effexor
Bupropion	Wellbutrin

© Cengage Learning®

promoting paroxetine for use in the pediatric age-range for the treatment of depression (Hensley, 2012).

It is important to note that adolescent girls are particularly vulnerable to depression when entering puberty (Phelps et al., 2002; Silberg et al., 1999). Clinicians should be sensitive to gender, family history of depression, impacting life events, loss, or death when assessing children for depression. Current trends and preliminary understandings of the research suggest that in addressing childhood depression, the clinician must consider both psychotherapy and medication (Badal, 1988, 2003). Ryan (2002) indicated that 30 to 40% of children do not have a sufficient response to the first SSRI treatment.

There is almost no literature on the effects of SSRIs on infants and preschoolers (McClure, Kubiszyn, & Kaslow, 2002a); however, evidence shows SSRI prescriptions are on the increase for this age group (Zito et al., 2000). The majority of researchers looked at the effects of fluoxetine (Prozac) on older children and adolescents, which has shown mixed results (Emslie et al., 1997). Some studies looking at the effects of paroxetine on children and adolescents are also promising (Findling et al., 2000; Keller et al., 2001), but more double-blind, placebo-controlled studies need to be done. Juveniles with a family history for manic or hypomanic symptoms are at higher risk for SSRI-induced manic or hypomanic episodes. If children or adolescents are treated with SSRI medications, treatment should be cautious and should observe the following conditions:

- SSRIs are used in addition to supportive psychotherapy or counseling to deal with psychological issues.
- SSRIs should be supported by education regarding the symptoms, the medication, and what relief the medication is to provide.
- Effective treatment involves parents or caregivers as much as possible.
- Effective treatment includes use of a depression scale (HAM-D or BDI-II) if the child is old enough to take one, to monitor symptoms.

- The acute phase of treatment should take place over 8 to 12 weeks followed by maintenance of 4 to 6 months.

McClure et al. (2002a) conclude that when medication is warranted, the SSRIs are the medication of first choice. Jureidini et al. (2004) disagree, however. They recently reviewed and critiqued seven published randomized, controlled trials of newer antidepressants for depressed children. These researchers found that pharmaceutical companies paid for the trials, the benefits of the drugs were small, and the adverse effects were downplayed, and they concluded antidepressant drugs could not be confidently recommended as a first-line treatment option. This is only one meta-analysis, but it points to the need for validity in published data and full disclosure of biases resulting from funding sources or researchers. Karger (2013) concluded that SSRI and even SNRI treatments for pediatric populations were/are too risky and this is from an international perspective. He stated that the SSRIs were more effective with anxiety disorders. Studies have been more compromised in pediatric populations with depression. Also, Craighead, Miklowitz, and Craighead (2013) summarized the work of Dr. Du of Shanghai who indicated that his studies demonstrate that SSRIs are safer in adolescents than in children. Dr. Du encouraged universal efforts of prevention to address the 17–20% of children who are depressed in all of our cultures.

From an integrative perspective, it is important to review all literature as it comes in, as well as review the researchers and the funding sources to check for possible bias. At the time of this writing, a new government-funded study of SSRIs and children was completed but not officially released in a peer-reviewed journal. The study was the Treatment for Adolescent with Depression Study (TADS), sponsored by the National Institute of Mental Health (NIMH). When we called NIMH to get a copy of the study, we were told the study needed to be peer-reviewed and the results would not be released until that process was complete. Nevertheless, *Time* magazine (Lemonick, 2004) and *The New York Times* (Harris, 2004) reported (without benefit of peer review) that the study supported the use of the medications with children. When we asked the NIMH representative how the popular press would have gotten the results to report *before* the peer review, she said she didn't know. Until a peer review of the study is concluded, the writers have no basis for these conclusions other than their own opinions of the study. Without including the results of peer review, readers are likely to come away with a "sound byte" interpretation of the results that may not be accurate. Readers can access the latest results of drug trials on the NIMH website http://www.nimh .nih.gov/studies/2mooddisordersdep.cfm. We did not try for the results in 2014.

THE PLACEBO PROBLEM

As we noted in Chapter Five, the placebo effects of compounds and the place and type of placebo in studies has yet to be explicated. According to Fisher and Fisher (1997), "A probe of the available scientific reservoir of pertinent studies does not reveal any serious evidence that antidepressants do more for childhood depression than do placebos" (p. 308). An earlier overview of studies by Thurber, Ensign, Punnett, and Welter (1995) concluded that the more adequate the experimental methods in each study, the less likely to be found superior to placebo were the drugs tested. Although Fisher and Fisher (1997) noted that the evidence is still limited for the effectiveness of many counseling/psychotherapy approaches to depressed children and adolescents, this does not excuse the prescribing of compounds for which very little evidence of efficacy and effectiveness exists.

In concluding this section, we remind the reader that clinicians are using off-label psychotropic medication for several other disorders. In each case, the clinician must weigh the benefit versus the potential adverse effects of the drug on the child. We must also speak to the child about his or her reaction and feelings about the medication and request feedback from the parents or guardians about the child's progress or struggles with the psychotropic medications. We believe it is an enormous responsibility to counsel children and adolescents who are on psychotropic medication where little research has been conducted on the efficacy, effectiveness, and safety of the drugs.

In April 2003, the recommendations were published of the Research Forum approved by the American Academy of Child and Adolescent Psychiatry (AACAP) on strategies for psychopharmacological studies on preschool children (Greenhill et al., 2003). The six workgroups of the Research Forum were (1) diagnosis/assessment, (2) research design, (3) ethics/institutional review board (IRB), (4) preschool protocol modifications, (5) FDA/regulatory industry, and (6) training/public issues. Finally, when our text was reviewed in 2005, most psychiatrists challenged us on our strident positions about pharmaceutical research, medicating children, split-treatment (working together—psychiatrist and mental health professional), and the general tone of our text. Now we wish to extend our empathy to all psychiatrists who work under tremendous pressure to cure the incurable and find the magic pill.

Review Questions

- Why is the black-box warning on antidepressants for children important?
- If a child is put on an antidepressant, what sort of monitoring is necessary for the child?
- What is the placebo problem with regard to children and antidepressants?

CONCLUSION

We have sought to highlight the complexity, controversy, and conundrums of child and adolescent psychopharmacology. By now, you are alert to factors from all four perspectives that impinge on this issue, generate "word magic," provide partial truths, or stimulate errors. In the colossal debate over ADHD, we discover not only errors but an inflexibility that may harm children rather than treat them. We recognize the power and influence of the pharmaceutical companies to market so many "off-label" psychotropic medications to children and adolescents with such confidence or, more accurately, grandiosity. Central to this dilemma are the shortages of mental health professionals and psychiatrists who exclusively treat children and adolescents. This shortage, coupled with the growing confidence of the effectiveness of psychopharmacology with some diagnoses, permitted pharmaceutical companies to market "off-label" drugs for children and adolescents on a grand scale while clinicians observe the phenomenon, almost powerless. Even the passage of the Best Pharmaceuticals Act for Children 12 years ago is not enough to slow this trend.

SUMMARY

The use of psychotropic medications with children and adolescents is very complex. Clearly there is no simple answer to this dilemma. Because most of the medications are prescribed off label, it is important that mental health professionals learn all that they can in order to protect the health and well-being of their clients who are children and adolescents. The information provided here spans the four perspectives to challenge the reader to consider medical, psychological, cultural, and social paradigms. The discussion of stimulant medications serves as a template for practitioners as they consider psychotropic applications with other disorders. When children or adolescents are placed on a psychotropic, it is always recommended that they receive counseling or other supportive services. The federal government through recent legislation is emphasizing how important and critical this issue is. Finally, the question is asked, "Do we as a society use psychotropic medication as the ultimate modality of behavior and anger management?"

CHAPTER TEN

Herbaceuticals

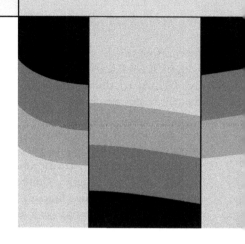

In this chapter we discuss what we call herbaceuticals, that is, plants or herbs that have or are thought to have value in affecting psychological symptoms. This chapter is structured into six sections. Section One deals with psychological issues surrounding herbaceutical use. The second deals with cultural issues, and the third with social issues. In Section Four, we examine the problems in assessing herbaceutical efficacy and use. Section Five covers the most commonly used herbaceuticals and Section Six provides an overview of the issue of legalizing cannabis for medicinal and recreational use.

Learning Objectives

- Understand why people use herbaceuticals and some of the problems with understanding their mechanisms of action.
- Know the herbs most commonly used in treating psychological symptoms, their mechanisms of action (if any), and side effects.
- Understand the debate over medical and recreational marijuana use.

The topic of herbaceuticals strikes at the heart of many issues already raised in this text. In the case of herbaceuticals, questions of efficacy, availability, potency, and responsibility are for the most part unanswered. We use the term *herbaceuticals* for herbal compounds used for medicinal purposes related to mental or physical well-being. It seems the most appropriate term, because to call these compounds "herbal drugs" implies some connection with

synthesized drugs sold as pharmaceuticals or street drugs used recreationally, neither of which is true. To call these compounds "medications" also misrepresents them, because they are treated differently from medications, as we will describe. We also briefly discuss the role of herbaceuticals as entheogens (from the Greek, meaning a way to realize the divine within oneself) but that will be the focus of Chapter Twelve (Ott, 1993). Ironically, the licit herbaceuticals we discuss here cannot, by law, advertise themselves as anything other than "dietary supplements." We address why later, in discussing social issues and perspectives. The use of herbaceuticals (called **phytotherapy**, from the Greek, meaning "plant therapy") is ancient, and many of these plants have been used for thousands of years, for a range of purposes, including mental, physical, and spiritual healing.

We have structured this chapter a bit differently from other chapters in the book. We begin by introducing general herbaceutical issues from the four integrative perspectives. Next we review what is known (and speculated) about a variety of herbal supplements, and then revisit the perspectives of the integrative model to examine specific issues. Finally, we use the perspectives of the integrative model review cannabis. There are no cases in this chapter, because the scope of our practices does not include consultation on herbaceuticals. For reasons we discuss, mental health clinicians who recommend herbal remedies do so at great risk for committing malpractice. Please note that we cite as much literature as possible in this chapter, because our knowledge regarding herbaceuticals is incomplete and the best we can do is keep up with and report to readers the literature that exists.

THE BEHAVIOR OF HERBACEUTICAL USE

What do we know about people's behavior regarding the use of herbaceuticals? Worldwide, it is estimated that up to 80% of all people have tried complementary and alternative medicine, including herbaceuticals (LaFrance et al., 2000). In a study of over 21,000 people in England (Harrison, Holt, Pattison, & Elton, 2004), more than 1 in 10 adults were taking herbal supplements regularly. Many people using herbal supplements do so because they cannot afford allopathic medicines (Mosihuzzaman, 2012). Alternative medicine is becoming more mainstream. In Cleveland, Ohio, where we work, the Cleveland Clinic recently added an institute for integrative medicine that includes Chinese herbal therapies (see http://my.clevelandclinic.org/wellness/integrative-medicine/treatments-services/default.aspx). From an integrative perspective, it is important to note that the widespread use of herbaceuticals worldwide is likely in part because many people do not have access to other medications for cost or distribution reasons. Herbaceutical approaches are firmly integrated into the medical systems in China, North and South Korea, as well as Vietnam (Northridge & Mack, 2002). Also, in many cultures people use herbaceuticals specifically to enhance well-being (Cocks & Moller, 2002; Perry, 2002). In Germany, herb use is more common than in the United States, and depression is treated with St. John's wort (*Hypericum perforatum*) four times as often as with fluoxetine (Gray, 1999). Herbaceutical use is also said to be increasing in England (Redvers, Laugharne, Kanagaratnam, & Srinivasan, 2001). We also know that more and more people with mental disorders are turning to herbaceuticals and dietary supplements. Users of these are more likely to view themselves as having mental health needs, to have received mental health care and to be dissatisfied with their overall healthcare (Niv et al., 2010).

Researchers indicate herbaceutical use is increasing worldwide (Boniel & Dannon, 2001). What are the estimates in the United States? Researchers estimate that 40% of Americans have tried "alternative therapies," with herbal therapies being the most common (Gray, 1999). The most rapidly growing herbal market in the United States is for products with supposed efficacy in treating symptoms of mental and emotional disorders (Beaubrun & Gray, 2000). An ongoing problem with herbaceutical use is that, as researchers estimate, 40 to 60% of those using herbal remedies do so without telling their physician (Gutherie, 1999). As you can see in examining various herbal preparations, all have potential for interactions with other drugs as well as for their own adverse effects. Most users in the United States are middle/upper-middle-class Caucasian women paying out-of-pocket (Klesper et al., 2000). In addition, older Mexican Americans suffering from poor health and depressive symptoms are more likely to use herbal supplements than is the general population (Loera, Black, Markides, Espino, & Goodwin, 2001). Increased use among Americans can be directly linked to a 1994 law that allowed herbal preparations to be sold unregulated as dietary supplements.

Do psychiatrists prescribe or recommend herbaceuticals to their patients? Interestingly, there are few data on this question, but a review of the literature seems to indicate significant differences depending on where the psychiatrists reside and practice. American medical practitioners are really not in a position to prescribe or recommend herbaceuticals, because the FDA does not regulate them, so in most cases the prescriber and the consumer have no idea what is actually in the product. Not many more data are available on physicians' attitudes toward herbaceuticals. One study, done with the faculty and students at the State University of New York Science Center, indicated that although most physicians do ask their patients about the use of herbaceuticals, most never research the herbaceuticals that patients report taking. These researchers did note that the younger the doctor, the more likely the doctor was to be aware of herbaceuticals (Silverstein & Spiegel, 2001).

It is interesting that American researchers raise questions about studies examining herbaceuticals that researchers rarely raise (but could raise) in regard to studies of drugs. Some researchers have noted that the medical community seems particularly critical of trials of herbaceuticals and applies to them more conservative standards than to drug compounds (Even, Friedman, & Dardennes, 2001). One problem that has arisen in the United States with regard to herbaceuticals is the "Don't ask, don't tell" syndrome (Boniel & Dannon, 2001). Basically, patients are reluctant to report their use of herbaceuticals with their doctor because they think the doctor would not approve. Similarly, most doctors don't ask patients if they are using herbaceuticals. This "silence" regarding herbaceuticals can be problematic, because they can interact badly with regular pharmaceuticals (Cupp, 1999; Gold, Laxer, Dergal, Lanctot, & Rochon, 2001).

A study of psychiatrists in Australia and New Zealand found that psychiatrists there were far more positive toward herbaceuticals, with 80% of respondents having used St. John's wort (Walter, Rey, & Harding, 2000). In European countries, where herbs such as St. John's wort are regularly prescribed (for example, Germany), psychiatrists have more positive attitudes about herbaceuticals. A crucial difference to consider is that the German government regulates the dosage and potency of herbaceuticals and promotes research and public education on them, so psychiatrists know exactly how much of the compound patients are being prescribed (Preston, O'Neal, & Talaga, 2002). Several studies from Germany indicate efficacy for St. John's wort (Kasper & Dienel, 2002).

SECTION ONE: PSYCHOLOGICAL ISSUES

Why Do People Take Herbaceuticals?

People report many reasons for turning to herbaceuticals. Table 10.1 summarizes some of the more common reasons given.

TABLE 10.1 Reasons People Report for Taking Herbaceuticals

Mistrusting traditional Western medicine

Believing that "natural" products are safer, less toxic than drugs

Sensing that herbaceuticals are more consistent with patient values or philosophy of health

Accepting anecdotal testimony about efficacy

Not needing a prescription

© Cengage Learning®

Mistrust of Traditional Western Medicine

Gutherie (1999) and Vermani, Milosevic, Smith, and Katzman (2005) noted mistrust of traditional Western medicine as one reason that patients seek alternative and complementary therapies. Many clients and members of the general public are becoming more aware of the adverse effects of medications as well as of questionable practices by pharmaceutical companies. This mistrust may be more pronounced regarding the medical subspecialty of psychiatry—particularly its diagnostic categories. Critics such as Colbert (2002), Breggin (1997), Healy (2002) and Ingersoll and Marquis (2014) all raise substantial questions regarding the accuracy of the *DSM* diagnoses, the degree to which the disorders have biological etiologies, and the extent to which they should be treated with traditional Western medicine. It is interesting too that people who take herbal medicines in some studies have a stronger internal locus of control (Sasagawa, Martzen, Kelleher, & Wenner, 2008).

The state of managed health care in the United States has also decreased consumer confidence in traditional Western medicine. Clients frequently report to us that their health maintenance organization (HMO) will not fill a prescription their doctor has given them, and offers them a different medication. They are usually aware that HMOs routinely make deals with pharmaceutical companies to carry particular drugs and not competing drugs that may have more efficacy in treating the same disorder.

In a nationwide survey, Astin (1998) also explored whether mistrust of traditional medicine was the reason people used herbaceuticals but found in his sample that the primary reasons people sought out alternative therapies were because such approaches were more congruent with their own beliefs, values, and philosophic orientations toward health and life. Rather than framing his participants' preference for herbaceuticals as a reaction to mistrust of traditional Western approaches, Astin sees it as proactive choice based on consciously chosen values. This is certainly the case for many whose spiritual or religious paths have a history of using herbaceuticals both medicinally and ritually. Religions like Wicca and Santeria are examples of spiritual paths with rich heritages of herbaceutical use (Hutton, 1999).

Belief That Natural Products Are Safer Than Drugs

Although people taking herbaceuticals often say they believe that natural products are safer than drugs (Gutherie, 1999; Walter & Rey, 1999), many hazards are actually associated with taking herbaceuticals (Mosihuzzaman, 2012). You do not have to look very far to find toxic compounds in nature. For example, belladonna, sassafras, licorice, and ephedra are all toxic in large enough amounts. In addition, because herbaceuticals are not regulated in most countries (including the United States), consumers really have no way of knowing exactly what they are taking in terms of contents, dosage, and potency of contents. Later in the chapter, we review the growing body of literature that reports on the interactions herbaceuticals can have with medications. Given that a significant percentage of clients taking herbaceuticals do not tell their doctors, these risks for problematic interactions increase (Izzo & Ernst, 2001).

Acceptance of Anecdotal Testimony About Efficacy

Both of us have treated clients who asked us about herbal supplements to treat symptoms of anxiety and depression. When we ask clients how they heard about these, they frequently say they know people who claim to have had success using herbal supplements to treat one or another symptom. It is possible that belief in anecdotal testimony facilitates some placebo effect. We caution readers that although anecdotal evidence may be a good starting point for research questions, it is not a good source for drawing conclusions. Case histories and individual clients' responses to different treatments help us refine how to research and evaluate those treatments. However, conclusions should not be overgeneralized based on one or two cases.

SECTION TWO: ISSUES OF CULTURE

Issues of culture related to herbaceuticals can be placed in two categories. The first is herbaceutical practices that derive from indigenous cultures and have been handed down to the present day. Examples include older Mexican Americans' reliance on herbaceuticals (Loera et al., 2001) and those cultures where herbaceuticals are an integrative part of medicine and wellness. Here, herbaceuticals could logically be extended to include **entheogens**, meaning "God-manifesting" agents. Despite the **current** prohibition in the United States, entheogens have been used (and continue to be used) here and in traditional societies as ways to facilitate the mystical vision (Smith, 2000). Despite the overgeneralizing rhetoric in the United States about the evils of mind-altering substances, ample evidence shows that in many cultures the moderate use of mind-altering plants is part of human evolutionary legacy as well as a strategy that can enhance well-being (Roberts & Winkelman, 2007; Siegel, 1989; Sullivan & Hagen, 2002).

The second category concerns the subcultures fighting over whether herbaceuticals can be a standard part of medical practice in the United States. This power issue interests not just medical practitioners but also pharmaceutical companies. Imagine what might happen if a plant such as St. John's wort caught on as an effective treatment for depression. Would the FDA seek to regulate its production and distribution? Would it become illegal to grow, as marijuana currently is? If not, would consumers with any gardening savvy pay for an antidepressant, when they could grow St. John's wort in a backyard at a fraction of the cost? In addition, would the medical lobby seek to restrict St. John's wort to prescription-only access? Although many believe there should be an over-the-counter anti-depressant (Volz & Laux, 2000), many others contest that possibility. From an integrative perspective, all these are important questions.

Another question implied in the power issue is, "How much protection can and should the government give its citizens?" People have come to expect regulation in how drugs are accessed as well as what is allowed in terms of advertising. The United States in particular has not defined the extent to which drugs should be regulated by prescription. Some researchers have suggested that compounds such as antidepressants could all be sold over the counter, because they are no more dangerous than many other over-the-counter substances (Healy, 1997). The prescription issue has particular relevance when considering such issues as marijuana used for medical purposes. Should citizens have the right to grow plants with psychotropic properties for their own use? Is government's role to protect people from themselves even when they don't want such protection?

SECTION THREE: ISSUES FROM THE SOCIAL PERSPECTIVE

Legal Issues

In pondering some of the questions ending the last section, you are likely aware that herbaceuticals use has legal aspects. Many people wonder why herbaceuticals sales picked up so much in the last 10 years. One answer is a 1994 law called the Dietary Supplement Health Education Act. The law, for which the supplements industry lobbied heavily, restricted the FDA's ability to control herbal products. Passage of that law allowed any product to be labeled a supplement as long as no claims were made that the product affected a disease. Whereas a manufacturer cannot claim something such as St. John's wort "alleviates depression," it can legally claim that a substance "helps facilitate emotional balance." As the Consumer's Union (1999) points out, the current law allows such products to be

marketed with absolutely no demonstrations of safety or efficacy. On the one hand, critics such as Pies (2000) believe that because herbal products can create adverse reactions in users, consumers need stricter FDA regulation of these products. On the other hand, advocates of access to herbaceuticals fear that regulation will turn into unnecessarily harsh, even draconian, restrictions, as happened with marijuana prohibition.

Another important legal issue concerns the types of liability U.S. physicians and mental health care providers may incur if they discuss unregulated compounds with clients. The cost of malpractice insurance in the United States has skyrocketed out of control (Vasankathumar, 2001), and attorneys and a public that seem eager to resort to litigation routinely scrutinize physicians. In such a climate, is it any wonder physicians are unlikely to recommend untested and unregulated herbaceuticals? Again, from an integrative perspective, it is unfair to blame physicians for what actually is an effort to achieve a "best practices" standard.

The legal and ethical issues become more complex for nonmedical mental health clinicians. We have already said clinicians are likely to be practicing ethically when discussing basic information about medication, helping the client work through issues related to medication, or acting as an information broker in helping the client get quality information about a medication. Although clinicians should try to answer clients' questions about herbaceuticals, clinicians should restrict themselves to the conclusions in peer-reviewed literature and should recommend that clients check with the doctor before starting any herbaceuticals compound. This conservative approach is important until more data on herbaceuticals are amassed and more standardization is achieved. As Rivas-Vasquez (2001) has pointed out, this is a high-risk area, and clinicians should tread carefully.

SECTION FOUR: PROBLEMS IN STUDYING MEDICINAL PLANTS

An important social issue we must also comment on is research practice related to herbaceuticals. Although approximately 5000 medicinal plants are

TABLE 10.2 Problems in Studying Medicinal Plants

Isolating compounds

Identifying species

Variations in composition

Variations in preparation

Adulteration and substitution

Chemical complexity

Problematic study designs

Language barriers

© Cengage Learning®

known, there are only current studies and published papers on about 100 (Northridge & Mack, 2002). Why the dearth of information? Clearly some of this lack is related to difficulties in studying plants that may have hundreds of active compounds and trying to decide which compounds produce the therapeutic effects. Table 10.2 lists some challenges in studying medicinal plants that may contribute to the dearth of literature. A brief discussion follows.

Isolating naturally occurring compounds is currently not a frontline research strategy in pharmaceuticals. The most popular research now focuses on drug–receptor interactions as well as on intracell changes. Further, isolating active compounds that produce a supposed therapeutic effect is very difficult and time consuming. In Chapter Seven, writing about the new antipsychotics, we noted an important question: How much dopamine antagonism versus serotonin antagonism is necessary for optimal antipsychotic effects? This is a difficult problem to solve even when there are only two primary variables. In plants with hundreds of active compounds, the variables multiply exponentially, and it is hard to know where to begin. Here, the chemical complexity of medicinal plants continues to be a problem. Plants contain thousands of chemicals. This complexity means each herbal preparation may have a variety of pharmacologic effects. For example, at least 40 chemical compounds

contribute to producing the aroma of coffee. That is 40 chemical compounds just for aroma alone, without even considering the pharmacologically active chemicals.

Medicinal plant species also vary, as do individual plants within a species, with each variation having its own combination and concentration of active elements. Inaccurate identification of species thus poses a potential problem for systematic study of medicinal plants. For example, the 250 varieties of the herb valerian vary in concentration of active compounds. Researchers would first have to determine which varieties had the most therapeutic effect and then isolate the active compounds to determine those that produce the effect.

Even if a researcher identifies the correct plants and can isolate the active elements, variations in composition result from genetic factors, climate, growing season, soil quality, rainfall, and postharvest storage conditions. Any of these can affect the composition of the plant. So researchers would also have to find ways to exercise control over as many of these variables as possible.

Once an herb is harvested, it can be prepared in many different formulations. For example, herbs can be dried and made into tea or concentrated and used as extract. In addition, extracts may be created with various solvents, including alcohol, oils, or water. Amount of active ingredients varies with preparation method.

Even for herbs harvested and prepared in a uniform manner, lack of standardization can affect the end product. Standardization depends on the integrity of the company selling and distributing the herb. Suppliers often adulterate and substitute other plant materials when the target plant is expensive. Tyler (1994) found that many preparations of ginseng have no ginseng but are filled with numerous other substances.

For the hardy researcher ready to tackle these challenges, there are more, including study design and access to current data. As with lithium, no one can patent a naturally occurring element, and this precludes making a lot of money on herbaceuticals. Thus, most herbaceuticals have few adequate studies to test their efficacy. Another problem is likely more pronounced for U.S. researchers, who are more likely than researchers in other countries to speak only one language. There are data on many herbaceuticals, but the data are in languages other than English. Although many noteworthy works on phytotherapy are now beginning to be translated into English (Blumenthal, 1998), the process is slow.

DIFFERENCES BETWEEN HERBS AND DRUGS

All the latter research problems point to some of the essential differences between herbal preparations and drugs. Although some may seem to be commonsense distinctions, they bear emphasizing, particularly in a society where people are so confused over what constitutes a "drug." Many critics of the current U.S. practice of labeling herbs such as St. John's wort as "dietary supplements" note that if such herbs may negatively interact with medicines, public safety is best served by regulating them as drugs (Stein, 2002). Table 10.3 summarizes important differences between herbs and drugs. This table is also followed by commentary.

As noted earlier, dosage of an herbal product is very difficult to determine, because there are few efficacy studies on varying dosages to determine the optimal dosage range. In addition, lack of standardization in preparing many herbal supplements makes it next to impossible to know the potency of the compound making up each dosage. Drugs

TABLE 10.3 Important Differences Between Herbs and Drugs

Dosage

Efficacy

Complexity of the compound

FDA role

Role of patents

Role of potency standards

are required to have efficacy studies as well as uniformity in dosage and potency. Under U.S. law, herbaceuticals do not. In addition, as noted, drugs must be regulated by the FDA, whereas herbaceuticals need not be. Drugs are usually monosubstances, whereas herbaceuticals may have many active elements. Finally, when a pharmaceutical company synthesizes a drug, it can get a patent on the compound, which lets the company monopolize the substance for a period of time (usually 17 years) in which to earn back the money it took to research the compound (plus, one assumes, profits).

These differences contribute to many problems with herbaceuticals, including lack of purity. Slifman et al. (1998) did a study of chemical analyses for many popular herbal compounds to see what was actually in them, and logged some disturbing results. The herbs studied had many contaminants. In some of the Chinese patent medicines studied, the researchers found mercury, arsenic, aspirin, and phenobarbital. In some of the medicines from India, the researchers found carbamazepine/Tegretol and diazepam/Valium!

Another related problem concerns unethical marketing. Bear in mind that under the 1994 Dietary Supplement Health Education Act, advertising can be legal without being ethical. One product marketed as an antitension supplement claimed to contain St. John's wort, 10 complementary herbs, and calcium. The product claimed these ingredients worked together for a synergistic effect. The product listed the following ingredients in each tablet:

300 mg St. John's wort
90 mg passion flower
70 mg hops
30 mg skullcap
40 mg black cohosh
30 mg wood betony
30 mg chamomile
15 mg lady's slipper
10 mg cayenne
5 mg chlorophyll
40 mg elemental calcium
10 mg elemental magnesium

Clearly, there is no way the company could have "known" the combination would have a calming effect, because most of the herbs listed had not been studied for any "calming" effect. Further, there would be no way of knowing what the effects of all these ingredients would be on the person taking the supplement. Should laws prohibit such advertising? It stands to reason that because the claims cannot be backed up by research, such claims should not be made to consumers.

SECTION FIVE: EXAMINING BETTER KNOWN HERBACEUTICALS WITH APPLICATION FOR PSYCHIATRIC PROBLEMS

In this section of the chapter, we share what we know about some of the more popular herbaceuticals thought to have uses for mental/emotional symptoms. Note that although some herbs have a good deal of research behind them at this point (such as St. John's wort), others have very little, and in some cases the jury is still out regarding efficacy. For each herb, we note the side effects we are aware of. Table 10.4 summarizes the herbs we cover in this section.

TABLE 10.4 Herbaceuticals Thought to Have Use in Mental/Emotional Disorders

Herb	Supposed Therapeutic Property
St. John's wort	Antidepressant
Kava	Anxiolytic
Valerian root	Anxiolytic
Passion flower	Anxiolytic/hypnotic
Hops	Anxiolytic/hypnotic
Melatonin	Hypnotic
Ginkgo	Cognitive enhancer
Ephedra	Stimulant

© Cengage Learning®

St. John's Wort

St. John's wort (*Hypericum perforatum*) is an aromatic perennial that is native to Europe and grows wild in Asia, North America, and South America. It has bright yellow flowers with red spots and is abundant in June. The red spots are supposed to symbolize the blood of John the Baptist, a Christian figure who was beheaded at the time of year the spots appear (early summer). *Perforatum* refers to the tiny perforation in each leaf of that subspecies; the leaves seen from directly overhead are positioned like a cross, in four directions on the stem; German ethno-botanist Bernhard Becker of Beendorf told the tale that St. John looked down and the devil was hiding beneath the plant; the plant opened up tiny holes to reveal the devil; a version from a less Druidic past says God's all-seeing eye bored the tiny holes. Other legends hold that June (when the plant flowers) is also the birthday of John the Baptist (the word "wort" is derived from the Old English *wyrt* and means "plant" or "vegetable"). St. John's wort has been used medicinally for over 2000 years. Paracelsus called it "arnica of the nerves" ("arnica" referring to perennial herbs) because of its soothing effects on nervous disorders (Bilia, Gallori, & Vincieri, 2002). Its use in treating mood disorders was pioneered by a German physician in 1939. Although traditionally prepared as tea, currently it is also prepared in ethanol and methanol extracts. The methanol extract is the extract used in the most systematic research on the herb and is prepared by a firm in Germany. Any research on St. John's wort in Germany uses this compound (labeled LI 160), as reflected in the literature. St. John's wort is hypothesized to have efficacy in treating depression. We review the studies supporting this hypothesis later; for now it's enough to say that a great deal of research supports the efficacy of St. John's wort in mild to moderate depression.

Mechanism of Action

St. John's wort has many elements that are biologically active, including naphthodianthrones, flavonoids, and xanthones. The two active ingredients, presumed to be naphthodianthrones, are hypericin and hyperforin. The word *hypericin* is a Greek word meaning "overcoming an apparition," and medical historians think the ancients believed the plant had the ability to ward off evil spirits. Modern researchers initially thought hypericin disabled MAO (like an MAO inhibitor), but now they think hypericin is more of a reuptake inhibitor of serotonin, dopamine, and norepinephrine (Wong, Smith, & Boon, 1998). In addition, hypericin seems to bind to GABA receptors, benzodiazepines receptors, and glutaminergic receptors. Hyperforin is also hypothesized to play a key role in the antidepressant activity of St. John's wort (Cervo et al., 2002); however, it is not known what its primary mechanism of action is at the time of this writing.

Efficacy of St. John's Wort

The consensus of opinion currently seems to be that St. John's wort has efficacy over placebo in treating mild to moderate depression (Sarris, Fava, Schweitzer, & Mischoulon, 2012). Several meta-analyses support this conclusion, including Gaster and Holroyd (2000); Kasper and Dienel (2002); Kim, Streltzer, and Goebert (1999); Laakmann, Jahn, and Schuele (2002); Linde et al. (1996); Linde and Mulrow (2000); and Whiskey, Werneke, and Taylor (2001). In addition, clinical trials have also supported the use of St. John's wort in mild to moderate depression (see Benner, Bjerkenstedt, & Edman, 2002; Ernst, 2002; Friede, Henneicke von Zepelin, & Freudenstein, 2001; Holsboer-Trachsler & Vanoni, 1999; Kelly, 2001; Lecrubier, Clerc, Didi, & Keiser, 2002; Volz, Murck, Kasper, & Moeller, 2002). The extract of St. John's wort used in most studies is labeled LI 160 and is the commonly prescribed compound for depression in Germany. LI 160 is distributed and regulated in Germany with regard to the potency and dosage of the compound. The recommended dosage is at least 900 mg per day. Of the trials that did not support efficacy, one of the more controversial was that by the Hypericum Depression Trial Study Group (2002), which found no differences among sertraline, St. John's wort, and placebo. This study was followed by no fewer than six commentaries (Gott & Wisner, 2002; Klaus, Mechart, Mulrow, & Berner, 2002; Kupfer & Frank, 2002; Spielmans,

2002; Volp, 2002; Wheatley, 2002), indicating a number of questions regarding the findings. Another trial (large-scale, multisite, placebo-controlled) also did not find St. John's wort significantly different from placebo (Shelton et al., 2001). All the studies showing significance for St. John's wort did so *only* with mild to moderate depression. These studies used participants whose depression was in the moderate to severe range, as measured by the Hamilton Depression Rating Scale. This discrepancy alone could account for the differences in findings.

With regard to studies comparing St. John's wort with standard antidepressants, four studies have compared St. John's wort to maprotiline/Ludiomil (a tricyclic derivative), imipramine/Tofranil and amitriptyline/Elavil. No significant differences were found in responses to the St. John's wort and these agents. One severe limitation in these studies was that the antidepressant doses were lower than would be normal in clinical practice (Wheatley, 1997). Another study (Friede et al., 2001) found St. John's wort at 500 mg per day as effective as fluoxetine/Prozac at 20 mg per day (the minimum therapeutic dosage in the United States) in treating mild to moderate depression. It is hoped that researchers will replicate this latter study.

In addition to treating mild to moderate depression, studies have suggested efficacy for St. John's wort in treating menopausal symptoms (Grube, Walper, & Wheatley, 1999) and Seasonal Affective Disorder (Wheatley, 1999). There is still debate about the efficacy of St. John's wort. Sarris (2013) and Sarris and Kavanaugh (2009) like most researchers found it had efficacy for mild to moderate depression. Grobler, Matthews, and Molenberghs (2013) claim that in many studies that show efficacy, there were missing data that when added and reanalyzed show St. John's wort performing no better than placebo. Obviously, the debate over this herbaceutical goes on.

Side and Interaction Effects of St. John's Wort

Although there is no systematic study of the side effects of St. John's wort, some reported side effects in studies can be shared here. Many researchers report that side effects are minimal (Gaster & Holroyd,

2000) and others that St. John's wort is well tolerated (Volz et al., 2002). Parker, Wong, Boon, and Seeman (2001) and Dannawi (2002) found that in sensitive patients, St. John's wort is associated with serotonin syndrome. This is a potentially life-threatening syndrome caused by increased accumulation of serotonin in the central nervous system. The symptoms of serotonin syndrome include disorientation, confusion, agitation, restlessness, fever, chills, diarrhea, hypertension, and sweating.

Far more likely than developing serotonin syndrome just from St. John's wort is that clients could develop the syndrome from combining St. John's wort with another serotonergic drug, as was the case in the Dannawi (2002) study. Parker and colleagues (2001) identified cases where the syndrome was associated only with St. John's wort. These researchers also found a case where St. John's wort was associated with hair loss. This is reminiscent of the case we shared in Chapter Five where the hair loss seemed caused by sertraline/Zoloft. In another study (Holsboer-Trachsler & Vanoni, 1999), gastrointestinal upset was one of the most frequently reported side effects, but in most cases it was rated as mild to moderate. Finally, one researcher noted that sexual dysfunction was a side effect of St. John's wort and could be treated with sildenafil (Viagra) (Asslian, 2000).

Although side effects are always a concern with a substance, they are eclipsed in importance by adverse interactions with other substances. All herbaceuticals exerting a psychotropic effect can have adverse interactions with other herbaceuticals or with other drugs the client may be taking. In one study, 19% of the people who reported taking herbaceuticals also reported an adverse reaction to them (Hailemaskel, Dutta, & Wutoh, 2001). Concern over adverse interactions between herbaceuticals and drugs have been voiced by researchers in Europe (Izzo & Ernst, 2001; Kistorp & Laursen, 2002), the United States (Keller & Lemberg, 2001; Pies, 2000), Canada (Asslian, 2000; Gold, Tullis, & Frost-Pineda, 2001), Israel (Boniel & Dannon, 2001), and Lebanon (Dannawi, 2002). Note that the presence of interaction effects implies pharmacodynamic activity in St. John's wort.

Drug interactions peculiar to St. John's wort include lowering blood concentrations of other drugs (particularly anticoagulants and anti-inflammatory drugs for arthritis). St. John's wort combined with certain oral contraceptives (ethinylestradiol/desogestrel) has been correlated with intermenstrual bleeding (Izzo & Ernst, 2001). These interactions seem related to the effects St. John's wort has on the **cytochrome P-450 enzyme** system, the liver enzyme system responsible for metabolizing most drugs. St. John's wort, like many FDA-approved pharmaceuticals, appears to elevate these enzymes, making them more efficient at metabolizing other drugs (Bilia et al., 2002).

Kava

The kava, or kava kava, shrub (*Piper methysticum*) is native to Polynesia and the Pacific Islands. It has been used there for millennia, primarily in liquid form made by grinding the dried rhizome (underground stem) and mixing with water and coconut milk. Captain James Cook and other European explorers in the 18th century described kava as having a calming effect. The crude drug can be derived from the rhizome, but now most formulations are made as ethanol–water or acetone extracts. Traditionally, kava is used socially similar to the way we use alcohol. At high doses kava, like alcohol, can cause intoxication.

Mechanism of Action

Kava is one of the few herbal treatments where the active ingredient is known. Meyer (1967) proved that the effects of kava were due to kavapyrones. These act as muscle relaxants and anticonvulsants, and they reduce excitability in the limbic system. They do so by inhibiting voltage-dependent sodium channels, increasing the number of GABA-A receptors, blocking NE reuptake, and suppressing release of glutamate (which metabolizes into glutamic acid, which, recall from Chapter Two, serves an excitatory function).

Efficacy of Kava as an Anxiolytic

Several double-blind, placebo-controlled studies support the use of kava as an anxiolytic (Kinzler, Kroner, & Helman, 1991; Volz, 1997; Warnecke, 1991). The only problem with these studies is that the patient population was not clearly defined by diagnosis. Two studies exist researching the effects of kava on symptoms of Generalized Anxiety Disorder (GAD). The first study (Wheatley, 2001) compared two doses of kava in patients suffering from GAD. Both dose schedules (120 mg once daily and 45 mg three times daily) were found effective. In the second, although overall differences from placebo were not significant, the authors felt the improvement warranted further investigation (Connor & Davidson, 2002). Rex, Morgenstern, and Fink (2002) compared kava with diazepam/Valium used on rats using a maze test. These authors concluded that the kava exerted an anxiolytic response in the rats similar to that induced by diazepam. They felt the study supported the use of kava as an anxiolytic. Sarris et al. (2013) found kava was well-tolerated and may be a moderately effective short-term option for the treatment of Generalized Anxiety Disorder. Finally, one meta-analysis (Witte, Loew, & Gaus, 2005) also found kava extract to have efficacy in nonpsychotic anxiety disorders.

Side Effects and Adverse Reactions

Although the few studies that exist note minimal side effects, there are some reports of rash, tiredness (Leak, 1999), and a rare occurrence of nausea (Wheatley, 1997). Although initial studies (few in number) seem to indicate kava is well tolerated, more research is needed to draw conclusions. The risk of adverse reactions for kava includes the possibility that it induces tolerance and dependence (Mischoulon, 2002), and there has been at least one report of acute liver failure tied to kava use (Brauer, Stangl, Siewert, Pfab, & Becker, 2003). Clearly, kava should not be mixed with other CNS depressants.

Ginkgo Biloba

The *Ginkgo biloba* tree is native to East Asia. Gingkos were first imported to Europe from Japan during the 18th century and now are common ornamental trees throughout Europe and North America. According to Wong et al. (1998), they are among the oldest species of deciduous trees on the planet.

Ginkgo fruit and seeds have been used in China for medicinal purposes for millennia. Ginkgo has been used to treat people with asthma, and leaves are used to dress wounds. Currently, most ginkgo products are derived from the dried leaves (the therapeutic extracts are labeled Egb 761 and LI 1370).

Mechanisms of Action

Gingko, like other herbs, contains a large number of substances that have been demonstrated to have a wide variety of pharmacologic properties. As with most herbs discussed so far, ginkgo has a wide variety of active ingredients we are only just learning about. A primary active ingredient seems to be flavonoids. Flavonoids are compounds found in numerous plants, and ingesting them is associated with decreased risk of several chronic diseases (Knekt et al., 2002). Flavonoids are effective antioxidants that decrease free radicals in the body. Free radicals are reactive chemicals that attack molecules by capturing electrons from the molecules and then modifying their chemical structure. Free radicals are believed to be one cause of Alzheimer's-type dementia. This connection provides a rationale for testing ginkgo on people suffering from Alzheimer's disease. If ginkgo has flavonoids that decrease the free radicals causing the damage to neurons, researchers hope their administration may slow the disease. Ginkgo leaves are harvested in May when the flavonoid content is highest.

Compounds called *ginkgolides* are another active ingredient in ginkgo. Researchers think ginkgolides inhibit platelet-activating factor. This effect may play a role in patients with vascular dementias, using the same mechanism as aspirin in forestalling additional strokes. It is also related to some of the adverse effects of ginkgo such as prolonged bleeding after chronic administration.

Efficacy of Ginkgo

So how well does ginkgo work with people suffering from Alzheimer's-type dementia? After several false starts and years of studies, it appears ginkgo does not have efficacy for treating this disorder, as once believed. More than 40 controlled studies were initially conducted in Europe testing ginkgo efficacy for treating dementia. Although these studies seemed to show positive effects, the patient populations were poorly defined, the numbers were small, the randomization poorly done, and the outcome measures were not standard (Kleijnen & Knipschild, 1992).

The LeBars study in 1997 corrected many of these shortcomings. This 52-week, randomized, double-blind, placebo-controlled study was done with 202 patients, who were diagnosed with either Alzheimer's disease (129) or vascular dementia (73). The patients were 45 to 90 years of age. Outcome measures included the Alzheimer's Disease Assessment Scale, Cognitive subscale (ADAS-Cog); the Geriatric Evaluation by Relatives Rating Instrument (GERRI); and the Clinical Global Impression of Change (CGIC).

On average, the ADAS-Cog and the GERRI showed significantly less decline in the ginkgo extract group than in the placebo. This difference was equivalent to a 6-month delay in progression of the disease. The results were comparable to the effects of 80 to 120 mg of tacrine/Cognex, a drug used to delay progression of Alzheimer's Disease. Although statistically significant, the results of the LeBars study were actually modest. In a later paper, LeBars and Kastelan (2000) noted that ginkgo is more likely to appear efficacious on broad dependent measures as opposed to more narrow cognitive assessments. Other studies using such narrow assessments do not find any significant differences between patients on ginkgo and those on placebo (Soloman, Adams, Silver, Zimmer, & DeVeaux, 2002). The evidence to date seems to show that the effects of ginkgo on cognition are minimal (Sommer & Schatzberg, 2002).

Valerian Root

Valerian root is another herb commonly prescribed in Europe. Valerian is a flowering perennial plant that grows in temperate climates worldwide. The root is believed to be a mild sedative/anxiolytic, although results of research have been conflicting. Valerian is on Germany's list of approved herbs, and supplements can be purchased in various formulations. For thousands of years the Greeks, Chinese, and the people of India used valerian as a mild sedative, and it is still used to flavor foods and beverages such as root beer. The rhizome and roots are harvested, dried, and served as tea or used to make an extract.

Mechanisms of Action

Valerian extract contains over 100 different constituents. Researchers do not know which of these is or are responsible for its effects, although some believe valerian may have an effect on GABA receptors and act like a mild benzodiazepine. Others have hypothesized that valerian inhibits the enzymatic breakdown of GABA, thus producing its tranquilizing effects (Houghton, 1999).

Efficacy of Valerian

In studies, 400 to 900 mg of valerian extract decreased sleep latency and nocturnal awakenings and improved subjective sleep quality. In some cases, the beneficial effects were seen only after two to four weeks of therapy (Balderer & Bobely, 1985; Leathwood & Chauffard, 1982; Leathwood, Chauffard, Heck, & Munoz-Box, 1982). It appears valerian can produce an anxiolytic effect, although the degree of that effect relative to the dose is still debated (Leak, 1999).

Side and Adverse Effects

The side effects of valerian have been reported to be headache, agitation, uneasiness, and possible liver toxicity (Yager, Siegfried, & DiMatteo, 1999). Julien noted the possibility that valerian could interact with SSRI antidepressants and cause serotonin syndrome. Studies on reaction time, alertness, and concentration indicate that the effects of valerian do not impair these functions on the morning after taking a dose (Kuhlmann, Berger, Podzuweit, & Schmidt, 1999). More research is obviously needed, but at this point valerian may prove promising as a mild anxiolytic.

Ephedrine

Ephedrine is a sympathomimetic alkaloid derived from any of several species of ephedra. The Asian species

Ephedra sinica typically has the highest concentration of ephedrine. Perhaps more than any other herbaceutical, ephedrine illustrates the dangers inherent in unregulated products that have powerful mechanisms of action. On February 17, 2003, major league baseball player Steve Bechler, 23, collapsed and died from heatstroke during spring training. The coroner in Broward County, Florida, believed that Bechler's use of an ephedrine-containing weight loss product contributed to his death. This tragedy reignited the debate over whether products containing ephedrine should be sold as over-the-counter supplements (Fox, 2003). In 2004, the FDA banned the sale in the United States of products containing ephedrine (Parry, 2004).

You may recall from Chapter Nine that ephedrine is an alkaloid (organic, nitrogen-containing compounds) found in the ma huang plant (*Ephedra sinica*), which has been used in Chinese medicine for thousands of years. The primary active constituent of ephedra is ephedrine, which served as the organic model for the first synthesized amphetamine. Ephedrine gained widespread medical use in the United States in the 1920s as a nasal decongestant, CNS stimulant, and asthma treatment, but its use decreased because of safety concerns. Ephedrine reappeared as a dietary supplement to weight loss products sold as herbal supplements. Although ephedrine-containing products account for less than 1% of herbaceuticals purchased, they are responsible for 64% of the adverse effects reported (Bent, Tiedt, Odden, & Shlipak, 2003).

Mechanisms of Action

Ephedrine is a psychostimulant that exerts its effects by releasing epinephrine, norepinephrine, and dopamine. It resembles amphetamine, although it has a much shorter half-life. Ephedrine has been shown to have pharmacodynamics similar to those of amphetamine (Angrist, Rotrosen, Kleinberg, Merriam, & Gershon, 1977; Ercil & France, 2003; Glennon & Young, 2000). Ephedrine is categorized as a sympathicomimetic agent, because it mimics the sympathetic nervous system. Recall from Chapter Two that the sympathetic nervous system prepares the body's fight–flight–freeze response. Ephedrine stimulates the cardiovascular system and dilates the bronchial tubes (hence its use in treating asthma attacks) (Van der Hooft & Stricher, 2002; Wooltorton & Sibbald, 2002). These effects also seem to be responsible for its appetite-suppressing qualities.

Adverse Effects

The primary adverse effects include stroke, heart attacks, cardiac arrhythmias, and seizures—all potential adverse effects seen in amphetamines as well (Geiger, 2002; Kaberi-Otarod, Conetta, Kundo, & Farkash, 2002; Van der Hooft & Stricher, 2002; Wooltorton & Sibbald, 2002). In addition to these adverse effects, there have also been reports of ephedrine-induced mania (Capwell, 1995), psychosis (Jacobs & Hirsch, 2000), and dependence (Gruber & Pope, 1998).

In the wake of the deaths from adverse effects, the FDA treated ephedrine as a potent psychostimulant to be regulated. Although the Dietary Supplements Health and Education Act of 1994 prohibits regulation of dietary supplements, the FDA may regulate if a supplement poses a significant or unreasonable risk of injury or illness. Given this authority, the FDA called for stricter regulations in 1997 (Maradino, 1997) and then banned ephedrine in 2003. A federal court upheld this decision in 2004 (Parry, 2004).

From an integrative perspective, regulation promises only a partial solution. Far less socially and individually dangerous drugs (such as cannabis) are completely prohibited in the United States, but people who want them find a way to get them. Thus, regulation may not solve the problem and may in fact increase the problem, adding immeasurably to the social damage surrounding its use. Many users of ephedrine-containing products seem to be athletes, and many are adolescents. From the intrapsychic perspective of the Integrative Model, these users report feeling that using the supplement gives them a "competitive edge" or brings them closer to an internalized ideal of thinness. Further, from the cultural perspective, subcultures can easily develop in groups of adolescent athletes where taking supplements becomes a norm, and this norm in turn increases use of supplements and the attendant risks. In one large scale study, researchers found that trainers had a significant influence on the attitudes and subjective norms of adolescent athletes and the researchers proposed ways to encourage attitudes that discouraged supplement use (Dunn et al., 2001).

Other Herbaceuticals

Passion Flower and Hops

Both passion flower and hops are purported to have sedative/anxiolytic properties, but there are little scientific data on either. Passion flower is a climbing vine native to North America. It has fallen into disuse in this country but is still one of the most common herbal hypnotics in Great Britain. Components of its extract appear to bind to GABA receptors.

Hops are the fruit of the hop plant, a vine native to Europe. Although used primarily for making beer, hops have been used as a tonic for over 1000 years. Their use as a sleeping aid resulted from the observation that hop pickers tired easily, possibly due to the transfer of hop resin from hands to mouth. Studies have not confirmed that hop resin, hop extract, or lipophilic hop concentrates have a sedative effect. There do not appear to be sufficient data to support its use as a sleep aid.

Melatonin

Melatonin is a hormone produced by the pineal gland. It binds to the suprachiasmic nucleus (SCN), which is the body's circadian pace maker or internal clock. The SCN normally produces an alerting signal that researchers think is blunted by melatonin. Melatonin is useful in initiating sleep but can cause a rebound in the SCN, causing wakefulness three to four hours after taking the melatonin. Various doses are used (1 to 100 mg), and anything over 5 mg raises the melatonin in the blood to levels higher than normal. The melatonin in health food stores is labeled to range between 1 and 5 mg, but the actual range is much more variable. Recent research has supported the use of melatonin as a safer alternative to hypnotics for adolescents (Eckerberg, Lowden, Nagai, & Akerstedt, 2012) and a recent meta-analysis supported the use of melatonin for primary sleep disorders (Ferracioli-Oda, Qawasmi, & Bloch, 2013).

SECTION SIX: AN INTEGRATIVE VIEW OF MARIJUANA

Although marijuana is not a licit herbaceutical in the United States, many people around the world still use it for everything from medical purposes, to enhancing sexual experience and well-being, to "finding God"—that is, as an entheogen. We have included this section for two reasons. First, I (Ingersoll) have taught dozens of courses and seminars on psychopharmacology, and in most of them students have questions about marijuana, its efficacy for medical use, and its actual dangers. Although it is not popular to say, many of these students are skeptical about the government media campaign against marijuana use and want to know where to find reliable information. The second reason we have included this section is because it illustrates the Integrative Model's capacity to capture the complexity of a topic, revealing the partial truths while also providing a critical view of the issues.

A Brief History of Marijuana Use

> There is something profoundly frightening to the orthodoxies of higher civilization about the shamanistically originated vision quest with drugs. (Wilson, 1993, p. 164)

Marijuana is an ancient drug that apparently has been used since prehistoric times. It is a product of the hemp plant (*Cannabis sativa,* Latin for "planted hemp"), a species that provides a useful fiber, an edible seed, oil, and a medicine (Weil & Rosen, 1993). Until recent times, it has been an important cultivated crop. As recently as 1943, farmers were paid to grow hemp; "Hemp for victory" was one of the industrial catchphrases of World War II. This was industrial hemp, not cultivated for its psychoactive properties, but marijuana was being used recreationally in society at the time. The United States at the time of this writing is clearly becoming more accepting of marijuana use (Benac, 2013) with 21 states allowing the use of medical marijuana and two states allowing recreational use (http://medicalmarijuana.procon.org/view.resource.php?resourceID=000881). Despite fears that this would unleash an epidemic of marijuana use especially among teenagers that does not seem to be the case (Lynne-Landsman, Livingston, & Wagenaar, 2013).

Marijuana is derived from the flowers and the tops of the leaves from male and female plants. Cannabis will grow almost anywhere, given adequate water and drainage. *Cannabis sativa* produces a sticky, yellowish resin, which seems to have evolved as a defense mechanism to protect itself from harmful predators. This resin contains the primary psychoactive ingredients of marijuana.

Cannabis is one of the few plants that legend says was not discovered by animals. Typically, humans seem to have learned which plants were safe for ingestion by watching animals eat them (and not fall over dead!). According to an Arab legend, in 1155 C.E. Haydar, an ascetic monk who founded an order of Sufis, discovered the plant dancing in the heat of a summer day (Siegel, 1989). Haydar mixed the plant with wine and found the drink made him laugh—little wonder. Medieval Muslim society disapproved of Haydar's discovery, but alas, the proverbial "cat" was out of the bag. The Sufis became heretics in Arab society, but the world was introduced to one of the most versatile and hotly debated plants; after all, how many plants have "wars" declared on them? A great deal of emotionalism surrounds marijuana today. Most of the debate does not even ask the most important questions, which we explore through the different perspectives of the Integrative Model.

Although we will never know if humans discovered the *Cannabis sativa* plant first, we do know many birds love marijuana seeds, which are rich in protein. For hundreds of years bird breeders have referred to marijuana seeds as "pigeon candy" and noted that birds fed on these seeds border on erotomanic behavior. This is not entirely surprising, because the seeds, and other parts of the plant, have been considered aphrodisiac at least since ancient Roman and Greek times (Grinspoon & Bakalar, 1997; Siegel, 1989). B. F. Skinner's famous pigeons, which played such a pivotal role in putting operant conditioning on the map, were fed a mixture that contained 10% hemp seeds. As Siegel (1989) wrote, people may never know "to what extent the foundations of Skinnerian psychology were made under the influence" (p. 155).

A Medical Model Perspective on Marijuana

From the medical model perspective, what do scientists know about marijuana? We begin by reviewing the active ingredients and their mechanisms of action. Obviously, like other herbaceuticals discussed in this chapter, cannabis varies a great deal in potency depending on the conditions under which it is grown and on the sex of the plant (Schwartz, 1987).

Delta-9-Tetrahydrocannabinol

The *Cannabis sativa* plant contains over 400 chemical agents, including over 60 cannabinoids. In 1964, researchers determined delta-9-tetrahydro-cannabinol (THC) to be the primary psychoactive ingredient in marijuana. It took another 20 years to determine that THC acted on a specific set of receptors in the brain called *cannabinoid receptors*. Two of these receptors have been discovered and are localized in the brain as well as throughout the body, particularly in the immune system (Herkenham et al., 1990; Matsuda, Lolait, Brownstein, Young, & Bonner, 1990). Cannabinoid receptors are located in the cortex, motor system, limbic system, and hippocampus. This appears to explain some of THC's effects on cognition, motor coordination, memory, and mood. Researchers have further determined that humans produce the equivalent of endogenous cannabinoids, which act on these receptors and appear to play a natural role in pain regulation, control of movement, cognition, memory (Watson, Benson, & Joy, 2000) and possibly as anti-inflammatory agents (Burstein & Zuerier, 2009).

Cannabinoid receptors exist primarily on presynaptic neurons and seem to inhibit the flow of calcium ions and facilitate the influx of potassium ions (Felder & Glass, 1998). With these mechanisms, cannabinoid receptors inhibit the release of other neurotransmitters from presynaptic neurons, and this inhibition likely causes THC's psychoactive effects. Some researchers hypothesize that cannabis is also related to dopamine release in the brain's pleasure centers (Voruganti, Slomka, Zabel, Mattar, & Awad, 2001). Watson et al. (2000) point out that scientists are just beginning to understand cannabinoid receptors and the different endogenous and exogenous cannabinoid compounds that may affect them. These authors point out that research on these compounds should not be restricted to THC proper, because a number of cannabinoids may have utility for a variety of uses.

Physiological Effects of THC

Being highly fat soluble, THC quickly enters the central nervous system. Heart rate and blood pressure both increase, and skin temperature falls. The drug calms aggressive behavior in animals, and further research is needed to determine whether this effect is also consistent in humans. Although the subjective high (which we later discuss from the intrapsychic perspective) lasts up to 12 hours, THC is metabolized slowly and can persist in the body for up to two weeks. Although this slow metabolism can lead to a reverse tolerance syndrome when the user becomes more sensitive to the drug, it also minimizes physical tolerance and dependence on THC. The only studies suggesting that marijuana is highly "addictive" (De Fonseca, Carrera, Navarro, Koob, & Weiss, 1997; Gianluigi, Pontieri, & Chiara, 1997) had three serious flaws. First, they used animal models, and results from such studies do not necessarily generalize across species. Second, the researchers disabled this natural process for the slow metabolism of the THC, creating an artificial reaction in the bodies of the lab animals. And third, the researchers did not even use THC but a synthetic compound (HU-210) believed similar to THC. Even these researchers, who seemed biased toward equating marijuana with heroin, admitted that probably only 9% of marijuana users would meet the criteria for dependence. These data were first summarized by Warner, Kessler, Hughes, Anthony, and Nelson (1995), who noted that 9% of the people who ever tried marijuana would develop dependence on it. This question of the dependence-inducing potential of cannabis requires further comment.

The Issue of Cannabis Dependence and Withdrawal

Although it is fashionable to use the word *addiction,* we find the word emotionally loaded and poorly operationalized, and used more to generate emotionalism than to explore a phenomenon rationally. Generally, it is thought bad to be "addicted" to something. Although *Webster's Unabridged Dictionary* (1989) defines addiction as having yielded to something that is habit forming, such as narcotics, the colloquial understanding seems to be any compulsive need to take a substance or engage in a behavior. However, as pointed out in Chapter Five, if addiction is defined as (1) tolerance to repeated administrations of a drug and (2) withdrawal on discontinuation, then we must conclude that SSRI antidepressants as well as benzodiazepines cause "addiction." These examples illustrate why we prefer to use words such as *tolerance* and *dependence*. Tolerance and dependence are more easily operationalized and explored using the scientific method. As in Chapter Five, dependence here is defined as a physical tolerance produced by repeated administration of a drug and a concomitant withdrawal syndrome (Stahl, 2000) or as a change in physiology or behavior after stopping a drug.

In surveys of which drugs are the most and least dependence inducing, marijuana is consistently found to be one of the least dependence inducing (Franklin, 1990). Although some marijuana users develop psychological dependence, most do not (Anthony, Warner, & Kessler, 1994; Watson et al., 2000). As noted earlier, the pharmacokinetics of cannabis cause it to be stored in the fat cells of the body and then slowly released over a relatively long period (long for a drug, that is). It is interesting that although advocates of marijuana prohibition downplay this mechanism, a similar mechanism in methylphenidate is described with enthusiasm as making it less likely that children on methylphenidate/Ritalin will become dependent on it (Volkow et al., 1995). Mechanisms that allow for slow metabolism seem to decrease the probability of physical dependence for compounds they operate in. Those rules apply regardless of whether the substance in question curries political favor. Heavy use of marijuana, like the heavy use of many substances, can, on stopping, result in mild withdrawal in symptoms such as sleeplessness and restlessness. One such study gave participants oral dosages of 180 to 210 mg of THC (the equivalent of THC that would be smoked in approximately four to eight marijuana cigarettes when less than one cigarette would be closer to what is generally used). Mild withdrawals followed discontinuation of these heavy doses (Jones, Benowitz & Bachman, 1976).

In a minority of chronic users (for example, those who smoked marijuana every day for years), withdrawal can include mental cloudiness, irritability, cramping, nausea, and aggression (Gold, Tullis, et al., 2001; Watson et al., 2000). When these effects occur, they are said to be short-lived (Haney, Ward, Comer, Foltin, & Fischman, 1999). *DSM-5* (APA, 2013) has added a section of Cannabis-Related Disorders including Cannabis Use Disorder, Cannabis Intoxication, and Cannabis Withdrawal. Cannabis withdrawal is cessation of cannabis use that has been heavy and prolonged (e.g. daily for at least a few months). The symptoms are not severe enough to require medical attention. How much of the withdrawal is psychological and how much is physical remains undetermined.

Even researchers who claim that there is physical dependence note that it is less severe than dependence on other drugs (Budney, Roffman, Stephens, & Walker, 2007). Psychological dependence is a state in which a person believes he or she cannot get through the day without a particular substance or activity. Researchers do know that, as with antidepressants, chronic cannabis exposure causes downregulation of cannabinoid receptors (Abood & Martin, 1992), which can be thought of as a type of physical tolerance. Recent studies on dependence and withdrawal seem consistent with what we have reported here. In one review of the literature, Smith (2002) concluded that studies to date do not provide strong evidence for the existence of a cannabis withdrawal syndrome similar to that with other drugs of abuse such as opioids. Research should continue in this area, and researchers should take care to preclude contaminating studies with political agendas.

Note that other characteristics are found in chronic and/or heavy users of marijuana, characteristics not likely to be found in moderate users. This group of heavy users includes people with AntiSocial Personality Disorder and Conduct Disorder (Watson et al., 2000). Some studies indicate that these characteristics, and the sequence of drug use, are better predictors of who will become dependent on any given substance than is the use of the substance alone (Eldredge, 1998; Morral, McCaffrey, & Paddock, 2002).

Is Cannabis a "Gateway" Drug?

Another interesting debate regarding cannabis is whether or not it is a gateway drug similar to alcohol and cigarettes. This gateway theory (also called the *stepping-stone theory*) has yet to be soundly supported (Watson et al., 2000). The theory basically is that using drugs such as alcohol, tobacco, and marijuana lead to the use of "harder" drugs such as cocaine and heroin. This notion mistakes correlation for causation. It is like noting that most people with pilot's licenses had driver's licenses first and then concluding that getting a driver's license somehow caused such people to get a pilot's license. In the same way, we could make the argument that diapers are "gateway pants." When researchers have found marijuana use to be correlated with later illicit substance use, they note that the other substance use is much more correlated with employment status and is short-term, subsiding by age 21 (Van Gundy, 2010).

Proponents of the gateway theory resort to unconvincing logical maneuvers to make their case. While defending the gateway theory from this criticism, Clayton and Leukefeld (1992) wrote, "We often act or react in our professional and personal lives according to observed correlations without solid and irrefutable evidence that two phenomena are causally related ... shouldn't we do the same with this information on smoking and other drug use?" Our short answer is no. If correlation is enough to pass as causation, then proponents of the gateway theory must account for other correlations. For example, why is it that where cannabis use carries no criminal penalties and is more available (such as in the Netherlands), there is a decreased tendency for people to use harder drugs (Korf, 2002; Model, 1993)? Further, proponents of the gateway theory would have to explain why Dutch studies note that the availability of cannabis has no relationship with heroin use or even with whether people continue to use cannabis (Sifaneck, 1995). The report on the gateway theory, by the think tank Rand Drug Policy Research Center (Morral et al., 2002), concludes there are other plausible explanations for hard drug use beside the gateway theory. For these researchers, it is not marijuana but individual propensities to use drugs that determine a person's risk of initiating hard drug use. Further, the researchers propose that the current prohibition policies that rely so heavily on the gateway theory are unnecessarily burdensome to society particularly in filling the courts and prisons with perpetrators of the victimless crime of marijuana possession.

It may be more helpful to examine patterns of drug use in heavy users, who are more at risk to develop dependence on marijuana or other drugs. One study that examined the sequence of drug use among serious users (Mackesy-Amiti, Fendrich, & Goldstein, 1997) found that progression of use in these users did not follow the standard gateway theory progression (alcohol, then marijuana, then harder illicit drugs). Rather, they found that many were more likely to use marijuana before alcohol and even harder drugs before marijuana. Their findings suggest that youths who are most at risk for serious drug use may be less likely to follow the sequence predicted by the gateway theory. Alcohol is still far more of a "gateway" drug than marijuana and some researchers promote the idea of focusing on preventing alcohol use in K-12 healthy-living programs (Kirby, 2012).

Proposed Medical Uses for Cannabis

Excellent reviews of the medicinal potential of cannabis are provided by Clark (2000); Gurley, Aranow, and Katz (1998); Mathre (1997); and Watson et al. (2000). Unless elsewhere noted, the following material is drawn from these sources. We noted earlier that cannabinoid receptors seem involved in analgesia (pain relief), and much evidence supports the use of cannabis for pain relief (Williamson & Evans, 2000). Evidence from studies on animals and humans indicates that cannabis can

provide significant pain relief. On a related note, cannabinoids seem to treat migraine headaches as well, because they maintain vasoconstriction (constriction of blood vessels). Patients with chronic pain are much less likely to develop dependence on cannabis than on a regimen of opioids. Cannabis also has efficacy as an antiemetic (antinausea) drug for patients undergoing chemotherapy and for patients suffering from wasting syndrome associated with AIDS. Researchers have also found that oncologists' attitudes toward medical marijuana are far more favorable than regulatory authorities have believed (Doblin & Kleinman, 1991). Although research in this area is relatively new, taking cannabis to reduce nausea and encourage appetite as well as to reduce pain are well-established uses. We discuss the subjective "high" produced by THC in discussing the intrapsychic perspective.

In addition to treating pain and nausea, medical marijuana may show efficacy in treating spasticity and movement disorders associated with spinal cord injuries, basal ganglia dysfunction, and multiple sclerosis. More data are needed to assess these claims however. Although many people have heard of medical marijuana in association with the treatment of glaucoma, it is not as efficacious as other therapies. Although cannabis does decrease intraocular pressure, the effects are short-lived and require high doses.

Finally, a line of research examines whether cannabinoids may act in the brain as neuroprotective agents. These agents would preclude or slow down a neurodegenerative disease such as Parkinson's disease or Alzheimer's disease. Hampson et al. (2000) examined this property of cannabinoids in rats and found that cannabidiol (a type of cannabinoid) was superior to other agents tested in preventing glutamate toxicity. In addition, both marijuana and synthesized cannabinoids have efficacy to protect the brain from neurotoxic responses after head injury or stroke (Nagayama et al., 1999). Again, regardless of what happens with marijuana as an herbaceutical, such lines of research hold promise for the development of neuroprotective pharmaceuticals.

Adverse Effects

What are the adverse effects of marijuana? First, it is not a drug that can be taken in lethal quantities, and no fatalities from marijuana are recorded. This is likely because there are no cannabinoid receptors in the brain stem or other parts of the brain controlling vital functions. There are adverse effects that should be considered; however, they are no more severe than any adverse effects for many of the prescription psychotropic medications we have discussed thus far if the drug is not taken by smoking. Table 10.5 summarizes categories of adverse effects of marijuana that we have evidence to support.

Respiratory Problems

If marijuana is smoked, the user has an increased probability of respiratory problems associated with smoking. As noted earlier, the tar content of marijuana cigarettes is significantly higher than that of tobacco cigarettes. In addition to tar, smoke from the cigarette is likely to cause airway irritation and inflammation in users. The degree of the problem stems from the combination of the user's susceptibility, amount used, and frequency of use (Roth et al., 1998; Tashkin, 1999). These effects can be totally avoided by ingesting marijuana baked in foods, unless the person taking it is so nauseous that he or she cannot keep any food down at all. In that case, some of the substance can be smoked and then once nausea subsides, more can be ingested.

TABLE 10.5 Adverse Effects of Marijuana

Respiratory problems related to smoking the drug

Cardiovascular side effects

Psychiatric side effects

Drug interactions

Infection from contaminated crop

Impairment of motor skills

Problems in pregnancy

© Cengage Learning®

Cardiovascular Side Effects

Marijuana is associated with a number of cardiovascular effects that can be significant (El-Mallakh, 1987; Hall & Degenhardt, 2014). Users can suffer from pronounced tachycardia, with an increase in heart rate of up to 50%. Users may also have transient hypertension. Although this hypertension is usually tolerated well in young users, it should be closely monitored in older users. One implication of this side effect is its propensity to lead the user to suffer panic and anxiety (Gurley et al., 1998). This is further discussed under psychiatric effects.

Psychiatric Effects

One of the most important factors in using psychoactive substances is referred to as "set and setting." *Set* refers to the psychological makeup and mind set of the user, and *setting* to the environment in which the psychoactive substance is to be used (Smith, 2000). Set and the human response to setting are two things that make it difficult to generalize from animal to human models. Some individuals' mind set and psychological makeup make them poor candidates for using particular psychoactive substances. These individuals are more prone to anxiety and panic under the influence of marijuana. Anxiety and panic can be a function of the setting as well.

Although cognitive effects are experienced during the high after smoking marijuana, studies thus far have found no long-term effects on intelligence (Fried, Watkinson, James, & Gray, 2002). There have been reports of marijuana triggering or exacerbating psychotic symptoms in people predisposed to such symptoms (Johns, 2001; Shufman & Witztum, 2000), but not in those who are at not at risk for developing psychotic symptoms.

Drug Interactions

Users of cannabis need to know it can have interactions with other drugs related to decreased intestinal motility (movement) and decreased stomach acid. Prescription use would need to take each of these effects into consideration. As with other herbaceuticals, to preclude any problematic interactions standard dosage and potency would have to be set.

Infection from Contaminated Crop

The adverse effect of infection from a contaminated crop is largely encouraged by the prohibition of marijuana and could be practically eliminated were the drug grown and processed under regulation. Marijuana can be contaminated with organisms, including fungal species found in the fecal matter of animals. Outbreaks of both hepatitis B and salmonella have been linked to contaminated marijuana (Gurley et al., 1998). Contaminated crop effects also include chemical contamination such as that from the U.S. government supporting the spraying of marijuana crops with dipyridylium (Paraquat), which is designed to sicken consumers and could be fatal depending on the amount ingested (Duke & Gross, 1993; Miron, 2004; Williamson, 1983).

Impairment of Motor Skills

Marijuana clearly impairs motor skills and reaction time (Ashton, 2001). The drug causes temporary impairment in perception, coordination, reaction time, and time perception (Sugrue et al., 1995). Users under the influence should not drive cars or operate other similarly dangerous machinery. Irresponsible behavior is a risk factor for automobile accidents and injuries.

Problems in Pregnancy

Marijuana use in pregnancy has been correlated with impaired fetal growth and shortened gestation (Zuckerman et al., 1989). Researchers believe that pregnant women underreport marijuana use but that these same women are likely to be polysubstance users.

The notion of medical marijuana raises the same problems inherent in the use of any herb. Problems of dosage, potency, plant gender, type, and so forth all need to be subjected to regulatory scrutiny. As with many other compounds, perhaps the simplest solution is to synthesize the cannabinoid, as has been done with dronabinol (Marinol). The biggest problem with dronabinol for people with severe nausea has been its oral formulation. This problem is being addressed in the United Kingdom, where GW Pharmaceuticals has developed and is currently testing a cannabis spray that is showing efficacy for chronic pain (Hoge, 2002).

Marijuana from the Psychological Perspective

Examining the evidence from the medical model perspective does not really begin to capture the complexity of the experience of marijuana use. Clearly, people do not smoke marijuana to cause respiratory distress, increased heart rate, and temporarily impaired motor skills. Why do so many people around the world, some legally and others illegally, use marijuana? There is not as much research on this question as on the medical uses of marijuana, and the answer is usually a form of word magic referring to "addiction," when in fact, as noted, only a minority of marijuana users develop any type of dependence on it. Many people smoke or ingest marijuana because they enjoy its **euphorant** effect. Some who use it for medical purposes also report this. Does this effect make marijuana an attractive drug of abuse? Yes, but several abusable, recreational drugs in our society are licit. Although prohibitionists argue that legalizing even medical marijuana will lead to more abuse of the drug, these fears have not been confirmed in societies more tolerant of cannabis use, and prohibitionist arguments in general have no support if their goal is to decrease drug consumption.

Many government officials would support medical use if the "high" could be taken out of it. This is a curious statement, given the drug's low potential for dependence—clearly much lower than legal drugs such as nicotine, caffeine, and alcohol. What is wrong with responsible enjoyment of the high that comes from smoking or ingesting marijuana? For that matter, anyone who has ever been on an oncology ward and listened to the suffering and retching of patients receiving chemotherapy would agree that if these people could enjoy a temporary drug-induced euphoria, why not let them? Certainly recreational use differs from medical marijuana use, although many see medical marijuana as the first step toward legalization (Crites-Leoni, 1998). However, the subjective reports of recreational users are an important component of an integrative analysis and is more important now that, since the first edition of this book, two states (Washington and Colorado) have legalized recreational use of marijuana and the federal government in 2014 passed an act agreeing that there would be no federal interference with these state initiatives (see http://www.upi.com/Top_News/US/2014/05/30/House-stops-feds-from-executing-raids-in-medical-marijuana-states/8451401465100/).

Perhaps the most thorough research on this topic was done by psychologist Charles Tart (1971/2000). His psychological study of marijuana intoxication is perhaps the best available. Current legal restrictions on research have precluded psychological studies on the drug, and researchers today rarely ask the question of what people enjoy so much about marijuana. From an integrative perspective this is an important question, though. First, note that not everybody enjoys the experience of being under the influence of marijuana. This section merely raises the question, for those who do enjoy it, should the drug continue to be prohibited? Tart has noted that the effects of the drug are variable and can be divided into three types: pure, potential, and placebo. Pure effects are almost always manifested regardless of set and setting (for example, alertness produced by amphetamine). Potential effects do not manifest unless numerous nondrug variables are in place related to set and setting. Placebo effects are brought on almost entirely by nondrug effects. The interesting thing about an integrative view of marijuana is that the medical model perspective describes pure effects, whereas potential effects relate more to the intrapsychic perspective.

Although medical users of marijuana experience relief from troubling symptoms, they also experience many of the things reported by Tart's participants. Following are just some of the reinforcing experiences these users associated with marijuana.

Changes in the Senses

Visually, users reported increased perceptual organization described as meaningful in terms of patterns, designs, and forms not perceived when not under the influence of marijuana. Users reported perceiving more subtle shades of colors and an enhanced visual depth. Commonly users report a sensual quality to vision while under the influence of marijuana. Although visual illusions or hallucinations are infrequent, they did occur occasionally.

In terms of auditory effects, several of Tart's participants reported subtle changes in sound as well as more acuity with regard to sounds. Other users report what would be akin to a three-dimensional sound space that for them took on a beautiful, indescribable quality. Other users reported synesthesias, "the experience of another sensory modality than the one actually stimulating the person" (Tart, 1971/2000, p. 74). An example of a synesthesia is "seeing sound" or "feeling a smell."

Enhancement of the sense of touch seems to be related to marijuana's purported sexual enhancement effects (Lewis, 1973; McGlothlin & West, 1968; Wilson, 1993). As the author Norman Mailer is reputed to have said, "Sex with pot is better than sex without pot" (in Wilson, 1993). Although many users felt less sexual drive under the influence of marijuana, others reported more attunement to their own body and to the body of their partner. They also noted that orgasm had new pleasurable qualities. Many participants in Tart's study felt they were better lovers under the influence of marijuana because they were less inhibited and more arousable, gentler and more giving, experienced prolonged duration of lovemaking, (for males) had longer-lasting erections, and were more in the present moment with the other. This ability to be in the present moment was interpreted as a deepening of intimacy.

Finally, subjective entheogenic experiences are associated with marijuana. Recall that an entheogen is a substance that supposedly accelerates or in some cases initiates experiences described as mystical or divine. As Smith (2000) noted, true mystical experiences must be incorporated into daily living, including mundane, sober daily consciousness. Altered states must transform into altered traits. Although entheogens are not a substitute for a spiritual practice, they may enhance a spiritual practice. Although marijuana is not as powerful an entheogen as a substance such as psilocybin, some users report spiritual experiences while under the influence. In Tart's study, users reported feeling in touch with the divine or more in touch with a spiritual perspective. Several users felt they meditated more effectively under the influence, and 33% of participants felt they had powerful religious experiences under the influence of marijuana, experiences that had long-term effects on them.

Marijuana From the Cultural Perspective

Marijuana has enjoyed popularity with different groups at different times in different societies. Herer (1992) noted that from approximately the 27th to the 7th century B.C.E., cannabis was incorporated into most cultures of the Middle East, Asia Minor, India, China, Japan, and Europe for uses ranging from the utilitarian to the recreational. We have already mentioned its rejection in 12th-century Muslim society, with the exception of Sufis. It was popular in 19th-century Europe, where in Paris intellectuals would gather with French doctor Jacques Moreau, who was studying the subjective effects of THC. Siegel (1989) has noted that human beings seem to manifest a fourth drive (in addition to hunger, thirst, and sex), seeking mind-altering or intoxicating states. Culture plays a large role in how this drive is going to be channeled. In U.S. society, many people are moderate users of alcohol. Most alcohol users do not drive under the influence, and they do not drink more than is good for them or enough to interfere with their obligations. Although this majority is not studied extensively, what is so different about someone who uses marijuana moderately in the same manner? In tolerating cannabis use, Dutch society has had none of the problems feared by prohibitionists in the United States. Given the lack of evidence for the effectiveness of prohibition, an increasing number of U.S. states, the United Kingdom, and Canada are minimizing criminal penalties for possession and use of marijuana.

Wilson (1993) and Eldredge (1998) have pointed out that in the United States the "war on drugs" has racist overtones. Marijuana smoking was strongly associated with Mexican immigrants during World War I. It is from this group that the slang "Mary Jane" is derived, because this is the Mexican Spanish translation of *marijuana*. Drug laws in many cases are far harsher on users in lower socio-economic income brackets, and the case could certainly be made that they become a useful measure of class control. For example, the penalties for possessing crack cocaine (derived from powder cocaine) are harsher than those for possessing powder cocaine (the parent compound of crack cocaine). Advocates of drug law reform note that users of powder cocaine are far more likely to be Caucasian and users of crack, to be African American. In addition, marijuana has been linked in the minds of many with countercultural movements that challenged authority during the Vietnam War era. The phrase "war on drugs" was coined by then-President Richard Nixon. The Carter administration was apparently considering legalization, but this was stopped by the Reagan administration, although prohibition has consistently been shown to be ineffective for both alcohol and marijuana. Some of the largest funders of the "war on drugs" are pharmaceutical companies. As commentator Ariana Huffington (2000) speculated, "It's not that they do not want us on drugs—they just want us on theirs" (p. 167). Pharmaceutical lobbies' influence on laws related to access to medical marijuana needs to be monitored.

Clearly U.S. culture has many issues to consider in relation to medical marijuana, and this review is a rough outline of just a few. Again, for medical purposes many problems could be overcome by allowing the prescription of synthetic cannabinoid inhalers, which would be treated like any other pharmaceutical with abuse potential (such as morphine).

From the cultural perspective, also consider that people in many oppressed groups use drugs (including marijuana) as an escape from a life that, in their opinion, is not worth living. This is one of the secrets (and fears) of American society: that its citizens may not find life worth living. If a majority of a society comes to this conclusion, they may decide they want to change the way the society is structured and this is a constant threat to those in power. Like it or not, we all must acknowledge that currently not all U.S. citizens have equal access to resources and many have little hope of attaining a decent standard of living. On the other side of the coin, other people, despite having material abundance, feel their lives have a meaningless quality. The promises of consumer culture leave them feeling empty. The question remains: If a government criminalizes the things its citizens use to relieve the pain of their daily existence, does it thus incur any responsibility to helping its citizens pursue other avenues toward happiness to decrease that pain? This was of course one of the themes in Aldous Huxley's (1932) dystopian novel *Brave New World* where the drudgery of daily life is eased by a mythic substance called *soma*.

Social/Legal Perspectives on Marijuana

Perhaps the biggest social/legal issue is the current drug laws, which have been described as "draconian" in publications as diverse as libertarian treatises (McWilliams, 1993) to commentaries in medical journals (Kassirer, 1997). Table 10.6 lists the groups who have recommended decriminalization of marijuana for medicinal purposes.

The laws that exist to prosecute people involved in marijuana possession, cultivation, or trafficking include people who, under their own state laws, may be growing or distributing medical marijuana through state-approved medical marijuana clubs. The laws of 15 U.S. states require life sentences for certain nonviolent marijuana offenses. Under federal law the death penalty can be sought for growing or selling a large amount of marijuana, even for a first offense. The 1986 Drug Abuse Act increased penalties for federal drug offenses and established mandatory minimum sentences, a move opposed by the American Bar Association and federal judges. The federal government can seize the property of "suspected drug traffickers" without even filing charges against them. For example, an entire farm can be seized if one marijuana plant is found on its grounds. Perhaps even more disturbing is a little known clause in the laws that allow informers to receive up to 25% of the assets seized in return for their testimony (Schlosser, 1997). The average time served in prison for a nonviolent drug offense is five years. Compare these

TABLE 10.6 Groups Supporting Medical Marijuana

American Bar Association

American Civil Liberties Union

American Public Health Association

National Nurses Society on Addiction

Conference of Episcopal Bishops

The People of the State of Alaska

The People of the State of Arizona

The People of the State of California

The People of the State of Canada

The People of the State of Colorado

The People of the State of Connecticut

The People of the State of Delaware

The People of the State of Hawaii

The People of the State of Illinois

The People of the State of Maine

The People of the State of Maryland

The People of the State of Massachusetts

The People of the State of Michigan

The People of the State of Minnesota

The People of the State of Montana

The People of the State of Nevada

The People of the State of New Hampshire

The People of the State of New Jersey

The People of the State of New Mexico

The People of the State of Oregon

The People of the State of Rhode Island

The People of the State of Washington, DC

penalties to the average penalty for kidnapping (4.5 years), assault (2 years), and sexual abuse (2.5 years) (McWilliams, 1993). Reviewing these averages, it is hard to avoid feeling as if we all were living in a surrealist novel. The laws passed to prohibit marijuana use appear far more dangerous than the drug itself. Despite prohibitionist fears that decriminalizing marijuana for medical use would increase crime and marijuana use in general, initial studies do not support this (Harper, 2012; Morris, TenEyck, Barnes, & Kovandzic, 2014).

CONCLUSIONS

What does an integrative investigation of marijuana as an herbaceutical tell us? How do the partial truths revealed help us draw conclusions? First, the Integrative Model does illustrate the complexity of the situation far more effectively than parochial debates in disciplines that rarely converse with each other. It is imperative to discuss marijuana from the medical model, psychological cultural, and social perspectives. An integrative approach to an issue such as medical marijuana could inform politicians of problems with the federal laws as they are written, particularly if medical marijuana is to receive federal approval. The integrative approach to medical marijuana also demythologizes the subjective high experienced with marijuana use. The psychological perspective requires us to hear the testimony of not just those in the minority whose use has led to personal or legal troubles, but from those who have had positive experiences using marijuana. This is an important complement to the information from the medical model perspective that, although useful, is incomplete.

SUMMARY

Herbaceuticals are not FDA-regulated substances in the United States and therefore, are not considered medicines proper. They are, however, increasingly used as an alternative and complementary approach to healing, even though federal laws prohibit their being advertised as a cure for any disorder. Mistrust of traditional medicine, cultural beliefs, increasing numbers of proactive consumers, and a belief in the safety of "natural" products all seem to be contributing to the increased use of these substances. Currently, research supports the efficacy of some compounds but not of others. It is important for mental health professionals to understand that just as they cannot make recommendations about psychotropic medications to clients, they should not recommend herbaceuticals either. They should, however, keep abreast of the literature on these substances, given their increasing use by consumers.

The herbaceutical with the best support for efficacy is St. John's wort, which is used to treat depression in Europe. Kava seems to be an effective anxiolytic as well. The literature on other substances such as ginkgo, valerian root, passion flower, hops, and melatonin is mixed but at this point does not seem to support their use as psychotropic agents. The most controversial substance in this chapter is marijuana. Although there appear to be some medical uses for it federal law still prohibits its use even if recommended by a physician. It is likely that the cultural and social issues (and the accompanying propaganda) will slow intelligent debate and discussion of both the proposed medical uses as well as the failure of prohibition.

STUDY QUESTIONS AND EXERCISES

1. What is the "don't ask, don't tell" syndrome related to herbaceuticals in the United States?

2. Discuss at least three reasons why people report preferring herbaceuticals to prescription medications. How would you counsel a client with this perspective who wanted to use St. John's wort rather than a prescription antidepressant?

3. What are some legal issues affecting the use of herbaceuticals in U.S. culture?

4. List and discuss some of the important differences between herbs and drugs.

5. What is the consensus of opinion on the efficacy of St. John's wort? Discuss one study that does *not* support its efficacy.

6. Discuss some of the dangers associated with ephedrine. How would you counsel a client who told you he or she wanted to use ephedrine-containing products? What legal and ethical issues are involved in your responses to the client?

7. What is your reaction to the integrative exploration of medical marijuana? What position do you take on the topic, and why?

8. Compare the dependence-inducing qualities of methylphenidate and marijuana. What conclusions do you reach in this exercise?

9. Debate whether or not the gateway theory of drug use is accurate.

10. Compare the side effect profile of marijuana with side effects of lithium and of an SSRI antidepressant. What conclusions do you reach about their relative usefulness, based on this exercise?

CHAPTER ELEVEN

Pharmacotherapy of Alcohol and Drug-Related Disorders

By Logan Lamprecht

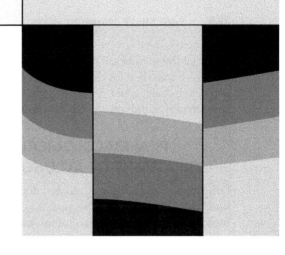

The pharmacotherapy of alcohol and drug dependence has dramatically changed over the past decade. Ongoing research concerning pharmacological options as a meaningful adjunct to the treatment experience of individuals attempting to rehabilitate from substance-related addictions and to maintain abstinence continues to demonstrate the efficacy of such therapeutic interventions when used appropriately and under the direction of medical professionals. In addition, the discovery of new medications along with combinations of pharmacotherapies to treat addiction from a multifaceted approach (management of physiological and psychological withdrawal symptoms, decreasing using behaviors, lowering craving urges, and maintenance of abstinence) have been shown to positively impact client treatment goals for abstinence and lifestyle change (Heilig & Egli, 2006; Karila et al., 2007; Williams, 2005).

This chapter is demarcated into five sections. Section One provides a brief overview concerning the development of pharmacological treatment options to supplement the therapy process for individuals struggling with alcohol and/or drug-related problems. Section Two presents statistical information regarding the prevalence of drug and alcohol-related problems over the past two decades and reports on current trends in treatment seeking behaviors. Section Three covers pharmacological information regarding the treatment of alcohol dependence. Section Four provides a detailed description of current pharmacotherapy treatments recommended for opioid dependence and presents

a review of the research regarding the efficacy of these treatments in practice. Section Five briefly covers salient viewpoints concerning cultural considerations about the implementation of medications to support treatment outcomes for patients who experience drug and/or alcohol-related problems of living.

SECTION ONE: BRIEF HISTORICAL SKETCH OF PHARMACOLOGICAL TREATMENTS FOR PATIENTS EXPERIENCING DRUG AND/OR ALCOHOL-RELATED CONCERNS

Learning Objectives

- Increased understanding about the development of pharmacological treatments for substance-abuse-related concerns.
- Know the approval process as well as approval dates for specific pharmacological medicines as determined by the Food and Drug Administration (FDA).
- Be able to conceptualize how pharmacological interventions were introduced as a pharmacological means for treating alcohol and/or drug addiction.

The historical context outlined in this section regarding the pharmacological treatment of substance-use disorders primarily focuses on alcohol and opioid-related dependence concerns and some of the historical antecedents and precursors that provided the foundation for research and evaluation of medications used for the primary purpose of promoting abstinence and decreasing the physiological and physical withdrawal symptoms from use.

PHARMACOLOGICAL TREATMENT OF ALCOHOLISM

Drugs approved for treating alcohol dependence are listed in Table 11.1. The first pharmacological drug used in the treatment of alcoholism was disulfiram, otherwise known as tetraethylthiuram disulfide (Antabuse) (Fuller et al., 1986; Williams, 2005). Disulfiram was used in the 1800s as a compounding chemical that aids in the creation of vulcanized rubber. Several alcohol-consumed laborers, upon being exposed to disulfiram experienced an immediate physiological reaction that included skin flushing, increased heart rate, and decreased blood pressure (Kurtzweil, 1996). The efficacy of disulfiram as a treatment option for alcoholism was later discovered by accident when a group of Danish researchers who were trying to determine the drug's potential to control for parasitic infestations in the

body realized that sensitization to the adverse consequences of alcohol consumption could represent a potent treatment option for alcoholism. Disulfiram was federally approved in 1948 in the United States and became the first drug to be approved by the Food and Drug Administration for the treatment of alcohol-related disorders. Pharmacodynamically, disulfiram blocks an enzyme that is necessary for the metabolism of ethanol in the body, which then produces extremely unpleasant physical consequences, including nausea and vomiting, whenever alcohol is ingested in the body.

The second of three drugs approved by the FDA in the United States is naltrexone (ReVia). Naltrexone was originally approved by the FDA in 1984 as a treatment for opioid addiction and was administered under the brand name Trexan. The FDA approved naltrexone in 1994 as a treatment option for alcohol-use disorders (Litten & Allen, 1999). It is manufactured under the name ReVia with its generic equivalent, Depade. Naltrexone has also recently become available in an extended-release option that is administered monthly to patients (Vivitrol). The primary pharmacodynamic purpose of naltrexone is to inhibit opioid receptors in the brain and to help to alleviate the endorphin-mediated reinforcing consequences of alcohol consumption (Herz, 1997). Contemporarily, the combined effects of naltrexone when prescribed adjacent to acamprosate, have shown promising results in terms of an effective treatment option for alcoholism (Garbutt, West, Carey, Lohr, & Crews, 1999).

The third drug approved more recently (2004) by the FDA for the treatment of alcohol-related disorders is acamprosate (Campral). The effectiveness of acamprosate was first demonstrated in Europe and has been a form of treatment for several years in many countries outside the United States, including Australia. The primary function of acamprosate, pharmacologically, is to support abstinence from alcohol by alleviating the physical and psychological discomfort symptoms that accompany individuals once they stop drinking behaviors (Mann, Lehert, & Morgan, 2004).

An additional pharmacological alternative being used for treating individuals with alcohol-related

TABLE 11.1 FDA-Approved Pharmacotherapies for Alcohol-Use Disorders

Generic Name	Brand Name	Recommended Daily Dosage
Naltrexone Hydrochloride	ReVia (oral)	50 mg/day to 100 mg/day
	Vivitrol (injection)	Monthly dose of 380 mg
Acamprosate	Campral	666 mg 3× daily or 2 g
Disulfiram	Antabuse	250 mg per day
Topiramate	Topamax	50 mg per day or up to 150 mg twice per day
Baclofen	Lioresal	60 mg per day

disorders is nalmefene (Revex). Nalmefene is an opioid receptor antagonist that was developed in the late 1970s and used primarily for the treatment of patients attempting to maintain abstinence from alcohol use (Garbutt et al., 1999). Although there are some studies that demonstrate the effectiveness of this drug, pharmacologically, when used to target alcohol-using behaviors, these studies are primarily contained within Europe and the drug has not been available for legal consumption in the U.S. pharmaceutical market since 2008. The drug has not been approved by the FDA.

Contemporary research also demonstrates some efficacy with additional pharmacotherapies as a treatment adjunct to alcoholism, including gamma-hydroxybutyric acid (GHB), baclofen (Kemstro), topiramate (Topomax), and fluoxetine (Prozac). This chapter briefly highlights some areas of research that explore the effectiveness of these medications for addressing pharmacological aspects of craving treatment in alcohol addiction.

PHARMACOLOGICAL TREATMENT OF OPIOID DEPENDENCE

The onset of pharmacotherapeutic treatments to target opioid dependence was primarily the result of the dramatic increase in intravenous abuse of heroin after World War II, particularly in New York City (Courtwright, Joseph, & Des Jarlais, 1989). By the late 1950s and early 1960s, abuse of heroin had escalated to epidemic proportions. Methadone (Dolophine), a long-lasting agonist with a half-life of between 24 and 36 hours, was created in Germany for analgesia before World War II. Isbell and Vogel (1949) demonstrated that methadone was an extremely effective medication for heroin addicts experiencing acute withdrawal symptoms due to prolonged heroin abuse. At the time of their research, Isbell and Vogel (1949) contended that patients who were addicted to heroin at the onset of treatment be submitted to a process where doses of methadone were slightly reduced over a timespan of 10 days or more. However, the research at the time showed that patients that

were discharged from treatment relapsed at extremely high rates. Due to the epidemic numbers of individuals that were addicted to heroin at the time, in 1958, the Joint Committee of the American Bar Association and the American Medical Association officially recommended the development of outpatient facilities to regulate the prescription of narcotics as a treatment modality on an experimental basis (Hunt & Odoroff, 1962).

Drugs used to treat opioid dependence are listed in Table 11.2. Methadone maintenance treatment (MMT) was initiated as a research endeavor at The Rockefeller University in 1964 and was funded by the Health Research Council of New York City in direct response to the alarming percentages of patients who were addicted to heroin post–World War II (Joseph, Stancliff, & Langrod, 2000; Payte, 2002). The research was headed by Dr. Dole, the chair of the Narcotics Committee Council located in New York, and Dr. Mary Kreek. They initially looked at the efficacy of daily administrations of morphine to patients experiencing heroin addiction. The research proved difficult due to the number of times morphine had to be injected into patients each day. After it was determined by the research that morphine was not a feasible treatment option, longer-lasting narcotics were introduced, including methadone. Instead of discontinuing methadone treatments as was previously noted in

TABLE 11.2 FDA-Approved Pharmacotherapies for Opioid Dependency

Generic Name	Brand Name	Recommended Daily Dosage
Methadone	Dolophine	80 to 150 mg daily
Levomethadyl acetate (LAAM)	Orlaam	40 to 140 mg daily
Buprenorphine	Butrans	8 to 12 mg daily
Buprenorphine/ Naloxone	Suboxone	16 mg/4 mg daily
Naltrexone	Depade	50 mg daily

© 2015 Cengage Learning®

experimental research conducted at the U.S. Public Health Hospital in Lexington, Kentucky, the research team had the patients remain on methadone so that its effectiveness could be explored (Dole, 1988). The research noted that as patients remained on the medication, they developed tolerance to the drug and were no longer sedated by the influence of opioids. One consequence of this outcome was that behavioral change was also noted, and patients began to plan for a productive, drug-free future, including employment and education. The patients in this particular study were able to obtain employment while remaining on a daily dose of 100 to 180 mg (Dole, 1988). This study contributed significantly to future studies that explored an ongoing and stabilized treatment process that required individuals to be on a consistent dose of methadone as a means of promoting positive treatment outcomes. Over the next few decades, the population of patients receiving regulated MMT grew from 6 (1964) to 44,000 (1998) (American Methadone Treatment Association [AMTA], 1998).

Several studies from 1965 through 1991 demonstrated a few central themes with respect to the treatment outcomes for opioid-dependent patients who submit to a regimented treatment program involving daily ingestion of methadone (Ball & Ross, 1991; Dole & Joseph, 1978; Gearing & Schweitzer, 1974). Some of these findings result in the following themes relative to patient outcomes post discharge from treatment:

- Significant improvements in productive behaviors, including employment and education seeking behaviors and a substantial decrease in number of arrests per 100 persons entering treatment (Gearing & Schweitzer, 1974)
- Death rates of patients terminating treatment is three times the amount of patients who are currently engaged in methadone treatment (Gearing & Schweitzer, 1974)
- A small number of patients (between 8 and 12%) were able to maintain successful treatment outcomes, including not relapsing and not being re-arrested (Dole & Joseph, 1978),

- A relatively high probability of relapse to heroin abuse (60% had relapsed within six months post-treatment discharge) (Dole & Joseph, 1978)
- Thirty-four percent of patients who were discharged from treatment in good standing were able to successfully maintain sobriety for between six months and one year (Dole & Joseph, 1978)
- After prolonged exposure to treatment (between 3 and 5 years), 92% of patients had successfully discontinued heroin use (Ball & Ross, 1991)
- Eighty-two percent of patients who had left short-term methadone treatment relapsed to heroin abuse within the first year (Ball & Ross, 1991)

It should be noted that according to the Bureau of Research and Evaluation at the University of Michigan, which surveyed 44 federally regulated methadone treatment programs, the primary determinants of successful outcomes (reduction of drug-using behaviors and/or abstinence) that were also consistent in each of the above studies were the dosage of methadone (amount consumed per day) and the amount of time the patient remained in treatment (Joseph et al., 2000).

As a result of significant research that examined the efficacy of methadone as a pharmacological treatment strategy for opioid dependence and opioid detoxification, methadone was approved by the FDA in 1972 as a primary means of treating opioid addiction.

Another primary psychopharmacological option used to reduce and treat opioid cravings and opioid-seeking behaviors is naltrexone (which has also been approved by the FDA for the treatment of alcohol dependence). Naltrexone was synthesized in 1965 and tested during the 1970s and 1980s for treating opioid dependence. The FDA approved the use of naltrexone for this purpose in 1984.

Dr. Abraham Wikler, a psychiatrist and neurologist, administered the narcotic-withdrawal ward at the Lexington Narcotic Hospital for several years. While there, he hypothesized that opioid craving and sustained drug abuse could be reduced if specific reinforcing effects were somehow diverted or thwarted at critical points (Wikler, 1948). Pharmacodynamically, naltrexone can effectively inhibit the cyclical nature of drug reinforcement and dependency by stopping opioid receptors. The metaphorical equivalent might be a bicycle tire moving at speed when suddenly, a solid object becomes lodged within the spokes, causing the wheel to come to an immediate stop (and its rider flying dangerously forward). With dependency, the receptors that have become sensitized and habituated to the euphoria caused by opioid ingestion and its accompanying behaviors require interruption. Naltrexone can assist with interrupting the physiologically conditioned responses within the body (particularly, the brain) associated with craving urges. Research has consistently shown positive treatment outcomes when opioid-dependent patients receive naltrexone, pharmacologically, in concert with psychosocial supports (Gonzalez & Brogden, 1988; Washton, Gold, & Pottash, 1984).

Another pharmacological option for treating opioid dependence is the drug known as buprenorphine (Butrans). Buprenorphine-related products were approved by the FDA in 2002 as a medication assisted treatment for opioid addiction (it should be noted that a buprenorphine product known as Buprenex has not received FDA approval as of this time). It is primarily used to decrease withdrawal symptoms and inhibits euphoric responses, physiologically, when used by the opioid-dependent patient. Patients who use buprenorphine are not required to participate in a federally regulated program such as a methadone clinic. Recent research has also shown the efficacy of buprenorphine when used in concert with naloxone (an opioid antagonist) (Suboxone). Bup/Nx (buprenorphine and naloxone) decreases withdrawal symptoms from opioids and does not lead to euphoria in the opioid-addicted person, and it significantly reduces the effects of other potentially problematic opioids for up to one day (Donovan, Knox, Skytta, Blayney, & DiCenzo, 2013). Suboxone continues to be a well-researched and prescribed form of medication-assisted treatment for opioid-use disorders.

This section provided the reader with a brief overview of the historical context surrounding medication-assisted therapies for the treatment of alcohol and opioid-use disorders, including FDA approval for recommended use in the United States. The next section provides a detailed narrative of statistical information regarding drug and alcohol dependency–related problems over the past few decades and presents the reader with a conceptual understanding of dependency for operational purposes.

Review Questions

- What are some of the historical antecedents to the pharmacological treatment of substance-use disorders?

- What is the timeline for FDA approval for some of the more prominently used pharmacological drugs for treating substance-use disorders in the United States?

- Why was methadone used to treat opioid dependence in place of morphine?

- What are two significant factors for methadone maintenance treatment and positive client outcomes?

SECTION TWO: CURRENT STATISTICAL IMPACT OF DRUG AND ALCOHOL ABUSE/DEPENDENCY AND TERMINOLOGY

Learning Objectives

- Understand the statistical impact of alcohol and drug dependency in the United States.

- Be familiar with the statistics regarding treatment seeking behaviors, including pharmacological treatment for illicit drug and alcohol-use disorders.

- Develop a working definition of alcohol and opioid dependence that draws from diagnostic criteria from historical narratives as well as the recently published *DSM-5*.

According to the newly revised *Diagnostic and Statistical Manual of Mental Disorders,* 5th Edition (2013a), the criteria for substance-use disorders has been changed to reflect the existence of a variety of behaviors associated with persistent use that interferes with daily activities of living. The *DSM-5* integrates the two *DSM-IV* disorders, abuse and dependence, into a coherent, single disorder called substance-use disorder (SUD) with mild, moderate, and severe sub-categories or classifications. Depending on how many criteria are met would denote whether or not the individual can be diagnosed with a substance-use disorder, or more specifically an opioid-use disorder (OUD) or alcohol-use disorder (AUD). The number of criteria met by the individual would determine the severity of the concern and provide recommendations for treatment. Some of these diagnostic criteria include: (a) significant use of time expended to obtain and use drugs and/or alcohol; (b) persistent desire or unsuccessful effort to decrease or appropriately manage alcohol and/or drug use; (c) recurrent alcohol and/or drug use leads to significant impairment in other tasks of daily life, such as employment, interpersonal, and/or educational; and (d) tolerance levels are reached, which requires increasingly larger amounts of consumption. A new criteria added to the diagnostic language in *DSM-5* is strong, craving urges for the individual to consume illicit drugs and/or alcohol.

The most recent statistic according to the National Survey on Drug Use and Health (2013) indicated that over 17.7 million Americans over the age of 12 (7.7% of the total population) were dependent on alcohol. In addition, it is estimated that nearly 20 million people needed some form of treatment for serious alcohol-related problems, but only 1.5 million of these individuals received treatment in the past year. For individuals who do enter treatment, it is estimated that between 40 and 70% of them experience relapse to drinking behaviors within one calendar year of terminating treatment (Finney, Hahn, & Moos, 1996).

Some additional statistics provided by the Substance Abuse and Mental Health Services Administration (SAMHSA) (2013) regarding alcohol use in the year 2012 in the United States include the following:

- Just over half of Americans aged 12 or older reported being current consumers of alcohol (135.5 million current drinkers)
- Nearly 25% of persons aged 12 or older reported binging on alcohol in the past 30 days
- In 2012, heavy drinking was reported by 6.5% of the population aged 12 or older (17 million people)—heavy drinking is defined as binge drinking on at least 5 days in the past 30 days
- In 2012, it was estimated that 14.9 million adults were alcohol dependent
- Cultural variables are significant factors for understanding alcohol-use disorders; gender and ethnicity play a significant role in determining the composition of the percentage of the total population that experiences alcohol-related problems (i.e., Whites and biracial individuals are more likely to abuse alcohol than all other ethnicities)
- The numbers of individuals who are alcohol dependent have remained consistent over the past decade (between 20 and 22 million people annually)

Williams (2005) noted that only about 20% of individuals who receive treatment for alcohol-related problems receive pharmacotherapy as a treatment adjunct. At the conclusion of this section, additional statistics regarding individuals receiving treatment for alcohol and/or substance abuse-related concerns will be briefly presented in a summative overview format.

The National Survey on Drug Use and Health (NSDUH) (2013) reported that in the year 2012, 23.9 million Americans over the age of 12 had abused an illicit drug and/or a psychotherapeutic medication in the past month. Of these 23.9 million people, 7.7 million needed help for illicit drug use, but only 1.4 million received any form of treatment, including psychosocial and/or pharmacological.

SAMHSA's 2013 national survey on drug use provided the following statistics related to illegal consumption of illicit drugs:

- Rate of current drug use among persons 12 or older increased from 8.1% in 2008 to 9.2% in 2012
- Cannabis is the most commonly abused illicit drug, with 18.9 million people abusing cannabis in the past month
- 1.6 million adults who currently abuse cocaine
- Nearly 700,000 adults who abuse heroin chronically, an increase of nearly 300,000 since 2007
- 2.6% of the adult population abused prescription-type psychotherapeutic drugs for nonmedical purposes in the past month
- An estimated 69.5 million Americans aged 12 or older were current users of a tobacco product (26.7% of the total population)
- 2.9 million persons aged 12 or older used an illicit drug for the first time within the past one year
- An estimated 22.2 million people aged 12 or older were classified with substance dependence or abuse in the past year (of this total, 2.8% were classified as dependent with respect to illicit drug use)
- Cultural demographic factors are a significant variable for understanding illicit drug use (i.e., adult males are two times as likely to abuse drugs than adult females)

The SAMHSA (2013) survey defined treatment need as having substance dependence or abuse or receiving substance-use treatment at a special facility, including inpatient settings, drug or alcohol rehabilitation or mental health facility, within the past year. In 2008, nearly 20% of all substance abuse treatment admissions were for primary opioid abuse or dependence (SAMHSA, 2009). In 2012, 23.1 million people needed treatment for an illicit drug or alcohol problem (nearly 9% of the total population). The survey noted that over 20 million people needed treatment for a substance abuse–dependency problem but did not receive any treatment as a special facility in 2012. The primary reason noted by participants for not seeking treatment was due to financial burdens and/or poor or inadequate insurance.

It is estimated that nearly a quarter of a billion dollars is spent annually in the United States on medical expenses, lost work productivity, expenses connected to drug-related criminal activity and on other expenses related to drug and alcohol problems. Nearly 18 billion annually is spent on drug and alcohol problems, and the majority of this amount is funded by public money, including Medicaid, Medicare, and local state and county-sponsored government programs that allocate monies for the treatment of drug and alcohol-related concerns for individuals without insurance. In their 2005 report on U.S. spending for substance abuse–related concerns, Mark, Coffey, Vandivort-Warren, Harwood, and King (2005) estimated annual costs of nearly $185 billion for alcohol abuse and 143 billion for drug abuse. In addition, they estimated that approximately 21 billion was spent in 2003 on the treatment of substance-use disorders (1.3% of all health care spending). Positive trends continue to be reported with respect to motivated individuals who receive a multifaceted treatment approach to address substance-use disorders (SAMHSA, 2007).

This section presented the reader with a brief overview of the statistical significance of the pervasive nature of substance-use disorders in the lives of many adolescent and adult Americans, including their widespread use, treatment-seeking probability, and financial costs to the public sector. The next section will provide an overview of alcoholism and pharmacotherapy treatments for promoting abstinence while simultaneously treating acute withdrawal symptoms.

Review Questions

- How does the *DSM-5* conceptualize substance-use disorders (as compared with the *DSM-IV*'s conceptualization of abuse and dependence)?
- What are your thoughts or reactions to the statistical significance of the pervasive nature of drug and alcohol abuse in America? What might explain the continued increase in the numbers of adult Americans who abuse alcohol and drugs annually?

- What are some of the sociopolitical forces that practitioners must consider when thinking about factors that prevent clients who are addicted to illicit drugs and alcohol from seeking and receiving meaningful and comprehensive treatment resources?

SECTION THREE: PHARMACOLOGICAL TREATMENT OF INDIVIDUALS WITH ALCOHOL-USE DISORDERS

Learning Objectives

- Be able to operationalize alcohol-related disorders for the purpose of understanding pharmacological treatment options in a mental health delivery context.
- Understand approved pharmacotherapy treatments for treating alcohol dependence, with the goal to address the impact of acute withdrawal symptoms and to promote continued abstinence of drinking behaviors.
- Be familiar with the pharmacodynamics (what the drug does to the body) and the pharmacokinetics (what the body does to the drug) of the drug, the patient and treatment outcomes.

For the purpose of this chapter, alcohol-related disorders will be conceptualized as an advancing neurological disease that is the direct result of changes in many of the neurotransmitter channels in the human brain that excite craving desires for the continued ingestion of alcohol. Persistent alcohol abuse then leads to the neuronal state becoming increasingly hyperexcited. Withdrawal symptoms are consequently associated with efforts made by the individual toward abstinence and are suggestive of instability between the glutamate and y-aminobutyric acid that impacts the biological signaling of many other neurotransmitters in the brain. Pharmacotherapy treatments for alcoholism focus on the neurotransmitter sections of the brain in order to stabilize these alterations and to lower using urges while simultaneously inhibiting reinforcement of alcohol use by introducing an aversive reaction to the drug upon ingestion. This operationalized understanding of alcoholism provides a meaningful bridge in understanding the incorporation of pharmacotherapy options into a comprehensive treatment strategy for individuals who are motivated to treat alcohol-use disorders and their accompanying behaviors.

Alcohol consumption has significant neurobiological effects on the body, including alteration of many of the organic proteins secreted in the body that are sensitive to the binding effects of alcohol once ingested, which include dopamine and adenosine. These neurotransmitter systems are intimately involved in the development of alcohol dependence and are primary treatment objectives with respect to pharmacotherapy. Chronic alcohol use leads to long-term transformative reconfigurations within the excitatory glutamatergic neurotransmitters and GABAergic systems within the body and become primary determinants that make up the initial onset of alcohol-dependent behaviors (Williams, 2005). After prolonged exposure to alcohol, their body reacts in a compensatory effort by upregulating the glutamatergic system while simultaneously downregulating the GABA system. This response is enacted in order to set in motion the body's physiological response to stabilize the inhibitory effects of alcohol as a result of chronic ingestion.

Treating alcoholism consists of two primary phases, including detoxification of the patient and rehabilitation efforts (Jung & Namkoong, 2006). During the beginning detoxification stages, the person can undergo acute psychological and physiological withdrawal symptoms. Rehabilitation efforts are primarily oriented around addressing relapse prevention strategies for the individual and to create a lifestyle that can support long-term abstinence from alcohol consumption.

This section will focus exclusively on FDA-approved medications that have demonstrated positive treatment outcomes with patients who experience alcohol-use related disorders (AUD). Evidence will be presented in terms of understanding the psychotherapeutic implications of the efficacy of the pharmacological interventions discussed in Section One of this chapter, including,

TABLE 11.3 Early and Late Symptoms of Alcohol Dependence Withdrawal

Anxiety

Depression

Fatigue

Irritability

Shakiness

Mood swings

Nightmares and tremors

Lucid thinking

Persistent headaches

Insomnia

Loss of appetite

Increased heart rate

Excessive perspiration

© 2015 Cengage Learning®

naltrexone, acamprosate, naltrexone administered in concert with acamprosate, and disulfiram. A brief overview will be provided concerning the "second" and "third" waves of pharmacological treatments for alcohol dependence (Heilig & Egli, 2006). Symptoms of alcohol withdrawal are summarized in Table 11.3.

DISULFIRAM TREATMENT

Disulfiram (Antabuse or Antabus) blocks the expression of an enzyme that is necessary for the metabolism of ethanol in the body and produces extremely unpleasant physiological responses in the body, including nausea and vomiting, when alcohol is ingested (Johansson, 1992). Once ethyl alcohol is consumed, it is quickly transformed into acetaldehyde, which is then oxidized by the liver and converted into the mitochondrial enzyme known as aldehyde dehydrogenase (ALDH) (1992). The disulfiram then competes with the

ALDH for binding sites with the nicotinamide adenine coenzyme and produces a permanent inhibition of ALDH enzyme activity. Once even small amounts of alcohol are introduced to the body after consuming disulfiram, the amount of acetaldehyde increases substantially, which consequently results in aversive physical reactions that inhibit continued alcohol consumption. Administration of this pharmacological option is recommended for individuals who are very motivated to engage in treatment and to abstain from alcohol-seeking behaviors.

Supervised disulfiram treatment has been shown to result in fairly positive outcomes for patients who experience alcohol dependence (Brewer, 1993; Laaksonen, Koski-Jannes, Salaspuro, Ahtinen, & Alho, 2008), particularly with respect to reduction of heavy drinking days and extending the time to the first drink of alcohol, when compared to acamprosate or naltrexone. The most controlled study was conducted by Fuller et al. (1986) and examined the efficacy of 250 mg of disulfiram per day against a placebo group with a group of 605 alcohol-dependent patients. The participants who received the FDA recommended daily dose of 250 mg of disulfiram consumed alcohol on fewer days than those that received the placebo. It should be noted that medication compliance was relatively low in this study, which complicated the generalizability of the research findings. A randomized study conducted by Diehl, Ulmer, and Mutschler (2010) demonstrated that nearly two times the amount of patients who were treated with disulfiram were able to successfully maintain abstinence over the course of treatment when contrasted with patients who were treated solely with acamprosate. This study did report that patients who were treated with acamprosate did report reduced cravings to use alcohol. However, disulfiram presents a difficult clinical challenge due to ambiguous clinical results with respect to its overall efficacy (Garbutt et al., 1999).

It should be noted that disulfiram is not a pharmacological cure for alcohol dependence. Pharmacotherapy that implements disulfiram into the treatment process should strongly consider psychosocial supports, such as supportive counseling or group psychotherapy. Disulfiram encourages patients to develop resources (internal and external) and the self-confidence necessary to maintain abstinence once the drug is discontinued. One of the most significant challenges with respect to disulfiram treatment is noncompliance due to the aversive nature of its reaction on the body. Therapeutic support can provide encouragement to patients who struggle to remain medication compliant.

NALTREXONE TREATMENT

Naltrexone became the second medication approved by the FDA after disulfiram as a pharmacological treatment for alcohol dependence. Naltrexone is available in oral form (ReVia) or intramuscular as an extended release injection administered once a month (Vivitrol). In addition, naltrexone is an antagonist at the opioid receptors, which essentially means that once ingested and metabolized in the body, it intercedes the various pleasurable consequences of alcohol, which leads to a decrease in craving urges connected to alcohol consumption (Kiefer, Jahn, & Tarnaske, 2003). The FDA recommended Naltrexone dose of 50 mg per day has demonstrated some efficacy in decreasing the compulsive, behavioral component of alcohol craving and increases compliance to alcohol detoxification treatment (Addolorato, Abenavoli, Leggio, & Gasbarrini, 2005a). Individualized dosing regimens have been suggested for select patients, ranging from 12.5 mg per day to 150 mg per day (Saitz & O'Malley, 1997). It should additionally be noted that patients treated with a 380 mg monthly dose of Vivitrol (extended release intravenous injection) demonstrated a significant reduction in heavy drinking behaviors when compared to alcohol-dependent patients who were treated with a placebo (Garbutt, Kranzler, & O'Malley, 2005). Naltrexone has also been shown to decrease desire for alcohol intake. Common side effects of naltrexone are nausea, infrequent headaches, dizziness, insomnia, vomiting spells, increase in anxious feelings, and restlessness (Addolorato et al., 2005; Litten & Fertig, 1996).

Naltrexone is administered to patients who are currently drinking alcohol in large quantities in order to decrease using urges. Some of the advantages of naltrexone are that it can be taken prior to detoxification and does not exhibit addictive properties (Sinclair, 2001). In addition, numerous landmark studies point to the treatment efficacy of naltrexone when used in conjunction with psychosocial supports to treat individuals who experience alcohol-use disorders at varying levels of severity (O'Malley et al., 1992; Volpicelli, Alterman, Hayashida, & O'Brien, 1992a). Volpiccelli et al. (1992) looked at 70 alcohol-dependent male outpatients at a VA hospital facility who were treated with 50 mg of naltrexone or a placebo daily for three consecutive months. It should be noted that in this study, all participating patients received four weeks of intensive abstinence oriented counseling. The participants in the study who received the naltrexone experienced fewer drinking days, were less likely to relapse into heavy drinking and self-reported decreased craving urges to use alcohol. The O'Malley et al. (1992) study demonstrated similar results over the course of six months of treatment, including follow-up measures. The group of patients who received the naltrexone dose exhibited fewer heavy drinking days and a decreasingly small number reported the reemergence of the full syndrome of alcoholism.

The pharmacotherapeutic effectiveness of naltrexone is directly associated with the interactive relationship between dopamine in the brain and the endogenous opioid neuropeptide systems in the body (Heinala et al., 2001). Endorphins are intimately involved in the unique expression of the reinforcing effects of alcohol consumption. Ingestion of ethanol encourages B-endorphin release in areas of the brain that encourage reward sensations. B-endorphins can also directly enhance DA (dopamine) excretion in the NAc (nucleus accumbens). Both processes are significant for alcohol-reward effects. The primary effects of B-endorphins are then negotiated via mu-opioid receptors. The administration of naltrexone into the body then operates as a competitive antagonist with opioid receptors and displays a strong affinity for the mu-receptor isoform. Thus, the primary treatment role for naltrexone is to decrease or stymy opioid receptors in the brain (antagonist) and to curb the endorphin-mediated reinforcing consequences of alcohol ingestion (Herz, 1997).

In the majority of studies concerning naltrexone administration, medication compliance is stressed. However, this is oftentimes a contraindicated variable that influences the feasibility of the research. Trials that included significant psychosocial supports, such as individual psychotherapy and intensive hospitalization, as an adjunct to the pharmacological treatment process demonstrated positive treatment outcomes with respect to decrease in drinking frequency and a reduction of heavy drinking behavior. The literature consistently points to the importance of implementing a comprehensive treatment approach that includes behavioral interventions, counseling and supportive psychotherapy and at times, depending on the motivation of the individual and the severity of the alcohol-use disorder, the introduction of pharmacotherapies to encourage abstinence, reduce drinking behaviors, and aid with acute withdrawal symptoms that would likely increase the likelihood of relapse within the first year of treatment (Kurtzweil, 1996).

ACAMPROSATE TREATMENT

Acamprosate (Capral) was approved by the FDA in 2004 for the treatment of alcohol-dependent individuals. Positive treatment outcomes were first demonstrated in Europe. Acamprosate is available for oral administration in a delayed-release formula at an FDA recommended dose of 2 mg per day (Mann et al., 2004). Acamprosate is a glutamate regulator agonist that encourages abstinence by alleviating or decreasing the physical and psychological discomfort symptoms, such as excessive perspiration, sleep disturbance, and increased anxiety, that frequently accompany individuals once they attempt to decrease or stop drinking behaviors. In other words, acamprosate's primary function is to reduce the accumulation of glutamate during continuous episodic alcohol withdrawal (Anton,

O'Malley, & Ciraulo, 2006). The drug, once ingested, is not metabolized and is discarded through the body by renal excretion (Mann et al., 2004). Acamprosate has been shown to effectively stabilize the excitatory and inhibitory pathways that adjust to chronic alcohol abuse, thus targeting symptoms associated with acute withdrawal.

Acamprosate has shown effectiveness in reducing the likelihood of relapse and supporting efforts toward abstinence with alcohol-dependent patients who have recently undergone detoxification (Mason, Goodman, Chabac, & Lehert, 2006). In total, acamprosate has been investigated in nearly 20 controlled, published research trials with nearly 4000 patients, and the outcomes consequent to these studies have reflected consistent treatment results, indicating the efficacy of acamprosate for helping alcohol-dependent patients maintain abstinence (Mann et al., 2004). Some of the targeted outcomes relative to alcohol-dependent behaviors include a meaningful decrease in alcohol craving, reduction of relapse tendencies and an increased number of alcohol-free days (Addolorato et al., 2005b). The most commonly reported side effect associated with acamprosate use is diarrhea (Paille et al., 1995). It should be noted that acamprosate has been a commonly used pharmacotherapy treatment option in other countries before it was approved by the FDA for pharmacotherapy consumption in America.

Research over the past decade has been conducted that examines the efficacy of naltrexone used in concert with acamprosate as a treatment option for alcohol-dependent individuals (Anton et al., 2006; Kiefer et al., 2003). The largest clinical pharmacotherapy trial conducted for alcohol-related use disorders in the United States, known as the COMBINE study, examined the impact of acamprosate, in isolation from and in conjunction with naltrexone, with over 1400 participants who were diagnosed with an alcohol abuse and/or dependence disorder. This study showed that naltrexone demonstrated efficacy in helping participants maintain abstinence for longer durations and additionally aided participants in reducing heavy drinking behaviors. Kiefer et al. (2003) studied the impact of naltrexone and acamprosate used in concert with one another to treat 160 alcohol-dependent individuals. The number of patients that had maintained abstinence at the conclusion of the 12-week treatment period was two times the amount for the group that received the pharmacological treatments in isolation from one another. Recent research additionally suggests that acamprosate is a more appropriate treatment option for alcohol-dependent individuals when the primary goal is complete abstinence, and naltrexone is better suited to effectively manage consumption (Bouza, Angeles, Magro, Munoz, & Amate, 2004).

COMBINED PHARMACOTHERAPY

There are several published studies that compare naltrexone, disulfiram, and acamprosate treatment for alcohol-use disorders. One of these studies conducted by Diehl et al. (2010) examined the treatment outcomes of 353 alcohol-dependent patients, including the long-term effectiveness of acamprosate and disulfiram with the goal of maintaining abstinence. Supervised disulfiram treatment led to longer periods of abstinence and extended the time to the first relapse of drinking when compared to acamprosate. Another study (Laaksonen et al., 2008) tracked alcohol-dependent individuals for nearly two-and-a-half years and examined the pharmacological impact of naltrexone, disulfiram, and acamprosate under two phases of supervised treatment. Disulfiram treatment was viewed more favorably than acamprosate and naltrexone with respect to impact on the number of heavy drinking days and extending the time to the first relapse.

ADDITIONAL PHARMACOTHERAPIES FOR ALCOHOL-USE DISORDERS

Another pharmacotherapy used in the treatment of alcohol-dependent individuals is known as nalmefene (Selincro), an opioid receptor antagonist that was developed in the early 1970s (Litten & Fertig, 1996). Nalmefene has a longer half-life than naltrexone. Dosages used to treat alcohol-dependent

individuals ranged from 20 to 80 mg per day. Litten and Fertig (1996) examined the effects of nalmefene on drinking behaviors and indicated a significant reduction in heavy drinking behaviors. More research is needed to understand the pharmacokinetic and pharmacodynamic relationship between the drinking behaviors in the alcohol-dependent patient and the ingestion and subsequent metabolism of the medication.

Additional research examines the efficacy of additional pharmacological treatment alternatives to address various aspects of alcohol-use disorders (Addolorato et al., 2005b; Heilig & Egli, 2006; Johnson et al., 2000). These pharmacotherapy options are classified as "second wave" and "third wave" future treatments for alcohol dependency (Heilig & Egli, 2006). Research has shown the potential for several psychotherapeutic medications to have positive treatment outcomes for individuals that are alcohol dependent. A few examples of second-wave treatments that are considered "near future" treatments due to some experimental research outcomes are: (a) fluoxetine (Prozac) and ondansetron (Zofran), SSRIs that appear to be well tolerated by alcohol-dependent individuals (Cornelius et al., 1997), and preliminary studies have demonstrated a reduction of drinking days that is attributable to marked improvement in depressive symptoms; (b) baclofen (Lioresal), a GABA receptor agonist that controls spasticity and has been shown to have some degree of efficacy in reducing intake behaviors, encouraging abstinence, relapse prevention, and reduction in alcohol-related cravings; and (c) topiramate (Topomax), an antiepileptic drug GABA receptor agonist that has shown some promise with respect to addressing obsessive and/or reward cravings. In all of these three experimental drug treatments, additional research is recommended, including comparisons with other approved drugs described above in this section.

The third wave of novel treatment approaches includes the following pharmacological interventions: (a) GHB (gamma-hydroxybutyric acid), an alcohol mimetic, endogenous compound with complex, neuromodulatory functions and has demonstrated some marginal therapeutic gains with respect to alcohol-dependent individuals and reduction of withdrawal symptoms; (b) Corticotropin-releasing factor, which looks to negotiate anxiety that often accompanies mood disturbances in people who experience alcohol dependency; and (c) Cannabinoid CB1 receptor antagonism, which has resulted in some efficacy with experiments conducted with rats, showing an elevation of this receptor that has been shown to contribute to phenotypes of excessive drinking behaviors.

This section outlined the pharmacological administration of medications to treat alcohol dependence, including the interaction of the drug in the body and the relationship of the interaction with behaviors consistent with individuals who suffer from an alcohol-use disorder. Dosing recommendations were provided, research efficacy was presented, and directions for future research concerning additional treatments were briefly introduced. The next section will discuss the pharmacological treatment of individuals who experience opioid dependence.

Review Questions

- How is alcohol dependence and/or alcohol-use disorders conceptualized within a treatment context?

- Briefly describe the three FDA-approved treatments for alcohol dependence, including the interaction of the drug in the body.

- What do comparative studies suggest regarding the integration of FDA-approved medications for alcohol-use disorders?

SECTION FOUR: PHARMACOTHERAPY OF INDIVIDUALS DIAGNOSED WITH SEVERE OPIOID DEPENDENCE

Learning Objectives

- Be able to understand the complexity of opioid dependence and/or opioid-use disorders, diagnostically.

- Become familiar with FDA approved pharmacological treatment approaches for opioid dependence.

- Understand recommended doses and pharmacodynamics and pharmacokinetics of the drug's interaction with the biological processes in the body of the opioid-dependent individual.

The World Health Organization [WHO] defined opioid dependence as a collection of cognitive, behavioral, and physiological features that constitute a complex diagnostic picture that contains six primary features: (a) strong desire or sense of compulsion to ingest opioids, (b) difficulties managing opioid use, (c) a strong physiological state of withdrawal, (d) increased tolerance to opioids, (e) progressive neglect of other activities of living and/or interests, including interpersonal, and (f) persistent opioid use in spite of clear, unequivocal evidence of blatantly harmful outcomes (WHO, 2009). The WHO created the "Guidelines for the Psychosocially Assisted Pharmacological Treatment of Opioid Dependence" in 2009. These guidelines provided minimum treatment requirements to inform the psychosocially supported pharmacological treatment of individuals who are opioid dependent. Opioid agonist treatment is defined as the administration of opioid agonists by trained and certified professionals within the federally authorized restraints of medical practice to individuals who are diagnosed with an opioid-use disorder in order to achieve desired treatment outcomes, usually including some form of drug abstinence. Opioid maintenance treatment used in concert with psychosocial assistance has consistently demonstrated the most efficacious treatment option. The most commonly administered opioid treatments are oral methadone liquid and sublingual buprenorphine tablets (WHO, 2009).

Opioid receptors are classified as G-protein coupled receptors and contain a variety of subtypes. The opioids effects of analgesia, euphoria, and sedation are facilitated by the mu-receptor. Opioid, once ingested, enlarge the secretion of DA (dopamine) in the body by lowering the production of gamma-aminobutyric acid (GABA) inhibition via mu-receptors in the ventral tegmental area of the brain (Johnson & North, 1992). Tolerance to opioids develops as a result of prolonged exposure to and desensitization of the opioid receptor. Consequentially, as a result of the alterations to multiple receptors, the cyclic adenosine monophosphate (cAMP)-producing enzymes become increasingly activated. When the opioid is withdrawn from the system, the cAMP becomes overstimulated, which results in opioid withdrawal (symptoms of opioid withdrawal are summarized in Table 11.4), compelling the opioid-dependent individual to ingest the substance to facilitate regulation (Williams, Christie, & Manzoni, 2001). Acute withdrawal symptoms are associated with watery eyes, excessive perspiration, increased irritability, sleep disturbance, nausea, vomiting, diarrhea, heightened blood pressure, bodily aches and chills, muscle spasms, and tremors, all of which can occur for several days.

Treatment of opioid dependence involves a multifaceted treatment delivery approach that emphasizes a variety of pharmacotherapeutic and behavioral interventions that address three treatment variables: (a) reduction and/or complete elimination of opioid use, (b) inhibiting future consequences that typically accompany opioid use, and (c) enhancing the quality of life and well-being of the opioid-dependent patient. Treating opioid dependence emphasizes pharmacological treatment of acute opioid withdrawal symptoms, agonist maintenance treatment to curtail the cessation of illegal opioids and psychosocial supports that oftentimes include a variety of therapeutic modalities, such as case management, psychotherapy, group and supportive environments such as NA, AA, or Al Anon.

The primary pharmacological treatments for opioid-dependent individuals consist of FDA-approved medications, methadone, naltrexone, buprenorphine and buprenorphine in combination with naloxone, also known as Suboxone or Subutex. These medications will be discussed in the following sections.

TABLE 11.4 Common Early and Late Opioid Withdrawal Symptoms

Agitation
Anxiety
Muscle aches
Increased tearing
Insomnia
Runny nose
Sweating
Yawning
Abdominal cramping
Diarrhea
Nausea
Vomiting

© 2015 Cengage Learning®

METHADONE MAINTENANCE TREATMENT (MMT)

Methadone (Dolophine) is a synthetic opioid and has been the primary form of medication-assisted treatment for opioid abuse and dependence for nearly four decades. Methadone is a treatment option available in the United States through federally approved and regulated MMT clinics. Methadone works primarily via mu-opioid receptors in the brain, where once ingested, it fuses itself to the receptors and when sufficient amounts of the drug are present, can inhibit or eliminate effects of other opioid agents, such as morphine or heroin (Payte, 2002). In essence, methadone, like buprenorphine (which will be discussed later in this section), tricks the brain into believing it is still getting the problem opiate, and the person consuming the medication likely feels normal or stabilized as opposed to feeling the euphoric consequences of opioid abuse. In addition, the person is not actively experiencing acute or complicated withdrawal symptoms, leading to a reduction in physiological and psychological craving urges. Once ingested, methadone is metabolized in order to produce a significant number of metabolites that are primarily inactive and nontoxic

(Moody, Alburges, Parker, Collins, & Strong, 1997). The subsequent elimination of half-life of methadone ranges from 24 to 36 hours at a relatively consistent rate but also demonstrates some variability (Loimer & Schmid, 1992). The residual methadone is then stored in the liver and secondary bodily tissue. In order to attain steady-state SMLs (serum methadone levels), on average, four to five half-lives are required, enabling the presence of the drug to balance the left over amount of drug remaining in the body (Benet, Kroetz, & Sheiner, 1996). When the methadone induction period is introduced, prior to approximating the steady state, half of each day's dose remains in the body and is subsequently combined with the following day's dosing, which leads to an increase in SMLs, even in the absence of a dose increase (Payte, 2002). The primary purpose of the induction process is to approximate the patient's opioid tolerance levels with respect to methadone, which aids in reducing withdrawal and craving urges.

The current dosing rate in the United States for the initial treatment is not to exceed 30 mg or 40 mg in total on the first day (Federal Register, 2001). During the first week of treatment, doses should not exceed more than 5 to 10 mg on any given day and the consummate week increase should not go beyond 20 mg. Once the patient reaches a steady state and methadone amounts exist in a sufficient concentration, he or she is placed onto a daily dose of between 80 and 120 mg as demonstrated by research (Payte, Zweben, & Martin, 2003). FDA guidelines for recommended dose range from 60 and 100 mg per day.

Methadone is ingested in a variety of formats, including pill form, as a liquid or a rapidly dissolving wafer and is consumed daily via supervised distribution in highly regulated clinic settings. Additionally, methadone can be administered immediately at the start of treatment. However, the opioid-dependent individual must be slowly weaned off of methadone in order to prevent withdrawal symptoms.

Daily maintenance doses of methadone have demonstrated a number of research-supported treatment outcomes, including: (a) increased functioning in daily life without the presence of debilitating symptoms commonly associated with opioid withdrawal (Payte, 1991; Dole, 1988), (b) reduction of morbidity and mortality commonly associated with continued abuse of heroin and other illicit opiates (Mattick, Breen, & Kimber, 2003), and (c) reduction of craving urges (Zweben & Payte, 1990). Despite the proven efficacy of methadone maintenance treatment, methadone's relatively abbreviated duration of analgesic effect, combined with its extended elimination half-life and its interaction potential with multiple drugs, increases the risk of poisonous and aversive reactions, including overdose-related fatalities USDHHS (2009).

As a result of research studies that demonstrate increased mortality connected to pharmacological ingestion of methadone (SAMHSA, 2009), the Substance Abuse and Mental Health Services (SAMHSA) asked the American Society of Addiction Medicine (ASAM) to develop an action group that could provide recommendations for the safe administration of methadone treatment, which included: (a) patient education, (b) availability of support services to encourage medication compliance in a supervised environment, (c) appropriate calculation of the initial dose that reflects a deliberate and thoughtful attempt to understand the individual patient's level of tolerance and psychosocial history, (d) close monitoring of the patient's response to treatment, dose adjustment during the stabilization stages of treatment, and (e) constant attention to patient functioning.

It should be noted that research suggests the following treatment recommendations as an adjunct to MMT (Gerra et al., 2003): (a) integration of psychosocial supports dramatically increases medication compliance and reduces the likelihood of fatal overdose; (b) patients who achieved stable employment and who report satisfactory interpersonal supports responded favorably to treatment; (c) patients treated at a methadone treatment facility responded to treatment as compared to patients who received two treatments per week in their home environment; and (d) therapy that address comorbidity for depression and anxiety significantly improved mood symptoms, leading to increased treatment effectiveness (McDowell, Levin, Seracini, & Nunes, 2000). Additionally, the longer a person is engaged, continuously in MMT (between six months and three years), the higher the likelihood he or she will avoid relapse. It should also be noted that secondary benefits to methadone maintenance include a decrease in HIV transmission and a reduction of criminal-related arrests (Keen & Oliver, 2004).

NALTREXONE PHARMACOTHERAPY

Naltrexone (ReVia) was originally approved by the FDA for the treatment of opioid dependence in 1984 and research has demonstrated efficacy as a treatment option that reduces the probability of relapse. Naltrexone is an opioid receptor antagonist, in that it syncs with opioid receptors and essentially blocks them from being activated by agonist compounds such as heroin or prescription opioids. Naltrexone, once ingested, is metabolized via the liver, which alters the chemical and turns it into the active metabolite 6-beta-naltrexol. The half-life and elimination phase of naltrexone are adequate to allow for once-daily oral dosing (or less frequently depending on the dosage size) (Miotto, McCann, Basch, Rawson, & Ling, 2002).

Consistent use of naltrexone reduces or eliminates, all together, the effects of getting high. Naltrexone, consequently, interrupts the cycle of euphoric reinforcement and addiction by stopping opioid receptors. It simultaneously reduces the effects of opioids if the person attempts to abuse the target opioid. There are many pharmacological advantages to using naltrexone as a treatment option for opioid dependence, including: (a) naltrexone is not associated with addictive properties and does not lead to physical dependence, thus reducing the likelihood for tolerance; (b) has been successfully administered as a meaningful component of opioid-detoxification (Buntwall, Bearn, Gossop, & Strang, 2000); and (c) it can be used as a meaningful and effective supplement to a comprehensive treatment plan designed to eliminate opioid use.

There are also substantial disadvantages to the pharmacological use of naltrexone in the treatment of opioid dependence. Some of these disadvantages include:

- Naltrexone cannot be ingested if a person is actively using opioids, and the individual must wait 6 to 10 days after withdrawal symptoms manifest (Miotto et al., 2002)
- Once naltrexone is discontinued, withdrawal symptoms can return, which increases the potential for recidivism
- Naltrexone does not directly treat aversive symptoms connected to opioid abuse
- Many patients who use naltrexone may not be sufficiently motivated to consume it on a regular basis, and
- If patients are taking naltrexone, the risk of overdose increases if the patient does experience a relapse episode during the course of their treatment

A number of studies demonstrate the efficacy of naltrexone as a significant treatment variable for the reduction and/or elimination of drug craving and opioid-seeking behaviors (Gonzalez & Brogden, 1988). In a dozen controlled studies between 1973 and 1984, over 85% of urine screens were free of target opioids for patients who were undergoing continuous naltrexone pharmacotherapy. In Washton, Gold, and Pottash (1984) landmark study demonstrating the efficacy of naltrexone for treating 114 opioid-detoxified patients, nearly two-thirds completed six months of treatment (that also included psychosocial supports) without experiencing opioid relapse. At 12 and 18 month follow-ups, slightly more than two-thirds of the patient population had remained abstinent.

An average daily dose of 50 mg naltrexone typically inhibits the effects of 25 mg intravenous heroin for a minimum of 24 hours (Yeo, 1997). When a patient initiates treatment, the beginning dose is typically around 10 mg and the amount is gradually increased by 10 mg each day until a 50-mg threshold is reached. The recommended length of treatment is between 6 and 12 months. Discontinuing naltrexone is recommended after a successful, sustained period of complete abstinence (Resnick, 1998).

BUPRENORPHINE TREATMENT

Buprenorphine (Butrans) is a mixed, opioid agonist-antagonist that behaves as a partial agonist at the mu-opioid receptor and as an antagonist at the kappa opioid receptor. When the mu receptor is activated, it sets into motion a series of nerve cell activities that constitute familiar opioid effects such as analgesia, euphoria, and suppression of the respiratory system. Buprenorphine partially stimulates the receptor and produces similar physiological responses in a less intense manner as compared to opioids such as heroin and morphine (Johnson & Strain, 1999). The consequence is that buprenorphine produces a moderate psychoactive response that decreases craving urges. Pharmacodynamically, once ingested, buprenorphine securely attaches itself to mu receptors in a more dramatic way than other problem opioids such as methadone. As a result, if an opioid-dependent patient consumes a problem opioid in addition to the buprenorphine, the pharmacological intervention will inhibit it, making it impossible for it to successfully reach the receptors and create the desired sensation and/or response in the body. In addition, if buprenorphine is administered to an individual who has already ingested another target opioid, then it essentially shoves the problem opioid off of the receptor. It is important to note that this kind of disruptive intervention, where the abused opioid is chemically detached from the receptor can produce withdrawal symptoms and many factors should be considered with care when administering the buprenorphine, such as the patient's level of physiological dependence and the timeline for when the abused opioid was ingested. As a partial agonist, withdrawal is mild to moderate compared to methadone and heroin, and buprenorphine can be used as maintenance or to transition a patient from an agonist, such as heroin or methadone, to an antagonist, like naltrexone (Donovan et al., 2013).

There are many advantages to using buprenorphine over methadone and naltrexone, including reduction of withdrawal symptoms and craving urges for opioids, and it inhibits the effects of other target opioids for at least one full day. In addition, patients do not have to engage in a federally regulated program such as a methadone clinic. Unlike naltrexone, buprenorphine can be ingested intravenously, sublingually (most common) or via the buccal route at the onset of withdrawal symptoms (Litten & Allen, 1999). Buprenorphine is available in two different formats, including in a buprenorphine hydrochloride (HCl) tablet known as Subutex and a synthesized, combination tablet, Suboxone, that consists of buprenorphine HCl and naloxone HCl in a ratio of 4:1 (Fudala et al., 1998). Suboxone was essentially developed due to the high potential for abuse for buprenorphine (Strain et al., 1997). In contrast to buprenorphine, naloxone is not easily metabolized and absorbed in the body and has a minimal effect when taking orally (Chiang & Hawks, 2003). Pharmacologically, buprenorphine has a limited risk for toxicity and overdose and low abuse rates are revealed in the research (DiPaula, Schwartz, Montoya, Barrett, & Tang, 2002).

There are three primary phases of buprenorphine maintenance therapy, including induction, stabilization, and maintenance. During the induction phase (Baxter, Scott, Vos, & Whiteford, 2013), medically supervised initiation of buprenorphine pharmacotherapy occurs. This phase requires the opioid-dependent individual to have successfully abstained from abusing opioids for a minimum of 12 hours. During this stage, the individual is in the early stages of acute opioid withdrawal. The stabilization phase is marked by the patient's efforts to discontinue to substantially reduce the abuse of the targeted problem opiate(s), has experienced a significant reduction of cravings and is experiencing minimal physiological side effects. During this phase, the buprenorphine will likely need to be adjusted to assist with stabilization. The maintenance phase of treatment is demarcated by the patient's progress toward recovery on a steady dose of buprenorphine or Suboxone. The length of time an individual remains in the maintenance phase is highly individualized. Medically supervised withdrawal or "detoxification" often takes place during this phase but in some unique cases, some individuals will remain on a stabilized dose of buprenorphine indefinitely.

The general recommendation for buprenorphine in maintenance treatment is between 8 and 24 mg daily. With ongoing opioid dependency, the dose should be increased gradually and on a case-by-case basis (WHO, 2009). In Soeffing, Martin, Fingerhood, Jasinski, and Rastegar (2009) study regarding buprenorphine maintenance treatment, 255 opioid-dependent patients were provided with at least one prescription for sublingual buprenorphine. The authors in this study determined treatment success as having six or more opioid negative blocks over the one year period in which the study spanned. At the completion of year one, 121 patients (47.5%) were opioid negative for six or more blocks and 16% were consistently negative for all 12 blocks of treatment.

There are several studies that have emerged in the last decade that help to illumine the efficacy of buprenorphine for treating opioid dependence by blocking the euphoria associated with opioid use and simultaneously preventing withdrawal (Donovan et al., 2013; Fiellin et al., 2002). It should be noted that in each of the studies that demonstrated buprenorphine effectiveness as a pharmacological treatment option for opioid dependence, counseling supports such as brief therapy were an integral part of the treatment process.

BUPRENORPHINE/NALOXONE TREATMENT (BUP/NX)

The final pharmacotherapy treatment approved by the FDA for use in the United States is Suboxone, which is an integrated medication approach that blends buprenorphine and naloxone (Bup/Nx) as a means of chemically treating opioid dependence. Suboxone combines buprenorphine, a synthetic opiate that enables the dependent individual to avoid the unpleasant feeling of drug withdrawal, and naloxone, which when integrated with street heroin effectively counteracts the euphoric effects of the heroin and facilitates the patient's movement into an active state of opiate withdrawal. By combining a partial opioid agonist with an opioid antagonist, a muted opioid effect is created that is capable of syncing with an opioid receptor in the brain. When the Suboxone is ingested by the opioid-dependent individual, he or she will experience a slight pleasurable sensation, but the majority of people report feeling "normal" during this phase of treatment. People who are diagnosed on the continuum of severity with respect to an opioid-use disorder do not report any euphoric consequence when taking Suboxone. With each administration of Suboxone, the person with opioid dependence essentially experiences a day-long sabbatical as a result of the buprenorphine becoming lodged within a person's brain opiate receptors, thus disallowing the full opioids access into the opiate receptors in the brain.

A study by McKeganey, Russell, and Cockayne (2013) regarding administration of Suboxone to patients who are opiate-dependent indicated that methadone and Suboxone proved to be equally effective in successfully preventing patients from returning to any heroin abuse in the 90 days prior to follow-up. Suboxone has been determined to assist in converting short- to long-term heroin abstinence. Recommended doses of 8 mg/2 mg to 24 mg/6 mg per day were explored in this research. Some of the noteworthy recovery-conducive outcomes that are reciprocally related to Suboxone treatment are:

- Improved cognitive performance compared to methadone use (Rapelli et al., 2007)
- Less severe side effects, physiological and psychological (O'Connor and Fiellin, 2000)
- Improved decision-making skills (Pirastu et al., 2005)
- Increased satisfaction with the use of Suboxone (Gordon, Burn, Campbell, & Baker, 2008)
- Enhanced respiratory functioning when compared with methadone (Law, Myles, Daglish, & Nutt, 2004)
- Cessation of heroin use (Johnson et al., 1995)
- More rapid stabilization (Doran, Holmes, Ladewig, & Ling, 2005)

- Fewer drug interactions (McCance-Katz et al., 2006)

The primary goal of Suboxone treatment is abstinence from opioid-using behaviors as opposed to maintenance. Patients are slowly tapered off from initial doses by 2 mg increments until she or he reaches the 1 mg threshold during the final week of pharmacotherapeutic treatment. As with other pharmacological treatments, educating patients about the drug, its usage, and other pertinent considerations is a vital part of the treatment process. Some recommendations regarding the use of buprenorphine include the following:

- Patients should be advised to let the sublingual buprenorphine tablets dissolve under their tongue to increase effectiveness of the drug.
- Avoid smoking for a minimum of 15 minutes before ingesting the medication.
- Consult your health care provider if any uncomfortable side effects are noticed.
- If taking pain-relieving medication for any medical procedure or injury, notify your practitioner as the interaction effects between the drugs could interfere with the treatment process.

This section highlighted the federally approved and research supported pharmacotherapies used as a comprehensive and individualized treatment approach to assist individuals experiencing opioid-use disorders on a wide continuum of severity. The concluding section of this chapter will provide the reader with a brief discussion of cultural considerations to hold in awareness when choosing, collaboratively with patients, a pharmacological response to the treatment of substance-use disorders.

Review Questions

- Describe, briefly, each of the federally approved medication maintenance programs for the treatment of opioid-use disorders.
- What are the pharmacokinetic and pharmacodynamic interactions with each of the drugs described above?

- As a practitioner, how might you present to a prospective client a multifaceted treatment approach to address opioid dependence?
- Describe pharmacological treatment considerations when working with clients who are not internally motivated to remain abstinent.

SECTION FIVE: CULTURAL CONSIDERATIONS FOR TREATING PATIENTS, PHARMACOLOGICALLY, WITH SUBSTANCE-USE DISORDERS

Learning Objectives

- Be encouraged to reflect on cultural complexity associated with chemical interventions that are designed to assist individuals experiencing severe substance-use disorders in changing lifestyle, maintaining abstinence, managing withdrawal symptoms that if left unattended to, could increase recidivism, and decrease drug-related cravings.
- Be knowledgeable about cultural factors that impact the treatment process, including intake, stabilization, and maintenance.
- Have understanding regarding cultural realities that face clients when seeking comprehensive substance abuse treatment options for problems of living.

What is implied in a comprehensive course of treatment that is targeted to address addictive, compulsive behaviors connected to a person's relationship with an illicit drug or substance? Essentially, the definitive criteria that frames substance-use disorders in the *DSM-5* (APA, 2013a), is suggestive of a significant lack of control to change behaviors associated with using patterns. Perhaps when clients enter treatment, they are already experiencing a great deal of disempowerment due to the very nature of their dependency relationship with a drug. In addition, the cultural landscape that encompasses drug and alcohol treatment is often-times very demeaning and stigmatizing.

STIGMATIZATION OF SUBSTANCE-USE ADDICTION AND TREATMENT

In a qualitative study conducted by Gourlay, Ricciardelli, and Ridge (2005), they interviewed 10 participants in Melbourne, Australia, who were receiving program-regulated methadone treatment for opioid dependence. One of the primary themes that emerged from the interviews was that the participants were conflicted with respect to their experience of receiving methadone treatment due to the perceived/experienced "highly stigmatized and disempowering" (2005, p. 1876) nature of the treatment context. For many of the participants, due to the stigmatized nature that engulfed individuals participating in a federally regulated methadone maintenance treatment program, the costs of participating and remaining engaged in treatment outweighed some of the perceived and/or expected benefits. The findings from this research are consistent with prior research that is suggestive of the negative impact of stigmatization as a barrier to participation in MMT (Matheson, 1998). Link and Phelan (2001) conceptualize the process of stigmatization as taking place when the person who is seeking treatment for a substance-use disorder is branded as a drug addict, consequently linking him- or herself into a negative, stereotyped discourse with cultural implications. Matheson (1998) highlighted the importance of treatment personnel to display positive and facilitative interpersonal conditions, including unconditional positive regard, nonjudgment, and warmth when engaged in service delivery in large part due to patients' internalized stigma consciousness.

MULTICULTURAL COMPETENT PRACTICE AND ADVOCACY

The multicultural counseling competencies (Sue, Arredondo, & McDavis, 1992) recommend that practitioners work to become self-aware about culturally shaped biases and attitudes that might inhibit the ability to effectively and sensitively provide treatment in an empathic and nonjudgmental manner. Practitioners who work with individuals

seeking treatment for substance-use disorders are encouraged to explore and understand internalized messages regarding people who experience drug addiction as well as people who participate in pharmacological treatment for dependence. It can be difficult to identify potentially limiting biases or to even acknowledge their existence. It is important to note that the nature of stigmatization effects people in different ways. This author recommends that critical reflection and journaling activities that encourage you to interrogate and understand your feelings and thoughts about people who suffer from substance-use problems, who seek drug treatment and who might potentially be resistant to engaging in the treatment process for a myriad of cultural factors. Other recommendations would be engaging in challenging conversations with colleagues and peers and remaining receptive and open to corrective feedback. Learning more about addiction, volunteering in community contexts that provide services to individuals who experience drug dependence, and even attending support groups might be other activities to promote increased sensitivity to the lived realities of drug- and alcohol-dependent individuals.

Sociopolitical factors are also at play in the erection of barriers to comprehensive treatment seeking behaviors (Appel, Ellison, Jansky, & Oldak, 2004). Some of these factors as reported by substance-dependent patients pretreatment include: (a) lack of or inadequate insurance, (b) deficient economic resources, (c) ignorance about treatment options, including pharmacotherapy that can assist in alleviating withdrawal symptoms and reduce craving, (d) suspicion about engaging in a highly regulated treatment process with culturally different people, (e) limited access to intake, including transportation concerns and location of treatment facilities, (f) child care concerns, and (g) lack of a personal identification card. As a mental health professional, how do we conceptualize our role in disrupting systemic disparities that disempower, disconnect, and marginalize large segments of the population that could benefit from participating in a comprehensive treatment program that includes psychosocial supports, such as supportive psychotherapy and group counseling as well as the possibility for a referral for pharmacotherapy? These are important concerns to address when broadening our definition of our professional role into the realm of social advocacy that requires a broader and more complicated look at institutionalized systems that disadvantage entire subsets of the total population based on cultural factors, including economic, racial, and unequal distribution of resources.

It is also important to consider the disordered nature of substance use from the client's vantage point, including special consideration of cultural factors. The Culture Formulation Interview format proposed in the *DSM-5* (APA, 2013a) is a useful resource for how a practitioner might explore the client's perception of her or his relationship with illicit drug and/ or alcohol use. When assessing for the client's perception of the problem behavior, I often encourage the client to explore cultural resources for a deeper understanding of the problem. Situating the problem in a culturally specific context aids in client understanding and recommending a sensitive course of treatment. It also empowers client to understand cultural and systemic forces that might have been previously denied from or not held in awareness. An example question might be, "How is your problem with heroin understood within your community?" When using the word "community," I add descriptors such as family (clan, tribe, family of choice, etc.), friends, spiritual and/or religious community and within whatever networks of an interpersonal nature where the client spends her or his time. This aids me in developing a culturally textured picture of how the client perceives the problem in her or his life as well as a detailed understanding of the messages the client internalizes (or distorts) from his or her participation in a culturally specific context.

While the research concerning pharmacological treatments for substance-use disorders has demonstrated some efficacy in terms of treating acute withdrawal symptoms, which can reduce recidivism and relapse, and promoting abstinent behaviors (Anton et al., 2006; Diehl et al., 2010; Jung & Namkoong, 2006; Karila et al., 2007; Kirchmayer et al., 2002; Laaksonen et al., 2008; Mason et al., 2006; Saitz & O'Malley, 1997; Veilleux, Covin,

Anderson, York, & Heinz, 2010), a comprehensive and multifaceted treatment delivery approach was recommended in all successful research studies that integrated assessment for pharmacotherapy (including individualized implementation for a prolonged period of time) and a number of psychosocial supports, including effective case management that can support substance-dependent patients with a number of primary and secondary treatment goals, including consistent adherence to pharmacological recommendations, and addressing psychosocial facets of the patient's life, including social, employment, and education, individual psychotherapy to promote lifestyle and behavioral change and other forms of supportive reinforcement such as group therapy and participating in supportive environments, including NA, AA, and/or Al Anon.

From an individual standpoint, empowering patients with education about substance-use disorders, the impact of the target drug on the body, teaching the client about behaviors that can promote treatment success, explaining the interaction of the medication on their body and highlighting medication compliance and follow through with other forms of behavioral supports while instilling hope in the patient's ability to be successful over the course of treatment are important practices for service delivery practitioners. Systemically, the multicultural competent practitioner is also sensitive to social issues that create barriers to help-seeking behaviors within the client's cultural-community context, including treatment follow-through. Possessing an advocacy consciousness enables the practitioner to not only implement strategies to encourage and empower clients toward their treatment goals but also to recognize the impact of social, political, economic, and cultural factors that shape and maintain barriers to treatment-seeking and treatment-compliant behaviors.

A PROBLEM CASE: THE CASE OF CARLOS

Carlos is a 39-year-old Latino man who is episodically homeless. He is rarely sober and his drug of choice is heroine. However, he gets by on weed,

Jack, crack, whatever he can sniff, and street gin. He has four kids by three women and has never held a job for more than four months. Every three or four years, his two daughters talk him into going to the local treatment center/methadone clinic to detox. Carlos knows this game because he eventually gets street drugs from another patient or acquires enough methadone to really enjoy himself during his stay.

Carlos returns to his street life and his family wonders what to do next. The girls learn of a treatment center in a neighboring city that uses a drug, Suboxone, which makes heroin addicts very sick if they attempt using while taking it. They convince Carlos to go to this center and he begins a regimen of Suboxone. Carlos believes he can still use even on the Suboxone. He tries and becomes very ill. He is sick and unable to eat for five days with cramping and other gastric problems. After his recovery, Carlos begins to reflect on his life on the streets and his addictions. He becomes a little more responsive to the entire treatment milieu at the center. Carlos does use again, but this in-patient experience begins his very long road to recovery.

Questions on the Case of Carlos

1. Can people recover from a heroin addiction/ dependence? How/Why?

2. What changed Carlos and how? Pharmacodynamics or pharmacokinetics?

3. How would you as a mental health professional work with Carlos?

4. What are your biases/countertransferences with addicted clients?

CLINICAL RECOMMENDATIONS

For mental health counselors and practitioners, many of the above questions from the case of Carlos encourage thoughtful consideration of how best to collaborate with Carlos in the treatment process in order to maintain his responsiveness to the treatment process. When a client makes the decision (and yes, it is decision on some level of consciousness) to engage in the treatment process to reduce or eliminate drug-using behaviors, it is important to understand and encourage the client's internal resources to facilitate meaningful change. This chapter has illustrated that pharmacotherapy options provide clients with a temporary reprieve from many of the physiological and/or psychological symptoms that accompany withdrawal from an addictive substance. This reprieve can free up energy and resources to address lifestyle and patterns of behavior that have reinforced dependency, oftentimes at the expense of relationships, personal goals, and well-being.

In the case of Carlos, it would be important to use a mixture of psychoeducation, instructing him about medication compliance and the physiological and treatment consequences of abusing problem opioids while consuming Suboxone, and supportive counseling to explore some of the reflective work he is doing that has encouraged increased engagement in the treatment process. As a participant in an in-patient setting, it would be important to closely monitor his responsiveness to the Suboxone treatments and attend to potential side effects that might complicate treatment. Recommendations for Carlos to participate in group therapy would also be important in order to promote therapeutic factors that can encourage and maintain abstinence and increasing coping behaviors. It is also apparent that he has supportive family members in his life. If the inpatient facility does not have a family treatment program as a component of Carlos's therapy, a recommendation would be made for him and supportive family members to attend Al Anon.

Review Questions

- Why is it important to understand client cultural factors when exploring treatment options with clients relative to their substance-use concerns?

- What levels of intervention can a multicultural competent practitioner attend to in order to address and potentially reduce barriers to treatment for drug and/or alcohol dependency?

- What is the impact of culturally specific stigma on individuals receiving or contemplating pharmacotherapy for substance-use disorders?

SUMMARY

The pharmacotherapy of alcohol and drug dependence continues to be a research-supported treatment variable that has demonstrated efficacy with respect to decreasing and/or eliminating consumption of alcohol and/or drugs, addressing acute withdrawal symptoms pharmacologically, and in maintaining abstinence post-treatment termination. Research continues to examine the effectiveness of medications, combinations of approved medications and new, experimental drugs that may positively affect core components of substance-use disorders. Mental health professionals have an ethical and professional responsibility to refer clients for intake for pharmacotherapies (primary intervention) upon collaboration with the client, to use appropriate education to inform clients of medications that can address substance-use concerns associated with withdrawal and abstinence, attention to side effects once the client has been prescribed a pharmacological option for the use concerns, and exploring the client feelings about treatment and compliance. In addition, clients need to be informed about the relationship between treatment efficacy and prolonged treatment as a means of encouraging abstinence and preventing acute withdrawal, which is often a precursor to relapse.

STUDY QUESTIONS AND EXERCISES

1. Describe your understanding of how opioid agonist treatment works to counter the chemical effects of problem opioids if ingested into the system.

2. Discuss some of the challenges that might co-exist with pharmacotherapy for substance-use disorders due to the prolonged nature of the treatment process, including medication compliance.

3. Describe the impact of buprenorphine in maintenance treatment. What is the role of the medicine in addressing withdrawal symptoms?

4. What are your thoughts about research that demonstrates efficacy of pharmacotherapy treatments of substance-use disorders while also incorporating psychosocial supports into the process? Do you think one has more of a therapeutic benefit than another? Explain.

5. Differentiate between pharmacological treatments for alcohol-use disorders (AUD) and opioid-use disorders (OUD) with marked severity. How are the FDA approved drugs different and similar to one another? What are your thoughts about how one course of treatment is recommended over another?

6. How might you work with a patient who is reluctant to engage in pharmacotherapy of opioid dependence due to internalized stigma about participating in a federally regulated methadone treatment clinic?

7. What strategies might you choose from when trying to collaborate with a patient in order to eliminate practical barriers to services, including economic, transportation, child care, and so on?

8. What steps should you consider when preparing a client to participate in a medication maintenance program? What therapeutic skills would be important to consider during this phase of treatment?

9. How do you explain the disproportionately low numbers of drug and alcohol-dependent individuals who are not receiving treatment? If you were to look systemically, how might you explain this glaring discrepancy?

10. If you were diagnosed with a substance-use disorder with moderate-to-severe symptomology, based on your knowledge after reading this chapter, would you take a pharmacological treatment for opioid and/or alcohol dependence? What factors would impact your decision? What might encourage you to take the step to engage in treatment? What might discourage or inhibit you to seek pharmacotherapy options?

CHAPTER TWELVE

Drug-Assisted Psychotherapy

By Ingmar Gorman

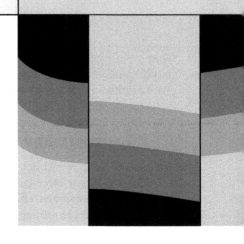

Learning Objectives

- To understand the psychological effects of 3, 4-methylenedioxy-N-methylamphetamine (MDMA) and psilocybin.
- To understand how the psychological effects of MDMA and psilocybin may be used psychotherapeutically.
- Be able to describe "set and setting" and to be able to articulate the importance of these factors.
- Be able to discuss the psychotherapeutic approach used in conjunction with MDMA-assisted psychotherapy for Post-Traumatic Stress Disorder (PTSD).
- Be able to describe the risks associated with the use of MDMA or psilocybin.

INTRODUCTION

Drug-assisted psychotherapy is defined by the use of a pharmacological substance's acute psychological and physiological effects to catalyze and enhance psychotherapy. This chapter will cover various substances used in drug-assisted psychotherapy, the psychopathologies being currently investigated in clinical trials, future avenues of research, and the benefits it may hold for people who are confronted with psychiatric illness. Although these studies are often associated with decades past, there is a current resurgence of research in the United States supported by modern psychotherapeutic and psychopharmacological understandings.

This chapter is dedicated to Alexander "Sasha" Shulgin (June 17, 1925–June 2, 2014), without whom current psychedelic research would not have been the same.

In this chapter, we will focus primarily on clinical research with the classical hallucinogen psilocybin (the compound found in magic mushrooms) and the empathogen 3, 4-methylenedioxy-N-methylamphetamine (MDMA). Other pharmacological agents such as lysergic acid diethylamide (LSD) and ibogaine will also be mentioned. Yet, a whole host of substances including the class of dissociatives, cannabis, peyote, ayahuasca, and others are worthy of further research but beyond the scope of the current chapter.

WHAT DO PSILOCYBIN AND MDMA DO?

The entactogen MDMA and the hallucinogen psilocybin belong to different classes of substances, and although distinct in their effects, they share a propensity to bring about an acute "altered" or "non-ordinary" psychological state. We can understand this alteration to refer to changes in our thoughts (cognitions), emotions (mood), and incoming sensory information (perception). An example of a day-to-day alteration in one's state is when a calm person becomes angry. Anger is associated with physiological changes such as increased perspiration, changes in facial expression, and other body language. When angry, a person is likely to appraise risks more optimistically and, in interpersonal contexts, blame others for his or her circumstances (Cox & Harrison, 2008).

"Non-ordinary" states are distinct in that they are alterations in psychological states which are uncommon or rare (Baruss & American Psychological Association, 2003). Examples of such states include sensations of oneness with the external world, profound feelings of well-being, or sacredness. However, delineating the effects of these substances by their frequency of occurrence is not entirely sufficient.

Another way to conceptualize similarities in the states induced by MDMA and psilocybin is to focus on their ability to increase the intensity of one's cognitions, emotions, and perceptions. In this way, Grof, Hofmann, and Weil (2008) have described hallucinogens as nonspecific amplifiers, which interact with the psychological factors and social context of the individual taking the substance. In other words, psilocybin can intensify how a person feels at a given moment, making the person sensitive to changes in his or her physical and social environment. For example, someone under the influence of psilocybin in an enclosed poorly lit room may begin to experience anxiety or claustrophobia, but after the window shades are opened to a view of a sunlit forest, the person may feel a profound alleviation of anxiety and a flooding feeling of well-being.

Describing these substances as catalysts of nonordinary states or as nonspecific amplifiers helps convey a sense of how varied the specific effects of these substances can be. To speak of changes in thought, emotion, and perception is nearly equivalent to speaking about changes in human experience generally. Although these definitions are limited, these terms help convey the difficulty in pinpointing the exact psychological effect of these substances.

HALLUCINOGEN TERMINOLOGY OVER TIME

The challenge of describing the effects of these substances is clearly reflected in the varied terminology that has emerged to label them over the course of time. The terms chosen often reflect the theoretical orientation of those originating the label. One of the earliest of such labels was "phantastica," coined in 1924 by the first person to discover the active alkaloid in the peyote cactus (Lewin, 1998).

With the discovery of lysergic acid diethylamide's (LSD's) psychoactivity in 1943, other terms entered the lexicon. These included: "psycholytic" translated as "soul dissolving" or "mind dissolving" introduced by Sandison in the 1960s, "psychedelic" translated as "soul manifesting" or "mind manifesting" introduced by Osmond in 1957 (Murray, 2003), and "psychodysleptic" emphasizing impairment of psychological function, and similar to "psychotomimetic" translated as "mimicking psychosis." "Oneirophrenica" or "oneirogen" emphasized dreamlike states as coined by Turner (1964), and "entheogen" (god-manifesting) emphasized the use of these substances strictly in a religious or spiritual context as coined by Ruck, Bigwood, Staples, Ott, and Wasson (1979).

Of these terms, "hallucinogen" is most dominant in the scientific field today, which emphasizes the hallucinatory effects of these drugs. This is considered to be a misnomer by many in the hallucinogen research world, as outright hallucinations are very rare. However, the utility of using the term "hallucinogen," aside from tradition, is that it can be used in reference to "classical hallucinogens." Classical hallucinogens can be further subdivided into tryptamines (e.g., psilocybin), ergolines (e.g., lysergic acid diethylamide), and phenethylamines (e.g., mescaline). In this chapter, hallucinogen and psychedelic will be used interchangeably, and will serve as a reference to the classical hallucinogens strictly.

THE SUBJECTIVE EFFECTS OF PSILOCYBIN

In their book, Stafford and Golightly (1967) describe the onset of hallucinogens as being associated with anxiety and suspense. These sensations are described as "weird" and "difficult to describe" by participants; however, these feelings often pass an hour after administration. Typical effects of psilocybin and other classical hallucinogens, include somatic symptoms (e.g., dizziness, nausea, drowsiness), perceptual symptoms (e.g., altered colors, sharpened sense of hearing), and psychological symptoms (changes in mood, distorted sense of time, dreamlike feelings, depersonalization) (Jacobs, 1984).

To better understand what happens with psilocybin after onset, we can briefly examine some recent research from the field. A study examining the mystical-like experiences of healthy humans who had been administered psilocybin found significant differences between psilocybin and placebo on a number of measures (Griffiths, Richards, McCann, & Jesse, 2006). Using a self-report instrument that captures elements of alteration in consciousness, such as positive shifts in consciousness or anxiety of losing control (Dittrich, 1998), participants reported feelings of oceanic boundlessness, dread of ego dissolution, and visionary restructualization. On another similar measure in the same study, participants reported feelings of internal unity, external unity, sacredness, noetic quality, transcendence of time and space, deeply felt positive mood, and ineffability.

Vollenweider and Kometer (2010) present quantitative data of the subjective effects of psilocybin using the five-dimensional altered states of consciousness rating scale (Dittrich, Lamparter, & Maurer, 2006). The intensity of the subjective responses was found to be dose-dependent and included elementary visual alterations, audio–visual synesthesia, vivid imagery, changes in meaning of percepts, experience of unity, and blissful states. Effects also included sensations of disembodiment and impaired control and cognition.

It is important to highlight that not everyone will experience the same exact effects, and variations in these effects may be partly explained by additional factors such as "set" and "setting," which will be explained later in this chapter. After these acute effects subside, usually after 4–6 hours, it is hypothesized that there are persistent effects such as a decrease in existential fear, feelings of well-being, improved mood, and an increase in healthier behaviors (anecdotally referred to as "afterglow"). These persistent effects are thought to be associated with therapeutic utility; however, they are currently not well understood or empirically verified.

THE SUBJECTIVE EFFECTS OF MDMA

The subjective effects of MDMA are commonly reported to include a sense of well-being, elevated mood, euphoria, a feeling of closeness with others, and increased sociability (Stevens, 2009). MDMA is not a hallucinogen, but rather classified as an empathogen or entactogen, emphasizing the emotional and social effects of the substance. However, individuals may experience psychological phenomena similar to those that occur under the influence of hallucinogens.

In a controlled study, Liechti, Gamma, and Vollenweider (2001) found significant differences between MDMA and placebo on positive mood, visual hallucinations or pseudohallucinations, synesthesia, changed meaning of percepts, facilitated recollection or imagination, and altered perception of space and time. These effects were not always positive and included mania-like experience, anxious derealization, thought disorder, and fears of loss of thought or body control. On another measure used in the study (Liechti et al., 2001), self-confidence, heightened mood, apprehension–anxiety, thoughtfulness–contemplativeness, extroversion, dazed state, sensitivity, and emotional excitation were elevated.

Within the context of therapy, MDMA has been reported to decrease fearfulness, while allowing for a clear-headed and alert state of consciousness (Greer & Tolbert, 1986; Mithoefer, Wagner, Mithoefer, Jerome, & Doblin, 2011). However, the complete picture of the subjective experience of MDMA is complex. Although the effects of MDMA are largely predictable and consistent across users, there is variability in the amount of anxiety (particularly the fear of loss of control) individuals may experience. Liechti et al. (2001) found increases in anxiety or no substantial decrease in anxiety, whereas others (Cami et al., 2000) have found sedation-like subjective effects in some participants.

CLINICAL RESEARCH WITH PSILOCYBIN AND MDMA

A Note About Psychoactive Biota Use Among Indigenous People

This chapter focuses entirely on psychiatric research from the 20th century onward. Such a discussion excludes a wealth of knowledge accumulated by indigenous cultures over many centuries. It would be an injustice to not acknowledge the historical and cultural antecedents to current research. Many of the pharmacological agents under investigation today were first used within indigenous contexts for religious and healing purposes. These include: psilocybin, ayahuasca, peyote, iboga, and others. It is, however, beyond the scope of the current chapter to include findings from anthropology, ethnobotony, ethnopharmacology, sociology, literature, and other important fields pertaining to indigenous and ancient plant use. If the reader is interested in additional resources on these topics, an excellent start would be "Plants of the Gods" by Schultes, Hoffman, and Rätsch (2001) or "Psychedelics Encyclopedia" by Stafford (1992).

A Short History of MDMA

Unlike psilocybin, there are no plants that contain MDMA and it is thus produced by laboratory synthesis. The plant sassafras does contain safrole, which is an oily liquid used as a precursor in the production of MDMA. Due to the complexity of its production, MDMA does not have an extensive history of human use. It has been misreported that MDMA was first synthesized in 1914 as an appetite suppressant. However, an investigation by Freudenmann, Öxler, and Bernschneider-Reif (2006) found no support for this claim when investigating Merck's historical archive in Darmstadt, Germany. Freudenmann et al. (2006) located a patent for MDMA dating back to 1912 with additional documentation highlighting a search for a new type of blood clotting agent. And although MDMA was resynthesized in 1927 and 1959, there was no evidence for human testing until 1960.

It wasn't until the mid-1970s that MDMA was rediscovered by the biochemist Alexander Shulgin (who died as this edition of the book was going to press), who observed that the substance can evoke "an easily controlled altered state of consciousness with emotional and sensual overtones, and with little hallucinatory effect" (Shulgin & Nichols, 1978, p. 77). Shulgin proceeded to introduce psychiatrists and psychologists to the drug, who found the substance to be an exceptional psychotherapeutic adjunct. Although no randomized clinical data were gathered from this period of underground therapy, it has been estimated that thousands of sessions took place throughout the decade. Some estimates indicate that up to 500,000 doses were administered in a psychotherapeutic setting within North America during its period of legality (Stolaroff & Multidisciplinary Association for Psychedelic Studies, 2004). It was said that the drug was exceptional in its utility to facilitate couples counseling.

THE NATURE OF EARLY DRUG-ASSISTED PSYCHOTHERAPY RESEARCH

When discussing the potential clinical benefits of drug-assisted psychotherapy, it is essential to properly contextualize current research of these substances. The current clinical studies using psilocybin and MDMA are in early stages of investigation. This means that small sample sizes are used to evaluate efficacy. Efficacy can be understood as a treatment providing positive results in a controlled research trial. Efficacy does not equate to effectiveness, which refers to finding positive therapeutic results in routine care outside the controlled experimental setting. It is therefore very important to highlight that none of the treatments discussed in this chapter have been evaluated for effectiveness. There is however early evidence supporting the efficacy of these treatments.

Small sample studies, such as some of those included in this chapter, are vulnerable to a Type I error and expectancy effects. A Type I error is the incorrect rejection of a true null hypothesis. In other words, it is the incorrect conclusion that a treatment should provide symptom relief, when it may not. An expectancy effect occurs when a participant or researcher expects a given result (symptom improvement) and this affects the outcome of the study (participant reports fewer symptoms). The issue with classical hallucinogen research from the 1960s and 1970s is that many early studies suffered from such flawed research designs. Although current research still encounters these issues, more modern research methodologies are allowing for increased confidence in the measured effects.

SET AND SETTING

We discussed how psilocybin and MDMA may be thought of as nonspecific amplifiers; substances that strengthen or intensify a person's thoughts, feelings, and perceptions, throughout the duration of the substance's effect. We have also briefly mentioned how these effects interact with a person's psychological, social, and physical context. Because these factors can influence a person's experience on the substance, guidelines for facilitating sessions with these drugs have evolved over the past 50 years, formally beginning with "set and setting" (Leary, Litwin, & Metzner, 1963).

"Set" can be understood as the current state of mind of the person taking the substance. This can include their personal psychological, social, and spiritual history and the context of the intoxication (intention or expectation of the drug's effect). "Setting" pertains to the environment or external factors, which include sounds, the appearance of the room, time of day, and so on. This is particularly significant when contrasting the therapist's office and a concert hall, where recreational use may occur. In addition to "set and setting," we may think of "cast" as the presence of other persons who accompany the individual under the acute effect of the drug. It is hypothesized that clinicians' and researchers' interaction with the individual before, during, and after the administration of the psychedelic is of particular importance. Clinicians will be familiar with this as the therapeutic alliance (Lambert, 2004), a topic which will be expanded on further in the chapter.

Empirical studies have attempted to examine the psychological factors (set) that may influence or predict the quality of a person's experience with psilocybin. A person's recent emotional excitability or their openness to experience has been shown to predict the positive or negative valence of a response to psilocybin (Studerus, Gamma, Kometer, & Vollenweider, 2012). And although clinical research has been able to measure consistent effects (e.g., Griffiths et al., 2006; Hasler, Grimberg, Benz, Huber, & Vollenweider, 2004), it is difficult to predict with absolute accuracy how an individual will respond to psilocybin.

It is thought that through proper screening, preparation, dosage, and the maintenance of a supportive setting, some of the variables that contribute to a negative response ("bad trips") can be controlled. However, it has also been hypothesized that an overemphasis on controlling a person's experience can contribute to negative responses as well. Drug-assisted psychotherapy has adapted to this dialectic by including an element of nondirectedness, to allow the participant greater agency in their experience when under the acute effects of the drugs. More will be mentioned on this topic in the "Psychotherapeutic Methods of Action" section of this chapter.

Due to the significance of "set, setting, and cast," Johnson, Richards, and Griffiths (2008) published a seminal article titled "Human Hallucinogen Research: Guidelines for Safety," which outlines a set of safeguards against factors that may contribute to an overwhelmingly distressing experience. Johnson et al. (2008) re-emphasized the importance of a trusting relationship between the participant or patient and the therapists, preparing the participant for what the psychedelic experience may entail, and a safe setting. In addition to these factors, we must not forget about the dose administered. Research has shown that psilocybin has an optimal dose range for inducing mystical-like experiences, which when exceeded, increases the likelihood of an anxious response (Griffiths et al., 2006).

PSILOCYBIN-ASSISTED PSYCHOTHERAPY IN BRIEF

Psilocybin occurs in various species of mushrooms and after ingestion is metabolized into psilocin, a serotonin receptor agonist (Presti & Nichols, 2006). In clinical research, psilocybin is given in doses ranging from 10 to 30 mg/kg, with effects including the aforementioned changes in perception, cognition, and affect. The duration of these effects often lasts between four and six hours. Psilocybin has a very low physiological toxicity profile, with no organ damage or negative neuropsychological effects

(Gable, 1993; Halpern & Pope, 1999; Hasler et al., 2004; Nichols, 2004; Strassman, 1984). However, as with other hallucinogens, there may be complications for individuals with a family history of psychosis.

The clinical application of psilocybin has focused on its utility in the treatment of anxiety related to cancer. A person diagnosed with cancer will often face physical, emotional, and existential challenges. Being confronted with the possibility of an untimely death can induce hopelessness, anxiety, depression, and these feelings can persist even after successful cancer treatment. Persons living with a cancer diagnosis often live with dread over the feeling of imminent death and may experience restlessness, fatigue, problems concentrating, and an inability to live their life to the fullest. It is thought that a mystical-like experience with psilocybin may help patients better understand their condition so that they may experience less anxiety.

The three institutions associated with this research are Habor-UCLA, New York University, and Johns Hopkins University. The study at Habor-UCLA has been completed and published (Grob et al., 2011), whereas the two remaining studies are ongoing. In a within-subject, double-blind, placebo-controlled study, researchers administered psilocybin to 12 subjects with advanced-stage cancer diagnosed with acute stress disorder, generalized anxiety disorder, anxiety disorder due to cancer, or adjustment disorder with anxiety. The study found significant decreases in depressive symptoms at six-month follow-up and significant decreases in trait anxiety scores at one month to six months post treatment. However, state anxiety scores demonstrated a nonsignificant increase at six months post treatment, with the authors speculating the deteriorating medical condition of the participants as being a factor.

MDMA-ASSISTED PSYCHOTHERAPY FOR POST-TRAUMATIC STRESS DISORDER

Post-Traumatic Stress Disorder (PTSD) is marked by intrusive symptoms such as nightmares, or distress on exposure to trauma-related cues; avoidance, characterized by efforts to avoid thoughts or reminders of the traumatic event; negative cognitions and mood, such as negative beliefs about the self and feelings of detachment from others; and alterations in arousal, characterized by difficulties falling asleep, outbursts of anger, difficulty in concentrating, and hypervigilance.

PTSD has often been shown to be a chronic illness, with patients receiving treatment experiencing symptoms for an average duration of 36 months, patients not receiving treatment experiencing symptoms for 64 months, and more than one-third of patients never fully recovering from PTSD (Kessler, Chiu, Demler, & Walters, 2005).

The reported lifetime prevalence of PTSD is approximately 8% in the United States (American Psychiatric Association, 2013a). Incidence among U.S. soldiers involved in the current Iraq War is estimated to be as high as 18%, with estimates of 75,000 to 225,000 soldiers suffering from PTSD. In 2004, the U.S. Veterans Administration spent $4.3 billion on PTSD disability for veterans who were mostly from the Vietnam War (MAPS, 2009).

The First Randomized Controlled Pilot Study

The first randomized controlled pilot study with MDMA to treat chronic, treatment-resistant PTSD was completed by Mithoefer et al. (2011). Participants in the study were enrolled only if they received a score of 50 on the Clinician-Administered PTSD Scale, a clinician-administered measure of PTSD (Weathers, Keane, & Davidson, 2001) and had at least one unsuccessful treatment with an SSRI and at least one unsuccessful treatment with psychotherapy. The participants included in the study suffered from chronic PTSD with an average duration estimated at over 19 years. Fifteen of the 20 participants had been previously prescribed an average of 4 different psychiatric drugs, and 15 had completed more than one course of psychotherapy (Mithoefer et al., 2011).

Individuals excluded from the study included those who did not suffer from a crime or combat-related traumatic event and women who were pregnant, nursing, or who were not taking birth control. Individuals with a history of psychotic, bipolar, dissociative identity, an eating disorder with purging, or borderline personality disorder were also excluded from the study. A list of contra-indicative medical complications was excluded, along with anyone who met the criteria for substance abuse or dependency, or anyone who had prior use with "ecstasy" more than five times or anytime within the preceding six months of the study (Mithoefer et al., 2011).

The CAPS served as the primary outcome measure, with efficacy measured via subsequent assessments after MDMA-assisted psychotherapy. In addition to the CAPS, the Impact of Events Scale-Revised (IES-R), a measure of psychological response to stress, and the Symptom Checklist 90-Revised (SCL-90-R), a measure of psychiatric symptom categories, were administered. Also, the Repeatable Battery for the Assessment of Neuropsychological Status (RBANS), the Paced Auditory Serial Addition Task (PASAT), and the Rey-Osterreith Complex Figure (RCFT) were used to assess potential neurocognitive changes (Mithoefer et al., 2011).

In the blinded segment of the study, participants underwent two experimental sessions with MDMA or placebo. First, physiological and psychological measures were taken, which were then followed by two 90-minute sessions with therapists. The participants then underwent their first MDMA session followed by a 90-minute therapy session the next morning. Psychological measures were administered four days after the experimental session, followed by three 90-minute therapy sessions for integration approximately once a week. Following the last integration session, one more experimental session with MDMA took place and the preceding stages were repeated. At the end of this process, psychological measures were once again assessed (Mithoefer et al., 2011). After the primary evaluation, the blind was broken for each participant. Participants assigned to the placebo control condition could enroll in an open-label crossover arm. All, save one of the eight participants in this condition, went on to enroll in the crossover arm with the active drug.

In the study, a clinical response was defined as a minimum of a 30% reduction in baseline CAPS total severity score. Ten of the 12 participants demonstrated such a reduction after MDMA treatment, whereas 2 of the 8 participants showed such a response in the placebo group. In addition, seven of the eight participants in the placebo control group who had chosen to partake in the crossover arm of the MDMA-assisted therapy, and all seven demonstrated a clinical response. Mithoefer et al. (2011, p. 10) also note that "all three subjects who reported being unable to work due to PTSD were able to return to work." No serious side effects took place and the neurophysiological and cognitive measures did not measure any impairment in functioning as resulting from the MDMA-assisted therapy.

Long-Term Follow-Up Study

A long-term follow-up (LTFU) evaluating the outcomes of the aforementioned was completed to assess the durability of these improvements (Mithoefer et al., 2013). The follow-up assessment was administered on an average of 45.4 months after the study's final MDMA session. Of the 16 participants who completed the CAPS, no statistically significant differences were found between the CAPS score at follow-up and the CAPS score obtained at the final end point for each individual prior to LTFU. However, two of these participants relapsed with a CAPS score above 50, indicating moderate-to-severe PTSD symptoms. The 19 participants who completed a questionnaire designed to assess perceived harms and benefits of the study indicated experiencing some benefit and did not report any harm. An open-label proof-of-principle study has been completed to test the use of an additional MDMA-assisted psychotherapy session to treat the participants who relapsed in the previous clinical trial. The participants have been treated and follow-up interviews are currently taking place.

HEALTHY VOLUNTEER RESEARCH

This textbook focuses on the use of psychopharmacology in the treatment of psychiatric disorders; yet, this chapter would not be complete without the inclusion of studies with healthy volunteers. Psychopathology is thought of as a condition in which illness must be extracted or removed from a person. Attention is rarely paid to the possibility of using psychopharmacology to prevent psychopathology or as a means to enhance the well-being of individuals not diagnosed with a psychiatric disorder.

Griffiths et al. (2006) published results of a double-blind study that reliably produced mystical-like experiences in a sample of 36 healthy volunteers. At two-month follow-up, participants reported having sustained positive changes in attitudes and behaviors, which was corroborated by two preselected community observers familiar with the participants. The participants attributed these changes to the mystical-like experience, which was reported to have substantial personal and spiritual significance. A 14-month follow-up study was conducted in which 58% of the volunteers rated the psilocybin experience as one of the top five most personally meaningful, and 57% reported it to be one of the top five most spiritually significant experiences of their lives (Griffiths, Richards, Johnson, McCann, & Jesse, 2008). Griffiths et al. (2011) found the positive changes in attitude and behavior to persist at 14-month follow-up. Commonly reported positive changes included better relationships with friends and family, increased physical and psychological self-care, and increased spiritual practice. The benefit reported by volunteers was related to the sequence of psilocybin doses they received. Participants who received ascending doses of psilocybin had more sustained positive changes in attitudes and behaviors than participants in the descending dosage condition.

In another recently published study (MacLean, Johnson, & Griffiths, 2011), researchers found evidence of personality change as a consequence of psilocybin administration in healthy adults. Measuring changes in the five broad domains of personality (also known as the Big Five), Maclean and colleagues found a significant increase in the domain of Openness. This personality change remained significantly altered in participants one year after the psychedelic experience in those participants who had a mystical experience. The construct of Openness consists of six facets: fantasy, aesthetics, feelings, ideas, values, and actions. It can generally be thought of as open-mindedness to new ideas and experiences.

Another extensive area of research in healthy humans pertains to understanding the basic neuropsychological, cognitive, and behavioral effects of MDMA and hallucinogens. A very large contribution in this regard has been made by Franz Vollenweider (Vollenweider & Kometer, 2010). Other important figures contributing to this research include: Baggott (Baggott, Coyle, Erowid, Erowid, & Robertson, 2011), Bedi (Bedi, Hyman, & de Wit, 2010), Carhart-Harris (Carhart-Harris et al., 2012), Dumont (Dumont et al., 2009), Gouzoulis-Mayfrank (Gouzoulis-Mayfrank & Daumann, 2006), and Kuypers and Ramaekers (Kuypers & Ramaekers, 2007).

THE USE OF MDMA AND HALLUCINOGENS IN CLINICAL TRAINING

It is suggested by some researchers that it is important for therapists who will be working with participants under the influence of psychedelics to have familiarity with nonordinary psychological states. The manual for MDMA-Assisted Psychotherapy for the Treatment of Posttraumatic Stress Disorder (MAPS, 2013a) includes the therapist's comfort with "intense emotional experience and its expression," "first-hand validation of and trust in the intelligence of the therapeutic process as it arises from an individual's psyche," as it helps "familiarize therapists with the terrain … of non-ordinary states," "help therapists to identify features of the experience that might be most helpful," allows the therapist "to be comfortable supporting people during times when the process is difficult and unsettling," and "provides the therapist with intrapersonal working knowledge of the integration process" (MAPS, 2013a). Such experience also alludes to the practice of psychotherapists to undergo therapy of their own to understand the psychotherapeutic process in themselves and others.

In a 40-year follow-up study, of the 20 psychotherapists interviewed, who conducted drug-assisted psychotherapy during the 1950s and 1960s with LSD, all showed high levels of agreement when asked whether their experiences with auto-intoxication, conducted during their training, were a valuable didactic experience for their work as psychotherapists (Winkler & Csémy, 2014). Similar findings have been established in the case of MDMA, where one study found that of the 20 psychiatrists interviewed with personal histories of MDMA, 85% had reported an increased ability to interact with others, 80% reported decreased defensiveness, 65% reported decreased fear, 60% decreased sense of separation from others, 50% increased awareness of emotions, and 50% reported decreased aggression (Liester, Grob, Bravo, & Walsh, 1992). It is important to emphasize that this does not suggest that therapists "need to have" prior experience with these substances, but that research suggests that it may have benefits.

To aid therapists in their understanding of the MDMA-induced state, a study has been approved in which therapists will receive MDMA as part of their training in MDMA-assisted psychotherapy (MAPS, 2009). The purpose is to "provide an in-depth understanding of how to maximize the therapeutic effects of MDMA-assisted psychotherapy," and "allow participants to better draw distinctions between common, self-limiting side effects of MDMA-assisted psychotherapy and those effects that require intervention" (MAPS, 2009, p. 7).

In a recent interview, Dr. Herb Kleber (White, 2013) discussed how in the late 1960s, he was interested in comparing therapists who had personal experiences with LSD to those who did not. There were anecdotal reports that therapists with the LSD experience had better outcomes in group therapy than those who did not. Dr. Kleber began the study but had to close the study prematurely due to Sandoz recalling the LSD after its widespread recreational use. In the interview, Dr. Kleber states, "… in general, most of the people did not seem to change very much. I was not terribly impressed with the outcome of the study." However, this research was never completed and therefore, no empirical evidence exists to support an interpretation.

MECHANISMS OF ACTION
Potential Mechanisms of Action in Psilocybin-Assisted Psychotherapy

Classical hallucinogens are also known as serotonergic hallucinogens as they act as 5-HT2A receptor agonists. This activation is necessary but not sufficient in the explanation of hallucinogens' effects (Nichols, 2004). Yet, their action is far more complex, causing alterations in glutamatergic, dopaminergic, and serotonergic transmission. Studies conducted by researchers in Zurich found that most of the subjective effects of psilocybin were attenuated by drug that inactivates 5-HT2A receptors (Carter et al., 2005). The evidence for contribution of dopaminergic receptors is weaker but the research in this area is incomplete. Recent neuroscientific advances have allowed for the neurobiological correlates of psychedelic states to be better understood.

Desynchronization of oscillatory rhythms in the posterior cingulate cortex (PCC) has been found to be one of the mechanisms associated with the subjective psychedelic experience with psilocybin (Muthukumaraswamy et al., 2013). The cerebral cortex is composed of interconnected neurons that make up networks that allow the brain to function. When these neurons fire in a particular pattern, brain waves may be observed using an electroencephalogram (EEG). Desynchronization is when this synchronization decreases. The function of the PCC is complex and unclear, but it is associated with the procession of emotion, memory, and is a central node in the default mode network (DMN). The DMN is a network of brain regions that are active when a person is not focused on the outside world and the brain is restfully awake.

A recent study using fMRI found evidence for the association between subjective effects of psilocybin and decreased connectivity and activity in the key connection hubs (thalamus, anterior and posterior cingulate cortex, medial prefrontal cortex), which enabled a state of unconstrained cognition (Carhart-Harris et al., 2012). These hubs are central to communication and integration across the brain, and thus play an important role in a diverse set of cognitive functions. In the past, it was thought that psychedelics increase brain activity, leading to their subjective psychological effects. This research shows evidence of the contrary.

Aldous Huxley and Huxley (1977) theorized that the brain functions as a reducing valve, acting to filter out unnecessary information and external stimuli, so we are not overwhelmed. The work of Dr. Carhart-Harris and colleagues indicates that psychedelics initiate a decrease in brain activity in areas responsible for constraining our sensory experience and our subjective experience of self-consciousness. As a result of this decrease, these senses are less constrained.

There is much more to learn about the neurobiological underpinnings of the psychedelic state. For a more detailed description of the effects of psychedelics, please see Vollenweider and Kometer (2010) and Nichols (2004).

Potential Mechanisms of Action in MDMA for PTSD

The psychopharmacological profile of MDMA is complex. It is associated with the release of serotonin, norepinephrine, and dopamine, and can act directly on adrenaline and serotonin receptors, and elevate vasopressin (Cami et al., 2000). The most common effects of MDMA include stimulant effects (cardiovascular, autonomic, and perceptual).

MDMA is relatively short acting (lasting four to six hours) and has been reported to facilitate introspection, interest and capability for intimacy, temporary freedom from anxiety, and emotional openness (Greer & Tolbert, 1986). The symptoms of increased and uncontrolled fear response and avoidance in PTSD can both be hurdles in the therapeutic process. Psychotherapies for PTSD such as cognitive-behavioral therapy involve the recall of traumatic memories, their updating, and integration (Ehlers & Clark, 2000).

The reduction of a fear response induced by MDMA may facilitate the revisiting of traumatic experiences during psychotherapy without associated emotional numbing (Mithoefer et al., 2011). Another proposed model is that MDMA increases the window of tolerance for engaging with trauma-related thoughts, memories, and feelings. The drug may deepen emotions, empathy, and contribute to a "clearer perspective of the trauma as a past event with a heightened awareness of the support and safety that exist in the present" (Gorman 2013a, p. 3).

Another mechanism of action implicated in MDMA-assisted therapy may be linked to changes in neurobiological abnormalities, particularly in the amygdala and ventral/medial prefrontal cortex, which has been hypothesized to result from PTSD. MDMA has been associated with increased blood in the ventromedial front and occipital cortex, and decreases in the left amygdala (Gamma et al., 2000).

The Psychotherapy in MDMA-Assisted Psychotherapy

The psychotherapy provided in clinical trials of MDMA-assisted psychotherapy for PTSD is a multifaceted integration of various treatment modalities. The following section outlines several components of the psychotherapy and how it may interact with the acute effects of MDMA. Although not comprehensive, these psychotherapy processes and techniques are considered to be key aspects of the treatment (Mithoefer, 2013).

One of the earliest goals at the beginning of MDMA-assisted psychotherapy is the establishment of the therapeutic alliance (Mithoefer, 2013). This alliance or relationship between the therapist and client has been one of the most consistent psychotherapy factors to be associated with therapeutic outcome (Lambert, 2004). In the case of persons living with PTSD, the alliance can be of particular importance due to the impact interpersonal trauma and shame may have on developing trust. Therapeutic alliance is developed in MDMA-assisted psychotherapy through introductory sessions with the therapists prior to MDMA administration. It may be further supported by the effects of MDMA.

This hormone oxytocin is thought to be affiliated with the establishment of trust and the facilitation of bonding in humans, and has been hypothesized to be a component of MDMA's psychophysiological effect. This is supported by indirect evidence showing levels of oxytocin to be elevated in the blood of healthy volunteers who had been administered MDMA and to be positively correlated with the prosocial effects of the drug (Dumont et al., 2009; Hysek et al., 2013). In this way, oxytocin may facilitate the establishment of the therapeutic alliance (Johansen & Krebs, 2009). However, conclusive evidence is yet to be collected.

The highly affective nature of PTSD symptoms and the content of trauma itself can present a challenge to establishing an alliance, and if left unaddressed, can impede the therapeutic process. Cloitre, Stovall-McClough, Miranda, and Chemtob (2004) found negative affect management to mediate the relationship between the therapeutic alliance and treatment outcome. In other words, the relationship between the patient and therapist is more likely to lead to better results if the patient is able to manage the negative feelings he or she experiences. In the case of MDMA-assisted psychotherapy, the pharmacological intervention can be thought of as a way of enhancing negative affect management. It allows the person to engage with traumatic content without a heightened fear response or dissociation, and within a highly supportive environment.

The potential for MDMA to manage negative affect is supported by preliminary neurobiological evidence. Extensive studies into the neurobiology of PTSD have found symptoms such as intrusive memories and hyperarousal to be associated with decreased hippocampal and medial prefrontal cortex signaling and increased amygdala activity (Ravindran & Stein, 2009). In contrast, healthy volunteers who were acutely administered MDMA showed decreased activity in the left amygdala, which is associated with fearful associations and memories (Gamma et al., 2000). A recent study by Carhart-Harris et al. (2014) found that the decrease in amygdala activity was associated with self-reported intensity of MDMA effects. The potential for MDMA to dampen an overactive amygdala remains a tentative hypothesis, which is currently being evaluated empirically in an fMRI substudy examining persons living with PTSD before and after MDMA-assisted psychotherapy treatment (MAPS, 2014).

In clinical studies for PTSD, participants are administered MDMA on only 2 or 3 occasions out of approximately 12 psychotherapy sessions. During these sessions, it is possible that the participants may experience increased anxiety and strong affective states. To support participants during these experiences, mindful diaphragmatic breathing techniques are taught prior to drug administration, which are similar to the relaxation exercises used in other psychotherapies such as Cognitive Behavioral Therapy (CBT) and Prolonged Exposure (PE).

MDMA-assisted psychotherapy shares other similarities to PE, Cognitive Processing Therapy (CPT), and Eye Movement Desensitization and Reprocessing (EMDR). This includes an emphasis on the importance of directive preparation sessions, which includes the establishment of the aforementioned therapeutic alliance, psychoeducation about PTSD, socialization to the treatment model, and preparing the participant for the process and consequences of exposure to traumatic material.

What makes MDMA-assisted psychotherapy distinct from the aforementioned treatments is an emphasis on the therapist's largely nondirective stance after the preparation sessions. A nondirective approach allows the participant to direct the pace and direction of the therapy session. This is done so that the participant can bring up traumatic content when optimally prepared to do so. To maintain an exposure component in MDMA-assisted psychotherapy, in cases where the participant avoids discussing the trauma entirely, the participant and therapist prior to the drug administration, have informally agreed that the therapist can bring up the traumatic content at a later point during treatment if needed. However, therapists in the current clinical studies have noted that participants discuss the trauma spontaneously, without the need for prompting by the therapist, in almost all (nearly 100) MDMA sessions.

A nondirective approach allows for several additional advantages. Participants may elect to discuss traumatic content not initially conceptualized in the case formulation. These experiences may be associated with intense shame or guilt, which the participant may not have been willing to share during intake. Providing the participant greater agency allows for unexpected, yet potentially important therapeutic content to surface.

Habituation to anxiety, fear, or other affective responses associated with the traumatic content is not the goal or process emphasized in MDMA-assisted psychotherapy. Rather, in MDMA-assisted psychotherapy, emphasis is placed on emotional connection, increased clarity into traumatic memories and a sense of mastery over the process and recall of traumatic events. Habituation can be understood as a form of learning, a consequence of repeated exposure, in which a person shows a decreased response to a stimulus. In the case of PTSD, this may be a repeated exposure to a traumatic event, with the aim of reducing a fear response and avoidance of stimuli associated with the event.

Part of the trauma processing relates to cognitive restructuring in which negative thoughts, beliefs, and distortions are challenged in a nondirective way to help the participant understand the meaning of their trauma. When a traumatic experience is reflected upon without psychophysiological dysregulation, aided by the MDMA, the traumatic memories can be safely recontextualized with the support of the therapist.

Perhaps the most central aspect of MDMA-assisted psychotherapy, particularly in the sessions in which the participant is under the effects of the MDMA, is the emphasis on the participant's inward focus. This is done with the participant closing his or her eyes and listening to appropriate music. As a consequence, the participant leads much of the therapy, with the therapists facilitating the participant's process. It is not assumed the therapist is the expert, but rather that the patient, with the help of the MDMA, will engage in the therapeutic process at least partially independently. In relation to cognitive restructuring, the participant may come to understand his or her trauma with a greater sense of agency and self-efficacy. In a traumatic event, the victim encounters powerlessness and helplessness over the situation. Allowing the person to regain some sense of power and control in MDMA-assisted psychotherapy is a reversal of this circumstance. In this situation, the therapists offer guidance and support when needed or requested.

The active role of the therapist becomes more prevalent during integration sessions. Participants discuss the content of the MDMA sessions, their reactions to it, and discuss the insights gained. The therapist must make clear to the participant that the process catalyzed by the MDMA session will continue for several weeks and participants are encouraged to discuss any distress that may arise. "Integration involves the ability to access and apply to daily life the lessons, insights, changes in perception, awareness of bodily sensations, and anything else that has been revealed during the MDMA sessions (MAPS, 2013a)." There are at least three integrative meetings planned after each MDMA-assisted psychotherapy session in which to address the sessions. Participants are also encouraged to use forms of self-expression, such as journaling or drawing, to confront or integrate material from the sessions. They also have option to view recordings of their sessions, though they are not required to do so.

IS IT THE DRUG, THE PSYCHOTHERAPY, OR BOTH?

Now that we have covered both MDMA- and psilocybin-assisted psychotherapy, we can begin to address a central question in this form of treatment. When drug-assisted psychotherapy successfully treats a patient, is it an effect of the substance, the psychotherapy, or the combination of the two. The importance of the therapist cannot be underestimated, as he or she can assist in the optimization of the aforementioned set and setting, assist in preparation before the substance is administered, and help with the integration of the experience afterward.

In his article, Bogenschutz (2013) succinctly describes the unique methodological issues encountered in clinical trials using psychedelics, and it is likely that these extend to MDMA as well. Psychedelics have both acute psychoactive effects and hypothesized persistent effects that last longer than the acute drug response. Bogenschutz (2013) highlights that the therapeutic brain changes induced may be dependent on the subjective experience of the patient. Unlike other psychopharmacological medications, the set and setting of the patient will impact the experience on the medication, which is hypothesized to impact the treatment outcome. Thus, a combination of psychotherapy and medication effect is being measured. This can be problematic because clinical trials focus on isolating variables, so that specific mechanisms of either drug or psychotherapy can be defined. We will address these questions by using two clinical illustrations.

CLINICAL EFFECT WITHOUT PSYCHOTHERAPY

Sewell, Halpern, and Pope (2006) interviewed individuals experiencing cluster headaches who had used psilocybin or LSD to treat their condition. Cluster headaches are chronic, occurring as regular attacks during a cluster period, and then subside into a remission period. The pain experienced in this neurological disorder is severe (rated as 11 out of 10 on pain scales), typically felt on one side of the head or around the eye (Nesbitt & Goadsby, 2012). The results of the interviews conducted by Sewell et al. (2006) indicated that individuals who used LSD and psilocybin to terminate cluster periods, required less than three doses to do so, and in doses that were subhallucinogenic (did not produce profound changes in cognition and perception). Several years later, it was found that the nonhallucinogenic 2-bromo-lysergic acid diethylamide (2-Bromo-LSD) could produce similar results as psilocybin or LSD. Although cluster headaches are not a psychiatric condition, this case illustrates how the psychedelic experience is not always necessary for treatment.

In 2006, a pilot study was published on the safety, tolerability, and efficacy of psilocybin in the treatment of OCD (Moreno, Wiegand, Taitano, & Delgado, 2006). Although treatments such as Cognitive-Behavior Therapy and other pharmacotherapy exist for OCD (Stein, Ipser, Baldwin, & Bandelow, 2007), the investigators sought to study anecdotal reports suggesting psilocybin may relieve symptoms of OCD. After

treatment with psilocybin, symptoms of OCD decreased by 23 to 100%, with improvement lasting beyond 24 hours post administration. In these studies, no formal psychotherapy was provided, although some participants reported the psychedelic experience to be psychologically and spiritually enriching. The reduction in symptoms after the acute effects of psilocybin brings us back to the question of mechanism of action. To this date, there has been no follow-up to this research. It is thus unknown whether the therapeutic effect of the psilocybin treatment was only pharmacologically mediated or a combination of pharmacologically and psychotherapeutically mediated.

BETWEEN PSYCHOPHARMACOLOGY AND PSYCHOTHERAPY

Ibogaine is not a classical hallucinogen, but shares some hallucinogen qualities. Ibogaine is referred to here as it sits in the center of the dialectic between pharmacological and psychotherapeutic action. The psychoactive effects of the substance have been described as introspective and dreamlike, with alterations in consciousness lasting beyond 20 hours. The experience has been characterized as unpleasant, with effects including ataxia and vomiting, making it potentially unattractive as a substance for recreational use (Brown, 2013). Mash (2010) provided an analysis of ibogaine experiences and identified the following themes reported by study participants: new insight (86.7%), need to become sober/abstinent now (68.3%), cleansed/healed/reborn (50%), second chance at life (40%), increased self-confidence (33.3%), and impending self-destruction if drug use continued (18.3%).

Unlike the other serotonergic hallucinogens, ibogaine also acts as an NDMA receptor antagonist and an agonist of the k-opioid receptor set (Glick & Maisonneuve, 1998). These properties may lend it to be of particular use in the treatment of addiction to a wide range of drugs including opiates, stimulants, nicotine, and alcohol (Brown, 2013). However, as other researchers have noted (Alper, Lotsof, Frenken, Luciano, & Bastiaans, 1999), there is a lack of systematic clinical research with ibogaine.

The therapeutic profile of ibogaine for substance-use disorder has been reported to include alleviation of withdrawal (Alper, Lotsof, & Kaplan, 2008; Alper et al., 1999) and cravings (Mash et al., 2000). These findings are supported by accumulated preclinical research with lab animals (Alper, 2001). These properties observed in lab rodents suggest a pharmacological rather than psychological mechanism of action. Thus, the psychedelic effects of ibogaine can be viewed as side effects (Carnicella, He, Yowell, Glick, & Ron, 2010). Undergoing a 20-hour experience with profound changes to cognition and perception is not practical if a similar effect can be achieved otherwise.

Two compounds related to ibogaine, noribogaine and 18-Methoxycoronaridine (18-MC), have been developed, which have demonstrated the antiaddictive profile of ibogaine in rodents, but are theorized to have fewer hallucinogenic side effects. Of these two, a preclinical study indicated noribogaine to be more effective in decreasing alcohol self-administration in rats (Carnicella et al., 2010). There have been no human trials at this point.

If a nonhallucinogenic analogue is developed with the same antiaddictive properties, would studies demonstrate the same treatment outcome as ibogaine? This empirical question brings us back to our discussion of mechanism of action. Treatment outcome, particularly in addiction, is supported not only by the removal of cravings and withdrawal symptoms, but by other psychological, social, and cultural factors. The hallucinogenic experience may increase confidence, readiness to change, greater understanding in motivations for use, and psychospiritual resources that may prevent relapse. It remains unanswered whether the hallucinogenic component of ibogaine contributes to efficacy. Yet, the length and the unpleasant quality of the ibogaine experience may be a barrier to those seeking treatment, suggesting that 18-MC or noribogaine may be more useful treatment tools.

To conclude this section, we see that in the case of cluster headaches, the purely pharmacological action of LSD and psilocybin was responsible for a therapeutic effect. In the study using psilocybin to treat persons living with OCD, no psychotherapy was provided, and clinical improvement was established, albeit for a short period of time. Whether the therapeutic effect on OCD could be prolonged with combination of psychotherapy remains uninvestigated. Finally, we discussed the antiaddictive properties of ibogaine and how both the psychological and pharmaceutical effects of the substance may contribute to recovery.

RISKS VERSUS BENEFITS
Safety of Psilocybin and other Classical Hallucinogens

The classical hallucinogens are considered to be physiologically safe and do not show the same dependency issues as other drugs associated with substance-use disorders. There is no evidence that these substances are toxic to any mammalian body organ and no deaths as a direct consequence of classical hallucinogens have been recorded. However, fatal accidents have occurred while under the influence of hallucinogens in uncontrolled settings by recreational users. The safety of classical hallucinogens is supported by a recent study by Krebs and Johansen (2013), who examined data from a U.S. national health survey to examine 130,000 participants of which 22,000 had taken a classical hallucinogen at some point in their lives. After controlling for risk factors, the study found no association between increased rates of psychiatric problems and psychedelic use. Counter to expectation, weak associations were found between the use of certain psychedelics and lower rates of mental health problems. It is important to note that these findings may be a result of chance and that these findings are not causal due to the retrospective nature of the research.

It is also important to take into consideration previous research which has found increased incidence of negative responses to hallucinogens in individuals with a family history of schizophrenia (Anastasopoulos & Photiades, 1962). There is a lack of firm empirical evidence demonstrating a direct causal link between the use of the classical hallucinogens and schizophrenia in humans. However, the common consensus is that hallucinogens may bring about a latent psychosis in individuals who are predisposed (e.g., genetically vulnerable) to schizophrenia. Participants who have such personal or family histories are excluded from studies using MDMA or hallucinogens.

Contraindications to hallucinogen administration include combining hallucinogens with a monoamine oxidase inhibitor (MAOI) or as previously mentioned, administering a hallucinogen to an individual with a family history of schizophrenia or other psychotic disorders. It is also important to state that the substances used in approved research trials in the United States have been synthesized with the oversight of multiple governing bodies, including the Drug Enforcement Agency. Individuals who seek out these substances off the black market run the risk of obtaining impure syntheses and potentially adulterated substances. In these circumstances, the possible negative consequences to a person's physical and psychological health cannot be underestimated.

Safety of MDMA

The greatest risk with MDMA pertains to cardiovascular issues associated with increased blood pressure and heart rate. Individuals with a serious cardiovascular condition are at risk when ingesting MDMA. These physiological changes are known to be predictable effects and are thus a serious concern for a vulnerable population. This issue is heightened in recreational settings, where the purity of the substance is in question or where users are overexerting themselves.

As with other pharmacological substances, there are dangers associated with MDMA's use in illegal contexts. Black market MDMA, commonly sold in tablets as *ecstasy* or in powder form as *molly,* may include other substances, contaminants, and adulterants, and thus, their interaction and effects on the body can be unpredictable. Use in uncontrolled settings only compounds these dangers. Prolonged dancing in poorly ventilated spaces after the ingestion of MDMA has been linked to hyperthermic reactions leading to medical complications and in some cases, death. However, excessive hydration associated with MDMA use can provoke severe hyponatremia induced by the syndrome of inappropriate antidiuretic hormone secretion. The greatest risk is in premenopausal women (Rosenson, Smollin, Sporer, Blanc, & Olson, 2007). The first fatalities associated with MDMA were related to severe pre-existing cardiac or respiratory disease. Cerebrovascular events have been reported as well, including stroke and subarachnoid hemorrhage, effects also reported after psychostimulant use (Gledhill, Moore, Bell, & Henry, 1993; Henry, Jeffreys, & Dawling, 1992). However, when considering the prevalence of illicit ecstasy use, the report of a serious adverse event is rare.

These dangers can be avoided within the context of therapy, as the use of pure MDMA can be assured, patients with medical contraindications can be excluded, and an appropriate environment can be provided. However, other potential dangers may still exist. Research with nonhuman animals has detected a reduction in brain serotonin after high, repeated doses of MDMA (Baumann, Wang, & Rothman, 2007). There are consistent findings of impaired memory in people reporting repeated, heavy use of ecstasy and other drugs (Reneman et al., 2006). To date, there has been only one prospective comparison of memory and serotonin uptake sites in people who later did or did not use ecstasy, finding difficulties in verbal memory but no changes in uptake sites (Schilt et al., 2007). A comparison of people with PTSD who received either placebo or MDMA failed to detect significant differences in performance on measures of cognitive function (Mithoefer et al., 2011). A comprehensive review of research on the neurotoxic effects of MDMA has been completed by Rogers et al. (2009).

Dependency

Data suggest that MDMA possesses an abuse potential that is greater than the classical hallucinogens but not as strong as stimulants such as cocaine and methamphetamine. Studies have shown that animals will self-administer MDMA, although they will not work as hard to obtain MDMA as they would for methamphetamine or cocaine (Fantegrossi, 2006; Wang & Woolverton, 2006).

Substance abuse is also low in representative samples (Lieb, Schuetz, Pfister, von Sydow, & Wittchen, 2002; von Sydow, Lieb, Pfister, Höfler, & Wittchen, 2002).

In the United States, 12% of high school seniors have admitted to trying MDMA at least once, with this number being twice as high according to research at undergraduate universities (Ruiz, Strain, & Langrod, 2007). In a study cited by MAPS (2006), of a sample of 74 drug-naïve participants, who received MDMA in a research setting, "none of the participants expressed any interest in taking MDMA as a recreational drug" (Liechti et al., 2001). This may be indicative of how intentions associated with use may be linked to abuse.

Risks Associated with Psychotherapeutic Use

Short-term side effects of MDMA administration include trismus (lockjaw), bruxism (teeth grinding), restlessness, anxiety, decreased appetite, tachycardia, palpitations, dry mouth, insomnia, difficulty concentrating, and impaired balance (Liechti et al., 2001; Peroutka, Newman, & Harris, 1988). MDMA may temporarily reduce immune functioning for two to three days, but this is likely to be below clinical significance and is similar to effects produced by other psychoactive drugs (Pacifici et al., 2000). Other side effects include mild alterations in perception and potential for complications due to comorbidity with substance abuse (MAPS, 2006). However, counterintuitively, preliminary data indicate that through addressing conditions that exacerbate it, MDMA may also be a potential adjunct in treating substance-use disorders (Jerome, Schuster, & Yazar-Klosinski, 2013). There is no evidence for lasting toxicity after MDMA administration in humans in Phase I studies utilizing 120-mg doses (Grob, Poland, Chang, & Ernst, 1996; Harris, Baggott, Mendelson, Mendelson, & Jones, 2002). This does not discount the possibility that neurotoxic effects may be occurring outside a controlled clinical context.

The Future of Psychedelic Research

As we have outlined in this chapter, current research into drug-assisted psychotherapy indicates preliminary clinical success. Although there is a need for more research with greater sample sizes, we may also begin to consider what future research questions may be posed.

The Future of MDMA Research

Grob and Danforth (MAPS, 2013b) will be launching a double-blind, placebo-controlled pilot study to assess the safety and feasibility of MDMA-assisted psychotherapy to treat social anxiety in adults on the autism spectrum. MDMA may be well suited to treat social anxiety as it produces decreases in fear and amygdalar responses to angry faces (Bedi, Phan, Angstadt, & de Wit, 2009). A recent study by Carhart-Harris et al. (2014) observed decreased communication between the medial temporal lobe and medial prefrontal cortex of healthy volunteers under the effects of MDMA while under fMRI. These changes in the limbic system are the opposite of what is observed in individuals who suffer from anxiety. Another rationale for the use of MDMA for social anxiety is the aforementioned elevation of oxytocin levels hypothesized to occur in the brain after MDMA administration. Increased levels of peripheral plasma oxytocin have been linked to prosocial feelings (Dumont et al., 2009).

Baggott (2013) proposes that a decrease in fear may be only a part of a more complex response to MDMA. In his research with healthy volunteers, participants were administered MDMA and completed a measure of authenticity. Those who received MDMA, compared to placebo, reported higher rates of authenticity operationalized as awareness and trusting of one's thoughts and feelings, acting in accordance with one's values, lack of interpretive distortions of self-relevant information, and acting with sincerity in relationship with close others. Thus, it may not be only a decrease in fear, but other psychological mechanisms that may lead to prosocial communicative behavior.

Another potentially promising application of MDMA is in the treatment of psychiatric conditions that exacerbate substance use disorders (Jerome et al., 2013). Currently, there are no published studies on the use of MDMA-assisted psychotherapy for this purpose. It is counter intuitive to use a drug that has the potential for abuse as a treatment for problematic substance use. However, MDMA may facilitate treatment by enhancing the psychotherapeutic process generally and more specifically by addressing psychological factors that contribute to substance misuse (Jerome et al., 2013). At this time, there are no studies being conducted to evaluate the feasibility of MDMA in the treatment of problematic substance use.

The Future of Psilocybin Research

Another novel area of study is the application of psilocybin as an adjunct to CBT for smoking cessation (Johnson, 2013). In this ongoing study, 50 participants with multiple unsuccessful quit attempts will receive the treatment. This consists of three psilocybin sessions, followed by eight weekly psychotherapy sessions to discuss the psilocybin experiences and provide support for smoking cessation. Although the study is yet to be completed, there are currently 12 of 50 participants who have been biologically confirmed as abstinent at 6 months post quit date. These biological markers include urinary nicotine and breath carbon monoxide levels.

There is renewed interest in the application of psilocybin in the treatment of addiction to alcohol. There is significant precedent for this research, as hundreds of articles were published focusing on LSD's potential to treat alcoholism in the 1960s. In a recent meta-analysis, T. S. Krebs & Johansen (2012) identified 546 participants in six randomized control trials published between 1966 and 1970. It was found that a single dose of LSD, accompanied with an alcohol treatment program, was associated with a decrease in problematic alcohol use at follow-up assessment, which ranged from 1 to 12 months after discharge from treatment programs. These effects were persistent at 3 months and 6 months, did not last at the 12-month period. Nonetheless, this is an impressive result for a single-dose treatment.

Bogenschutz (2013) is currently completing a small open-label pilot study examining the effects of psilocybin in 10 alcohol-dependent participants. The treatment provided uses two-dose sessions and incorporates Motivational Enhancement Therapy into 12 sessions over a 12-week period. Particular attention is paid to the role of spirituality in relation to the participant's alcohol use. It is hypothesized that the treatment will contribute to increases in motivation, self-efficacy, and spirituality, which are important factors in recovery from substance misuse. The study's primary outcome will be decreases in participant's drinking behavior. Once completed, it is likely that a study with a larger participant pool will be launched.

More generally, we can contrast the current paradigm for psychiatric treatment and the model of drug-assisted psychotherapy. Under the former paradigm, a person visits a psychiatrist, he or she is evaluated, and if deemed appropriate, he or she will be prescribed a medication. The person will then take the medicine daily, and is followed up with on a semiregular basis. The drug-assisted psychotherapy model, in contrast, requires a person to receive several sessions of psychotherapy in preparation for receiving the medicine. When ready, the person receives the drug in the context of a psychotherapy session, and then several integration psychotherapy sessions take place. Depending on the treatment, this cycle may repeat approximately one to three times. As such, this treatment may be considered a "brief therapy" with a psychopharmacological agent as an adjunct.

The medicine or adjuvant is thought to be beneficial through a synergistic relationship with the psychotherapy provided. However, it remains unclear how exactly the medicine aids in the psychotherapeutic process. Further investigations into this area will allow researchers to improve the psychotherapy, to offer maximum potential benefit to the participant. How current (often competing) evidence-based psychotherapies will be compatible with these medicines is unknown. Will an existing psychotherapeutic model work best in conjunction with these substances or will a novel model of psychotherapy emerge? These questions will continue to be investigated as research in this field continues.

Legal Status of MDMA and the Classical Hallucinogens

The classical hallucinogens and MDMA are classified as Schedule-I controlled substances in the United States, meaning "the drug or other substance has a high potential for abuse," "the drug or other substance has no currently accepted medical use in treatment in the United States," and "there is a lack of accepted safety for use of the drug or other substance under medical supervision (Office of Diversion Control, 2012)." It is therefore important to note that research presented in this chapter has been conducted under legal clinical and preclinical contexts. All published research is reviewed and approved or cleared by ethics review and multiple regulatory authorities. Considering the medical and psychotherapeutic potential of these substances and the relative safety demonstrated in the clinical data presented here, questions regarding the validity of the aforementioned scheduling should be raised.

Review Questions

- In what ways can the effects of MDMA and psilocybin be thought of as similar? In what ways are they different?
- What is set and setting? Why is it important?
- Which psychiatric ailments are currently being investigated with psilocybin-assisted psychotherapy? How may this treatment be helpful?
- Which psychiatric ailments are currently being investigated with MDMA-assisted psychotherapy? How may this treatment be helpful?
- Are the effects of drug-assisted psychotherapy purely pharmacological, psychotherapeutic, or both? Why may this be a challenging question to answer?
- Describe some of the psychotherapeutic approaches used in MDMA-assisted psychotherapy for PTSD.
- What are the risks associated with MDMA and psilocybin, respectively?
- Do you think MDMA and psilocybin are accurately scheduled substances?

CHAPTER THIRTEEN

Psychotropic Medication and the Elderly

By Elliott Ingersoll and Laura McIntyre

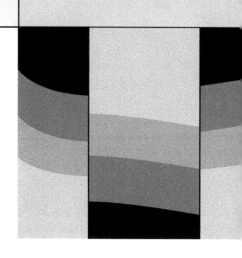

INTRODUCTION: THE NEW OLD AGE

Psychotropic medication and its use with elderly clients as a population is of particular interest to clinicians due to several unique cultural, psychological, social, and physiological factors. Living longer and better is likely an instinct and human desire as old as time, and can be attributed in part recently to more and better education about health and nutrition as well as to strides made in health knowledge and application through technology. It makes sense to address trends in areas regarding older adults that may influence use of psychotropic medications. Odd as it may seem, at a time when people are living longer than ever and requiring more geriatric psychiatrists (Grossberg, 2010) there are fewer geriatric psychiatry fellowships nationwide (Bragg, Warshaw, Cheong, Meganathan, & Brewer, 2012), and we are starting to fill the gap with other professionals like nurses (Beck, Buckwalter, Dudzik, & Evans, 2011).

Old age is typically a degenerative process of the body and mind that precedes physical death as we know it. As joyless as that sounds, as a construct it seems to also be culturally defined, and varies across cultures. Most developed countries have settled on age 65 as defining of the term elderly; however, as Susan Jacoby (2011) discusses in her book, *Never Say Die: The Myth and Marketing of the New Old Age* (2011), we are now finding ourselves in a storm of marketing and media tempting new categories of older adults to "beat old age" and live as fast, sexy, and exciting as their younger counterparts. "50 is the new 40" and so forth, are common marketing ploys to sell methods to live a higher quality of life the older we get (including better quality through pharmaceuticals). This is all modeled and tested on perfect models of old age, like people in their 60s and 70s. The problem is that most aspiring "oldsters" are in younger old age and not exactly representative of elderly populations such as those that mental health professionals work with in nursing homes. Whether these new standards of "successful aging" become ingrained in society or not, there is a need to address the use of psychotropic medications by clinicians to treat symptoms, behavior, degenerative mechanisms, and illnesses that could be attributed to typical aging or concurrent experiences during the aging process. This is challenging because literature on the use of psychotropic medications in the elderly can be flawed and misleading, for reasons explained in this chapter.

This chapter is divided into five sections. Section One describes *DSM-5* changes to delirium and dementia as well as medications to treat the two most common dementias. Section Two examines the state of psychosocial interventions for elderly clients. Section Three discusses pharmacologic treatment of dementia and other issues with psychotropic medications and the elderly. Section Four covers aging and assisted living. Finally, Section Five looks at side effects issues peculiar to the elderly.

SECTION ONE: *DSM-5* CHANGES TO DELIRIUM AND DEMENTIA

Learning Objectives

- Be able to describe *DSM-5* changes pertaining to Neurocognitive Disorders.
- Understand implications of changes in diagnostic criteria as it pertains to the elderly and clinical assessment and treatment.
- Understand use of etiological subtypes and cognitive domains in *DSM-5*.

The American Psychiatric Association (APA) has made several across-the-board changes in the *DSM-5*. Some changes in diagnosis appear to be a general move from attributing causation to a more dimensional perspective, instead highlighting developmental and life-span issues, which include several measures (where there is available data) of gender, race, and culture (including examining life-span functioning issues regarding disorders). Additionally, *DSM-5* incorporates the latest research and clinical expertise (including some exploration of biomarkers discussed with etiology, though like genetic testing, this is still an emerging concept), differential diagnoses to distinguish disorders from others comparatively, and examines risks and prognostic factors (American Psychiatric Association, 2013a).

Neurocognitive Disorders (NCDS)

Neurocognitive Disorders (NCDS) are a new addition as the categories in the *DSM-5* for what were previously Delirium, Dementia, Amnestic, and other Cognitive Disorders. NCD seems a preferred term anyway, to distinguish dementias not associated with degenerative aging (such as impairment secondary to a medical condition). On the other hand the term dementia will continue to be used in some settings. As we will see, several of the *DSM-5* changes are highly significant to working with the elderly adult population and not always for the better.

Major and Mild NCDs

The word "dementia" is Latin for "madness," and it seems the editors of *DSM-5* attempted, in a way, to reduce some of the stigma that seems to follow the word by replacing the word with two phrases: major neurocognitive disorder (major NCD) and mild neurocognitive disorder (mild NCD). There is no single disease called "dementia" (Gottfries, 1988). Dementias may arise from Alzheimer's disease, Parkinson's disease, Huntington's chorea, and Pick's disease to name a few. Their primary characteristics are declining cognitive function rather than a deficit, as previously utilized in diagnosis. In this sense, it separates them from neurodevelopmental disorders (NDs) in which the defining feature, a cognitive deficit, may be present from birth or developmentally impairing. It should be mentioned here that it is possible to develop an NCD against an existing ND. NCDs are unique in that we do know much more about the etiology of these than any other *DSM* disorder. Major and mild NCDs are generally distinguished in a subtle but significant way, by severity of cognitive impairment and severity of impairment of independence.

Major NCD concerns more severe impairments and stays consistent with medical terminology for the sake of appropriate treatment plans and to facilitate ongoing research. Major NCD brings together previous diagnoses including dementia and amnestic disorder, but is essentially dementia. The etiology of dementias is more well-known compared to most *DSM* disorders. The main purpose for a mild NCD category is a matter of debate. Some say it is more for nonmedical mental health professionals working with elderly clients who are still functioning somewhat independently. In this case, it allows for exploration of more effective treatment plans that focus on daily functioning and independence, maintaining and even preventing further decline in cognitive impairments. It could be considered an "early detection and intervention," system. For some clients it can allow them to make the most of the time they have before suffering a major NCD. For others it can help them maintain or improve functioning and stave off decline. That said, mild NCDs may be an early stage of a later major NCD. As Frances (2013) pointed out, the biggest problem with this new category of mild NCDs is that you are going to be creating millions of patients who may be suffering from nothing more than normal aging and for whom medications can only deliver side effects. He maintained that including mild NCD is basically giving a diagnostic label to a normal part of aging. He wrote that "I would heartily endorse MND if there were a treatment for it or if it provided a really good way of predicting the future. But there is no treatment and little predictive power ... accepting mental aging makes more sense than diagnosing it ..." (p. 180). Truth be told, we have no effective treatments for the dementias and to medicate more people is at this point in time reckless.

Etiological Subtypes

Etiological subtypes (which again, utilize the term dementia when appropriate) for major NCD and mild NCD include Alzheimer's disease, Frontotemporal lobe degeneration, Lewy body disease, Vascular disease, Traumatic brain injury and Substance or medication-induced dementias, HIV infection, Prion disease (e.g., bovine spongiform disorder), Parkinson's disease, Huntington's disease, as well as other causes.

MEDICATIONS FOR ALZHEIMER'S DISEASE AND PARKINSON'S DISEASE

The majority of medication for dementia is for Alzheimer's type dementia (AD), the most common type. AD is a cortical dementia as well as a progressive neurodegenerative disease that involves the irreversible loss of cholinergic neurons. It comes in two variations, an early-onset familial form that seems mostly genetic and a far more common late-onset form that is less rooted in genetics (or may not be at all due to genetic vulnerability) (Balin & Hudson, 2014). In 2013, AD is thought to cost the United States over $200 billion annually (Alzheimer's Association, 2013). Although we still do not know the full etiological picture for this dementia, the predominant problem is what are called neuritic senile plaques (NSP) and neurofibrillary tangles (NFT). NST are composed of beta-amyloid deposits that are key to the neuron death. NFT are made of modified tau protein. Genetic analyses have identified mutations in several genes that result in increased production and deposit of beta-amyloid. The beta-amyloid accumulates due to what is thought to be a problem between production and removal of beta-amyloid. The hypothesis of etiology derived from these findings is called Amyloid Cascade Hypothesis (Hardy & Higgins, 1992) and has been the most popular theory of etiology for 20 years (Balin & Hudson, 2014). The main alternate hypothesis centers on tau protein. Tau protein normally binds and contributes to the structure of microtubules (components of cytoskeleton of eukaryotic cells). An AD tau is hyperphosphorylated (meaning a biochemical site related to signaling mechanisms is saturated). This is what leads to the NFTs which disrupt neuronal transport and lead to cell death (Massoud & Gauthier, 2010). The ultimate strategy would be to develop a neuroprotective agent to modify the effects of beta-amyloid or a medication to flush it from the system before it builds to dangerous levels. Thus far, all we have are drugs to treat symptoms, not underlying causes. The symptoms are far more than cognitive decline. They include behavioral disorders, movement difficulties, mood and anxiety symptoms and what can only be described as radical personality changes.

CAN ALZHEIMER'S DISEASE BE PREVENTED?

Before we address medications, it is important to clarify whether there are any preventative efforts clients can engage to preclude AD. Popular lore is full of stories about being physically active, mentally active, using ginkgo but are they true? There is mounting evidence that the hippocampus is one of the last brain structures to fully mature and the first to be affected by AD. Could it be that environmental exposures during early life could influence later life onset of AD? Studies have suggested education, complexity of occupation, and an engaged lifestyle have protective effects (Carrillo et al., 2013). Exercise has also been associated with a reduced risk of dementia (Ahlskog, Geda, Graff-Radford, & Petersen, 2011). Exercise was linked to vascular health which was thought to have been preventative but the clinical trials to prevent AD with vascular health are contradictory. The first studies used blood pressure medication to see if that slowed cognitive decline. Three studies have shown that proper use of antihypertensive agents in hypertension and after a cerebrovascular event is associated with a reduction in the incidence of cognitive impairment (Tzourio et al., 2003). The recently completed HYpertension in the Very Elderly Trial (HYVET) study, however, showed that treatment of people over 80 is associated with a reduction in vascular problems but not cognitive impairment (Peters et al., 2008).

Well what about lifestyle? Worldwide, lower levels of education, physical inactivity, suffering from depression, and smoking were all correlated with AD risk (Barnes & Yaffe, 2011). In the United States physical inactivity, depression, smoking, and hypertension had the highest correlations with AD. Other risk factors include sleep-disordered breathing. *DSM-5* (APA, 2013) lists three sleep apneas that may be risk factors for AD: Obstructive Sleep Apnea, Central Sleep Apnea, and Sleep-Related Hypoventilation. The influence of diet is more controversial as some studies suggest that omega-3 fatty acids (Schaefer et al., 2006) or adherence to the "Mediterranean diet" could reduce one's risk of AD. However, in a State-of-the-Science Conference held by the National Institutes of Health (NIH) in 2010 there was not sufficient evidence found to say that these diet variables could decrease the risk of AD (Daviglus et al., 2011).

There are several planned and ongoing prevention trials for AD that focus on different populations including asymptomatic individuals and presymptomatic individuals with genetic risk factors. The Anti-Amyloid Treatment for Asymptomatic AD Trial (A4 Trial) is to be conducted by the National Institute on Ageing (NIA). This will study clinically normal beta-amyloid positive individuals who will receive an anti-amyloid therapy for a 3-year period.

The therapeutic agent for this trial is solanezumab/Alzforum which is basically an antibody directed at the beta-amyloid peptide. One trial of solanezumab/Alzforum funded by Eli Lilly with over 2000 patients, half of whom received solanezumab/Alzforum intravenously every 4 weeks for 18 months failed to show improvement in the primary outcomes (Doody et al., 2014). As we will see this is a variation on initial work done with cannabis compounds. A hypothetical biomarker model of AD is gaining credence. Amyloid imaging and cerebrospinal fluid (CSF) total tau (t-tau) and p-tau, and structural MRI to determine how close in time a particular person is to relevant cognitive events. For example, one recent study concluded that a reduction in the CSF levels of one type of beta-amyloid (beta-amyloid 42) is an early upstream marker of AD (Buchhave et al., 2012). With prevention research raising as many questions as answers, we will not turn to medications to treat the symptoms of AD (remembering there is no cure at this time).

ACETYLCHOLINESTERASE INHIBITORS

Acetylcholinesterase inhibitors (AChE-Is) are the most common drugs used to treat Alzheimer's disease (AD). The most common are donepezil/Aricept, rivastigmine/Exelon, and galantamine/Razadyne. For the most part, these agents have similar efficacy (Molino, Colucci, Fasanaro, Traini, Amenta, 2013; Tan et al., 2014). All these drugs bind to the enzyme (acetylcholinesterase) that breaks down acetylcholine (Ach) much in the same way MAO inhibitors attach to monoamine oxidase to prevent the breakdown of norepinephrine. The side effects include gastrointestinal distress, abdominal cramping, and in some cases anorexia. The main limitations to these medications is that there is only modest improvement at best and in all cases, if the patient lives long enough, the disease process will overtake what the medication can do. A newer treatment for AD is memantine/Namenda, which is an NMDA receptor antagonist that acts on the Glutamate (Glu) system. The homeostasis of the

Glu system is very delicate so NMDA antagonists (as mentioned in the chapters on mood stabilizers and antipsychotics) are hard to titrate. More research is needed before we can draw general conclusions on this compound.

Donepezil/Aricept is a piperidine derivative that reversibly inhibits acetylcholinesterase (remember from Chapter Five that not all inhibitors are reversible—e.g., MAO Inhibitor?). Birks and Harvey (2006) did a meta-analytic review of donepezil/Aricept efficacy across 24 trials with almost 6000 participants. Their findings showed significant improvement versus placebo at 24 weeks and 52 weeks on several measures related to cognition. They concluded that people with symptoms anywhere from mild to severe treated for periods of 12, 24, or 52 weeks experienced benefits in cognitive function. Positron Emission Tomography (PET) scans evaluated acetylcholinesterase (AChE) activity in 14 people with AD before and after treatment with donepezil/Aricept. The results showed modest inhibition of AChE with treatment, mostly in the cingulate cortex and this correlates with tests of executive function. As in all areas we have covered in this book, there are some who question the way efficacy is reported in donepezil/Aricept studies. Killin, Russ, Starr, Abrahams, and Della Sala (2014) noted that the effect size of donepezil/Aricept on cognition is larger in industry-funded trials than in independent trials. This is not explained by the longer duration of the industry-funded trials, suggesting perhaps the studies that are industry funded are methodologically designed to inflate the significance. There seems to be consensus that donepezil/Aricept is helpful but there is also consensus that it should not be given until symptoms develop. It is not a prophylactic.

Rivastigmine/Exelon is a carbamate derivative that reversibly inhibits both AChE and butyrylcholinesterase (BuChE). It is the only acetylcholinesterase inhibitor that also inhibits BuChE. BuChE is widely distributed in the central nervous system and might play a role in the function of acetylcholine neurons and neuronal degeneration. It is not clear how BuChE inhibition relates to rivastigmine/Exelon's efficacy. Birks, Grimley Evans, Iakovidou, Tsolaki, and Holt (2009) evaluated nine trials with almost 5000 subjects and found rivastigmine/Exelon at 6 to 12 mg daily is associated with significant improvement versus placebo. Winblad et al. (2007) studied the transdermal formulation and found it had similar efficacy to the tablets but with a 2/3 reduction in reports of nausea. Adler, Muller, and Articus (2014) also found that the transdermal formulation decreased caregiver burden and increased treatment adherence.

Galantamine/Razadyne is a tertiary alkaloid drug that reversibly inhibits AChE. It also binds to the nicotinic Ach receptors enhancing Ach function. The relevance of that to its efficacy though is at this time unclear. Cusi et al. (2007) reviewed 10 trials with almost 7000 participants with mild to moderate AD. The results suggest galantamine/Razadyne was significantly better than placebo. There was not a significant dose-response effect, doses above 8 mg daily were consistently significant. Comparative studies of these three AChE inhibitors led to conflicting results, which makes it hard to recommend one over another. Massoud and Gauthier (2010) recommend using tolerability of the compound as a guide as to which one to use. More recently Tan et al. (2014) found cognitive effects of all drugs to be significant. Memantine/Namenda (described next) was included in this study and the authors concluded there were more dropouts with AChE than with memantine/Namenda (which works via a different mechanism).

Memantine/Namenda is an N-methyl-D-aspartate (NMDA) receptor antagonist. Studies have shown that increased glutamate may lead to excitotoxicity and play a central role in AD (Sucher, Awobuluyi, Choi, & Lipton, 1996). By blocking the glutamate receptor the theory is that this will decrease the excitotoxicity. Massoud and Guthier (2010) summarized findings on the drug. In six trials with moderate-to-severe cases data showed significant benefits versus placebo at 6 months on measures of cognition. A trial comparing memantine/Namenda with donepezil/Aricept showed additional benefits in patients with moderate-to-severe symptoms. As noted, Tan et al. (2014) found that there were fewer dropouts with memantine/Namenda.

The other most common neurodegenerative disease is Parkinson's disease (PD). It occurs in about 1% of people 65–69 years old worldwide. PD is characterized by a progressive loss of dopamine (DA) neurons in a unique combination of brain regions, particularly the substantia nigra. As with Alzheimer's we can only treat the symptoms and in many cases the disease process will overtake what we can do with medication. The primary drugs used to treat PD all try to make up for the loss of DA neurons. Several DA agonists are used to treat PD including levodopa/Carbadopa, apomorphine/Apokan, lisuirde/Revenil, and pramipezole/Mirapex. The most common is levodopa/Carbadopa. Most agonists bind at D1 or D2 receptors. DA receptor stimulation in the dorsal striatum is the primary mechanism by which the drugs partly alleviate the motor features that are associated with PD. PD also affects 5-HT and NE neurotransmitters that may account for PD-related depression (Brichta, Greengard, & Flajolet, 2013). Levadopa is a precursor to DA and thus stimulates the production of DA in the brain. It is sometimes given with levodopa/Carbadopa to ease side effects like nausea. Unfortunately as time goes on each dose becomes less effective. Catechol-o-methyltransferase (COMT) inhibitors (like tolcapone/Tasmar) can help extend the effectiveness of levodopa/Carbadopa and prolong its effects but these medications may have severe side effects on the liver. In addition, there are side effects to levodopa, including induced dyskinesias (drug-induced abnormal movement). Newer therapies being investigated to treat these are glutamate and adenosine receptor antagonists (Blandini & Armentero, 2012).

Other drugs that have modest anti-Parkinsonian actions are amantadine/Symmetrel and memantine/Namenda. As noted memantine/Namenda is an NMDA antagonist and we described its actions above. Amantadine/Symmetrel is actually an antiviral and its mechanism of action in PD is unknown. Amantadine is actually an antiviral agent that has modest anti-Parkinsonian action. We do not know its mechanism of action but Advokat, Comaty, and Julien (2014) suggest it may "… alter dopamine release or reuptake, or it may have anticholinergic properties" (p. 569).

Given that the AChE-Is have been called "cognitive enhancers" and since "cognitive enhancement" has frequently been linked (if only in popular thought) with stimulants, what about treating symptoms of dementia with stimulants? The idea is not a new one and psychostimulants including caffeine and amphetamines have been used to treat various aspects of dementia and related problems from the early 20th century to the present (Rasmussen, 2008). In 1984 Loew posed the question as to whether stimulants might be a neglected option in treating what was then referred to as senility. Roccaforte and Burke (1990) reviewed the limited literature of the effects of stimulants on cognition, motivation, and depression. They concluded that the extant literature was promising enough to require more study. Galynker et al. (1997) did a pilot study to evaluate the effect of methylphenidate/Ritalin on the negative symptoms of dementia. Dementia from AD and vascular dementia were treated. They concluded that in both types of dementia, negative symptoms appeared responsive to methylphenidate/Ritalin. Padala, Burke, Bhatia, and Petty (2007) presented four cases of apathy that were treated with a regimen of methylphenidate/Ritalin. They noted significant improvement in apathy, motivation, and persistence. Following up on that, Padala et al. (2010) noted that methylphenidate/Ritalin was effective in treating apathy and depression in a 12-week treatment study. It is also interesting that in the Padala study no one dropped out due to adverse effects. Finally Rahman and colleagues (2006) tried to reduce abnormal risk-taking behavior in people with frontotemporal dementia using methylphenidate/Ritalin. They concluded that methylphenidate/Ritalin was effective in "normalizing" decision making in the test subjects without impairing other aspects of cognition.

There have been attempts to understand the relationship of caffeine to cognition and whether it could serve to decrease dementia symptoms. In a meta-analysis Santos, Costa, Santos, Vaz-Carneiro, and Lunet (2010) found that caffeine may serve as a mild neuroprotective agent but the differences in methodology made it difficult to conclude anything with certainty. Biessels (2010) concluded the same thing stating that there are not enough studies now to make anything more than general statements. Referencing the Cardiovascular Risk Factors, Aging and Incidence of Dementia (CAIDE) study,

Eskelinen (Eskelinen & Kivipelto 2010; Eskelinen, Ngandu, Tuomilehto, Soininen, & Kivipelto, 2009) noted that coffee drinking may be associated with a decreased risk of AD and that this may be mediated by the caffeine and/or other mechanisms like the antioxidant capacity of coffee.

A lesser-known research area is studying the neuroprotective properties of cannabis as well as the use of cannabis to ease some symptoms of dementia. Marchalant, Baranger, Wenk, Khrestchatisky, and Rivera (2012) suggested that because cannabinoids can positively affect age-related processes like neuroinflammation, neurogenesis, and memory, epidemiologic studies should be done on long-term, chronic cannabinoid users to assess their risk for developing AD compared to the general population. Aggarwal and Carter (2010) note that information (or misinformation as the case may be) disseminated by governmental organizations would lead most readers to the conclusion that cannabis has no benefits for the brain and nervous system. This is not the case at all. There are many peer-reviewed studies that support the hypothesis that the cannabinoids in marijuana have neuroprotective properties and can be used to treat neurotoxicity and neuroinflammation. Cannabis may limit the formation of neuritic plaques in the brain and perhaps slow the process of AD. Eubanks et al. (2006) reported that delta 9-THC, both in the test tube and in computer models, inhibited acetylcholinesterase (AChE—the enzyme that breaks down Ach) and prevents AChE amyloid plaque collection. They concluded that "THC is a considerably superior inhibitor of amyloid-B-peptide aggregation …" (p. 773). Other studies have shown that cannabidiol (CBD) and a synthetic cannabinoid (WIN-55, 212-2) can prevent brain cell death caused by exposure to amyloid plaques in animal models (Marchalant, Rosi, & Wenk, 2007; Marchalant et al., 2009).

In another study, Marchalant, Cerbai, Brothers, and Wenk (2008) reported that the number of activated microglia (active in immune defense) increase during normal aging. Stimulation of endocannabinoid receptors reduced the number of microglia in the hippocampi of young rats. The same holds true for older rats and if researchers get clearance to do human studies we may find that stimulation of the cannabinoid receptors could provide clinical benefits in age-related diseases like AD. Finally, Iuvone et al. (2004) demonstrated that CBD exerts a combination of neuroprotective, antioxidative, and antiapoptotic effects against beta-amyloid toxicity. At the time of this writing, it seems that the biggest barriers to research are all legal related to the federal criminalization of cannabis. As researcher Gary Wenk (2014) noted, if you are not connected to the only legal, grant-funded marijuana farm at the University of Missouri, it gets very expensive very quickly to conduct independent research as the time you put in just for legal clearance is itself a significant obstacle. As state decriminalization of marijuana expands, perhaps the federal prohibition will end, at least enough to allow unfettered, scientific research to resume.

Review Questions

- What are some general changes to the *DSM-5* that could benefit the elderly as a population?
- What are the changes to Delirium and Dementia in *DSM-5*?
- What are the primary drugs to treat Alzheimer's disease and how do they work?
- What are the primary drugs used to treat Parkinson's disease and how do they work?
- What are alternatives and/or preventative treatments for dementia?

SECTION TWO: THE STATE OF PSYCHOSOCIAL INTERVENTIONS FOR ELDERLY CLIENTS

Learning Objectives

- Describe several psychosocial interventions to treating elderly clients.
- Understand the need for further research and valid data to expand literature on nonpharmaceutical approaches.

Functioning of elderly people in a clinical context is clearly affected by social and coping skills and support. Looking through an integral lens at treating for mental health disorders, including organic disorders, we know that exploring all facets and dimensions of a client's experiences seems the most thorough way to diagnose and treat if needed, and also to decide if medication could be helpful, when psychosocial interventions can help or whether a combination would be more appropriate. There is growing evidence that psychosocial interventions can empower elderly clients to adapt to a variety of concerns unique to them psychosocially, and also adjust to illnesses and mental health disorders such as depression or cognitive impairments that are often correlated with aging. Proper clinical assessment of older clients' psychosocial experiences and changes they are experiencing is important for clinicians, as is empathically trying to understand the clients' belief systems.

Frank (2014) notes that depression in elderly people has been underreported for decades. Major Depressive Disorder (MDD) affects up to 20% of people older than 65. The point prevalence for MDD in people with Mild Cognitive Impairment (MCI) is approximately the same as in those without MCI (Polyakova et al., 2014). The elderly as a population represent 12% of the population but account for 20% of completed suicides. Males aged 75 and over have the highest rates of suicide in industrialized societies and in many countries suicide rates rise with age (Cattell, 2000). Some psychotropic medications are more highly correlated with suicide as hypnotics and benzodiazepines may increase the suicide risk almost 10-fold (Carlsten & Waren, 2009). Additionally, men account for 81% of suicides of people aged 65 and older. When assessing for later life depression, risk factors are female gender status, unmarried status, stressful life events, lack of social support, and concurrent medical illnesses. All of this is important when considering effective treatments. Many older clients have substantial comorbid conditions such as heart failure, diabetes, and cancer. Chronic disease is a risk factor for developing depression. Some clinicians estimate that antidepressants seem to have equivalent efficacy in younger and older adults but be reminded this may be only about 50% and many older people are not going to

tolerate the side effects for a limited return (Nelson & Devenand, 2011). Others note that when you add in cognitive impairment the antidepressant efficacy drops to 40% at best (Thase, Entsuah, & Rudolph, 2001). This is not just a medical question though. Whereas therapeutically our ethical commitment is on the side of life, it behooves all clinicians working with this population to really think through their own perspective on suicide. Is it always bad? Wrong? If so, why? Too often these existential questions are glibly overlooked exacerbating an already difficult situation when the client thinks the clinician is clueless about suffering, the meaning of life, and the quality of life.

Particularly because the elderly may not respond to medication, psychosocial interventions are important. One such intervention is Problem Adaptation Therapy (PATH). PATH involves the same therapeutic factors thought to be effective in most theories of psychotherapy including relationship and client strength factors but more specifically PATH focuses on the client's ecosystem. This includes the client, the home, and the caregivers if relevant. PATH incorporates environmental adaptation tools and invites participation from caregivers, hence this is more specific and focused than just supportive therapy (Kiosses, Arean, Teri, & Alexopoulos, 2009). PATH is an intervention conducted at the home to reduce depressive symptoms and disability in elderly clients with cognitive impairments and disability. Kiosses, Arean, Teri, and Alexopoulos (2010) found that PATH was more efficacious than Supportive Therapy (ST) in decreasing depressive symptoms in elderly clients.

Interpersonal Psychotherapy (IPT) is recommended for elderly clients as a treatment for depression and is shown to be significant in improving general mental and social functioning when used in place of general medical practitioner care. Like its name suggests, it is an intervention that focuses on interpersonal efficacy and functioning. It also uses techniques that focus on communication, to increase social support and puzzle out symptoms. A modified version is Interpersonal Psychotherapy for Mild Cognitive Impairment (IPT-MCI), which includes the client and a caregiver in sessions to promote a richer relationship between them. This can be especially helpful for "old-old" clients who may be experiencing more cognitive and medical issues, and with whom medication may be less effective and have more adverse side effects.

Problem-Solving Therapy for Mild Executive Dysfunction (PST-MED) is a 12-week session for ambulatory elderly clients, which teaches a five-step problem-solving model. The model is taught over the first five weeks of treatment and then the last seven sessions are dedicated to refining problem-solving skills (Alexopoulos et al., 2011; Arean et al., 2010). Participants set treatment goals, discuss and evaluate different ways to reach them, create plans and evaluate how well the plans worked. The results suggest that this not only assisted with planning but also reduced depressive symptoms in a considerable number in subjects with depression and cognitive dysfunction (Arean et al., 2010).

Cognitive Behavioral Therapy (CBT) has been shown to be a very effective treatment for depression in older adults (Doubleday, King, & Papageorgiuo, 2002) after screening for specific cognitive impairments, sensory impairments, and disability. Generally, even with a wider variability of measurable cognitive ability and considering decline of some cognitive abilities in later life, older people can be memory-trained and do well on sustained-attention tasks. According to McKeith et al., (1999), "'fluid intelligence' (the ability to acquire and manipulate new information, i.e., 'wit') declines with age whereas 'crystallized intelligence' (the cumulative product of information acquired as a result of fluid intelligence, i.e., 'wisdom') does not." Though research is still emerging, CBT can be utilized with a variety of issues pertaining to elderly people but may need some modifications as we currently see in other psychosocial interventions.

Group therapy is an effective treatment option for older adults, especially those who do not respond favorably to psychotropic medications or individual therapy. Though it has some inherent challenges like accessibility, group therapy can be empowering and transforming for elderly clients when they can socialize with other older adults and share age-related issues (Sochting, O'Neal, Third, Rogers, & Ogrodniczuk, 2013). There are many modalities of group therapy with music group therapy being one of the more effective. Group music interventions are noninvasive and inexpensive ways to reduce symptoms of depression.

These approaches also work with clients suffering from mild-to-moderate dementia. Because of the nature of the brain and what might be called musical intelligence (even if that is just the part of the brain shaped by the music you have listened to all your life), musical memories persist longer than some types of memories making this an evocative treatment approach. Chu and colleagues (2014) collected data on participants' prior musical experience, training (if any), and preferences. Other members of the team collected responses to dependent measures and took salivary cortisol samples as a measure of stress reduction. Although the cortisol levels pre and post were not significant, depressive symptoms were significantly decreased and cognitive functioning significantly delayed.

Other newer nonpharmacological interventions include aromatherapy (Thorgrimsen, Spector, Wiles, & Orrell, 2003), where aromatherapy showed benefit for people with dementia in one small trial. Also there are multisensory therapies, some using a therapeutic PARO robot. Paro is designed to look like a baby seal and was developed by a Japanese industrial automation pioneer Takanori Shibata. It has shown success in elevating mood in facilities where live animals would not be possible. Paro is equipped with five sensors: tactile, light, audition, temperature, and posture sensors with which it can perceive people and its environment. It can respond to sensory input by things like blinking, wagging its tail, and turning in the direction of a voice (Sabanovic, Bennett, Chang, & Huber, 2013). Research attempting to support significant efficacy over pharmacological interventions is also emerging, such as a Penn State College of Medicine pilot study that studied rates of psychotropic drug prescriptions for clients with dementia over 60 years of age in long-term care involved in a Group-based Creative Expression Storytelling Program compared to similar clients in a standard care activity program. The study attempted to explore whether there is a correlation between using the group-based creative program and reduced prescribing of psychotropic medications for clients with dementia (Houser, 2012).

The need to recognize psychosocial interventions as effective in treating a variety of aging issues often seems outweighed by a tendency to overdetermine symptoms in older adults. A number of noncognitive symptoms can be classified under such diagnoses as dementia without a full clinical evaluation, which could lead to nonpharmaceutical interventions as a primary approach. This often leads to diagnosis and treatment (not to mention how clients will understand their symptoms, which could be conflicting for them) using the medical model of disease rather than a more integrative approach to treatment, as well as inappropriate prescribing. Psychosocial interventions could be imagined as a valuable part of multidisciplinary preventative health programs for elderly people and that as people live longer, there are many promising and emerging alternatives to typical primary and secondary clinical treatments.

Review Questions

- Describe several psychosocial interventions for the elderly.
- Why should clinicians consider psychosocial interventions as a primary approach to treatment with the elderly as opposed to pharmacological approaches?
- What are the advantages of clinicians using an integral lens when considering treatment or utilizing preventative, multidisciplinary programs to care for older adults?

SECTION THREE: PHARMACOLOGIC TREATMENT OF DEMENTIA: FROM THE 20TH CENTURY AND INTO THE 21ST CENTURY

Learning Objectives

- Understand trends of psychotropic medication use and why it is relevant to the elderly.
- Describe several commonly prescribed psychotropic medications clinicians utilize to treat elderly clients.
- Describe several drawbacks to available literature regarding psychotropic drugs.

Psychotropic medications are very commonly prescribed for elderly clients (many are now saying overprescribed) in both community based and managed care (which includes several settings such as geriatric units, acute care geriatric units, and nursing homes). It is not only important for clinicians working with aging adults to be aware of rates of prescription, but important to gauge the accuracy of the literature available regarding pharmacological treatment. Whether benefits outweigh the risks of those treatments is of particular significance to clinicians working with elderly clients. In general, psychotropic prescription rates are increasing. Trends for elderly population in outpatient and in managed care settings show a high rate of psychotropic medication use, especially for women and clients in institutions. It should be noted that geriatric patients being treated for mental illness are more likely to have comorbid disorders and more likely to be overmedicated (Laroche, Charmes, Nouaille, Picard, & Merle, 2006; Procyshyn, Barr, Brickell, & Honer, 2010). Advokat et al. (2014) state emphatically "The elderly are frequently prescribed medication that they do not need or that cause them significant problems either because of extensions of expected pharmacological effects or through adverse interactions with other medications. Inappropriate medication use in the elderly is a major functional and safety issue …" (p. 556). The other big problem is, like many overmedicated children, the elderly are increasingly likely to be on multiple psychotropic medications. Sabzwari, Qidwai, and Bhanji (2013) warn that increasing polypharmacy with psychotropic medications seems to be correlated with increased risk for iatrogenic (preventable harm arising from medical treatment) error.

One problem in nursing homes is that patients are inappropriately medicated more because of staff distress than patient need. Zuidema, Jonghe, Verhey, and Koopmans (2011) looked at staff distress and the nursing home environment and their effects on psychotropic drug use. They found that both staff distress and negative aspects of the nursing home environment were positively correlated with more drugs being used for the patients. Human beings it seems have a healthy denial of death (one can't ruminate on it all day) that merges with an unhealthy "blind eye" turned toward how poor most nursing home environments really are. If you doubt this ask yourself how you felt the last time you visited a nursing home. If you haven't visited one recently, why not? Why not go "hang out" and talk with residents? In Oberlin Ohio, a unique quality of life program allows graduate students from a local music academy live rent free in nursing homes and pay for room and board by doing concerts and tending to the instruments there. It is innovative programs like this that will bridge the distance we have created between our elderly and the rest of our society.

One solution to polypharmacy in nursing homes was proposed by Smeets et al. (2013) in the form of a program with the acronym PROPER (PRescription Optimization of Psychotropic drugs in the Elderly nuRsing home patients with dementia). This was a multicenter cluster randomized, controlled, pragmatic trial using parallel groups with a duration of 18 months with 4 six-monthly assessments. The intervention consisted of structured and repeated medication review supported by education and continuous evaluation. It involved pharmacists, physicians, and nurses. There were three parts to this: (1) preparation and education, (2) conduct, (3) evaluation and guidance. The ongoing (at the time of this writing) trial is expected to decrease overmedication simply by making it an object of awareness for all involved. Simple as this sounds it makes sense. We always tell our students that all psychotherapy is helping clients make aspects of themselves and their lives objects of awareness. The same holds true for ethical practice in any profession.

COMMONLY PRESCRIBED PSYCHOTROPIC MEDICATIONS IN ELDERLY POPULATION

DEPRESSION

According to the Centers for Disease Control (CDC) the highest rate of suicide deaths for males and females is in the 50–54 age group with about 20 suicides per 100,000. The next highest is the 54–59 age group, and adults 65 and older have a suicide rate of about 15 per 100,000 but for males alone it is 32 per 100,000. For males 85 and older the rate jumps to approximately 47 suicides per 100,000 people (CDC, 2014). Older adults prefer to receive their mental health treatment from their primary health care provider but Advokat, Comaty, and Julien warn that may not be the best approach. As Frances (2013) noted, general practitioners often *do* have strong relationships with their patients but are not specifically trained in psychiatry and especially geriatric psychiatry. Team approaches can be useful but often are too expensive given the shortage of professionals to treat the elderly. In studying patients with depression older than age (Reynolds et al., 2011), the team cautioned that adding an antidepressant to a cognitive enhancer like donepezil/Aricept requires careful weighing of risks and benefits. This again points to the increase in complexity when treating comorbid conditions. Efficacy has also been demonstrated for escitalopram/Lexapro, and duloxetine/Cymbalta (Dolder, Nelson, & Stump, 2010). Of course there are downsides too. Some researchers have found SSRI use in the elderly is correlated with increased risk of falls (likely due to dizziness) (Sterke, Ziere, van Beeck, Looman, & van der Cammen, 2012).

ANXIETY

We know Anxiety Disorder continues to be a problem in old age (Blay & Marinho, 2012). We have already touched on the concern that certain anxiolytics (benzodiazepines) can be problematic in the elderly as they are correlated with higher suicide rates and falls. We also know that elderly patients coming to emergency rooms are more likely to be prescribed benzodiazepines (Spanemberg et al., 2011). Although many books on psychopharmacology do not ask the obvious question, we will. If benzodiazepines are so problematic for elderly clients why prescribe them? Whereas many clients prefer benzodiazepines to SSRI antidepressants (and they do have more efficacy for anxiety than SSRIs), in several studies, long-term use of benzodiazepines in elderly clients is associated with poorer outcomes in anxiety and sleep (Beland et al., 2010; Nordfjaern, 2013), psychomotor impairment (Bulat, Castle, Rutledge, & Quigley, 2008), and increased risk of falling (Quigley, Barnett, Bulat, & Friedman, 2014). In some cases patients may be taking these because these were the only drugs available when they were first treated for anxiety. In other cases some people may get genuine benefits and in others tolerance and dependence may be a reason the patients request for the medications. Many recommend new guidelines like not using benzodiazepines for more than 30 days or limited prescriptions to those benzodiazepines like alprazolam/Xanax that have shorter half-lives (Lindsey, 2009).

PSYCHOSIS/AGITATION

The behavioral and psychological symptoms of dementia (BPSD) include delusions, apathy, depression, agitation, and irritability. The most difficult of these for caregivers are delusions, agitation, and irritability (Fauth & Gibbons, 2014). The Omnibus Budget Reconciliation Act (OBRA) of 1987 was legislation that aimed to combat misuse of psychotropic medications as well as protect clients in long-term care/nursing homes from unnecessary "physical or chemical restraints imposed for purposes of discipline or convenience" (Omnibus Budget Reconciliation Act, 1987). Additionally, the Health Care Financing Administration (HCFA) regulates nursing homes that use Medicaid and Medicare programs and has created a set of guidelines and regulations to further OBRA in an attempt to reduce inappropriate prescribing.

Atypical antipsychotics have been used more than neuroleptics recently because it was thought that the EPS in neuroleptics is too problematic for the elderly. Well that concern is now being replaced with concern over the atypicals as the severity of their side effect profile becomes more known and problematic (Gurevich, Guller, Berner, & Tal, 2012). In addition in 2005 the FDA issued a black-box warning against the use of atypicals for BPSD in the elderly (FDA, 2005). The warning stated that "Of a total of seventeen placebo controlled trials performed with olanzapine

(Zyprexa) aripiprazole (Abilify), risperidone (Risperdal), or quetiapine (Seroquel) in elderly demented patients with behavioral disorders, fifteen showed numerical increases in mortality in the drug-treated group compared to the placebo-treated patients" (p. 1). In some ways given the severe side effects of the atypical antipsychotics it is hard to believe they would not cause some level of damage. Despite the warning and the controversy that surrounds it, treatment of BPSD with atypicals continues though may be declining for another reason. The Centers for Medicare and Medicaid Services (CMS) have always targeted excessive use of antipsychotics in the absence of an appropriate diagnosis or necessity. Beginning in May 2012 an initiative called Partnership to Improve Dementia Care initiated training and research on humane methods to deal with BPSD. The use of atypical antipsychotics will continue to be part of the CMS quality review of facilities (Advokat et al., 2014).

We are still in need of better research with more representative sampling for medicating elderly clients. As early as 1997, Satlin and Wasserman lamented that the literature regarding pharmacological treatment of the elderly is fallible for a variety of reasons, including:

- Many studies utilize younger-old clients, 55–65 years of age to represent a population of people in trials receiving antidepressant therapy when a larger population of older people are actually the ones receiving them.
- Many subjects in studies are the picture of health when many older adults are actually suffering from physiological illnesses. The advantage of this in research is clear but it is not a true representation.
- Many studies are inclusive of clients with only mild/moderate symptoms.

Finally, discussing prescription rates for the elderly seems to merit concern about compliance with psychotropic medication prescribing, but there are two sides to the coin. Elderly clients may be unwitting targets for misleading, dangerous, and even fatal attempts to keep them in compliance with taking drugs pushed on them with tempting direct-to-consumer (DTC) advertising, still legal in the United States. Most DTC drug advertisements zone is on seniors to sell expensive, newer drugs that promise seniors they will treat, but not cure, their ailments. With physicians being coerced, the FDA being laissez-faire regarding ads backing up claims and "Big Pharma" valuing profit over lives, seniors are at a disadvantage and are at risk (Lurie, 2005).

This leads us to a short summary of the primary ethical issues in geriatric psychiatry that must be examined in case of elderly clients being treated with psychotropic medication. The first issue is autonomy versus family or group centrism. Does a medication provide more autonomy for the client? If so does that offset the risk of adverse effects. Even individuals who desire autonomy must sometimes accept that they will require help from family or other caregivers. This raises the ethical concern of who can be told what about medications. Rabins and Black (2010) note that "… in the absence of objections raised by the elder, there is implicit agreement that the involvement of family members is ethically appropriate … however since this contradicts regulations in the USA (HIPPA) and the principle of autonomy … judgment and caution should be exercised" (p. 268). Another issue is caregiving, which straddles the autonomy family centric dilemma. One of the biggest conflicts is when the provider has therapeutic relationships with the provider of care and the recipient of care. If those parties have conflicting goals, consideration should be given to drawing in another professional so that each party has their own clinician/advocate.

Another important concern for nonmedical and medical mental health professions is elder abuse. The elderly are a vulnerable group at increased risk for abuse. According to Lachs and Pillemer (2004), there are three main elements of abuse: harm, a trust relationship, and intent. Clinicians are charged with assessing whether abuse may have occurred and this requires the clinician to make judgments that require ethical considerations. Rabins and Black (2010) give an example of questioning intent when a caregiver becomes frustrated and makes a verbal statement that harms the ill person. They ask, if the perpetrator of harm is suffering from exhaustion and poor judgment? This, they say can be as incapacitating temporarily as dementia can be long-term. Note that careful and repeated consideration of challenging situations and regular discussion is the best approach. This leads to the ethical imperative for the caregiver: self-care. We know that caregivers of people with dementia take psychotropic drugs (benzodiazepines and antidepressants) more frequently than caregivers of patients without dementia (Camargos et al., 2012). This is attributed to the particular stress of caring for someone suffering from dementia. Can clinicians help caregivers find resources that allow for them to renew their energies after long periods caring for a loved one? This is also an ethical imperative for medical and nonmedical mental health professionals.

Another important ethical imperative in working with the elderly is surrogate decision making. Cognitive impairment disrupts decision-making capacity and the ability to consent to medical procedures and other relevant choices. For medical procedures, decisions should be made by a caregiver or substitute whom the patient has previously chosen and identified in advance (preferably through the appropriate legal documents). There are two legal standards for surrogate decision making. The first is "… substituted judgment used if the patient's wishes are known to the surrogate or 'best interest', used if the patient's wishes are not known" (Rabins & Black, 2010, p. 270). The use of advance directives can be one way of maximizing a client's autonomy. These document a person's values and wishes from general to specific ways. There can be many reasons people do not execute such directives: lack of education, cultural norms, or just the healthy denial of existential givens like illness and dying that all of us have. The final ethical imperative Rabins and Black (2010) cover is end-of-life issues. The older we get the more we should intentionally make our end-of-life wishes known but, as Jacoby (2011) points out, when 80 is the new 50 why rush things? There is also a large body of research that illustrates that people who have advance directives change their minds after developing a life-threatening illness. If that person has appointed a durable power of attorney that person can act in "best interest."

Review Questions

- What do prescription rates look like in general? For elderly people?
- What are some commonly prescribed psychotropic drugs for older adults?
- Why should we take literature regarding pharmacological treatment of the elderly with a grain of salt, as clinicians?
- What are the primary ethical issues to consider when working with elderly clients?

SECTION FOUR: AGING AND ASSISTED LIVING

Learning Objectives

- Describe several challenges to elderly clients living in managed care/assisted living settings.
- How has legislation attempted to change inappropriate prescribing?

Deinstitutionalization in the late 1960s was prompted by the federal government, ending Medicaid payment for state psychiatric hospitals and institutions for the treatment of mental health. Their point was twofold: to end poor conditions in these facilities and throw the cost back onto states for such care. Theoretically, better functioning and independence to help former patients adapt to community living should have been a focus of treating people with mental disorders, though many psychiatric patients were instead dumped into various other settings like nursing homes and geriatric units. Inappropriate prescribing of psychotropic drugs in managed care settings is a recent concern along with issues of abuse, social stigma, and the unique needs of the elderly with regards to side effects of psychotropic

medications (discussed in the next section of this chapter). Assisted living carries risks like abuse, stigma, inadequate care, and improperly trained staff. In many instances even when staff are trained the staff to patient ratio is rarely optimal. For the most part we know that direct care staff (trained or not) are far more comfortable than assisted living administrators in dealing with resident's mental health needs. Whereas administrators are more often concerned about liability (such as getting sued for *not* chemically restraining a resident who may fall or otherwise injure himself) the direct care staff are more focused on the resident (Dakin, Quijana, & McAlister, 2011). If there are not enough direct care staff, prescribed psychotropic drugs that have differential or adverse side effects for older adults in managed care facilities may not even be noticed, let alone monitored properly. Between 35 and 53% of assisted living clients were receiving one or more psychotropic medications, but only 45% of nursing home nurses had proper psychiatric training (Lindsey, 2009).

Review Questions

- What are the obstacles for older adults needing treatment in assisted living settings?
- What are the significant legislative attempts made to combat issues of abuse and inappropriate prescribing of psychotropic medications in nursing homes? What else can be done?

SECTION FIVE: SIDE EFFECTS PECULIAR TO THE ELDERLY

Learning Objectives

- Describe various side effects peculiar to the elderly as a population.
- Understand the implications of adverse side effects for the elderly.

Older adults are especially prone to adverse side effects and can be more frail and sensitive to side effects that may be more tolerated by their younger counterparts. Age-related physiological changes can cause differences in pharmacokinetics and pharmacodynamics, as well as cause adverse side effects and exacerbate both existing psychiatric disorders and concurrent medical problems. People older than 70 are 3.5 times more likely to be admitted to hospitals due to adverse side effects than their younger counterparts, and the risk for these reactions rises drastically with the number of medications they are taking as well as with their age (Lindsey, 2009).

PSYCHOTROPIC SIDE/ADVERSE EFFECTS IN ELDERLY CLIENTS

As you can tell from this chapter, there is still debate about which medications cause the most problematic side effects for elderly clients. Given that most Americans, and especially the elderly, are on more than one medication, it becomes difficult to discern which medications or combinations of medications are responsible for which adverse events. It is interesting that in reviewing side effects in the elderly in studies conducted in the United States, the benzodiazepines come in for far more criticism than other classes of psychotropic medications. Studies conducted outside the United States more often implicate multiple classes of psychotropic medications as well as nonpsychotropic medications. For example, one research team in Brazil (de Paula, Bochner, & Montilla, 2012) found that antibiotics were as or more likely to cause falls. Another study in Australia concluded antidepressants, anxiolytics, hypnotics, and antipsychotics (or a combination) are all associated with falls and fractures in females but not males (Vitry, Hoile, Gilbert, Esterman, & Luszcz, 2010). This may relate to the extreme and confused nature of U.S. policies on any drugs that may be potentially abused. It is also of interest that social use of alcohol is far more accepted in European societies and in the United States. Even though alcohol use among the elderly can be a problem, many elderly people have moderately enjoyed a cocktail at the end of the day and all of a sudden something like moving into assisted living is supposed to end this

(ask yourself how many bars you've seen in assisted living facilities).

There are also multiple dermatologic adverse effects that the elderly may be more susceptible to. Adverse Cutaneous Drug Reactions (ACDRs) are the most frequent adverse events in patients receiving psychotropic medications (Mitkov, Trowbridge, Lockshin, & Caplan, 2014). Whereas some of these are benign and easily treated, others (like Stevens–Johnson syndrome) can be life-threatening. For the benign reactions, clinicians will want to weigh the risks of discontinuation versus taking the patient off the medication if they are suffering from suicidality or suffering from severe symptoms (Bliss & Warnock, 2013). Common ACDRs include pruritus (an unpleasant sensation in the skin that provokes itching), which can be caused by antidepressants, mood stabilizers, and antipsychotics. Exanthematous reactions are an idiosyncratic, T-cell mediated, delayed hypersensitivity reactions that can cause extreme, red macules (flat discolored area) and papules (a solid, discolored elevation of the skin). Urticaria (hives) and angioedema (swelling similar to hives but under the skin) are the second most common ACDRs. Fixed drug eruptions (lesions that appear within hours of taking the medication and can be mild to severe) and photosensitivity vary in severity and can be caused by antidepressants, mood stabilizers, and antipsychotics. Alopecia (hair loss) is associated with various antidepressants, mood stabilizers, and antipsychotics. These are just some of the more common dermatologic reactions and the interested reader should go to Bliss and Warnock (2013) for a complete list.

Review Questions

- What are psychotropic medication side effects as they pertain to older adults?
- What are the implications for prescribing psychotropic drugs to elderly clients?
- How can clinicians weigh the benefits and risks for prescribing as opposed to alternative treatments?

Clearly as we are all living longer, we will continue to struggle more with psychological issues. The field of geriatric psychiatry is still in its developing stages and currently is perhaps overemphasizing pharmacological interventions. Although more research is needed on the efficacy of psychosocial interventions, we clearly have enough evidence that in many cases psychosocial interventions are preferable to medications (like benzodiazepines). The biggest hurdle in this area may be convincing Medicare to allot more funding for psychosocial interventions, particularly in assisted living facilities.

As noted in the beginning of this chapter, the past several decades have seen a significant increase in the population of older adults and associated mental health problems throughout the world. We are beginning to recognize the multifaceted nature of the problem and the fact that this is going to call for a complex set of solutions (Lim & Aizenstein, 2014). The "one-size-fits-all" approach that is adopted by pharmaceutical company marketing is a poor response to the most radical demographic shift our species has ever experienced. If we put quality-of-life concerns first, backed by using interventions that have efficacy, we stand a good chance of increasing the quality of services we can deliver to elderly clients. As emphasized throughout this book, being mindful of what psychotropic medications can and cannot deliver is the first step to freeing funding and energy for complementary interventions. If all goes well, we will all get to see old age and I am sure we all want to have access to interventions that help us maintain an optimal quality of life.

Glossary

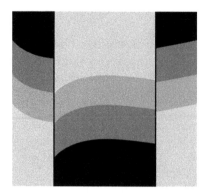

acetate A salt or ester of acetic acid, which is the essential component in vinegar.

adherence The degree to which a client adheres to a medication regimen particularly with regard to dosage and time of day taken.

allopathic treatment model A type of treatment that works by introducing agents (usually medications) that act in a manner opposite to the symptoms. In this book, the allopathic model represents what we are calling the *medical model perspective.*

amine hypothesis of depression The hypothesis that depression is caused by a lack of amine-based neurotransmitters such as norepinephrine and that antidepressant medication somehow corrects this "chemical imbalance." This has been found to be too simplistic to explain the dynamics of antidepressant medication.

anhedonia One of the so-called vegetative signs of depression, meaning a loss of pleasure or joy in all things.

antagonists Drugs whose main mechanism of action is to block a receptor site without exerting any particular action.

antihistamines A class of drugs that block histamine receptors in the body and decrease the influence of histamine.

antihypertensive A class of drugs whose effects decrease blood pressure.

antischizophrenic An early word used to describe medications that decreased the symptoms of Schizophrenia. Later replaced by the word *antipsychotic.*

anthropomorphizing Giving a nonhuman entity like a neuron human qualities. It is a literary device to try to increase understanding but may obscure it if not used properly.

anxiolytic "Anxiety reducing"; medications used to treat anxiety.

arborization The process of dendritic growth in which dendrites grow to make connections with other neurons.

associative tolerance This is where one would display tolerance to a drug in some but not all settings. What seems to be the case is that contextual cues associated with drug onset act as conditioned stimuli that can bring about tolerance.

atypical antipsychotics A class of antipsychotic medications that work very differently from the older or "typical" antipsychotics. The atypical antipsychotics include clozapine and the serotonin-dopamine antagonists.

autonomic nervous system The system of nerves that innervates the blood vessels, heart, viscera, smooth muscles, and glands. This system controls involuntary functions and is divided into the sympathetic and parasympathetic nervous systems (see glosses).

autonomic side effects Side effects that are affecting the autonomic nervous system.

autoreceptors These receptors, when stimulated, send a message back inside the neuron to decrease the output of whatever neurotransmitter the neuron produces.

bradykinesia Fatigue when performing repetitive movements.

brain stem A component of the central nervous system also called the "reptilian brain," because it is evolutionarily the oldest section of the brain. The brain stem controls many vital functions such as respiration and heart rate.

Broca's area A cerebral area in the inferior frontal gyrus associated with the movement necessary for speech. Named after Paul Broca, the 19th-century neurologist, who concluded that the left frontal lobe was implicated in articulation of speech.

bromide A salt of hydrobromic acid consisting of two elements, one of which is bromine.

catecholaminergic hypothesis of depression The first variation of the amine hypothesis of how antidepressants work. Created by Ernst Albert Zeller and his research team, the hypothesis was that catecholamine neurotransmitters (especially norepinephrine—NE) played a role in depression possibly by the person with depression being deficient in NE. When serotonin (5-HT) was also suspected the catecholamine hypothesis was broadened to the amine hypothesis.

category error Using the wrong knowledge tool to pursue an issue or answer a question. An example is using a blood test to find out who a person's favorite actress is. In a category error, the tool or questions are not illegitimate, but the wrong tool is selected. Category errors are common when disciples of one approach to reality (such as scientists) believe their tools are the right tools for all approaches.

central nervous system The brain and spinal cord.

cognitive triad of depression Three elements that according to Aaron Beck's cognitive therapy are present in depression: negative views about self, negative views about the world, and negative views about the future.

comorbidity Term used when a child, adolescent, or adult has more than one diagnosis in Axis I of the section of a five-axis diagnosis.

compliance The overall extent to which a client takes medication as prescribed.

contraindications Conditions that prohibit the use of a medication. For example, lithium is contraindicated in patients with kidney or liver disease because such diseases make it difficult for the body to metabolize and eliminate lithium.

corpus striatum A striped mass of white and gray matter located in the front of the thalamus in each brain hemisphere. This area is related to regulating motor behavior and the brain's reward centers.

cultural perspective One of four perspectives referred to in this book. This one reflects shared worldviews and beliefs that are loosely referred to as *culture*. These could also include what we might refer to as "subcultures"; for example, the subculture of the pharmaceutical industry or the subculture of the helping professions in general.

cultural psychiatry A special field of psychiatry concerned with the cultural aspects of human behavior, mental health, psychopathology, and treatment. It promotes culturally competent treatment and aims to expand human knowledge of human behavior.

cytochrome P-450 enzyme system The enzyme system in the human liver that governs most of the metabolism of psychotropic medications that is done by the liver.

delirium A disturbance in consciousness (usually temporary) characterized by restlessness, excitement, and sometimes hallucinations.

Delphic motto The Delphic injunction "Know thyself" is inscribed over the archway leading into the Temple of Delphi, which was dedicated to the god Apollo and occupied by the Delphic oracle.

delusions False beliefs that persist despite a preponderance of evidence to the contrary.

dendrites The branching processes of a neuron with receptors on them that conduct signals toward the cell.

dendritic growth The constant growth of dendrites to form synapses or connections with other neurons. Also sometimes called *arborization*, because its appearance is similar to the branching growth of a tree (from *arbor*, Latin for tree).

dependence In reference to drug dependence, dependence is defined physically and mentally. Physical dependence is the tolerance built up to the effects of a drug so that more and more of the drug become necessary to get the same effect. This type of dependence is also associated with withdrawal symptoms on discontinuation of the drug. Psychological dependence is the conviction that one cannot get through the day without taking some of the drug on which one is psychologically dependent.

depolarized The state of a neuron when it fires. This state is characterized by an influx of positive ions and a pumping out of negative ions.

developmental lines The simultaneous occurrence of several aspects of human growth and development. Cognitive, emotional, linguistic, psychomotor, and gender development (to name a few) occur simultaneously in the toddler.

Developmental Pharmacology The study of brain development in children and adolescents after the infusion of a psychotropic medication focusing on brain development in two key areas, including the impact on brain plasticity or the brain's ability to shape itself in response to environmental or chemical input and the impact on sensitive periods, which are developmental epochs when neural representation is happening before hard wiring occurs.

Diffusion How organisms exchange food, waste, gasses, and heat with their surroundings. The rate of diffusion is represented by Fick's law, which states that diffusive flux goes from regions of high concentration to regions of low concentration.

direct-to-consumer (DTC) advertising Advertising for psychotropic medications that is aimed at the consumer of the medication (the client or patient) rather than the prescriber of the medication (the physician). This type of advertising was prohibited by law until the 1980s.

disinformation False information intentionally spread to advance a political agenda.

dopamine hypothesis of Schizophrenia The hypothesis that Schizophrenia was somehow caused by too much dopamine in the brain, the overactivity of dopamine, or the oversensitivity of dopamine receptors. This theory, although useful for understanding some antipsychotic medications, is too simplistic to account for the spectrum of symptoms seen in Schizophrenia.

double-blind, randomized, placebo-controlled trials The "gold standard" of design for clinical trials of medication. These trials are conducted in a manner so that the participants and doctors do not know who is getting the medication and who is getting the placebo (double blind), assignment of drug conditions is random (randomized), and a placebo is used. A placebo is a compound that might appear to be a drug but that is thought to exert no influence on the symptoms being examined. A placebo can be active or inert. Studies with active placebos produce smaller effect sizes.

downregulation The decrease in the number and sensitivity of receptors on a neuron in response to the presence of a drug.

Dysthymia A category of mood disorder in the *Diagnostic and Statistical Manual* of the American Psychiatric Association that refers to a low-grade, chronic depression that persists for two years or longer.

dystonia A neurological disorder marked by involuntary muscle spasms that can cause painful twisting of the body.

dystonic reaction A reaction to a psychotropic medication that manifests as various dystonias.

ego-dystonic symptoms Symptoms that are in contrast to the way a client views himself or herself. These are typically easier to treat than symptoms that the client identifies with (ego-syntonic).

encephalon Generally referring to the brain.

enculturation The process through which people, starting in childhood, acquire a cultural system through their environment, particularly from parents and schools. This does not always mean that the individuals acculturate to the major culture.

endocrine glands Glands such as the thyroid, adrenal, and pituitary glands that secrete certain substances, particularly hormones, directly into the blood.

entheogen Literally, "god-manifester"; a drug that has been highly correlated with mystical insights, such as psilocybin or LSD.

epiphenomenon Any secondary phenomenon—in the context of this book, referring to the mind as a secondary phenomenon to the brain.

equanimity A state of mental or emotional composure, especially under stressful circumstances. It can be cultivated in various meditative practices and is viewed as one of the tools whereby a person can develop a healthy detachment (not dissociation) from powerful emotions, which allows the person so detached to have more choices in how to respond to such emotions. Equanimity is a disposition introduced by Buddhism as one of the four sublime states. In the Buddhist context, it is the practice of approaching an interaction with respect and caring while remaining unattached to how the interaction unfolds and how one is treated.

ethnopharmacotherapy A newer subdiscipline of psychopharmacology that explores how objectively different groups of people respond differently to medications. The differences explored include race, ethnicity, sex, and gender.

etiology The cause or origin of a disease.

euphorant A drug that induces euphoria.

euthymia A clinical term meaning neither manic nor depressed. Derived from a Greek root meaning joyous and tranquil.

extrapyramidal system the system in the brain related to motor skills that includes the cerebellum, subthalamus and basal ganglia

extrapyramidal motor system This system is made up of the subthalamus and the basal ganglia and is involved in fine motor movement. This system is seriously disrupted by the older antipsychotic medications called *neuroleptics*.

extrapyramidal symptoms or side effects Side effects caused by drugs interfering with dopamine neurons in these nervous system structures. Usually refers to side effects of neuroleptic drugs (also called *typical* or *first-generation antipsychotics*).

first-messenger effect The effect of a drug molecule or neurotransmitter binding to a receptor.

flat affect The lack of emotional expression that is one of the negative symptoms of Schizophrenia. Flat affect is also a side effect of neuroleptic or typical antipsychotic medication.

G protein A family of receptors so named because they bind guanine nucleotides. This family plays an important role in second-messenger systems described in this book.

glucose A simple sugar that is the principal source of energy for all living organisms.

hallucinations The experience or perception of physical stimuli when none appears to exist (such as hearing voices when no voices are within hearing range). Hallucinations are one of the positive symptoms of Schizophrenia.

homeostasis A state of balance.

Huntington's Chorea A hereditary chorea (disease of the nervous system characterized by jerky, uncontrolled movements) characterized by gradual deterioration of the brain and loss of movement.

hyperpolarization the state of a neuron characterized by being negatively charged (more negative ions inside the cell and positive ions outside). This negative charge decreases the probability that a cell will fire.

hypertension Medical term for high blood pressure.

hypnotic A classification of drugs used to induce or assist with sleep.

illusion Similar to a hallucination, the misperception of stimuli that actually exist.

ketoacidosis A feature of uncontrolled diabetes that combines two sets of symptoms: ketosis and acidosis. Ketosis is an accumulation of substances called *ketone bodies* in the blood. These bodies are made when there is not enough insulin in the blood and the body must break down fat instead of sugar (glucose) for energy. Acidosis is increased acidity of the blood.

Kluver-Bucy syndrome Emotional and behavioral changes associated with damage to the amygdala and inferior temporal cortex. Symptoms include characterized by diminished fear and aggression as well as amnesia and hyper sexuality. The syndrome can also result from Pick's disease, a progressive dementia beginning in middle life thought to be caused by an abnormal buildup of the tau protein.

lability The quality of being labile or prone to sudden emotional changes ("swings") from one extreme to the other.

lifetime prevalence An estimate at a given time of all the individuals who have ever suffered from a particular disorder.

lipophilicitous The quality of being fat soluble.

locus coeruleus A cluster of neurons that release norepinephrine and appear to have projections to most norepinephrine neurons in the brain.

loose associations A positive symptom of Schizophrenia in which mental associations are not governed by logic but idiosyncratically.

lysergic acid diethylamide (LSD) A hallucinogen characterized as a nonspecific amplifier of intrapsychic contents; discovered in 1943.

macromolecule A very large molecule composed of hundreds or thousands of atoms.

magic bullet Colloquially, an ideal drug that targets only a problematic area or tissue without disturbing surrounding areas or tissues.

major tranquilizer Colloquially—and inaccurately—antipsychotic medications.

mammalian brain The portion of the brain that encompasses the midbrain and limbic system characteristic of brains in mammals (colloquial).

medical model perspective One of four perspectives referred to in this book, this is the perspective of scientific materialism and the dominant perspective in biological psychiatry. This perspective uses scientific method to explore observable, measurable aspects of the individual. Although this perspective has been very successful in allopathic medicine, it has been less successful in treating mental and emotional disorders.

megalomania A highly exaggerated and/or delusional concept of one's self-importance.

mesencephalon Midbrain.

midbrain Referring to mesencephalon.

minimal brain dysfunction (MBD) This diagnosis from the 1960s vaguely attempted to categorize some symptoms of both ADHD and ODD. This diagnosis prompted the development of a norm for methodology to evaluate the effects of drugs, particularly stimulants on children.

minor tranquilizer Anxiolytic medications such as the benzodiazepines; colloquial.

misinformation Typically, a misunderstanding that arises from one of several factors. Not to be confused with "disinformation," which is the intentional spread of false information.

mitochondrion (plural, mitochondria) An organelle (cell organ) in the cell cytoplasm that has its own DNA inherited from the maternal line and that produces enzymes essential for energy.

molecular structure In psychopharmacology, the arrangement of molecules in a particular drug compound.

mood stabilizer An ill-defined category of psychotropic medication whose main purpose is treating bipolar mood disorders and aggressive, acting-out behaviors. The phrase is actually attributed to the marketing arm of Abbott labs rather than any research that supported the idea of such "stabilization."

Multimodal Treatment Study, The A study sponsored by the National Institute on Mental Health (NIMH) to examine children with ADHS who received stimulant medication only, received behavioral therapy only, or received both stimulant and behavioral therapy. In general, almost all children improved in their symptoms, but the children with the combined treatment demonstrated greater gains.

negative feedback loop A description, from behavioral theory, of a cycle that is thought to underlie depression. It assumes some stressors have disrupted normal behavior, and the reinforcers that normal behavior used to bring have stopped. This can set up a cycle of self-criticism and further withdrawal or depressive behaviors that then bring new reinforcement to make up for the reinforcers that were lost. This is called a *negative feedback loop (secondary gain)* when the depressive behaviors cause the people in the support network to gather together around the crisis of the person's depression.

negative symptoms of Schizophrenia Symptoms of Schizophrenia that are characterized by the absence of a quality that normally exists, such as a range of emotion, volition, and sociability.

neocortex Literally, "new brain"; the outermost layer of the brain to develop latest in the evolutionary history of the brain.

neuroleptic Older or "typical" antipsychotic medications, most of which work through dopamine antagonism. Literally, "neuron clasping."

neurons Specialized impulse-conducting cells that are the functional units of the nervous system.

noradrenergic Activity related to norepinephrine; synonymous with *noradrenalin*.

nucleus (plural, nuclei) Mass of gray matter in the brain or spinal cord.

off-label use A drug being used for a purpose not reviewed or approved by the Food and Drug Administration.

on-label use A drug used in a manner that the Food and Drug Administration has approved. Approval means that evidence for efficacy and effectiveness has been presented with regard to the on-label use.

overdetermined In reference to symptoms of many mental or emotional disorders, we say that the disorders and symptoms are "overdetermined," meaning that they likely are caused by multiple variables ranging from biological, to psychological, to cultural, to spiritual.

paranoia One of the positive symptoms of Schizophrenia; manifests as an unwarranted mistrust of others.

parasympathetic nervous system A subdivision of the autonomic nervous system that is active during conservation of energy.

parenteral Administered by injection.

Pediatric Rule In 1998 the FDA came out with this rule to *require* pharmaceutical companies to assess the safety and effectiveness of new drugs. On October 17, 2002, the U.S. District Court of Columbia ruled that the FDA did not have authority to issue this rule.

peripheral nervous system The nervous system lying outside the brain and spinal cord and containing the somatic and autonomic nervous systems.

permeable Capable of being permeated. In psychopharmacology, usually refers to cell membranes through which drug molecules can pass.

Persistent Depressive Disorder A new *DSM-5* label (for what used to be called "Dysthymia" under *DSM-IV*) in the new section called "Depressive Disorders."

pharmacodynamics The mechanisms of how drugs act on the body.

pharmacokinetics The mechanisms of how the body reacts to and acts on drug molecules introduced into it.

phenomenological The subjective experience of phenomena.

phospholipid biolayer Two layers of lipid molecules that form a polar membrane. Phospholipids are the major components of cell membranes so named because they contain an organic molecule from the phosphate group.

phytotherapy From the Greek, meaning "plant therapy." Used in reference to herbaceuticals.

placebo response Response similar to a response to a drug that occurs when the patient is given a placebo (a substance thought to be inert with regard to the symptoms under study). This is not a well-researched area although in many drug trials, the placebo response is almost as strong as the response to the medication.

pleasure centers (of the brain) Neural pathways in the brain thought to mediate rewards. These pathways are typically dopaminergic in quality.

polypharmacy Mixing several medications to alleviate symptoms.

positive symptoms Symptoms of Schizophrenia that are present and are not normal (such as hallucinations, delusions, and paranoia).

postsynaptic In the sequence of events in neural transmission, refers to the part of the sequence enacted after the neurotransmitters pass through the cleft and bind to receptors.

precursor compounds Compounds that are combined to make neurotransmitters (for example, tryptophan is a precursor compound necessary for production of serotonin).

presynaptic In the sequence of events in neural transmission, refers to the part of the sequence enacted before neurotransmitters pass through the cleft and bind to receptors.

prophylactic Having some preventive quality.

protein kinase C A second-messenger-system-dependent protein kinase (substance that helps create enzymes) that plays a pivotal role in how a cell responds to extracellular stimuli.

psychic energizers A psychodynamic concept prevalent in U.S. psychiatry in the 1950s. If a drug was thought to be a psychic energizer, it was believed to somehow liberate repressed id energy that the ego could then use.

psychological perspective One of four perspectives referred to in this book; the perspective that represents the subjective experience of the client. This includes thoughts, feelings, and worldviews as well as such things as mystical or intuitive experiences. Although this perspective registers changes in brain activity, to date we cannot conclude that the experiences divulged through exploring this perspective are "caused by" the brain.

psychotropic From the Greek; "acting on" or "moving toward" the mind.

Pulmonary system The pulmonary system includes the lungs and the muscles of breathing that pump air in and out of the lungs.

pyramidal cells Large neurons shaped like pyramids found in the hippocampus and frontal cortex and implicated in motor function.

relativism A philosophical position that any one position or perspective is just as good as any other position or perspective. As Ken Wilber points out, this is an irrational position in that it is self-contradictory, because it assumes that the proposition that no position is any better than another itself presumes to be better than alternative propositions.

reptilian brain Colloquially, the brain stem, the part of the human brain hypothesized to appear earliest in evolution.

resting state The state of a cell when it is polarized (its electrical charge is balanced).

second-messenger effects Effects that occur through second-messenger systems that include the impact of G-proteins and enzymes after a neurotransmitter binds to a receptor.

self-efficacy A construct pioneered by Albert Bandura that is related to a person's belief that he or she can accomplish things in life and do some things well. People with low self-efficacy believe they cannot do what they need to get what they want in life.

side effects Effects distinct from main effects. Side effects are just effects unnecessary to the proposed therapeutic action of a drug. They occur to the extent that a drug is "dirty" or affects areas other than the desired area.

social perspective One of four perspectives referred to in this book, the social perspective deals with the measurable aspects of groups, namely, institutions of society related to psychopharmacology. These include institutions such as the Food and Drug Administration.

somatic nervous system The part of the peripheral nervous system that connects with sense receptors and skeletal muscles.

somatosensory cortex The region of the cortex whose primary input is from the somatosensory nuclei.

state-dependent learning A phenomenon through which memory retrieval is most efficient when an individual is in the same state of consciousness as they were when the memory was formed.

sympathetic nervous system The part of the autonomic nervous system that is active during arousal, such as in fight, flight, or freeze responses.

synapse The combination (juncture) of the presynaptic neuron, the synaptic cleft, and the postsynaptic neuron.

tardive dyskinesia Late-appearing, abnormal movement. One of four extrapyramidal side effects attributed to some antipsychotic medications.

telencephalon The anterior (front) section of the forebrain, consisting of the cerebrum and olfactory lobes.

teratogen Literally, an agent that may produce monsters or monstrous growths. Medically speaking, agents correlated with the presence of birth defects.

teratogenesis The development of birth defects. The adjective *teratogenic* refers to agents that may produce monsters or monstrous growths. Medically this is understood as referring to agents that are correlated with the presence of birth defects.

thought disorder A positive symptom of Schizophrenia. Can manifest as a disorder in the stream, content, or form of thoughts.

tolerance The clinical state of reduced responsiveness to a drug that can be produced by a variety of mechanisms, all of which result in the person needing increased doses of the drug to achieve effects previously attained by lower doses.

toxic environment A phrase we first came across in workshops with psychologist James Garbarino, who used the word to describe environments typified by high rates of poverty, little access to resources, and high rates of violence.

typical antipsychotics Although several classes of drugs fall into this category, they all exert their effects by dopamine antagonism. Also known as neuroleptic or first-generation antipsychotics.

upregulation The increase in number and sensitivity of receptors on a neuron in response to the presence of a drug.

urate Salt of uric acid.

vegetative symptoms Generally, symptoms relating to bodily processes that are performed involuntarily or unconsciously. In psychopharmacology, symptoms that express physically (poor appetite, sleep disturbance) rather than psychologically.

visual cortex The section of the cortex associated with input from the visual system.

Wernicke's area A section of the left temporal lobe in the human brain that is involved in comprehending words and producing meaningful speech.

word magic In this book, using words to create an illusion of certainty where only speculation exists.

word salad A positive symptom of Schizophrenia that manifests as linguistic disorganization so pronounced it can impair effective communication.

References

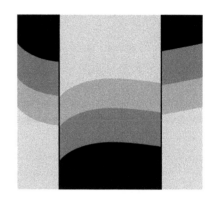

Abidi, S., & Bhaskara, S. M. (2003). From chlorpromazine to clo-zapine: Antipsychotic adverse effects and the clinician's dilemma. *Canadian Journal of Psychiatry, 48,* 749–755.

Abood, R., & Martin, B. R. (1992). Neurobiology of marijuana abuse. *Trends in Pharmacological Sciences, 13,* 480–485.

Addolorato, G., Abenavoli, L., Leggio, L., & Gasbarrini, G. (2005a). *How many cravings? Admissions.* Rockville, MD: Substance Abuse and Mental Health Services.

Addolorato, G., Cuore, R., Armuzzi, A., Gasbarrini, G., De Lor-enzi, G., Ancona, C., et al. (2005b). Pharmacological approaches to the management of alcohol addiction. *European Review for Medical and Pharmacological Sciences, 6,* 89–97.

Adler, G., Muller, B., & Articus, K. (2014). The transdermal for-mulation of rivastigmine improves caregiver burden and treat-ment adherence of patients with Alzheimer's disease under daily practice conditions. *International Journal of Clinical Practice, 68,* 465–470.

Advokat, C. D., Comaty, J. E., & Julien, R. M. (2014). *Julien's primer of drug action: A comprehensive guide to the actions, uses, and side effects of psychoactive drugs.* New York: Worth.

Aggarwal, S. K., & Carter, G. T. (2010). Cannabinoids and neuro-protection. In J. Holland (Ed.), *The pot book: A complete guide to cannabis; its role in medicine, politics, science and culture* (pp. 295–301). Santa Cruz, CA: MAPS.

Ahlskog, J. E., Geda, Y. E., Graff-Radford, N. R., & Petersen, Y. C. (2011). Physical exercise as a preventive or disease-modifying treatment of dementia and brain aging. *Mayo Clin-ical Practice, 86,* 876–884.

Akamine, Y., Yasui-Furukori, N., Ieiri, I., & Uno, T. (2012). Psy-chotropic drug-drug interaction involving P-Glycoprotein. *CNS Drugs, 26,* 959–973.

Akiskal, H. S., & Benazzi, F. (2006). The DSM-IV and ICD-10 categories of recurrent [major] depressive and bipolar II dis-orders: Evidence that they lie on a dimensional spectrum. *Journal of Affective Disorders, 92,* 45–54.

Akiskal, H. S., & McKinney, W. T. (1973). Depressive disorders: Toward a unified hypothesis. *Science, 182,* 20–29.

Alexander, C. N., & Langer, E. J. (1990). *Higher stages of human development.* New York: Oxford University Press.

Alexopoulos, G. S., Raue, P. J., Klosses, D. N., Mackin, R. S., Kanellopoulos, D., McCulloch, C., et al. (2011). Problem solving therapy and supportive therapy in older adults with major depression and executive dysfunction: Effect on disabil-ity. *Archives of General Psychiatry, 68,* 33–41.

Alloy, L. B., Urosevic, S., Abramson, L. Y., Jager-Hyman, S., Nusslock, R., Whitehouse, W. G., et al. (2012). Progression along the bipolar spectrum: A longitudinal study of predictors of conversion from bipolar spectrum conditions to bipolar I and bipolar II. *Journal of Abnormal Psychology, 121,* 16–27.

Almeida, V., Levin, R., Peres, F. F., Niigaki, S. T., Calzavara, M. B., Zuardi, A. W., et al. (2013). Cannabidiol exhibits anxio-lytic but not antipsychotic property evaluated in the social interaction test. *Progress in Neuro-Psychopharmacology & Biologi-cal Psychiatry, 41,* 30–35.

Alper, K. R. (2001). Ibogaine: a review. *The Alkaloids: Chemistry and Biology, 56,* 1–38.

Alper, K. R., Lotsof, H. S., Frenken, G. M., Luciano, D. J., & Bas-tiaans, J. (1999). Treatment of acute opioid withdrawal with ibogaine. *The American Journal on Addictions/American Academy of Psychiatrists in Alcoholism and Addictions, 8*(3), 234–242.

Alper, K. R., Lotsof, H. S., & Kaplan, C. D. (2008). The ibogaine medical subculture. *Journal of Ethnopharmacology, 115*(1), 9–24. doi:10.1016/j.jep.2007.08.034

Alramadhan, E., Hanna, M. S., Hanna, M. S., Goldstein, T. A., Avila, S. M., & Weeks, B. S. (2012). Dietary and botanical anxiolytics. *Medical Science Monitor, 18,* RA40–RA48.

Alzheimer's Association. (2013). *2013 Alzheimer's disease facts and figure.* Chicago: Author.

American Academy of Child & Adolescent Psychiatry. (2001, January 9). *AACAP work force fact sheet.* Retrieved May 30, 2014, from http://www.aacap.org/App_Themes/AACAP/docs/Advocacy/federal_and_state_initiatives/workforce/work_force_fact_sheet_2012.pdf

American Academy of Child & Adolescent Psychiatry. (2007). Practice parameter for the assessment and treatment of chil-dren and adolescents with attention-deficit-hyperactivity dis-order. *Journal of the American Academy of Child and Adolescent Psychiatry, 46,* 894–921.

American Academy of Child & Adolescent Psychiatry. (2009). Practice parameter on the use of psychotropic medication in children and adolescents. *Journal of the American Academy of Child and Adolescent Psychiatry, 48*(9) 961–973.

American Academy of Child & Adolescent Psychiatry. (2011). ADHD: Clinical practice guideline for the diagnosis, evaluation, and treatment of attention-deficit-hyperactivity disorder in children and adolescents. *Pediatrics, 128,* 1007–1021.

American Academy of Child & Adolescent Psychiatry. (2012). Practice parameter for the assessment and treatment of children and adolescents with attention-deficit-hyperactivity disorder. *Journal of the American Academy of Child and Adolescent Psychiatry, 54,* 678–682.

American Academy of Pediatrics. (2001). Clinical practice guidelines: Treatment of the schoolaged child with attention deficit/hyperactivity disorder. *Journal of Pediatrics, 108,* 1033–1044.

American Academy of Pediatrics. (2011). ADHD: Clinical practice guideline for the diagnosis, evaluation, and treatment of attention-deficit hyperactivity disorders. *Pediatrics, 128,* 1–18.

American Methadone Treatment Association. (1998). *1998 methadone maintenance program and patient census in the U.S.* New York, NY: AMTA.

American Psychiatric Association. (1994). *Diagnostic and statistical manual of mental disorders* (4th ed.). Washington, DC: Author.

American Psychiatric Association. (2000a). *Diagnostic and statistical manual of mental disorders* (4th ed., text rev.). Washington, DC: Author.

American Psychiatric Association. (2000b). *Practice guidelines for the treatment of psychiatric disorders: Compendium 2000.* Washington, DC: Author.

American Psychiatric Association. (2013). *Diagnostic and statistical manual of mental disorders* (5th ed.). Washington, DC: Author.

American Psychological Association. (1995). *Curriculum for level one training in psychopharmacology.* Washington, DC: Author.

American Psychological Association. (2011). Practice guidelines regarding psychologists' involvement in pharmacological issues. *American Psychologist, 66,* 835–849.

Amstutz, U., Ross, C. J., Castro-Pastrana, L. I., Rieder, M. J., Shear, N. H., Hayden, M. R., et al. (2013). HLA-A 31:01 and HLA-B 15:02 as genetic markers for carbamazepine hypersensitivity in children. *Clinical Pharmacology and Therapeutics, 94,* 142–149.

Anastasopoulos, G., & Photiades, H. (1962). Effects of LSD-25 on relatives of schizophrenic patients. *The Journal of Mental Science, 108,* 95–98.

Anderla, G. (1973). *Information in 1985: A forecasting study of information needs and resources.* Paris: Organization for Economic Cooperation and Development.

Anderla, G. (1974). *The growth of scientific and technical information: A challenge.* Washington, DC: National Science Foundation.

Andersen, L. S. (2005). A personal communication with Carl F Rak.

Andreasen, N. (2000). Schizophrenia: The fundamental questions. *Brain Research Reviews, 31,* 106–112.

Andreasen, N. (2001). *Brave new brain.* New York: Oxford University Press.

Androutsos, C. (2012). Schizophrenia in children and adolescents: Relevance and differentiation from adult schizophrenia. *Psychiatrike, 23,* 82–93.

Angrist, B., Rotrosen, J., Kleinberg, D., Merriam, V., & Gershon, S. (1977). Dopaminergic agonist properties of ephedrine: Theoretical implications. *Psychopharmacology, 55,* 115–120.

Angst, J., Azorin, J. M., Bowden, C. L., Perugi, G., Vieta, E., Gamma, A., et al. (2011). Prevalence and characteristics of undiagnosed bipolar disorders in patients with a major depressive episode: The BRIDGE study. *Archives of General Psychiatry, 68,* 791–798.

Anthony, J. C., Warner, L. A., & Kessler, R. C. (1994). Comparative epidemiology of dependence on tobacco, alcohol, controlled substances, and inhalants: Basic findings from the national comorbidity survey. *Experimental and Clinical Psychopharmacology, 2,* 244–268.

Anton, R. F., O'Malley, S. S., & Ciraulo, D. A. (2006). Combined pharmacotherapies and behavioral interventions for alcohol dependence: The COMBINE study. A randomized controlled trial. *JAMA, 295*(17), 2003–2017.

Appel, P. W., Ellison, A. A., Jansky, H. K., & Oldak, R. (2004). Barriers to enrollment in drug abuse treatment and suggestions for reducing them: *American Journal of Drug and Alcohol Abuse, 30,* 129–153.

Aquila, R. (2002). Management of weight gain in patients with schizophrenia. *Journal of Clinical Psychiatry, 63*(Suppl. 4), 33–36.

Arean, P. A., Raue, P., Mackin, R. D., Kanellopoulos, D., McCulloch, C., & Alexopoulos, M. D. (2010). Problem solving therapy and supportive therapy in older adults with major depression and executive dysfunction. *American Journal of Psychiatry, 167,* 1391–1398.

Arif, S. A., & Mitchell, M. M. (2014). Iloperidone: A new drug for the treatment of schizophrenia. *American Journal of Health-System Pharmacy: AJHP: Official Journal of the American Society of Health-System Pharmacists, 68,* 301–308.

Armstrong, D., & Winstein, K. J. (2008). Antidepressants in scrutiny over efficacy. *The Wall Street Journal.* Retrieved May 14, 2014, from http://online.wsj.com/news/articles/SB120051950205895415

Armstrong, T. (1997). *The myth of the ADD child: 50 ways to improve your child's behavior and attention span without drugs, labels, or coercion.* New York: Plume.

Aronson, J. K., & Reynolds, D. J. M. (1992). ABC of monitoring drug therapy: Lithium. *British Medical Journal, 305,* 1273–1276.

Asburg, M., & Traskman, L. (1981). Studies of CSF 5-HIAA in depression and suicidal behaviour. *Advances in Experimental Medicine and Biology, 133,* 739–752.

Asghar, S. A. (2002). Case report of 5 bipolar disorder patients (rapid cycling) followed for 3 years, treated with lamotrigine. *European Psychiatry, 5*(Suppl. 1), 109.

Ashburner, J., & Friston, K. J. (2001). Why 'voxel-based morphometry' should be used with imperfectly registered images. *Neuroimage, 14,* 1238–1243.

Ashton, C. H. (2001). Pharmacology and effects of cannabis: A brief review. *British Journal of Psychiatry, 178,* 101–106.

Asslian, P. (2000). Sildenafil for St. John's wort-induced sexual dysfunction. *Journal of Sex and Marital Therapy, 26,* 357–358.

Associated Press. (2009). *Eli Lilly settles Zyprexa lawsuit for $1.42 billion.* Retrieved May 4, 2014, from http://www.nbcnews.com/id/28677805/ns/health-health_care/t/eli-lilly-settles-zyprexa-lawsuit-billion/#.U2aoEvldU3k

Astin, J. A. (1998). Why patients use alternative medicine: Results of a national study. *Journal of the American Medical Association, 279,* 1548–1553.

Atack, J. R. (2000). Lithium, phosphatidylinositol signaling, and bipolar disorder. In H. K. Manji, C. L. Bowden, & R. H. Belmaker (Eds.), *Bipolar medications: Mechanisms of action* (pp. 1–30). Washington, DC: American Psychiatric Press.

August, G. J., Realmuto, G. M., MacDonald, A. W., Nugent, S. M., & Crosby, R. (1996). Prevalence of ADHD and comorbid disorders among elementary school children screened for disruptive behavior. *Journal of Abnormal Child Psychology, 24,* 571–595.

Aupoint, O., Doerfler, L., Connor, D. F., Stille, C., Tisminetzke, M., & McLaughlin, T. J. (2013). A collaborative care model to improve access to pediatric mental health services. *Administration Policy in Mental Health, 40,* 264–273.

Avery, R. J., Eisenberg, M. D., & Simon, K. I. (2012). The impact of direct-to-consumer television and magazine advertising on antidepressant use. *Journal of Health Economics, 31,* 705–718.

Avissar, S., & Schreiber, G. (1989). Muscarinic receptor subclassification and G-proteins: Significance for lithium action in affective disorders and for the treatment of extrapyramidal side effects of neuroleptics. *Biological Psychiatry, 26,* 113–130.

Avorn, J., & Kesselheim, A. (2011). A hemorrhage of off-label use. *Annals of Internal Medicine, 154,* 556–557.

Avram, M. J., & Donnelley, M. B. (2013). The pharmacokinetics and pharmacodynamics of zaleplon delivered as a thermally generated aerosol in a single breath to volunteers. *Journal of Clinical Pharmacology, 1,* 152–159.

Awad, G., Hassan, M., Loebel, A., Hsu, J., Pikalov, A., & Rajagopalan, K. (2014). Health-related quality of life among patients treated with lurasidone: Results from a switch trial in patients with schizophrenia. *BMC Psychiatry, 14,* 53.

Azzaro, A. J., Ziemniak, J., Kemper, E., Campbell, B. J., & VanDenBerg, C. (2007). Pharmacokinetics and absolute bioavailability of selegiline following treatment of a healthy subjects with the selegiline transdermal system (6mg/24h): A comparison with oral selegiline capsules. *Journal of Clinical Pharmacology, 47,* 1256–1267.

Babyak, M., Blumenthal, J. A., Herman, S., Khatri, P., Doraiswamy, M., Moore, K., et al. (2000). Exercise treatment for major depression: Maintenance of therapeutic benefit at 10 months. *Psychosomatic Medicine, 62,* 633–638.

Badal, D. W. (1988). *Treatment of depression and related moods: A manual for psychotherapists.* Northvale, NJ: Jason Aronson.

Badal, D. W. (2003). *Treating chronic depression: Psychotherapy and medication.* Northvale, NJ: Jason Aronson.

Bader, A., & Adesman, A. (2010). Complementary and alternative therapies for children and adolescents with ADHD. *Current Opinion in Pediatrics, 24,* 760–769.

Baggott, M. J. (2013). *Beyond fear: MDMA and emotion.* Retrieved from http://www.maps.org/conference/ps13matthewbaggottmdma/

Baggott, M. J., Coyle, J. R., Erowid, E., Erowid, F., & Robertson, L. C. (2011). Abnormal visual experiences in individuals with histories of hallucinogen use: A Web-based questionnaire. *Drug and Alcohol Dependence, 114*(1), 61–67. doi:10.1016/j.drugalcdep.2010.09.006

Balderer, G., & Bobely, A. A. (1985). Effect of valerian on human sleep. *Psychopharmacology (Berl[in]), 87,* 406–409.

Baldessarini, R. J., Tondo, L., & Hennen, J. (1999). Effects of lithium treatment and its discontinuation on suicidal behavior in bipolar manic depressive disorders. *Journal of Clinical Psychiatry, 60*(Suppl. 2), 441–448.

Baldessarini, R. J., Tondo, L., Hennen, J., & Viguera, A. C. (2002). Is lithium still worth using? *Harvard Review of Psychiatry, 10,* 59–75.

Baldwin, D. S., & Talat, B. (2012). Should benzodiazepines still have a role in treating patients with anxiety disorders? *Human Psychopharmacology, 27,* 237–238.

Balin, B. J., & Hudson, A. P. (2014). Etiology and pathogenesis of late-onset Alzheimer' disease. *Current Allergy Asthma Report, 14,* 417–426.

Ball, J. C., & Ross, A. (1991). *The effectiveness of methadone maintenance treatment: Patients, programs, services and outcome.* New York: Springer Publishing.

Ballenger, J. C. (1995). Benzodiazepines. In A. F. Schatzberg & C. B. Nemeroff (Eds.), *The American Psychiatric Press textbook of psychopharmacology* (pp. 231–246). Washington, DC: American Psychiatric Press.

Ballenger, J. C., & Post, R. M. (1980). Carbamazepine (Tegretol) in manicdepressive illness: A new treatment. *American Journal of Psychiatry, 137,* 782–790.

Balon, R. (1999). Positive aspects of collaborative treatment. In R. Balon & M. B. Riba (Eds.), *Psychopharmacology and psychotherapy: A collaborative approach* (pp. 1–32). Washington, DC: American Psychiatric Association.

Banaschewski, T. (2009). Editorial: Mood irritability—do we need to refine the diagnostic validity of oppositional defiant disorder and pediatric bipolar disorder? *The Journal of Child Psychology and Psychiatry, 50,* 201–202.

Bandelow, B., Boerner, R. J., Kasper, S., Linden, M., Wittchen, H. U., & Moller, H. J. (2013). The diagnosis and treatment of generalized anxiety disorder. *Deutsches Ärzteblatt International, 110,* 300–310.

Barber, J. P., & Luborsky, M. L. (1991). A psychodynamic view of simple phobia in prescriptive matching: A commentary. *Psychotherapy, 28,* 469–472.

Barclay, L. (2002). Aripiprazole may change schizophrenia treatment. *Medscape Wire, 1,* 2–4.

Barkley, R. A. (1998). *Attention-deficit hyperactivity disorder: A handbook for diagnosis and treatment* (2nd ed.). New York: Guilford Press.

Barkley, R. A., DuPaul, G. J., & Conner, D. F. (1999). Stimulants. In J. Werry & M. Aman (Eds.), *Practitioner's guide to psychoactive drugs for children and adolescents* (2nd ed., pp. 213–247). New York: Plenum.

Barkley, R. A., Karlsson, J., Strzelecki, E., & Murphy, J. V. (1984). Effects of age and Ritalin dosage on the mother-child interactions of hyperactive children. *Journal of Consulting and Clinical Psychology, 52,* 750–758.

Barlow, D. H., & Durand, V. M. (2002). *Abnormal psychology: An integrative approach.* Belmont, CA: Wadsworth.

Barnard-Brak, L., & Brak, V. (2011). Pharmacotherapy and academic achievement among children with Attention-deficit hyperactivity disorder. *Journal of Child and Adolescent Psychopharmacology, 21,* 597–603.

Barnes, D. E., & Yaffe, K. (2011). The projected effect of risk factor reduction on Alzheimer disease prevalence. *Lancet Neurology, 10,* 819–828.

Baroni, A., Lunsford, J. R., Luckenbaugh, D. A., Toubin, K. E., & Leibenluft, E. (2009). Assessment review: The diagnosis of Bipolar I disorder in children and adolescents. *Journal of Child Psychology and Psychiatry, 50,* 203–215.

Barrickman, L. L., Perry, P. J., Allen, A. J., & Kuperman, S. (1995). Bupropion versus methylphenidate in the treatment of ADHD. *Journal of the American Academy of Child and Adolescent Psychiatry, 34,* 649–657.

Baruss, I., & American Psychological Association. (2003). *Alterations of consciousness: An empirical analysis for social scientists* (1st ed.). Washington, DC: American Psychological Association.

Baskin-Somers, A. R., Wallace, J. F., MacCoon, D. G., Curtin, J. J., & Newman, J. P. (2010). Clarifying the factors that undermine behavioral inhibition system functioning in psychopathology. *Personality Disorders: Theory, Research & Treatment, 4,* 203–217.

Bassarath, L. (2003). Medication strategies in childhood aggression: A review. *Canadian Journal of Psychiatry, 48,* 367–373.

Baumann, M. H., Wang, X., & Rothman, R. B. (2007). 3,4-Methylenedioxymethamphetamine (MDMA) neurotoxicity in rats: a reappraisal of past and present findings. *Psychopharmacology, 189*(4), 407–424. doi:10.1007/s00213-006-0322-6

Baumeister, A. A., Hawkins, M. F., & Uzelac, S. M. (2003). The myth of reserpine-induced depression: Role in the historical development of the monoamine hypothesis. *Journal of the History of the Neurosciences, 12,* 207–220.

Baxter, A. J., Scott, K. M., Ferrari, A. J., Norman, R. E., Vos, T., & Whiteford, H. A. (2014). Challenging the myth of an "epidemic" of common mental disorders: Trends in the global prevalence of anxiety and depression between 1990 and 2010. *Depression and Anxiety, 21,* 23–35.

Baxter, A. J., Scott, K. M., Vos, T., & Whiteford, H. A. (2013). Global prevalence of anxiety disorders: A systematic review and meta-regression. *Psychological Medicine, 43,* 897–910.

Baxter, L. E., Campbell, A., DeShields, M., Levounis, P., Martin, J. A., McNicholas, L., et al. (2013). Safe methadone induction and stabilization: Report of an expert panel. *Journal of Addiction Medicine, 7*(6), 377–386.

BBC News. (2002). *Medical plea key to Buck's defense.* Retrieved April 6, 2014, from http://news.bbc.co.uk/2/hi/health/1913066.stm

Beasley, C. M., Dornseif, B. E., Bosomworth, J. C., Sayler, M. E., Rampey, A. H., Heiligenstein, J. H., et al. (1991). Fluoxetine and suicide: A metaanalysis of controlled trials of treatment for depression. *British Medical Journal (Clinical Research Edition), 303,* 685–692.

Beaubrun, G., & Gray, G. E. (2000). A review of herbal medicines for psychiatric disorders. *Psychiatric Services, 51,* 1130–1134.

Beaumont, G. (1973). Sexual side effects of clomipramine. *Journal of International Medical Research, 1,* 469–472.

Beck, A. T. (2008). The evolution of the cognitive model of depression and it sneurobiological correlates. *American Journal of Psychiatry, 165,* 969–977.

Beck, A. T., Rush, A. J., Shaw, B. F., & Emery, G. (1979). *Cognitive therapy of depression.* New York: Guilford Press.

Beck, C., Buckwalter, K. C., Dudzik, P. M., & Evans, L. K. (2011). Filling the void in geriatric mental health: The geropsychiatric nursing collaborative as a model for change. *Nursing Outlook, 59,* 236–241.

Bedi, G., Hyman, D., & de Wit, H. (2010). Is ecstasy an "empathogen"? Effects of ±3,4-methylenedioxymethamphetamine on prosocial feelings and identification of emotional states in others. *Biological Psychiatry, 68*(12), 1134–1140. doi:10.1016/j.biopsych.2010.08.003

Bedi, G., Phan, K. L., Angstadt, M., & de Wit, H. (2009). Effects of MDMA on sociability and neural response to social threat and social reward. *Psychopharmacology, 207*(1), 73–83. doi:10.1007/s00213-009-1635-z

Beland, S. G., Preville, M., Dubois, M. F., Lorrain, D., Grenier, S., Voyer, P., et al. (2010). Benzodiazepine use and quality of sleep in the community dwelling elderly population. *Aging & Mental Health, 14,* 843–850.

Bell, C. C., & Mehta, H. (1980). The misdiagnosis of black patients with manicdepressive illness. *Journal of the American Medical Association, 72,* 141–145.

Bell, C. C., & Mehta, H. (1981). The misdiagnosis of black patients with manicdepressive illness: Second in a series. *Journal of the American Medical Association, 73,* 101–107.

Bell, R. D., Alexander, G. M., Schwartzman, R. K., & Yu, J. (1982). The methylphenidateinduced stereotypy in the awake rate: Local cerebral metabolism. *Neurology, 32,* 377–381.

Bella, V. L., & Piccoli, F. (2003). Olanzapineinduced tardive dyskinesia. *British Journal of Psychiatry, 182,* 81–82.

Belmaker, R. H. (2014). Lurasidone and bipolar disorder. *The American Journal of Psychiatry, 171,* 131–133.

Benac, N. (2013). U.S. becoming more accepting of medical marijauana. *CMAJ: Canadian Medical Association Journal, 185,* 745–746.

Bender, A. E., & Alloy, L. B. (2011). Life stress and kindling in bipolar disorder: Review of the evidence and integration with emerging biopsychosocial theories. *Clinical Psychology Review, 4,* 383–398.

Benet, L. Z., Kroetz, D. L., & Sheiner, L. B. (1996). Pharmacokinetics. In J. G. Hardman & L. E. Limbird (Eds.), *Goodman and Gilman's the pharmacological basis of therapeutics* (pp. 3–27). New York: McGraw-Hill.

Benner, R., Bjerkenstedt, L., & Edman, G. V. (2002). Hypericum perforatum extract (St. John's wort) for depression. *Psychiatric Annals, 32,* 21–26.

Bennett, C. F., Brown, R. T., Carver, J., & Anderson, D. (1999). Stimulant medication for the child with attention deficit/hyperactivity disorder. *Pediatric Clinics of North America, 46,* 924–944.

BenPorath, D. (2002). Stigmatization of individuals who receive psychotherapy: An interaction between helpseeking behavior and the presence of depression. *Journal of Social and Clinical Psychology, 21,* 400–413.

Bent, S., Tiedt, T. N., Odden, M. C., & Shlipak, M. G. (2003). The relative safety of ephedra compared with other herbal products. *Annals of Internal Medicine, 138,* 468–471.

Berardinelli, C., & Mostade, J. (2003). *Supervision of psychopharmacology.* Unpublished presentation given at John Carroll University, University Heights, OH.

Berger, A., Edelsberg, J., Treglia, M., Alvir, J. M. J., & Oster, G. (2012). Change in healthcare utilization and costs following initiation of benzodiazepine therapy for long-term treatment of generalized anxiety disorder: A retrospective cohort study. *BMC Psychiatry, 12,* 177–184.

Berger, F. M. (1970). The discovery of meprobamate. In F. Ayd & B. Blackwell (Eds.), *Discoveries in biological psychiatry* (pp. 115–129). Philadelphia: Lippincott.

Berk, M., Ichim, L., & Brook, S. (1999). Olanzapine compared to lithium in mania: A doubleblind, randomized, controlled trial. *International Clinical Psychopharmacology, 14,* 339–343.

Berman, R., Cappielle, A., Anand, A., Oren, D., Heninger, G., Charney, D., et al. (2000). Antidepressant effects of ketamine in depressed patients. *Biologial Psychiatry, 47,* 351–354.

Bernstein, G. A., Borschardt, C. M., & Perwien, A. R. (1996). Anxiety disorders in children and adolescents: A review of the past 10 years. *Journal of American Academy of Child and Adolescent Psychiatry, 35,* 1110–1119.

Bernstein, G. A., & Shaw, K. (1997). Practice parameters for the assessment and treatment of children and adolescents with anxiety disorders. *Journal of the American Academy of Child and Adolescent Psychiatry, 36*(Suppl. 1), 69–84.

Bested, A. C., Logan, A. C., & Selhub, E. M. (2013). Intestinal microbiota, probiotics and mental health: From Metchnikoff to modern advances: Part II—contemporary contextual research. *Gut Pathogens, 5,* 470–474.

Bhugra, D., & Bhui, K. (2001). *Crosscultural psychiatry: A practical guide.* New York: Oxford University Press.

Bichsell, S. (2001). Schizophrenia and severe mental illness. In E. R. Welfel & R. E. Ingersoll (Eds.), *The mental health desk reference: A practice based guide to diagnosis, treatment, and professional ethics* (pp. 142–154). New York: Wiley.

Biederman, J., Mick, E., Faraone, S. V., & Burback, M. (2001). Patterns of remission and symptom decline in conduct disorder: A four-year prospective study of an ADHD sample. *Journal of the American Academy of Child and Adolescent Psychiatry, 40,* 290–298.

Biederman, J., Wilens, T. E., Mick, E., Faraone, S. V., & Spencer, T. (1998). Does attentiondeficit hyperactivity disorder impact the developmental course of drug and alcohol abuse and dependence? *Biological Psychiatry, 44,* 269–273.

Biessels, G. J. (2010). Caffeine, diabetes, cognition and dementia. *Journal of Alzheimer's Disease, 20*(Suppl. 1), S143–S150.

Bilia, A. R., Gallori, S., & Vincieri, F. F. (2002). St. John's wort and depression: Efficacy, safety, and tolerability—an update. *Life Sciences, 70,* 3077–3096.

Birks, J., Grimley Evans, J., Iakovidou, V., Tsolaki, M., & Holt, F. E. (2009). Rivastigmine for Alzheimer's disease. *The Cochrane Database of Systematic Reviews,* isuue 2, 191–199.

Birks, J., & Harvey, R. J. (2006). Donepezil for dementia due to Alzheimer's disease. *The Cochrane Database of Systematic Reviews,* issue 1, 146–159.

Birmaher, B. (1998). Should we use antidepressant medication for children and adolescents with depressive disorders? *Pediatric Clinics of North America, 46,* 926–944.

Bishop, T. F., Keyhani, S., & Pincus, H. A. (2014). Acceptance of insurance by psychiatrists and the implications for access to mental health care. *JAMA, 71,* 176–181.

Bland, R. (1997). Epidemiology of affective disorders: A review. *Canadian Journal of Psychiatry, 42,* 367–377.

Blandini, F., & Armentero, M. T. (2012). New pharmacological avenues for the treatment of L-DOPA-induced dyskinesias in Parkinson's disease: Targeting glutamate and adenosine receptors. *Expert Opinion on Investigational Drugs, 21,* 153–168.

Blay, S. L., & Marinho, V. (2012). Anxiety disorders in old age. *Current Opinion in Psychiatry, 25,* 463–467.

Bliss, S. A., & Warnock, J. K. (2013). Psychiatric medications: Adverse cutaneous drug reactions. *Clinics in Dermatology, 31,* 101–109.

Bloom, F. E., Nelson, C. A., & Lazerson, A. (2001). *Brain, mind, and behavior* (3rd ed.). New York: Worth.

Bloom, F. E., Nelson, C. A., & Lazerson, A. (2005). *Brain, mind and Behavior* (3rd ed). Freeman: New York.

Blumenthal, M. (Ed.). (1998). *The complete German commission E monographs: Therapeutic guide to herbal medicines.* Austin, TX: American Botanical Council.

Bodenheimer, T. (2000). Uneasy alliance: Clinical investigators and the pharmaceutical industry. *New England Journal of Medicine, 342,* 1539–1544.

Bogenschutz, M. P. (2013). Studying the effects of classic hallucinogens in the treatment of alcoholism: rationale, methodology, and current research with psilocybin. *Current Drug Abuse Reviews, 6*(1), 17–29.

Bolliger, C. T., van Biljon, X., & Axelsson, A. (2007). A nicotine mouth spray for smoking cessation: A pilot study of preference, safety and efficacy. *Respiration, 74,* 196–701.

Bond, W. S. (1990). Therapy update: Ethnicity and psychotropic drugs. *Clinical Pharmacology, 10,* 467–470.

Boniel, T., & Dannon, P. (2001). The safety of herbal medicines in the psychiatric practice. *Harefuah, 140,* 780–783.

Boothroyd, A. (1997). Auditory development of the hearing child. *Scandinavian Audiology, 26*(Suppl. 46), 9–16.

Bostic, J. Q., Wilens, T., Spencer, T., & Biederman, J. (1997). Juvenile mood disorders and office psychopharmacology. *Pediatric Clinics of North America, 44,* 1487–1503.

Boston University Medical Center. (2002). *Barbiturate drugs.* Retrieved November 16, 2002, from http://web.bu.edu/cohis/cuboaboo/hypnotio/barb.htm

Botteron, K. N., & Geller, B. (1999). Disorders, symptoms, and their pharmacotherapy. In J. S. Werry & M. G. Aman

(Eds.), *Practitioner's guide to psychoactive drugs for children and adolescents* (pp. 183–209). New York: Plenum.

Boulenger, J. P., Lundbeck, A. S., Loft, H., & Olsen, C. K. (2014). Efficacy and safety of vortioxetine (Lu AA210004), 15 and 20 mg/day: A randomized, double-blind, placebo-controlled duloxeting-referenced study in the acute treatment of adult patients with major depressive disorder. *International Clinical Psychopharmacology, 29,* 138–149.

Bouza, C., Angeles, M., Magro, A., Munoz, A., & Amate, J. M. (2004). Efficacy and safety of naltrexone and acamprosate in the treatment of alcohol dependence: A systematic review. *Addiction, 99*(7), 811–828.

Bowden, C. L. (1995). Predictors of response to divalproex and lithium. *Journal of Clinical Psychiatry, 56*(Suppl. 3), 25–30.

Bowden, C. L. (1998). Treatment of bipolar disorder. In A. F. Schatzberg & C. B. Nemeroff (Eds.), *Textbook of psychopharmacology* (2nd ed., pp. 733–743). Washington, DC: American Psychiatric Press.

Bowden, C. L., Brugger, A. M., Swann, A. C., Calabrese, J. R., Janicak, P. G., Petty, F., et al. (1994). Efficacy of divalproex vs. lithium and placebo in the treatment of mania (The Depakote Mania Study Group). *Journal of the American Medical Association, 271,* 918–924.

Bowskill, S. V., Patel, M. X., Handley, S. A., & Flanagan, R. J. (2012). Plasma amisulpride in relation to prescribed dose, clozapine augmentation, and other factors: Data froma therapeutic drug monitoring service, 2002–2010. *Human Psychopharmacology, 27,* 507–513.

Boyd, E. A., & Bero, L. A. (2000). Assessing faculty financial relationships with industry: A case study. *Journal of the American Medical Association, 284,* 2209–2214.

Bradley, C. (1937). The behavior of children receiving benzedrine. *American Journal of Orthopsychiatry, 9,* 577–585.

Bragg, E. J., Warshaw, G. A., Cheong, J., Meganathan, K., & Brewer, D. E. (2012). National survey of geriatric psychiatry fellowship programs: Comparing findings in 2006/2007 and the 2001/2002 from the American Geriatrics Society and Association of Directors of geriatric academic program' geriatric workforce policy studies center. *The American Journal of Geriatric Psychiatry, 20,* 169–178.

Bramble, D. (2003). Annotation: The use of psychotropic medications in children: A British view. *Journal of Child Psychology and Psychiatry, 44,* 169–179.

Brauer, R. B., Stangl, M., Siewert, J. R., Pfab, R., & Becker, K. (2003). Acute liver failure after administration of the herbal tranquilizer kavakava (Piper methysticum). *Journal of Clinical Psychiatry, 64,* 216–218.

Breggin, P. R. (1997). *Brain disabling treatments in psychiatry: Drugs, electroshock, and the role of the FDA.* New York: Springer.

Brent, J. S. (1998). A timesensitive method for assisting adults in transition. *Journal of Humanistic Psychology, 38,* 7–24.

Bressi, C., Procellana, M., Marinaccio, P. M., Nocito, E. P., & Magri, L. (2010). Short-term psychodynamic psychotherapy versus treatment as usual for depressive and anxiety disorders: A randomized clinical trial of efficacy. *The Journal of Nervous and Mental Disease, 198,* 647–652.

Brewer, C. (1993). Recent developments in disulfiram treatment. *Alcohol and Alcoholism, 28*(4), 383–395.

Brichta, L., Greengard, P., & Flajolet, M. (2013). Advances in the pharmacological treatment of Parkinson's disease: Targeting neurotransmitter systems. *Trends in Neuroscience, 36,* 543–554.

Britten, N. (1998). Psychiatry, stigma, and resistance. *British Medical Journal, 10,* 963–973.

Brody, A. L., Saxena, S., Stoessel, P., Gillies, P., Fairbanks, L. A., Alborzian, S., et al. (2001). Regional brain metabolic changes in patients with major depression treated with either paroxetine or interpersonal therapy: Preliminary findings. *Archives of General Psychiatry, 58,* 631–640.

Brown, R. T., & Sammons, M. T. (2002). Pediatric psychopharmacology: A review of new developments and recent research. *Professional Psychology: Research and Practice, 33,* 135–147.

Brown, R. T., & Sawyer, M. G. (1998). *Medications for schoolage children: Effects on learning and behavior.* New York: Guilford Press.

Brown, T. K. (2013). Ibogaine in the treatment of substance dependence. *Current Drug Abuse Reviews, 6*(1), 3–16.

Brown University, Manisses Communications Group. (2002). Examining psychotropic medication use in pediatric patients. *Child and Adolescent Psychopharmacology Update, 4,* 3–5. Retrieved September 2002, from http://www.medscape.com/viewarticle/423374print

Brown University Psychopharmacology Update. (2003). Debate continues about atypical antipsychotics and diabetes. *Brown University Psychopharmacology Update, 14,* 1. Providence, RI: Manisses Communications.

Browne, C. A., & Lucki, I. (2013). Antidepressant effects of ketamine: Mechanisms underlying fast-acting novel antidepressants. *Frontiers in Pharmacology, 4,* 1–18.

Brubaker, L. (2012). Conflict of interest: What is the role of our professional societies? *Neurology and Urodynamics, 31,* 1217–1218.

Brushwood, D. B. (2003). Maximizing the value of electronic prescription monitoring programs. *The Journal of Law, Medicine and Ethics, 31,* 41–54.

Bryden, K. E., Carrey, N. J., & Kutcher, S. P. (2001). Update and recommendations for the use of antipsychotics in earlyonset psychoses. *Journal of Child & Adolescent Psychopharmacology, 11,* 113–130.

Buchhave, P., Minthon, L., Zetterberg, H., Wallin, A. K., Blennow, K., & Hansson, O. (2012). Cerebrospinal fluid levels of beta-amyloid 1-42 but not of tau, are fully changed already 5 to 10 years before the onset of Alzheimer dementia. *Archives of General Psychiatry, 69,* 98–106.

Buck, M. (2000). *The FDA modernization act of 1997: Impact on pediatric medicine.* Retrieved February 14, 2002, from http://www.medscape.com/viewarticle/410910

Budney, A. J., Roffman, R., Stephens, R. S., & Walker, D. (2007). Marijuana dependence and its treatment. *Addiction Science & Clinical Practice, 12,* 10–19.

Buelow, G., Herbert, S., & Buelow, S. (2000). *Psychotherapist's resource on psychiatric medications: Issues of treatment and referral.* Belmont, CA: Brooks/Cole.

Bulat, T., Castle, S., Rutledge, M., & Quigley, P. (2008). Clinical practice algorithms: Medication management to reduce fall risk in the elderly—Part 4, Anticoagulants, anticonvulsants, anticholinergics/bladder relaxants, and antipsychotics. *Journal of the American Association of Nurse Practitioners, 20,* 174–176.

Buntwall, N., Bearn, J., Gossop, M., & Strang, J. (2000). Naltrexone and lofexidine buprenorphine and antivirals. The nonnucleoside reverse-transcriptase inhibitors buprenorphine and naloxone. *Drug and Alcohol Dependence, 70,* 539–547.

Burstein, S. H., & Zurier, R. B. (2009). Cannabinoids, endocannabinoids, and related analogs in inflammation. *The AAPS Journal, 11,* 109–119.

Bushman, B. J., & Anderson, C. A. (2001). Media violence and the American public: Scientific facts versus media misinformation. *American Psychologist, 56*(6–7), 477–489.

Buskila, D., & Sarzi-Puttini, P. (2006). Biology and therapy of fibromyalgia. Genetic aspects of fibromyalgia syndrome. *Arthritis Research & Therapy, 8,* 218.

Buston, K. (2002). Adolescents with mental problems: What do they say about health services? *Journal of Adolescence, 25,* 221–242.

Cade, J. F. (1949). Lithium salts in the treatment of psychotic excitement. *Medical Journal of Australia, 36,* 349–352.

Calabrese, J. R., Bowden, C. L., Sachs, G. S., Asher, J. A., Monaghan, E., & Rudd, G. D. (1999). A doubleblind placebocontrolled study of lamotrigine monotherapy in outpatients with bipolar I disorder. *Journal of Clinical Psychiatry, 60,* 79–88.

Calabrese, J. R., Shelton, M. D., Rapport, D. J., & Kimmel, S. E. (2002). Bipolar disorders and the effectiveness of novel anticonvulsants. *Journal of Clinical Psychiatry, 63*(Suppl. 3), 5–9.

Camargos, E. F., Souza, A. B., Nascimento, A. S., Morais-E-Silva, A. C., Quintas, J. L., Louzada, L. L., et al. (2012). Use of psychotropic medications by caregivers of elderly patients with dementia: Is this a sign of caregiver burden? *Arquivos De Neuro-Psiquiatria, 70,* 169–174.

Cami, J., Farré, M., Mas, M., Roset, P. N., Poudevida, S., Mas, A., et al. (2000). Human pharmacology of 3,4-methylenedioxymethamphetamine ("ecstasy"): psychomotor performance and subjective effects. *Journal of Clinical Psychopharmacology, 20*(4), 455–466.

Campbell, M., & Cueva, J. E. (1995). Psychopharmacology in child and adolescent psychiatry: A review of the past seven years. Part I. *Journal of the American Academy of Child and Adolescent Psychiatry, 34,* 1124–1132.

Campbell, M., Kafantaris, V., & Cueva, J. E. (1995). An update on the use of lithium carbonate in aggressive children and adolescents with conduct disorders. *Psychopharmacology Bulletin, 31,* 93–102.

Campbell, M., Rapoport, J., & Simpson, G. (1999). Antipsychotics in children and adolescents. *Journal of the American Academy of Child and Adolescent Psychiatry, 38,* 537–545.

Canadian Medical Association. (2013). Pharma influence widespread at medical schools: Study. *Canadian Medical Assocation Journal, 185,* 1121–1122.

Capwell, R. R. (1995). Ephedrineinduced mania from an herbal diet supplement. *American Journal of Psychiatry, 152,* 647.

Carey, N., Jones, S. L., & O'Toole, A. W. (2013). Do you feel powerless when a patient refuses medication? *Journal of Psychosocial Nursing and Mental Health Services, 28,* 19–25.

Carhart-Harris, R. L., Erritzoe, D., Williams, T., Stone, J. M., Reed, L. J., Colasanti, A., et al. (2012). Neural correlates of the psychedelic state as determined by fMRI studies with psilocybin. *Proceedings of the National Academy of Sciences, 109*(6), 2138–2143. doi:10.1073/pnas.1119598109

Carhart-Harris, R. L., Murphy, K., Leech, R., Erritzoe, D., Wall, M. B., Ferguson, B., et al. (2014). The effects of acutely administered 3,4-methylenedioxymethamphetamine on spontaneous brain function in healthy volunteers measured with arterial spin labeling and blood oxygen level-dependent resting state functional connectivity. *Biological Psychiatry.* doi:10.1016/j.biopsych.2013.12.015

Carlson, G. A. (1996). Compared to attention deficit hyperactivity disorder. *American Journal of Psychiatry, 153,* 1128–1130.

Carlson, N. R. (2012). *Physiology of behavior* (11th ed.). Boston: Pearson.

Carlsson, A., Fuxe, K., & Ungerstedt, U. (1968). The effect of imipramine on central 5-hydroxytryptamine neurons. *Journal of Pharmacy and Pharmacology, 20,* 150–151.

Carlsson, A., & Lindqvist, M. (1963). Effect of chlorpromazine or haloperidol on the formation of 3methoxytyramine and normetanephrine in mouse brain. *Acta Pharmacologica, 20,* 140–144.

Carlsten, A., & Waren, M. (2009). Are sedatives and hypnotics associated with increased suicide risk of suicide in the elderly? *BMC Geriatrics, 9,* 20–22.

Carnicella, S., He, D.-Y., Yowell, Q. V., Glick, S. D., & Ron, D. (2010). Noribogaine, but not 18-MC, exhibits similar actions as ibogaine on GDNF expression and ethanol self-administration. *Addiction Biology, 15*(4), 424–433. doi:10.1111/j.1369-1600.2010.00251.x

Caroff, S. N., & Mann, S. C. (1993). Neuroleptic malignant syndrome. *Medical Clinics of North America, 77,* 185–202.

Carrey, N., Mendella, P., MacMaster, F. P., & Kutcher, S. (2002). Developmental psychopharmacology. In S. Kutcher (Ed.), *Practical child and adolescent psycho* (pp. 38–69). Cambridge, UK: Cambridge University Press.

Carrillo, M. C., Brashear, H. R., Logovinsky, V., Ryan, J. M., Feldman, H. H., Siemers, E. R., et al. (2013). Can we prevent Alzheimer's disease? Secondary "prevention" trials in Alzheimer's disease. *Alzheimer's & Dementia, 9,* 121–131.

Carter, O. L., Burr, D. C., Pettigrew, J. D., Wallis, G. M., Hasler, F., & Vollenweider, F. X. (2005). Using psilocybin to investigate the relationship between attention, working memory, and the serotonin 1A and 2A receptors. *Journal of Cognitive Neuroscience, 17*(10), 1497–1508. doi:10.1162/089892905774597191

Casey, D. A. (1993). Neuroleptic-induced extrapyramidal syndromes and tardive dyskinesia. *Psychiatric Clinics of North America, 16,* 589–610.

Castellanos, F. X., Lee, P. P., Sharp, W., Jeffries, N. O., Greenstein, D. K., Blumenthal, J. D., et al. (2002). Developmental trajectories of brain volume abnormalities in children and adolescents with attention-deficit/hyperactivity disorder. *Journal of the American Medical Association, 288,* 1740–1748.

Cattell, H. (2000). Suicide in the elderly. *Advances in Psychiatric Treatment, 6,* 102–108.

Celada, P., Bortolozzi, A., & Artigas, F. (2013). Serotonin 5-HT1A receptors as agents to treat psychiatric disorders: Rationale and current status of research. *CNS Drugs, 27,* 703–716.

Centers for Disease Control. (2014). *Injury center: Violence prevention.* Retrieved April 19, 2014, from http://www.cdc.gov/violence prevention/suicide/statistics/aag.html#C

Cervo, L., Rozio, M., Ekalle-Soppo, C. B., Guiso, G., Morazzoni, P., & Caccia, S. (2002). Role of hyperforin in the antidepressant-like activity of hypericum extracts. *Psychopharmacology, 164,* 423–428.

Chalmers, D. J. (1995). The puzzle of conscious experience. *Scientific American, 273,* 80–86.

Chan, K. W., Hui, L. M., Wong, H. Y., Lee, H. M., Chang, W. C., & Chen, Y. H. (2014). Medication adherence, knowledge about psychosis, and insight among patients with a schizophrenia spectrum disorder. *The Journal of Nervous and Mental Disease, 202,* 25–29.

Chang, K. D. (2008). The bipolar spectrum in children and adolescents: Developmental issues. *Journal of Clinical Psychiatry, 69*(3), e9.

Chapla, N., Gallucci, G., Trimzi, I., & Meier, B. R. (2013). Addicted to sleep: A case of Ambien abuse. *Delaware Medical Journal, 85,* 109–111.

Chen, H., Mehta, S., Aparasu, R., Patel, A., & Ochoa-Perez, M. (2014). Comparative effectiveness of monotherapy with mood stabilizers versus second generation (atypical) antipsychotics for the treatment of bipolar disorder in children and adolescents. *Pharmacoepidemiology and Drug Safety, 23,* 299–308.

Chengappa, K. N., Gershon, S., & Levine, J. (2001). The evolving role of topiramate among other mood stabilizers in the management of bipolar disorder. *Bipolar Disorder, 3,* 215–232.

Chiang, C. N., & Hawks, R. L. (2003). Pharmacokinetics of the combination tablet of buprenorphine and naloxone. *Drug and Alcohol Dependence, 70,* 539–547.

Chimos, S., Evarts, S. D., Littlehale, S. K., & Rothman, D. J. (2013). Manging conflicts of interest in clinical care: The "race to the middle" at U.S. Medical schools. *Academic Medicine: Journal of the Association of American Medical Colleges, 88,* 1464–1470.

Chimos, S., Patterson, L., Raveis, V. H., & Rothman, D. J. (2011). Managing conflict of interest in clinical care: A national survey at U.S. Medical schools. *Academic Medicine: Journal of the Association of American Medicine, 86,* 293–299.

Chodera, A., Nowakowska, E., & Bartczak, G. (1994). Tolerance to a new class of non-benzodiazepine anxiolytics. *Polish Journal of Pharmacology, 46,* 479–481.

Chollet, J., Saragoussi, D., Clay, E., & Francois, C. (2013). A clinical research practice datalink analysis of antidepressant treatment patterns and health care costs in generalized anxiety disorder. *Value in Health, 16,* 1133–1139.

Chomsky, N. (2002). *Distorted morality: America's war on terror?* [Lectures on DVD]. New York: Silent Films.

Chu, H., Yang, C. Y., Lin, Y., Ou, K. L., Lee, T. Y., O'Brien, A. P., et al. (2014). The impact of group music therapy on depression and cognition in elderly persons with dementia: A randomized controlled study. *Biological Research for Nursing, 16,* 209–217.

Church of Scientology. (1994). *The scientology handbook: Based on the works of L. Ron Hubbard.* Los Angeles, CA: Bridge Publications.

Churchland, P. S. (1995). *Neurophilosophy: Toward a unified science of the mind/brain.* Cambridge, MA: MIT Press.

Churchland, P. S. (1999). Toward a natural science of the mind. In Z. Houshmand, R. B. Livingston, & B. A. Wallace (Eds.), *Consciousness at the crossroads: Conversations: Conversations with the Dalai Lama on brain science and Buddhism* (pp. 17–32). Ithaca, NY: Snow Lion Press.

Cipriani, A., Koesters, M., Furukawa, T. A., Nose, M., Purgato, M., Omori, I. M., et al. (2012). Duloxetine versus other anti-depressive agents for depression. *The Cochrane Database of Systematic Reviews,* issue 10, 123–126.

Clark, P. (2000). The ethics of medical marijuana: Government restrictions vs. Medical necessity. *Journal of Public Health Policy, 21,* 40–60.

Clayton, R. R., & Leukefeld, C. G. (1992). The prevention of drug use among youth: Implications of legalization. *Journal of Primary Prevention, 12,* 289–303.

Cloitre, M., Stovall-McClough, K. C., Miranda, R., & Chemtob, C. M. (2004). Therapeutic alliance, negative mood regulation, and treatment outcome in child abuse-related posttraumatic stress disorder. *Journal of Consulting and Clinical Psychology, 72*(3), 411–416. doi:10.1037/0022-006X.72.3.411

Cocks, M., & Moller, V. (2002). Use of indigenous and indigenised medicines to enhance personal well being: A South African case study. *Social Science and Medicine, 54,* 387–397.

Coffey, B. (1990). Anxiolytics for children and adolescents: Traditional and new drugs. *Journal of Child and Adolescent Psychopharmacology, 1,* 57–83.

Cohen, D., Gerardin, P., Mazet, P., Purper-Ouakil, D., & Flament, M. F. (2004). Pharmacological treatment of adolescent major depression. *Journal of Child and Adolescent Psychopharmacology, 14,* 19–31.

Colbert, T. C. (2002, June 14). *Drugs or psychotherapy? What's the answer?* Symposium conducted in Beachwood, Ohio. College of Neuropsychopharmacology, Puerto Rico.

Collett, B. R., Ohan, J. L., & Myers, K. M. (2003). Tenyear review of rating scales. V: Scales assessing attentiondeficit/hyperactive disorder. *Journal of the Combination Treatment Compared with Conventional Lofexidine Treatment for in-Patient American Academy of Child and Adolescent Psychiatry, 42,* 1015–1037.

Connor, K. M., & Davidson, J. R. (2002). A placebo-controlled study of kava kava in generalized anxiety disorder. *International Clinical Psychopharmacology, 17,* 185–188.

Connors, C. K. (1972). Pharmacotherapy. In H. C. Quay & J. S. Werry (Eds.), *Psychopathological disorders of childhood* (pp. 316–347). New York: Wiley.

Connors, D. (1996). Bupropion hydrochloride in attention deficit disorder with hyperactivity. *Journal of the American Academy of Child and Adolescent Psychiatry, 35,* 1314–1321.

Consumer's Union. (1999). Herbal Rx: The promises and pitfalls. *Consumer Reports, 64,* 44–48.

Coppen, A., & Healy, D. (1996). Biological psychiatry in Britain. In D. Healy (Ed.), *The psychopharmacologists* (pp. 265–286). London: Chapman & Hall.

Cornelius, J. R., Salloum, I. M., Ehler, J. G., Jarrett, P. J., Cornelius, M. D., Perel, J. M., et al. (1997). Fluoxetine in depressed alcoholics: A double-line placebo-controlled trial. *Archives of General Psychiatry, 54,* 700–705.

Cornwell, B. R., Salvadore, G., Furey, M., Marquardt, C. A., Brutsche, N. E., Gillon, C., et al. (2012). Synaptic potentiation is critical for rapid antidepressant response to ketamine in treatment-resistant major depression. *Biological Psychiatry, 72,* 555–561.

Correll, C. U., Manu, P., Olshanskiy, V., Napolitano, B., Kane, J. M., & Malhotra, A. K. (2009). Cardiometabolic risk of second-generation antipsychotic medications during first-time use in children and adolescents. *JAMA, 302,* 1765–1763.

Corrigan, P., River, P., Lundin, R., Wasowski, K., Campion, J., Methsien, J., et al. (2000). Stigmatizing attributions about mental illness. *Journal of Community Psychology, 28,* 91–102.

Cortese, L., Bressan, R. A., Castle, D. J., & Mosolov, S. N. (2013). Management of schizophrenia: Clinical experience with asenapine. *Journal of Psychopharmacology, 27*(Suppl. 4), 14–22.

Cott, J., & Wisner, K. L. (2002). Effect of Hypericum perforatum (St. John's wort) in major depressive disorder: A randomized controlled trial: Comment. *Journal of the American Medical Association, 288,* 448.

Courtwright, D., Joseph, H., & Des Jarlais, D. (1989). *Addicts who survived: An oral history of narcotic use in American, 1923–1965.* Knoxville, TN: University of Tennessee Press.

Cousin, D. A., Butts, K., & Young, A. H. (2010). The role of dopamine in bipolar disorder. *Bipolar Disorders, 11,* 787–806.

Cox, D. E., & Harrison, D. W. (2008). Models of anger: contributions from psychophysiology, neuropsychology and the cognitive behavioral perspective. *Brain Structure & Function, 212*(5), 371–385. doi:10.1007/s00429-007-0168-7

Coyle, J. T. (2000). Psychotropic drug use in very young children. *Journal of the American Medical Association, 283,* 1059–1060.

Cozolino, L. (2010). *The neuroscience of psychotherapy* (2nd ed.). New York: Norton.

Craighead, W. E., Miklowitz, D. J., & Craighead, L. W. (Eds.). (2013). *Psychopathology: History, diagnosis, and empirical foundation* (2nd ed.). New York: John Wiley & Sons.

Crews, W. D., & Harrison, D. W. (1995). The neuropsychology of depression and its implications for cognitive therapy. *Neuropsychology Review, 5,* 81–123.

Crites-Leoni, A. (1998). Medicinal use of marijuana: Is the debate a smoke screen for movement toward legalization? *Journal of Legal Medicine, 19,* 273–304.

Cuffs, Y. L., Hargraves, J. L., Rosal, M., Briesacher, B. A., Schoenthaler, A., Person, S., et al. (2013). Reported racial discrimination, trust in physicians, and medication adherence among inner-city African-Americans with hypertension. *American Journal of Public Health, 103,* e55–e62.

Cuijpers, P., Sijbrandij, M., Koole, S. L., Andersson, G., Beekman, A. T., & Reynolds, C. G. (2013). The efficacy of psychotherapy and pharmacotherapy in treating depressive and anxiety disorders: A meta-analysis of direct comparisons. *World Psychiatry, 12,* 137–148.

Cummings, C. M., & Fristad, M. A. (2007). Medications prescribed for children with mood disorders: Effects of a family-based psychoeducation program. *Experimental and Clinical Psychopharmacology, 15,* 555–562.

Cupp, M. J. (1999). Herbal remedies: Adverse effects and drug interactions. *American Family Physician, 59,* 1661–1662.

Cusi, C., Cantisani, T. A., Celeni, M. G., Incorvaia, B., Righetti, E., & Candelise, L. (2007). Galantamine for Alzheimer's disease and mild cognitive impairment. *Neuroepidemiology, 28,* 116–117.

Dakin, E., Quijano, L. M., & McAlister, C. (2011). Assisted facility administrator and direct care staff views of resident mental health concerns and staff training needs. *Journal of Gerontological Social Work, 54,* 53–72.

Dalawari, P., Patel, N. M., Bzdawka, W., Petrone, J., Liou, V., & Ambrecht, E. (2013). Racial differences in beliefs of physician prescribing practices for low-cost pharmacy options. *Administration of Emergency Medicine, 46,* 396–403.

Dalrymple, K. L. (2012). Issues and controversies surrounding the diagnosis and treatment of social anxiety disorder. *Expert Review of Neurotherapeutics, 12,* 993–1015.

Damasio, A. (1995). *Descartes' error: Emotion, reason and the human brain.* New York: Putnam.

Damasio, A. (2000). *The feeling of what happens: Body and emotion in the making of consciousness.* New York: Harvest.

Damasio, A. (2010). *Self comes to mind: Constructing the conscious brain.* New York: Pantheon.

Damkier, N. J., Jublin, H., & Taylor, D. (2011). Optimizing clozapine treatment. *Acta Psychaitrica Scandinavica, 123,* 411–422.

Danion, J. M., Rein, W., Fleurot, O., & the Amisulpride Study Group. (1999). Improvement of schizophrenic patients with primary negative symptoms treated with amisulpride. *American Journal of Psychiatry, 156,* 610–616.

Dannawi, M. (2002). Possible serotonin syndrome after combination of buspirone and St. John's wort. *Journal of Psychopharmacology, 16,* 401.

Dardennes, R., Even, C., Bange, F., & Heim, A. (1995). Comparison of carbamazepine and lithium in the prophylaxis of bipolar disorders: A meta-analysis. *British Journal of Psychiatry, 166,* 378–381.

Dargani, N. V., & Malhotra, A. K. (2014). Safety profile of iloperidone in the treatment of schizophrenia. *Expert Opinion on Drug Safety, 13,* 241–246.

Daumit, G. L., Crum, R. M., Guallar, E., Powe, N. R., Primm, A. B., Steinwachs, D. M., et al. (2003). Outpatient prescriptions for atypical antipsychotics for African Americans, Hispanics, and Whites in the United States. *Archives of General Psychiatry, 60,* 121–128.

Davari-Ashtiani, R., Beheshti, S., Shahrbabaki, M. E., Razjouryan, K., Amini, H., & Mazhabdar, H. (2010). Buspirone versus methylphenidate in the treatment of attention deficit hyperactivity disorder: A double-bline and randomized trial. *Child Psychiatry and Human Development, 41,* 723–728.

David, A., & Kemp, R. (1997). Five perspectives on the phenomenon of insight in psychosis. *Psychiatric Annals, 27,* 791–797.

Davighus, M. L., Plassman, B. L., Pirzada, A., Dall, C. C., Dowen, P. E., & Burke, J. R. (2011). Risk factors and preventive interventions for Alzheimer's disease: State of the science. *Archives of Neurology, 68,* 1185–1190.

Davis, M. C., Fuller, M. A., Strauss, M. E., Konicki, P. E., & Jaskiw, G. E. (2013). Discontinuation of clozapine: A 15- year naturalistic retrospective study of 320 patients. *Acta Psychiatrica Scandinavica, 16,* 445–449.

De Araujo, A. A., de Araujo, D. D., do Nascimento, G. G., Ribeiro, S. B., Chaves, K. M., deLima Silva, V., et al. (2014). Quality of life in patients with schizophrenia: The impact of socio-economic factors and adverse effects of atypical antipsychotic drugs. *The Psychiatric Quarterly, 5,* 314–319.

De Fonseca, F. R., Carrera, M. R. A., Navarro, M., Koob, G. F., & Weiss, F. (1997). Activation of corticotropin-releasing factor in the limbic system during cannabinoid withdrawal. *Science, 276,* 2050–2054.

De Mello Schier, A. R., de Oliveira Ribeiro, N. P., de Oiverira e Silva, A. C., Cecilio Hallak, J. E., Crippa, J. A. S., Nardi, A. E., et al. (2012). Cannabidiol, a cannabis sativa constituent as an anxiolytic drug. *Revista Brasileira De Psiquiatria, 34*(Suppl.), S104–S117.

De Melo Coelho, F. G., Gobbi, S., Andreatto, C. A., Corazza, D. I., Pedroso, R. V., & Galduroz, R. F. (2013). Physical exerticise modulates peripheral levels of brain derived neurotrophic factor (BDNF): A systematic review of experimental studies in the elderly. *Archives of Gerontology and Geriatrics, 56,* 10–15.

De Paula, T. C., Bochner, R., & Montilla, D. E. (2012). Clinical and epidemiological analysis of hospitalizations of elderly due to poisoning and adverse effects of medications, Brazil from 2004 to 2008. *Revista Brasileira De Epdemiologia, 15,* 828–844.

Del Ra, A. C., Spielmans, G. I., Fluckiger, C., & Wampold, B. E. (2013). Efficacy of new generation antidepressants: Differences seem illusory. *PLoS One, 8,* 1–9.

de Silva, V. A., & Hanwella, R. (2012). Efficacy and tolerability of venlafaxine versus specific serotonin reuptake inhibitors in treatment of major depressive disorder: A meta-analysis of published studies. *International Clinical Psychopharmacology, 27,* 8–16.

Dean, A. J., Witham, M., & McGuire, T. (2009). Predictors in safety-related enquiries about psychotropic medication in young people and families accessing a medicines information service. *Journal of Child and Adolescent Psychopharmacology, 19,* 179–185.

Debner, A. (2001a, April 10). Many children can't get mental care. *Boston Globe,* p. B1.

Debner, A. (2001b, May 8). Doctors see crisis in youth psychiatry. *Boston Globe,* p. B2.

Decina, P., Schlegel, A. M., & Fieve, R. R. (1987). Lithium poisoning. *New York State Journal of Medicine, 87,* 230–231.

Delbello, M. P., Schwiers, M. L., Rosenberg, H. L., & Strakowski, S. M. (2002). A double-blind, randomized, placebo-controlled study of quetiapine as adjunctive treatment for adolescent mania. *Journal of the American Academy of Child and Adolescent Psychiatry, 41,* 1216–1223.

Delgado, P. L., & Gelenberg, A. J. (2001). Antidepressant and antimanic medications. In G. O. Gabbard (Ed.), *Treatments of psychiatric disorders* (3rd ed., pp. 1137–1180). Washington, DC: American Psychiatric Publishing.

Dell'osso, B., & Lader, M. (2013). Do benzodiazepines still deserve a major role in the treatment of psychiatric disorders? A critical reappraisal. *European Psychiatry, 28,* 7–20.

Delva, N. J., & Hawken, E. R. (2001). Preventing lithium intoxication: Guide for physicians. *Canadian Family Physician, 47,* 1595–1600.

Demyttenaere, K. (2001). Compliance and acceptance in antidepressant treatment. *Journal of Psychiatry in Clinical Practice, 5,* 529–535.

Demyttenaere, K., Mesters, P., Boulanger, B., Dewe, W., Delsemme, M., Gregoire, J., et al. (2001). Adherence to treatment regimen in depressed patients treated with amitriptyline or fluoxetine. *Journal of Affective Disorders, 65,* 243–252.

Demyttenaere, K., & Jaspers, L. (2008). Bupropion and SSRI-induced sexual side effects. *Journal of Psychopharmacology, 22,* 792–803.

Dennett, D. C. (1991). *Consciousness explained.* Boston: Little, Brown.

Dennison, U., Clarkson, M., O'Mullane, J. O., & Cassidy, E. M. (2011). The incidence and clinical correlates of lithium toxicity: A retrospective review. *Irish Journal of Medical Science, 180,* 661–665.

DeQuardo, J. R., & Tandon, R. (1998). Do atypical antipsychotic medications favorably alter the long-term course of schizophrenia? *Journal of Psychiatric Research, 32,* 229–242.

Derry, S. (2007). Atypical antipsychotics in bipolar disorder: Systematic review of randomized trials. *BMC Psychiatry, 7,* 40.

DeRuiter, J., & Holston, P. L. (2012). Drug patent expirations and the "patent cliff." *U.S. Pharmacist.* Retrieved May 13, 2014, from http://www.uspharmacist.com/content/s/216/c/35249/

Dhillon, S. (2012). Aripiprazole: A review of its use in the management of mania in adults with bipolar I disorder. *Drugs, 72,* 133–162.

Diaz, E., Woods, S. W., & Rosenheck, R. A. (2005). Effects of ethnicity on psychotropic medications adherence. *Community Mental Health Journal, 41,* 521–537.

Diehl, A., Ulmer, L., & Mutschler, J. (2010). Why is disulfiram superior to acamprosate in the routine clinical setting? A retrospective long-term study in 353 alcohol-dependent patients. *Alcohol Alcohol, 45*(3), 271–277.

DiMaggio, J. (2006). *Marilyn, Joe & Me: June DiMaggio tells it like it was.* New York: Penimen.

DiPaula, B. A., Schwartz, R., Montoya, I. D., Barrett, D., & Tang, C. (2002). Heroin detoxification with buprenorphine on an inpatient psychiatric unit. *Journal of SubstanceAbuse Treatment, 23,* 163–169.

Dittrich, A. (1998). The standardized psychometric assessment of altered states of consciousness (ASCs) in humans *Pharmacopsychiatry, 31*(Suppl. 2), 80–84. doi:10.1055/s-2007-979351

Dittrich, A., Lamparter, D., & Maurer, M. (2006). *5D-ASC: Questionnaire for the assessment of altered states of consciousness. A short introduction* (3rd ed.). Zurich: PSIN PLUS.

Djulbegovic, B., Lacevic, M., Cantor, A., Fields, K. K., Bennett, C. L., Adams, J. R., et al. (2000). The uncertainty principle and industry sponsored research. *The Lancet, 356,* 365–368.

Doblin, R. E., & Kleinman, M. A. R. (1991). Marijuana as anti-emetic medicine: A survey of oncologists' experiences and attitudes. *Journal of Clinical Oncology, 9,* 1314–1319.

Dodd, C. (2001). *Dodd and Dewine introduce bill to provide better drug safety.* Retrieved September 2002, from www.senate.gov/~dodd/press/Release/01/0504.htm

Dolder, C. R., & Jeste, D. V. (2003). Incidence of tardive dyskinesia with typical versus atypical antipsychotics in very high-risk patients. *Biological Psychiatry, 53,* 1142–1145.

Dolder, C. R., Nelson, M., & Stump, A. (2010). Pharmacological and clinical profile of newer antidepressants: Implications for the treatment of elderly patients. *Drugs Aging, 27,* 625–643.

Dole, V. P. (1988). Implications of methadone maintenance for theories of narcotic addiction. *JAMA, 260,* 3025–3029.

Dole, V. P., & Joseph, H. (1978). Long-term outcome of patients treated with methadone maintenance. *Annals of the New York Academy of Sciences, 311,* 181–196.

Donovan, D. M., Knox, P. C., Skytta, J. A. F., Blayney, J. A., & DiCenzo, J. (2013). Buprenorphine from detox and beyond: Preliminary evaluation of a pilot program to increase heroin dependent individuals' engagement in a full continuum of care. *Journal of Substance Abuse Treatment, 44,* 426–432.

Doody, R. S., Thomas, R. G., Farlow, M., Iwatsubo, T., Vellas, B., Joffe, S., et al. (2014). Phase 3 trials of solanezumab for mild-to-moderate Alzheimer's disease. *The New England Journal of Medicine, 370,* 311–321.

Dooley, M., & Plosker, G. L. (2000). Zaleplon: A review of its use in the treatment of insomnia. *Drugs, 60,* 413–445.

Doolittle, W. F. (2013). Is junk DNA bunk? A critique of ENCODE. *Proceedings of the National Academy of Sciences of the United States of America, 110,* 5294–5300.

Doran, C. M., Holmes, J., Ladewig, D., & Ling, W. (2005). Review: Buprenorphine induction and stabilization in the treatment of opiate dependence. *Heroin Addiction and Related Clinical Problems, 7,* 7–18.

Dossey, L. (2001). *Healing beyond the body: Medicine and the infinite reach of the mind.* Boston: Shambhala.

Doubleday, E. K., King, P., & Papageorgiuo, C. (2002). Relationship between fluid intelligence and ability to benefit from cognitive-behavioural therapy in older adults: A preliminary investigation *British Journal of Clinical Psychology, 41,* 423–428.

Dougherty, L. R., Tolep, M. R., Bufferd, S. J., Olino, T. M., Dyson, M., Traditi, J., et al. (2013). Preschool anxiety disorders: Comprehensive assessment of clinical, demographic, temperamental, familial and life stress correlates. *Journal of Clinical Child and Adolescent Psychiatry, 42,* 577–589.

Dubovsky, S. L. (2014). Pharmacokinetic evaluation of vortioxetine for the treatment of major depressive disorder. *Expert Opinion on Drug Metabolism & Toxicology, 5,* 45–52.

Dubyna, J., & Quinn, C. (1996). The self-management of psychiatric medications: A pilot study. *Journal of Psychiatric and Mental Health Nursing, 3,* 297–302.

Duffy, A. (2010). The early natural history of bipolar disorder: What have we learned from longitudinal high risk research? *Canadian Journal of Psychiatry, 55,* 477–485.

Duggal, H. S. (2007). New-onset transient hallucinations possibly due to eszopiclone: A case study. *Primary Care Companion Journal of Clinical Psychiatry, 9,* 467–468.

Duke, S. B., & Gross, A. C. (1993). *America's longest war: Rethinking our tragic crusade against drugs.* New York: Putnam.

Duman, R. S., Heninger, G. R., & Nestler, E. J. (1997). A molecular and cellular theory of depression. *Archives of General Psychiatry, 54,* 597–608.

Dumont, G. J. H., Sweep, F. C. G. J., van der Steen, R., Hermsen, R., Donders, A. R. T., Touw, D. J., et al. (2009). Increased oxytocin concentrations and prosocial feelings in humans after ecstasy (3,4-methylenedioxymethamphetamine) administration. *Social Neuroscience, 4*(4), 359–366. doi:10.1080/17470910802649470

Dunn, M. S., Eddy, J. M., Wang, M. Q., Nagy, S., Perko, M. A., & Bartee, R. T. (2001). The influence of significant others on attitudes, subjective norms and intentions regarding dietary supplement use among adolescent athletes. *Adolescence, 36,* 583–591.

Dunner, C. L. (2007). Efficacy and tolerability of adjunctive ziprasidone in treatment-resistant depression: A randomized, open-label pilot study. *The Journal of Clinical Psychiatry, 68,* 1071–1077.

DuPaul, G. J., & Rappaport, M. D. (1993). Does methylphenidate normalize the classroom performance of children with attention deficit disorder? *Journal of the American Academy of Child and Adolescent Psychiatry, 32,* 190–198.

Eberle, A. J. (1998). Valproate and polycystic ovaries. *Journal of the American Academy of Child and Adolescent Psychiatry, 37,* 1009.

Eckerberg, B., Lowden, A., Nagai, R., & Akerstedt, T. (2012). Melatonin treatment effects on adolescent students sleep timing and sleepiness in a placebo-controlled crossover study. *Chronobiology International, 29,* 1239–1248.

Edwards, J. H. (2002). Evidenced-based treatment for child ADHD: "Real world" practical implications. *Journal of Mental Health Counseling, 24,* 126–129.

Ehlers, A., & Clark, D. M. (2000). A cognitive model of posttraumatic stress disorder. *Behaviour Research and Therapy, 38*(4), 319–345.

Eisner, B. (1994). *Ecstasy: The MDMA story.* Berkeley, CA: Ronin.

Ekinci, O., & Ekinci, A. (2013). Association between insight, cognitive insight, positive symptoms and violence in patients with schizophrenia. *Nordic Journal of Psychiatry, 67,* 116–123.

ElBatsh, M. M., Assareh, N., Marsden, C. A., & Kendall, D. A. (2012). Anxiogenic-like effects of chronic cannabidiol administration in rats. *Psychopharmacology, 221,* 239–247.

Eldredge, D. C. (1998). *Ending the war on drugs: A solution for America.* Bridgehampton, NY: Bridgeworks.

El-Mallakh, R. (1987). Marijuana and migraine. *Headache, 27,* 442–443.

Emiliano, A. B., & Fudge, J. L. (2004). From galactorrhea to osteopenia: Rethinking serotonin-prolactin interactions. *Neuropsychopharmacology, 29,* 833–846.

Emsell, L., & McDonald, C. (2009). The structural neuroimaging of bipolar disorder. *International Review of Psychiatry, 21,* 297–313.

Emslie, G. J., Rush, A. J., Weinberg, W. A., Kowarch, R. A., Hughes, C. W., Carmody, T., et al. (1997). A double-blind, randomized, placebo-controlled trial of fluoxetine in children and adolescents with depression. *Archives of General Psychiatry, 54,* 1031–1037.

Epstein, A. J., Busch, S. H., Busch, A. B., Asch, D. A., & Barry, C. L. (2013). Does exposure to conflict of interest policies in psychiatry residency affect antidepressant prescribing? *Medical Care, 51,* 199–203.

Epstein, H. T. (2001). An outline of the role of brain in human cognitive development. *Brain and Cognition, 45,* 44–51.

Epstein, J. N., Langberg, J. M., Lichtenstein, P. K., Altaye, M., Brinkman, W. B., House, K., et al. (2010). Attention-deficit/hyperactivity disorder outcomes for children treated in community-based pediatric settings. *Archives of Pediatric and Adolescent Medicine, 164,* 160–165.

Ercil, N. E., & France, C. P. (2003). Amphetamine-like discrimination stimulus effects of ephedrine and its stereoisomers in pigeons. *Experimental & Clinical Psychopharmacology, 11,* 3–8.

Erikson, E. (1968). *Identity, youth, and crisis.* New York: Norton.

Ernst, M. E., (2002). The risk-benefit profile of commonly used herbal therapies: Ginkgo, St. John's wort, Ginseng, Echinacea, Saw Palmetto, and Kava. *Annals of Internal Medicine, 136,* 42–53.

Ernst, M. E., Kelly, M. W., Hoehns, J. D., Swegle, J. M., Buys, L. M., Logemann, C. D., et al. (2000). Prescription medication costs: A study of physician familiarity. *Archives of Family Medicine, 9,* 1002–1007.

Ernst, M. E., Malone, R. P., Rowan, A. B., George, R., Gonzalez, N. M., & Silva, R. R. (1999). Anti- psychotics (neuroleptics). In J. S. Werry & M. Aman (Eds.), *Practitioner's guide to psychoactive drugs for children and adolescents* (pp. 297–325). New York: Plenum.

Eskelinen, M. H., & Kivipelto, M. (2010). Caffeine as a protective factor in dementia and Alzheimer's disease. *Journal of Alzheimer's Disease, 20*(Suppl.), S167–S174.

Eskelinen, M. H., Ngandu, T., Tuomilehto, J., Soininen, H., & Kivipelto, M. (2009). Midlife coffee and tea drinking and the risk of late-life dementia: A population based CAIDE study. *Journal of Alzheimer's Disease, 16,* 85–91.

Essali, A., Haasan, A. H. N., Li, C., & Rathbone, J. (2009). Clozapine versus typical neuroleptic medication for schizophrenia. *The Cochrane Database of Systematic Reviews,* issue 21, 1469–1479.

Essali, A., Rihawi, A., Altujjar, M., Alhafez, B., Tarboush, A., & Hasan, A. (2013). Anticholinergic medication for non-clozapine neuroleptic-induced hypersalivation in people with schizophrenia. *The Cochrane Database of Systematic Reviews,* issue 12, 149–153.

Essali, M., Deirawan, H., Soares-Weiser, K., & Adams, C. E. (2011). Calcium channel blockers for neuroleptic-induced tardive dyskinesia. *The Cochrane Database of Systematic Reviews,* issue 12, 139–143.

Ettinger, R. H. (2011). *Psychopharmacology.* Boston: Prentice Hall.

Eubanks, L. M., Rogers, C. J., Beuscher, A. E., Koob, G. F., Olson, A. J., Dickerson, T. J., et al. (2006). A molecular link between the active component of marijuana and Alzheimer's disease pathology. *Molecular Pharmaceutics, 3,* 773–777.

Even, C., Friedman, S., & Dardennes, R. (2001). Anti- depressant trials generally have methodological defects. *British Medical Journal, 323,* 574.

Express Scripts. (2001). *Fact sheet: Express scripts drug trend report.* Retrieved November 14, 2001, from http://www.express-scripts.com/

Eyding, D., Leigemann, M., Grouven, U., Harter, M., Krump, M., Kaiser, T., et al. (2010). Reboxetine for acute treatment of major depression: Systematic review and meta-analysis of published and unpublished placebo and selective serotonin reuptake inhibitor or controlled trials. *British Medical Journal, 341,* c4737–c4759.

Fantegrossi, W. E. (2006). Reinforcing effects of methylenedioxy amphetamine congeners in rhesus monkeys: are intravenous self-administration experiments relevant to MDMA neurotoxicity? *Psychopharmacology, 189*(4), 471–482. doi:10.1007/s00213-006-0320-8

Faraone, S. V., Phiszka, S. R., Olvera, R. L., Skolnik, R. S., & Biederman, J. (2001). Efficacy of adderall and methylphenidate in attention deficit hyperactivity disorder: A reanalysis using drug-placebo and drug-drug response curve methodology. *Journal of Child and Adolescent Psychopharmacology, 11,* 171–180.

Fauth, E. B., & Gibbons, A. (2014). Which behavioral and psychological symptoms of dementia are the most problematic? Variability by prevalence, intensity, distress ratings, and associations with caregiver depressive symptoms. *International Journal of Geriatric Psychiatry, 29,* 263–271.

Fawcett, J., & Busch, K. A. (Eds.). (1998). *Textbook of psychopharmacology* (2nd ed.). Washington, DC: American Psychiatric Association.

FDA. (2005). *Public health advisory: Deaths with antipsychotics in elderly patients with behavioral disturbances.* Retrieved from April 19, 2014, http://www.fda.gov/drugs/drugsafety/postmarketdrugsafetyinformationforpatientsandproviders/drugsafetyinformationforheathcareprofessionals/publichealthadvisories/ucm053171.htm

FDA. (2013a). *FDA drug safety podcast.* Retrieved May 26, 2014, from http://www.fda.gov/drugs/drugsafety/drugsafetypodcasts/ucm379162.htm

FDA. (2013b). *Update: Bupropion Hydrochloride Extended-Release 300 mg bioequivalence studies.* Retrieved May 14, 2014, from http://www.fda.gov/drugs/drugsafety/postmarketdrugsafetyinformationforpatientsandproviders/ucm322161.htm

Federal Register. (2001). Opioid drugs in maintenance and detoxification treatment of opiate addiction: Final rule. *CFR Part 8, 66*(11), 4085.

Felder, C. C., & Glass, M. (1998). Cannabinoid receptors and their endogenous agonists. *Annual Review of Pharmacology and Toxicology, 38,* 179–200.

Feldman, R. S., Meyer, J. S., & Quenzer, L. F. (1997). Sedative and hypnotic drugs. In A. L. Sinauer (Ed.), *Principles of neuropsychopharmacology* (pp. 702–703). Sunderland, MA: Sinauer.

Fenton, W. S., & McGlashan, T. H. (1997). We can talk: Individual psychotherapy for schizophrenia. *American Journal of Psychiatry, 154,* 1493–1495.

Fernandez, H. H., & Friedman, J. H. (2003). Classification and treatment of tardive syndromes. *Neurologist, 9,* 16–27.

Ferracioli-Oda, E., Qawasmi, A., & Bloch, M. H. (2013). Meta-analysis: Melatonin for the treatment of primary sleep disorders. *Los One, 8,* 637–640.

Ferrier, I. N. (1998). Lamotrigine and gabapentin: Alternatives in the treatment of bipolar disorder. *Neuro- Psychobiology, 38,* 192–197.

Fields, R. D. (2009). *The other brain: From dementia to schizophrenia, How new discoveries about the brain are revolutionizing medicine and science.* New York: Simon & Schuster.

Fields, R. D. (2010). Changes in the brain's white matter. *Science, 330,* 768–769.

Fields, R. D. (2011). The hidden brain. *Scientific American Mind, 22,* 53–65.

Fiellin, D. A., Pantalon, M. V., Pakes, J. P., O'Connor, P. G., Chawarski, M., & Schottenfeld, R. S. (2002). Treatment of heroin dependence with buprenorphine in primary care. *American Journal of Drug and Alcohol Abuse, 28*(2), 231–241.

Finberg, J. P. (2014). Update on the pharmacology of selective inhibitors of MAO-A and MAO-B; focus on modulation of CNS monoamine neurotransmitter release. *Pharmacology & Therapeutics, 3,* 34–45.

Findling, R. L., McNamara, N. K., Branicky, L. A., Schluchter, M. D., Lemon, E., & Blumer, J. (2000). A double-blind pilot study of risperidone in the treatment of conduct disorder. *Journal of the American Academy of Child and Adolescent Psychiatry, 39,* 509–516.

Finney, J. W., Hahn, A. C., & Moos, R. H. (1996). The effectiveness of inpatient and outpatient treatment for alcohol abuse: The need to focus on mediators and moderators of setting effects. *Addiction, 91*(12), 1773–1796.

Fisher, R. L., & Fisher, S. (1997). Are we justified in treating children with psychotropic drugs? In S. Fisher & R. P. Greenberg (Eds.), *From placebo to panacea: Putting psychiatric drugs to the test* (pp. 307–322). New York: Wiley.

Fisher, S., & Greenberg, R. P. (Eds.). (1997). *From placebo to panacea: Putting psychiatric drugs to the test.* New York: Wiley.

Fitzgerald, K. T., & Bronstein, A. C. (2013). Selective serotonin reuptake inhibitor exposure. *Topics in Companion Animal Medicine, 28,* 13–17.

Flaherty, J. A., & Meagher, R. (1980). Measuring racial bias in inpatient treatment. *American Journal of Psychiatry, 137,* 679–682.

Flam, F. (1994). Hints of language in junk DNA. *Science, 266,* 1320.

Flanagan, R. J. (2008). Fatal toxicity of drugs used in psychiatry. *Human Psychopharmacology, 23,* 43–51.

Fleischhacker, W. W., Czobor, P., Hummer, M., Kemmler, G., Kohnen, R., & Volavka, J. (2003). Placebo or active control trials of antipsychotic drugs? *Archives of General Psychiatry, 60,* 458–464.

Food and Drug Administration [FDA]. (2003). *FDA public health advisory: Reports of suicidality in pediatric patients being treated with antidepressant medication for major depressive disorder.* Retrieved November 1, 2003, from www.fda.gov/cder/drug/advisory/mdd.htm

Forsythe, P., Kunze, W. A., & Bienenstock, J. (2012). On communication between gut microbes and the brain. *Current Opinion in Gastroenterology, 28,* 557–562.

Fortinguerra, F., Clavenna, M., & Bonati, M. (2014). Psychotropic drug use during breastfeeding: A review of the evidence. *Pedatrics, 124,* 547–556.

Fowler, J. S., Logan, J., Azzaro, A. J., Fielding, R. M., Zhu, W., Poshusta, A. K., et al. (2010). Reversible inhibitors of monoamine oxidase-a (RIMAs): Robust, reversible inhibition of human brain MAO-A by CX157. *Neuropsychopharmacology, 35*(3), 623–631.

Fox, M. (2003). Baseball player's death re-ignites ephedra debate. *Reuters Daily News,* p. 2, C1.

Frances, A. (2013). *Saving normal: An insider's revolt against out-of-control psychiatric diagnosis, DSM-5, big pharma, and the medicalization of ordinary life.* New York: Morrow.

Frank, C. (2014). Pharmacologic treatment of depression in the elderly. *Canadian Family Physician, 60,* 121–131.

Franklin, D. (1990). Hooked-not hooked: Why isn't everyone an addict? *Health, 1,* 39–52.

Frazier, J. A., Ahn, M. S., DeJong, S., Bent, E. K., Breeze, J. L., & Guiliano, A. J. (2005). Magnetic resonance imaging studies in early-onset bipolar disorder: A critical review. *Harvard Review of Psychiatry, 13,* 125–140.

Freedman, A. M., & Schatzberg, A. F. (1997). A placebo-controlled, double-blind randomized trial of an extract of Ginkgo biloba for dementia. *Journal of the American Medical Association, 278,* 1327–1332.

Freeman, T. W., Clothier, J. L., Pazzaglia, P., Lesem, M. D., & Swann, A. C. (1992). A double-blind comparison of valproate and lithium in the treatment of acute mania. *American Journal of Psychiatry, 149*(1), 108–111.

Freud, S. (1925). Inhibitions, symptoms, and anxiety. In J. Strachey (Ed.), *The standard edition of the complete psychological works of sigmund freud* (pp. 77–178). London: Hogarth Press.

Freud, S., & Carter, D. (2011). *On cocaine.* New York: Hersperus.

Freudenmann, R. W., Öxler, F., & Bernschneider-Reif, S. (2006). The origin of MDMA (ecstasy) revisited: the true story reconstructed from the original documents. *Addiction, 101*(9), 1241–1245. doi:10.1111/j.1360-0443.2006.01511.x

Fried, P., Watkinson, B., James, D., & Gray, R. (2002). Current and former marijuana use: Preliminary findings of a longitudinal study of effects on IQ in young adults. *Canadian Medical Association Journal, 166,* 887–891.

Friede, M., Henneicke von Zepelin, H. H., & Freudenstein, J. (2001). Differential therapy of mild to moderate depressive episodes (ICD-10 F 32.0; F 32.1) with St. John's wort. *Pharmacopsychiatry, 34*(Suppl. 1), 38–41.

Friedman, J. H. (2003). Atypical antipsychotics in the EPS-vulnerable patient. *Psychoneuroendocrinology, 28,* 39–51.

Friedman, R. A. (2012, September 24). A call for caution on antipsychotic drugs. *New York Times,* Health Section, pp. 1–2. Retrieved April 13, 2014, from http://www.nytimes.com/2012/09/25/health/a-call-for-caution-in-the-use-of-antipsychotic-drugs.html

Frood, A. (2007). Inhaling cannabis without the smoke. *Nature News, 10.* Retrieved May 6, 2014, from http://www.nature.com/news/2007/070508/full/news070508-11.html

Frye, M. A., Ketter, T. A., Kimbrell, T. A., Dunn, R. T., Speer, R. M., Osuch, E. A., et al. (2000). A placebo-controlled study of lamotrigine and gabapentin monotherapy in refractory mood disorders. *Journal of Clinical Psychopharmacology, 20,* 607–614.

Fudalla, P. J., Macfadden, W., Boardman, C., & Chiang, C. N. (1998). Effects of buprenorphine for the management of opioid withdrawal. *Drug and Alcohol Dependence, 50,* 1-8.

Fuller, M. A., Shermock, K. M., Secic, M., & Grogg, A. L. (2003). Comparative study of the development of diabetes mellitus in patients taking risperidone and olanzapine. *Pharmocotherapy, 23,* 1037–1043.

Fuller, R. K., Branchey, L., Brightwell, D. R., Derman, R. M., Emrick, C. D., Iber, F. L., et al. (1986). Disulfiram treatment of alcoholism: A Veterans Administration cooperative study. *Journal of the American Medical Association, 256,* 1449-1455.

Furman, R. (1993). Kuhn, chaos and psychoanalysis. *Child Analysis, 4,* 133–150.

Furman, R. (2000). Attention deficit/hyperactivity disorder: An alternative viewpoint. *Journal of Infant, Child and Adolescent Psychotherapy, 2,* 125–144.

Gabbard, G. O. (1994). *Psychodynamic psychiatry in clinical practice: The DSM-IV edition.* Washington, DC: American Psychiatric Press.

Gabbard, G. O. (2001a). Mind and brain in psychiatric treatment. In G. O. Gabbard (Ed.), *Treatment of the DSM-IV psychiatric disorders* (3rd ed., pp. 3–21). Washington, DC: American Psychiatric Press.

Gabbard, G. O. (Ed.). (2001b). *Treatments of psychiatric disorders* (3rd ed., Vols. I and II). Washington, DC: American Psychiatric Association.

Gable, R. S. (1993). Toward a comparative overview of dependence potential and acute toxicity of psychoactive substances used nonmedically. *The American Journal of Drug and Alcohol Abuse, 19*(3), 263–281.

Galbally, M., Roberts, M., Buist, A., & Perinatal Psychotropic Review Group. (2010). Mood stabilizers in pregnancy: A systematic review. *Australian and New Zealand Journal of Psychiatry, 44,* 967–977.

Galynker, I., Leronimo, C., Miner, C., Rosenblum, J., Vilkas, N., & Rosenthal, R. (1997). Methylphenidate treatment of negative symptoms in patients with dementia. *The Journal of Neuropsychiatry and Clinical Neurosciences, 9,* 231–239.

Gamma, A., Buck, A., Berthold, T., Liechti, M. E., Vollenweider, F. X., & Hell, D. (2000). 3,4-Methylenedioxymethamphetamine (MDMA) modulates cortical and limbic brain activity as measured by [H(2)(15)O]-PET in healthy humans. *Neuropsychopharmacology: Official Publication of the American College of Neuropsychopharmacology, 23*(4), 388–395. doi:10.1016/S0893-133X(00)00130-5

Garbarino, J. (1998). Children in a violent world: A metaphysical perspective. *Family and Conciliation Courts Review, 36,* 360–367.

Garbutt, J. C., Kranzler, H. R., & O'Malley, S. S. (2005). Efficacy and tolerability of long-acting injectable naltrexone for alcohol dependence: A randomized controlled trial. *Journal of the American Medical Association, 293*(13), 1617–1625.

Garbutt, J. C., West, S. L., Carey, T. S., Lohr, K. N., & Crews, F. T. (1999). Pharmacological treatment of alcohol dependence: A review of the evidence. *Journal of the American Medical Association, 281*(14), 1318–1325.

Gardiner, H. W., & Kosmitzki, C. (2001). *Lives across cultures: Cross cultural human development* (2nd ed.). Boston: Allyn and Bacon.

Garland, E. J. (2002). Anxiety disorders. In S. Kutcher (Ed.), *Practical child and adolescent psychopharmacology* (pp. 187–229). Cambridge, UK: Cambridge.University Press.

Garver, D., Lazarus, A., Rajogopalan, K., Lamerato, L., Katz, L. M., Stern, L. S., et al. (2006). Racial differences in medication switching and concomitant prescriptions in the treatment of bipolar disorder. *Psychiatric Services, 57,* 332–338.

Gaster, B., & Holroyd, J. (2000). St. John's wort for depression: A systematic review. *Archives of Internal Medicine, 160,* 152–156.

Gearing, F. R., & Schweitzer, M. D. (1974). An epidemiologic evaluation of long-term methadone maintenance treatment for heroin addiction. *American Journal of Epidemiology, 100*(2), 101–112.

Geiger, J. D. (2002). Adverse events associated with supplements containing ephedra alkaloids. *Clinical Journal of Sport Medicine, 12,* 263.

Geller, B., Luby, J. L., Joshi, P., Wagner, K. D., Emslie, G., Walkup, J. T., et al. (2012). A randomized controlled trial of risperidone, lithium, or divalproex sodium for initial treatment of bipolar I disorder, manic or mixed phase, in children and adolescents. *Archives of General Psychiatry, 69,* 515–528.

Gelman, S. (1999). *Medicating schizophrenia: A history.* New Brunswick, NJ: Rutgers University Press.

Gentile, S. (2010). Neurodevelopmental effects of prenatal exposure to psychotropic medications. *Depression and Anxiety, 27,* 275–286.

Genung, V. (2013). Psychopharmacology column: A review of psychotropic mediation lactation risks for infants during breastfeeding. *Journal of Child and Adolescent Psychiatric Nursing, 26,* 214–219.

Gerra, G., Ferri, M., Polidori, E., Santoro, G., Zaimovic, A., & Sternieri, E. (2003). Long-term methadone maintenance effectiveness: Psychosocial and pharmacological variables. *Journal of Substance Abuse Treatment, 25,* 1–8.

Ghaemi, S. N., Berv, D. A., Klugman, J., Resenquist, K. J., & Hsu, D. J. (2003). Oxcarbazepine treatment of bipolar disorder. *Journal of Clinical Psychiatry, 64,* 943–945.

Ghaemi, S. N., Ko, J. Y., & Goodwin, F. K. (2002). "Cade's disease" and beyond: Misdiagnosis, antidepressant use, and a proposed definition for bipolar spectrum disorder. *Canadian Journal of Psychiatry, 47,* 125–134.

Gianluigi, T., Pontieri, F. E., & Chiara, G. (1997). Cannabinoid and heroin activation of mesolimbic dopamine transmission by a common opioid receptor mechanism. *Science, 276,* 2048–2049.

Gigliucci, V., O'Dowd, G., Casey, S., Egan, D., Gibney, S., & Harkin, A. (2013). Ketamine elicits sustained antidepressant-like activity via a serotonin-dependent mechanism. *Psychopharmacology, 228,* 157–166.

Gimenez, M., Ortiz, H., Soriano-Mas, C., Lopez-Sola, M., Farre, M., Deus, J., et al. (2014). Functional effects of chronic paroxetine versus placebo on the fear, stress and anxiety brain circuit in social anxiety disorder: Initial validation of an imaging protocol for drug discovery. *European Neuropsychopharmacology, 24*(1), 105–116.

Glazer, W. M., Morgenstern, H., & Doucette, J. (1994). Race and tardive dyskinesia among outpatients at a CMHC. *Hospital Community Psychiatry, 45,* 38–42.

Gledhill, J. A., Moore, D. F., Bell, D., & Henry, J. A. (1993). Subarachnoid haemorrhage associated with MDMA abuse. *Journal of Neurology, Neurosurgery, and Psychiatry, 56*(9), 1036–1037.

Glennon, R. A., & Young, R. (2000). Amphetamine-stimulus generalization to an herbal ephedrine product. *Pharmacology, Biochemistry, & Behavior, 65,* 655–688.

Glick, S. D., & Maisonneuve, I. S. (1998). Mechanisms of antiaddictive actions of ibogaine. *Annals of the New York Academy of Sciences, 844,* 214–226.

Gochman, P., Miller, R., & Rapoport, J. L. (2011). Childhood-onset schizophrenia: The challenge of diagnosis. *Current Psychiatry Reports, 13,* 321–322.

Gold, J. L., Laxer, D. A., Dergal, J. M., Lanctot, K. L., & Rochon, P. A. (2001). Herbal-drug interactions: A focus on dementia. *Current Opinion in Clinical Nutrition and Metabolic Care, 4,* 29–34.

Gold, M. S., Tullis, M., & Frost-Pineda, K. (2001). Cannabis use, abuse, and dependence. In G. O. Gabbard (Ed.), *Treatment of psychiatric disorders* (3rd ed., pp. 703–719). Washington, DC: American Psychiatric Association.

Goldman-Rakic, P., & Brown, R. M. (1982). Postnatal development of monoamine content and synthesis in the cerebral cortex of rhesus monkeys. *Developmental Brain Research, 4,* 339–349.

Goldstein, A. P., & Conoley, J. C. (1998). Student aggression: Current status. In A. P. Goldstein & J. C. Conoley (Eds.), *School violence intervention: A practical handbook* (pp. 3–19). New York: Guilford Press.

Goldstein, L. E., Spron, J., Brown, S., Kim, H., Finkelstein, J., Gaffey, G. K., et al. (1999). New-onset diabetes mellitus and diabetic ketoacidosis associated with olanzapine treatment. *Psychosomatics, 40,* 438–443.

Goleman, D. (1993, December 15). Use of antidepressants in children at issue. *New York Times,* p. 7.

Gonzales, J. P., & Brogden, R. N. (1988). Naltrexone: A review of its pharmacologic and pharmacokinetic properties and therapeutic efficacy in the management of opioid dependence. *Drugs, 35*(3), 192–213.

Goodwin, F. K., & Ghaemi, S. N. (1999). The impact of the discovery of lithium on psychiatric thought and practice in the USA and Europe. *Australian New Zealand Journal of Psychiatry, 33*(Suppl. 1), 54–64.

Goodwin, F. K., & Jamison, K. R. (1990). *Manic depressive illness.* New York: Oxford University Press.

Gordis, E. (2000). Why do some people drink too much? The role of genetic and psychosocial influences. *Alcohol Research and Health, 24,* 17–26.

Gordon, A., & Price, L. H. (1999). Mood stabilizers and weight loss with topiramate. *American Journal of Psychiatry, 156,* 968–969.

Gordon, D., Burn, D., Campbell, A., & Baker, O. (2008). *The 2007 user satisfaction survey of Tier 2 and 3 service users in England.* National Treatment Agency for Substance Misuse. Retrieved January 2, 2014 from http://www.nta.nhs.uk/uploads/nta_2007_user_satis_survey_tier2and3_service_users_england.pdf

Gorman, I. (2013a). *An analysis of the working alliance in MDMA-assisted therapy.* Retrieved May 23, 2014, from https://www.youtube.com/watch?v=BGCteSuae8

Gorman, J. M. (2006). Gender differences in depression and response to psychotropic medication. *Gender Medicine, 3,* 93–109.

Gottfries, C. G. (1988). Dementia: Classification and aspects of treatment. *Psychopharmacology Series, 5,* 187–195.

Gould, E., Beylin, A., Panapat, P., Reeves, A., & Shors, T. J. (1999). Learning enhances adult neurogenesis in the hippocampal formation. *Nature Neuroscience, 2,* 260–265.

Gourlay, J., Ricciardelli, L., & Ridge, D. (2005). Users' experiences of heroin and methadone treatment. *Substance Use and Misuse, 40,* 1875–1882.

Gouzoulis-Mayfrank, E., & Daumann, J. (2006). Neurotoxicity of methylenedioxyamphetamines (MDMA; ecstasy) in humans: How strong is the evidence for persistent brain damage? *Addiction, 101*(3), 348–361. doi:10.1111/j.1360-0443.2006.01314.x

Gowing, L., Ali, R., & White, J. (2002). Effects of buprenorphine for the management of opioid withdrawal. *Cochrane Database of Systematic Reviews,* issue 2, CD002025.

Grande, I., Pons, A., Baeza, I., Torras, A., & Bernardo, M. (2011). QTc prolongation: Is clozapine safe? Study of 82 cases before and after clozapine treatment. *Human Psychopharmacology, 26,* 397–403.

Gray, G. E. (1999). A psychiatric perspective on herbal remedies. *Directions in Psychiatry, 19,* 349–359.

Gray, J. A. (1987). *Neuropsychological theory of anxiety: An investigation of the septal-hippocampal system* (2nd ed.). Cambridge, England: Cambridge University Press.

Green, R. W., & Albon, J. S. (2001). What does the MTA study tell us about effective psychosocial treatment for ADHD? *Journal of Clinical Child Psychology, 30,* 114–121.

Greenberg, G. (2013). The psychiatric drug crisis. *The New Yorker.* Retrieved April 13, 2014, from http://www.newyorker.com/online/blogs/elements/2013/09/psychiatry-prozac-ssri-mental-health-theory-discredited.html

Greenberg, R. P., & Fisher, S. (1997). Mood-mending medicines: Probing drug, psychotherapy, and placebo solutions. In S. Fisher & R. P. Greenberg (Eds.), *From placebo to panacea: Putting psychiatric drugs to the test* (pp. 115–172). New York: Wiley.

Greenblatt, D. J. (1991). Benzodiazepine hypnotics: Sorting the pharmacokinetic facts. *The Journal of Clinical Psychiatry, 52*(Suppl.), 4–10.

Greenblatt, D. J., Harmatz, J. S., Walsh, J. K., Luthringer, R., Staner, L., Otmani, S., et al. (2011). Pharmacokinetic profile of SKP-1041, a modified release formulation of zaleplon. *Biopharmaceutics & Drug Disposition, 32,* 189–197.

Greenhill, L. L. (1998). Childhood attention deficit hyperactivity disorder: Pharmacological treatments. In P. Nathan & J. Gorman (Eds.), *A guide to treatments that work* (pp. 42–64). New York: Oxford University Press.

Greenhill, L. L., Jensen, P. S., Abikoff, H., Blumer, J. L., DeVeaugh-Geiss, J., Fisher, C., et al. (2003). Developing strategies for psychopharmacological studies on preschool children. *Journal of the American Academy of Child and Adolescent Psychiatry, 42*, 406–414.

Greer, G. (1985). Using MDMA in psychotherapy. *Advances, 2*, 57–62.

Greer, G., & Tolbert, R. (1986). Subjective reports of the effects of MDMA in a clinical setting. *Journal of Psychoactive Drugs, 18*(4), 319–327.

Griffiths, R. R., Johnson, M. W., Richards, W. A., Richards, B. D., McCann, U., & Jesse, R. (2011). Psilocybin occasioned mystical-type experiences: immediate and persisting dose-related effects. *Psychopharmacology, 218*(4), 649–665. doi:10.1007/s00213-011-2358-5

Griffiths, R. R., Richards, W. A., Johnson, M., McCann, U., & Jesse, R. (2008). Mystical-type experiences occasioned by psilocybin mediate the attribution of personal meaning and spiritual significance 14 months later. *Journal of Psychopharmacology, 22*(6), 621–632. doi:10.1177/0269881108094300

Griffiths, R. R., Richards, W. A., McCann, U., & Jesse, R. (2006). Psilocybin can occasion mystical-type experiences having substantial and sustained personal meaning and spiritual significance. *Psychopharmacology, 187*(3), 268–283; discussion 284–292. doi:10.1007/s00213-006-0457-5

Grilly, D. M. (1994). *Drugs and human behavior* (3rd ed.). Boston: Allyn and Bacon.

Grilly, D.M., & Salomone, J. (2011). *Drugs, brain and behavior* (6th ed.). Upper Saddle River, NJ: Pearson.

Grinspoon, L., & Bakalar, J. B. (1997). *Psychedelic drugs reconsidered.* New York: Lindsmith Center.

Grob, C. S., Danforth, A. L., Chopra, G. S., Hagerty, M., McKay, C. R., Halberstadt, A. L., et al. (2011). Pilot study of psilocybin treatment for anxiety in patients with advanced-stage cancer. *Archives of General Psychiatry, 68*(1), 71. doi:10.1001/archgenpsychiatry.2010.116

Grob, C. S., Poland, R. E., Chang, L., & Ernst, T. (1996). Psychobiologic effects of 3,4-methylenedioxymethamphetamine in humans: methodological considerations and preliminary observations. *Behavioural Brain Research, 73*(1–2), 103–107.

Grobler, A. C., Matthews, G., & Molenberghs, G. (2013). The impact of missing data on clinical trials: A re-analysis of a placbo controlled trial of hypericum perforatum (St. John's wort) and sertraline in major depressive disorder. *Psychopharmacology, 11*, 345–351.

Grof, S. (1998). *The transpersonal vision: The healing potential of non-ordinary states of consciousness.* Boulder, CO: Sounds True.

Grof, S. (2000). *Psychology of the future: Lessons from modern consciousness research.* Albany: SUNY Press.

Grof, P. (2006). Responders to long-term lithium treatment. In M. Bauer, P. Grof, & B. Mueller-Oerlinghausen (Eds.), *Lithium in neuropsychiatry: The comprehensive guide* (pp. 157–178). London: Informa.

Grof, P., & Alda, M. (2001). Discrepancies in the efficacy of lithium. *Archives of General Psychiatry, 57*, 191.

Grof, P., Alda, M., Grof, E., Fox, D., & Cameron, P. (1993). The challenge of predicting response to stabilising lithium treatment: The importance of patient selection. *British Journal of Psychiatry, 163*(Suppl. 21), 16–19.

Grof, P., & Muller-Oerlinghausen, B. (2009). A critical appraisal of lithium's efficacy and effectiveness: The last 60 years. *Bipolar Disorders, 11*(Suppl. 2), 10–19.

Grof, S., Hofmann, A., & Weil, A. (2008). *LSD psychotherapy.* Ben Lomond, CA: Multidisciplinary Association for Psychedelic Studies.

Grootens, K. P., van Veelen, N. M., Peuskens, J., Sabbe, B. G., Thys, E., Buitelaar, J. K., et al. (2009). Ziprasidone vs olanzapine in recent-onset schizophrenia and schizoaffective disorder: results of an 8-week double-blind randomized controlled trial. *Schizophrenia Bulletin, 37*, 352–361.

Grossberg, G. T. (2010). Geriatric psychiatry—an emerging specialty. *Missouri Medicine, 107*, 401–405.

Grube, B., Walper, A., & Wheatley, D. (1999). St. John's wort extract: Efficacy for menopausal symptoms of psychological origin. *Advances in Therapy, 16*, 177–186.

Gruber, A. J., & Pope, H. G. (1998). Ephedrine abuse among 36 female weightlifters. *American Journal on Addictions, 7*, 256–261.

Gunaratana, B. H. (2002). *Mindfulness in plain English.* Boston: Wisdom Publications.

Gurevich, A., Guller, V., Berner, Y. N., & Tal, S. (2012). Are atypical antipsychotics safer than typical antipsychotics for treating behavioral and psychological symptoms of dementia? *The Journal of Nutrition, Health & Aging, 16*, 557–561.

Gurley, R. J., Aranow, R., & Katz, M. (1998). Medicinal marijuana: A comprehensive review. *Journal of Psychoactive Drugs, 30*, 137–147.

Gurvich, T., & Cunningham, J. A. (2000, March 1). Appropriate use of psychotropic drugs in nursing homes. *American Family Physician, 61*(5), 1437–1446.

Gutgesell, H., Atkins, D., Barst, R., Buck, M., Franklin, W., Humes, R., et al. (1999). AHA scientific statement: Cardiovascular monitoring of children and adolescents receiving psychotropic drugs. *Journal of the American Academy of Child & Adolescent Psychiatry, 38*, 1047–1050.

Gutherie, S. K. (1999, September 24). *Herbaceuticals in psychiatry.* Unpublished lecture given at the Medical College of Ohio, Toledo.

Haile, C. N., Murrough, J. W., Iosifescu, D. V., Chang, L. C., Al Jurdi, A. I., Foulkes, A., et al. (2014). Plasma brain derived neurotrophic factor (BDNF) and response to ketamine in treatment resistant depression. *International Journal of Neuropsychopharmacology, 17*, 331–336.

Hailemaskel, B., Dutta, A., & Wutoh, A. (2001). Adverse reactions and interactions among herbal users. *Issues in Interdisciplinary Care, 3*, 297–300.

Hall, W., & Degenhardt, L. (2014). The adverse health effects of chronic cannabis use. *Drug Testing and Analysis, 6,* 39–45.

Halpern, J. H., & Pope, H. G., Jr. (1999). Do hallucinogens cause residual neuropsychological toxicity? *Drug and Alcohol Dependence, 53*(3), 247–256.

Hamilton, J. A. (1986). An overview of the clinical rationale for advancing gender related psychopharmacology and drug abuse research. In B. A. Ray & M. C. Baude (Eds.), *Women and drugs: A new era for research* (pp. 14–20). Washington, DC: U.S. Government Printing Office. (NIDA [National Institute on Drug Abuse] manuscript).

Hamlin, V., McCarthy, E. M., & Tyson, V. (2010). Pediatric psychotropic medication initiation and adherence: A literature review based on social exchange theory. *Journal of Child and Adolescent Psychiatric Nursing, 23,* 151–172.

Hampson, A. J., Grimaldi, M., Lolic, M., Wink, D., Rosenthal, R., & Axelrod, J. (2000). Neuroprotective antioxidants from marijuana. *Annals of the New York Academy of Sciences, 899,* 274–282.

Haney, M., Ward, A. S., Comer, S. D., Foltin, R. W., & Fischman, M. W. (1999). Abstinence symptoms following smoked marijuana in humans. *Psychopharmacology, 141,* 395–404.

Hansen, F., de Oliveira, D. L., Amaral, F. U., Guedes, F. S., Schneider, T. J., Tumelero, A. C., et al. (2011). Effects of chronic administration of tryptophan with or without concomitant fluoxetine in depression-related and anxiety-like behaviors on adult rat. *Neuroscience Letters, 499,* 59–63.

Hardy, J. A., & Higgins, G. A. (1992). Alzheimer's disease: The amyloid cascade hypothesis. *Science, 256,* 184–185.

Harmer, C. J., Bhagwagar, Z., Perrett, D. J., Volim, B. A., Cowen, P. J., & Goodwin, G. M. (2003). Acute SSRI administration affects the processing of social cues in healthy volunteers. *Neuropscychopharmacology, 28,* 148–152.

Harmer, C. J., & Cowen, P. J. (2013). "It's the way you look at it"—a cognitive neuropsychological account of SSRI action in depression. *Philosophical Transactions of the Royal Society, 368,* 1–8.

Harper, S. (2012). Do medical marijuana laws increase marijuana use? Replication study and extension. *Annals of Epidemiology, 22,* 207–212.

Harris, D. S., Baggott, M., Mendelson, J. H., Mendelson, J. E., & Jones, R. T. (2002). Subjective and hormonal effects of 3, 4-methylenedioxymethamphetamine (MDMA) in humans. *Psychopharmacology, 162*(4), 396–405. doi:10.1007/s00213-002-1131-1

Harris, G. (2004). Study shows medication helps teens in depression. *New York Times,* p. A10.

Harrison, R. A., Holt, D., Pattison, D. J., & Elton, P. J. (2004). Who and how many people are taking herbal supplements? A survey of 21,923 adults. *International Journal for Vitamin and Nutrition Research, 74,* 183–186.

Harrison, T. S., & Keating, G. M. (2005). Zolpidem: A review of its use in the management of insomnia. *CNS Drugs, 19,* 65–89.

Hartberg, C. B., Sundet, K., Rimol, L., Haukvik, U. K., Lange, E. H., Nesvag, R., et al. (2011). Subcortical brain volumes relate to neurocognition in schizophrenia and bipolar disorder and healthy controls. *Progress in Neuro-Psychopharmacology & Biological Psychiatry, 35,* 1122–1130.

Hartong, E. G., Moleman, P., Hoogduin, C. A., Broekman, T. G., & Nolan, N. A. (2003). Prophylactic efficacy of lithium versus carbamazepine/Tegretol in treatment-naive bipolar patients. *The Journal of Clinical Psychiatry, 63,* 144–151.

Hasimoto, K., Malchow, B., Falkai, P., & Schmitt, A. (2013). Glutamate modulators as potential therapeutic drugs in schizophrenia and affective disorders. *European Archives of Psychiatry & Clinical Neuroscience, 263,* 367–377.

Hasler, F., Grimberg, U., Benz, M. A., Huber, T., & Vollenweider, F. X. (2004). Acute psychological and physiological effects of psilocybin in healthy humans: a double-blind, placebo-controlled dose effect study. *Psychopharmacology, 172*(2), 145–156. doi:10.1007/s00213-003-1640-6

Hausmann, L. R., Gao, S., Lee, E. S., & Kwoh, C. K. (2013). Racial disparities in the monitoring of patients on chronic opioid therapy. *Pain, 154,* 46–52.

Healy, D. (1997). *The antidepressant era.* Cambridge, MA: Harvard University Press.

Healy, D. (2002). *The creation of psychopharmacology.* Cambridge, MA: Harvard University Press.

Healy, D. (2008). *Mania: A short history of bipolar disorder.* Baltimore, MD: Johns Hopkins Press.

Healy, D. (2013). *Pharmageddon.* Berkeley, CA: University of California Press.

Healy, D., Herxheimer, A., & Menkes, D. B. (2007). Antidepressants and violence: Problems at the interface of medicine and law. *International Journal of Risk and Safety in Medicine, 19,* 17–33.

Healy, M. (2014, February 18). New test suggests antidepressant paxil may promote breast cancer. *Los Angeles Times,* p. 2.

Heilig, M., & Egli, M. (2006). Pharmacological treatment of alcohol dependence: Target symptoms and target mechanisms. *Pharmacology & Therapeutics, 111,* 855–876.

Heimann, S. W. (1999). High-dose olanzapine in an adolescent. *Journal of the American Academy of Child and Adolescent Psychiatry, 38,* 496–498.

Heinala, P., Alho, H., Kiianmaa, K., Lonnqvist, J., Kuoppasalmi, K., & Sinclair, J. D. (2001). Targeted use of naltrexone without prior detoxification in the treatment of alcohol dependence: A factorial double-blind, placebo controlled trial. *Journal of Clinical Psychopharmacology, 21*(3), 287–292.

Heinrich, M., & Gibbons, S. (2001). Ethnopharmacology in drug discovery: An analysis of its role and potential contribution. *Journal of Pharmacy and Pharmacology, 53,* 425–432.

Hellerstein, D. J., Batchelder, S., Hyler, S., Arnaout, B., Corpuz, V., Coram, L., et al. (2008). Aripiprazole as an adjunctive treatment for refractory unipolar depression. *Progress in Neuro-Psychopharmacology & Biological Psychiatry, 32,* 744–750.

Henry, J. A., Jeffreys, K. J., & Dawling, S. (1992). Toxicity and deaths from 3,4 methylenedioxymethamphetamine ("ecstasy"). *Lancet, 340*(8816), 384–387.

Hensley, S. (2012). *Glaxo to plead guilty to three charges in sweeping healthcare settlement*. Retrieved May 28, 2014, from http://www.npr.org/blogs/health/2012/07/02/156116607/glaxo-pleads-guilty-to-3-charges-in-sweeping-health-settlement

Herer, J. (1992). *The emperor wears no clothes: Hemp & the marijuana conspiracy* (rev. ed.). Van Nuys, CA: HEMP Publishing.

Herkenham, M. L., Little, M. D., Johnson, M. R., Melvin, L. S., deCosta, B. R., & Rice, K. C. (1990). Cannabinoid receptor localization in the brain. *Proceedings of the National Academy of Science, 87,* 1932–1936.

Hernandez, F., Nido, J. D., Avila, J., & Villanueva, N. (2009). GSK3 inhibitors and disease. *Mini-Reviews in Medicinal Chemistry, 9,* 1024–1029.

Herz, A. (1997). Endogenous opioid systems and alcohol addiction. *Psychopharmacology, 129*(2), 99–111.

Hester, R. K., Delaney, H. D., & Campbell, W. (2011). Moderatedrinking.com and moderation management: Outcomes of a randomized clinical trial with non-dependent problem drinkers. *Journal of Consulting and Clinical Psychology, 79,* 215–224.

Higgit, A. C., Lader, M. H., & Fonagy, P. (1985). Clinical management of benzodiazepine dependence. *British Medical Journal, 291,* 688–689.

Hirschfeld, R. M. A., Calabrese, J. R., Weissman, M. M., Reed, M., Davies, M. A., Frye, M. A., et al. (2003). Screening for bipolar disorder in the community. *Journal of Clinical Psychiatry, 64,* 53–59.

Hodge, K., & Jespersen, S. (2008). Side-effects and treatment with clozapine: A comparison between the views of consumers and their clinicians. *International Journal of Mental Health Nursing, 17,* 2–8.

Hoge, W. (2002). *Britain to relax marijuana laws*. Retrieved October 14, 2004, from http://www.hempfarm.org/Papers/Britains_Relax.html

Hollon, M. F. (1999). Direct-to-consumer marketing of prescription drugs: Creating consumer demand. *Journal of the American Medical Association, 281,* 1227–1228.

Holsboer-Trachsler, F., & Vanoni, C. (1999). Clinical efficacy and tolerance of the hypericum special extract LI 160 in depressive disorders: A drug monitoring study. *Schweizerische Rundschau für Medizin Praxis, 88,* 1475–1480.

Hood, S. D., Norman, A., Hince, D. A., Meichar, J. K., & Hulse, G. K. (2014). Benzodiazepine dependence and its treatment with low dose flumazenil. *British Journal of Clinical Pharmacology, 77,* 285–294.

Houghton, P. J. (1999). The scientific basis for the reputed activity of valerian. *Journal of Pharmacy and Pharmacology, 51,* 505–512.

House, A. E. (1999). *DSM-IV diagnosis in the schools*. New York: Guilford Press.

Houser, W., & Milton, S. Hershey Medical Center. (2012, July). *Effects of involvement in a group-based creative expression program on psychotrpoic drug use in persons with dementia*. (Clinical trial number NCT01382693). Retrieved August, 26, 2014, from http://clinicaltrials.gov/show/NCT01382693

Howland, R. H. (2009). Prescribing psychotropic medications during pregnancy and lactation: Principles and guidelines. *Journal of Psychosocial Nursing and Mental Health Services, 47,* 19–23.

Hubble, M., Duncan, B. L., & Miller, S. A. (2001). *The heart and soul of change: What works in therapy*. Washington, DC: American Psychological Association.

Huedo-Medina, T. B., Kirsch, I., Middlemas, J., Klonizakis, M., & Siriwardena, N. (2012). Effectiveness of non-benzodiazepine hypnotics in treatment of adult insomnia: Meta-analysis of data submitted to the food and drug administration. *British Medical Journal, 345,* 343–355.

Huffington, A. (2000). *How to overthrow the government*. New York: Regan Books.

Hunt, G. H., & Odoroff, M. E. (1962). Follow up study of narcotic drug addicts after hospitalization. *Public Health Reports, 77,* 41–54.

Hurley, S. C. (2002). Lamotrigine update and its use in mood disorders. *Annals of Pharmacotherapy, 36,* 860–873.

Hurley, L. L., Akinfiresoyle, L., Nwulia, E., Kamiya, A., Kulkami, A. A., & Tizabi, Y. (2013). Antidepressant-like effect of curcumin in WKY rat model of depression is associated with an increase in hippocampal BDNF. *Behavioural Brain Research, 239,* 27–30.

Hutton, R. (1999). *The triumph of the moon: A history of modern pagan witchcraft*. Oxford, UK: Oxford University Press.

Huxley, A. (1932). *Brave new world*. New York: Perennial.

Huxley, A., & Huxley, A. (1977). *The doors of perception? and, heaven and hell*. St Albans: Triad.

Hypericum Depression Trial Study Group. (2002). Effect of Hypericum perforatum (St. John's wort) in major depressive disorder: A randomized controlled trial. *Journal of the American Medical Association, 287,* 1807–1814.

Hysek, C. M., Schmid, Y., Simmler, L. D., Domes, G., Heinrichs, M., Eisenegger, C., et al. (2013). MDMA enhances emotional empathy and prosocial behavior. *Social Cognitive and Affective Neuroscience*. doi:10.1093/scan/nst161

IMS Health. (2014). *Medicine use and shifting cost of healthcare*. Retrieved May 8, 2014, from http://www.imshealth.com/cds/imshealth/Global/Content/Corporate/IMS%20Health%20Institute/Reports/Secure/IIHI_US_Use_of_Meds_for_2013.pdf

Ingersoll, R. E. (2000). Teaching a course in psychopharmacology to counselors: Justification, structure, and methods. *Counselor Education and Supervision, 40,* 58–69.

Ingersoll, R. E. (2001). The nonmedical therapist's role in pharmacological interventions with adults. In E. R. Welfel & R. E. Ingersoll (Eds.), *The mental health desk reference* (pp. 88–93). New York: Wiley.

Ingersoll, R. E. (2002). An integral approach for teaching and practicing diagnosis. *Journal of Transpersonal Psychology, 34,* 115–127.

Ingersoll, R. E., Bauer, A. L., & Burns, L. (2004). Children and psychotropic medication: What role should advocacy counseling play? *Journal of Counseling and Development, 82,* 342–348.

Ingersoll, R. E., & Burns, L. (2001). Prevalence of adult disorders. In E. R. Welfel & R. E. Ingersoll (Eds.), *The mental health desk reference* (pp. 3–9). New York: Wiley.

Ingersoll, R. E., & Marquis, A. (2014). *Understanding psychopathology: An integral exploration*. Upper Saddle Hill, NJ: Pearson.

Interactive Medical Networks (producer). (2001). *What makes a drug a mood stabilizer? A video symposium.* Carrolton, TX: Interactive Medical Networks.

International Committee of Medical Journal Editors. (2001). *Uniform requirements for manuscripts submitted to biomedical journals.* Retrieved from www.icmje.org

Isaacs, T. (2013). *Huge fines, settlements and lawsuits are routine business for big pharma.* Retrieved September 11, 2013, from http://www.naturalnews.com/041261_Big_Pharma_settlements_fines.html

Isbell, H., & Vogel, V. H. (1949). The addiction liability of methadone and its use in the treatment of morphine abstinence syndrome. *American Journal of Psychiatry, 105*(12), 909–914.

Iuvone, T., Esposito, G., Esposito, R., Santamaria, T., De Rosa, M., & Izzo, A. A. (2004). Neuroprotective effect of cannabidiol, a non-psychoactive component from Cannabis Sativa, on B-amyloid-induced toxicity in PC12 cells. *Journal of Neurochemistry, 89,* 134–141.

Izzo, A. A., & Ernst, E. (2001). Interactions between herbal medicines and prescribed drugs: A systematic review. *Drugs, 61,* 2163–2175.

Jacobs, B. L. (Ed.). (1984). *Hallucinogens, neurochemical, behavioral, and clinical perspectives.* New York: Raven Press.

Jacobs, K. M., & Hirsch, K. A. (2000). Psychiatric complications of ma-huang. *Psychosomatics: Journal of Consultation Liaison Psychiatry, 41,* 58–62.

Jacobson, J. P. R., Medvedev, I. O., & Caron, M. G. (2012). The 5-HT deficiency theory of depression: Perspectives from a naturalistic 5-HT deficiency model, the tryptophan hydroxylase 2arg439His knockin mouse. *Philosophical Transactions of the Royal Society London Biological Sciences, 367,* 2444–2459.

Jacoby, S. (2011). *Never say die: The myth and marketing of the new old age.* New York: Pantheon Books.

Jackson, G. E. (2006). A curious consensus: "Brain scans prove disease?" *Ethical Human Psychology and Psychiatry, 8,* 55–60.

Jairam, R., Prabjuswamy, M., & Dullur, P. (2012). Do we really know how to treat a child with bipolar disorder or one with severe mood dysregulation? Is there a magic bullet? *Depression Research and Treatment,* 1–9.

Jamison, K. R. (1989). Mood disorders and patterns of creativity in British writers and artists. *Psychiatry, 52,* 125–134.

Jamison, K. R. (1993a). Mood disorders, creativity, and the artistic temperament. In J. J. Schildkraut (Ed.), *Depression and the spiritual in modern art: Homage to Miro* (pp. 15–32). New York: Wiley.

Jamison, K. R. (1993b). *Touched with fire: Manicdepressive illness and the artistic temperament.* New York: Macmillan.

Jamison, K. R., & Akiskal, H. S. (1983). Medication compliance in patients with bipolar disorder. *Psychiatric Clinics of North America, 6,* 175–192.

Jaska, P. (1998). *Fact sheet on attention deficit hyperactivity disorder (ADHD/ADD).* Retrieved February 26, 2003, from www.add.org/content/abc/factsheet.htm

Javitt, D. C. (2010). Glutamatergic theories of schizophrenia. *The Israel Journal of Psychiatry and Related Sciences, 47,* 4–16.

Jensen, P. S., Bhatara, V. S., Vitiello, B., Hoagwood, K., Feil, M., & Burke, L. (1999). Psychoactive medication practices for U. S. Children: Gaps between research and clinical practice. *Journal of the American Academy of Child and Adolescent Psychiatry, 38,* 557–565.

Jensvold, M. F., Halbreich, U., & Hamilton, J. A. (Eds.). (1996). *Psychopharmacology and women: Sex, gender, and hormones.* Washington, DC: American Psychiatric Association.

Jerome, L., Schuster, S., & Yazar-Klosinski, B. B. (2013). Can MDMA play a role in the treatment of substance abuse? *Current Drug Abuse Reviews, 6*(1), 54–62.

J&J to pay $2B, including $18 million to N.J., over how it marketed antipsychotic drug. (2013). *Bloomberg News.* Retrieved April 13, 2014, from http://www.nj.com/business/index.ssf/2013/11/johnson_johnson_pleads_guilty.html

Johansen, P., & Krebs, T. (2009). How could MDMA (ecstasy) help anxiety disorders? A neurobiological rationale. *Journal of Psychopharmacology, 23*(4), 389–391. doi:10.1177/0269881109102787

Johansson, B. (1992). A review of pharmacokinetics and pharmacodynamics of disulfiram and its metabolites. *Acta Psychiatrica Scandivavica, 86,* 15–26.

Johns, A. (2001). Psychiatric effects of cannabis. *British Journal of Psychiatry, 179,* 116–122.

Johnson, B. A., Roache, J. D., Javors, M. A., DiClemente, C. C., Cloninger, C. R., Prihoda, T. J., et al. (2000). Ondansetron for reduction of drinking among biologically predisposed alcoholic patients: A randomized controlled trial. *JAMA, 284*(8), 963–971.

Johnson, M. (2013). *Facilitation of cognitive behavioral therapy for smoking cessation using the 5-HT2A agonist psilocybin.* San Diego: College on Problems of Drug Dependence.

Johnson, M., Richards, W., & Griffiths, R. (2008). Human hallucinogen research: guidelines for safety. *Journal of Psychopharmacology (Oxford, England), 22*(6), 603–620. doi:10.1177/0269881108093587

Johnson, R. E., Eissenberg, T., Stitzer, M. L., Strain, E. C., Liebson, I. A., & Bigelow, G. E. (1995). A placebo controlled clinical trial of buprenorphine as a treatment for opioid dependence. *Drug and Alcohol Dependence, 40,* 17–25.

Johnson, R. E., & Straing, E. C. (1999). Other medications for the treatment of opioid dependence. In E. C. Straing & M. Stitzer (Eds.), *Methadone treatment for opioid dependence* (pp. 281-322). Baltimore, MD: John Hopkins University Press.

Johnson, S. W., & North, R. A. (1992). Opioids excite dopamine neurons by hyper-polarization of local interneurons. *The Journal of Neuroscience, 12*(2), 483–488.

Johnstone, T. B. C., Hogenkamp, D. J., Coyne, L., Su, J., Halliwell, R. F., Tran, M. B., et al. (2004). Modifying quinolone antibiotics yields new anxiolytics. *Nature Medicine, 10,* 31–33.

Jones, D. S., & Perlis, R. H. (2006). Pharmacogenetics, race and psychiatry: Prospects and challenges. *Harvard Review of Psychiatry, 14,* 92–108.

Jones, K., Lacro, R. V., Johnson, K. A., & Adams, J. (1989). Patterns of malformations in the children of women treated with carbamazepine during pregnancy. *New England Journal of Medicine, 320,* 1661–1666.

Jones, P. B., Barnes, T. R., Davies, L., Dunn, G., Lloyd, H., Hayhurst, K. P., et al. (2006). Randomized controlled trial of the effect on quality of life second vs first generation antipsychotic drugs in schizophrenia: Cost utility of the latest antipsychotic drugs in schizophrenia study (CUtLASS 1). *Archives of General Psychiatry, 63,* 1079–1087.

Jones, R. T., Benowitz, N., & Bachman, J. (1976). Clinical studies of cannabis tolerance and dependence. *Annals of the New York Academy of Sciences, 282,* 221–239.

Jope, R. S., & Bijur, G. N. (2002). Mood stabilizers glycogen synthase kinase 3B and cell survival. *Molecular Psychiatry,* 7(Suppl. 1), S35–S45.

Jorm, A. F. (2000). Mental health literacy: Public knowledge and beliefs about mental health disorders. *British Journal of Psychiatry, 177,* 396–401.

Jorm, A. F., Christensen, H., Griffiths, K. M., & Rodgers, B. (2002). Effectiveness of complementary and selfhelp treatments for depression. *Medical Journal of Australia, 176*(Suppl. 1), 84–96.

Joseph, H., Stancliff, S., & Langrod, J. (2000). Methadone maintenance treatment: A review of historical and clinical issues. *Mt. Sinai Journal of Medicine, 67,* 347–364.

Joukamaa, M., Heliovaara, M., Knekt, P., Aromaa, A., Raitasalo, R., & Lehtinen, V. (2006). Schizophrenia, neuroleptic medication and mortality. *The British Journal of Psychiatry, 188,* 122–127.

Judd, L. L., Squire, L. R., Butters, N., Salmon, D. P., & Paller, K. A. (1987). Effects of psychotropic drugs on cognition and memory in normal humans and animals. In H. Y. Meltzer (Ed.), *Psychopharmacology: The third generation of progress* (pp. 1467–1475). New York: Raven.

Julien, R. M. (2001). *A primer of drug action: A concise nontechnical guide to the actions, uses, and side effects of psychoactive drugs, revised and updated.* New York: Worth.

Julien, R. M., Advokat, C. D., & Comaty, J. E. (2011). *A primer of drug action* (12th edition). New York: Worth.

Julien, R. M., Advokat, C. D., & Comaty, J. E. (2011). *A primer of drug action: A concise, nontechnical guide to the actions, uses, and side effects of psychoactive drugs* (12th ed.). New York: Worth.

Jung, Y. C., & Namkoong, K. (2006). Pharmacotherapy for alcohol dependence: Anticraving medications for relapse prevention. *Yonsei Medical Journal, 47*(2), 167–178.

Jureidini, J. N., Doecke, C. J., Mansfield, P. R., Haby, M. M., Menkes, D. B., & Tonkin, A. L. (2004). Efficacy and safety of antidepressants for children and adolescents. *British Medical Journal, 328,* 879–883.

Kaberi-Otarod, J., Conetta, R., Kundo, K. K., & Farkash, A. (2002). Ischemic stroke in a user of thermadrene: A case study in alternative medicine. *Clinical Pharmacology, and Therapeutics, 72,* 343–346.

Kafantaris, V., Coletti, D. J., Dicker, R., Padula, G., & Kane, J. M. (2001). Adjunctive antipsychotic treatment of adolescents with bipolar psychosis. *Journal of the Academy of Child and Adolescent Psychiatry, 40,* 1448–1456.

Kalat, J. W. (2001). *Introduction to psychology* (6th ed.). Belmont, CA: Wadsworth.

Kales, H. C., Nease, D. E., Sirey, J. A., Zivin, K., Kim, H. M., KIavanaugh, J., et al. (2013). Racial differences in adherence to antidepressant treatment later in life. *American Journal of Geriatric Psychiatry, 21,* 999–1009.

Kamath, J., & Handratta, V. (2008). Desvenlafaxine succinate for major depressive disorder: A critical review of the evidence. *Expert Review of Neurotherapeutics, 8,* 1787–1803.

Kane, J. M., & Correll, C. U. (2010). Past and present progress in the pharmacologic treatment of schizophrenia. *The Journal of Clinical Psychiatry, 71,* 1115–1124.

Kane, J. M., Eerdekens, M., Lindenmayer, J. P., Keith, S. J., Lesem, M., & Karcher, K. (2003). Long-acting injectable risperidone: Efficacy and safety of the first long-acting atypical antipsychotic. *American Journal of Psychiatry, 160,* 1125–1132.

Kane, J. M., & Marder, S. R. (1993). Psychopharmaco logic treatment of schizophrenia. *Schizophrenia Bulletin, 19,* 287–302.

Karila, L., Gorelick, D., Weinstein, A., Noble, F., Benyamina, A., Coscas, S., et al. (2007). New treatments for cocaine dependence: A focused review. *International Journal of Neuropsychopharmacology, 11,* 425–438.

Kasper, S., & Dienel, A. (2002). Cluster analysis of symptoms during antidepressant treatment with hypericum extract in mildly to moderately depressed out-patients: A meta-analysis of data from three randomized, placebo-controlled trials. *Psychopharmacology, 164,* 301–308.

Kassirer, J. P. (1997). Federal foolishness and marijuana. *New England Journal of Medicine, 336,* 366–367.

Kauffman, J. M. (2009). Selective serotonin reuptake inhibitor (SSRI) drugs: More risks than benefits? *Journal of American Physicians and Surgeons, 14,* 7–12.

Kay, J. (2009). Toward a neurobiology of child psychotherapy. *Journal of Loss and Trauma, 14,* 287–303.

Kazeem, G. R., Cox, C., Aponte, J., Messenheimer, J., Brazell, C., Nelson, A. C., et al. (2009). High-resolution HLA genotyping and severe cutaneous adverse reactions in lamotrigine-treated patients. *Pharmacogenetics and Genomics, 19,* 661–665.

Kean, S. (2014, May 4). Beyond the damaged brain. *New York Times,* opinion section, p. 8.

Keck, P. E., & McElroy, S. L. (1998). Antiepileptic drugs. In A. F. Schatzberb & C. B. Nemeroff (Eds.), *Textbook of psychopharmacology* (2nd ed., pp. 431–454). Washington, DC: American Psychiatric Press.

Keck, P. E., & McElroy, S. L. (2002). Clinical pharmacodynamics and pharmacokinetics of antimanic and mood stabilizing medications. *Journal of Clinical Psychiatry, 63*(Suppl. 4), 3–11.

Keen, J., & Oliver, P. (2004). Commissioning pharmacological treatments for drug users: A brief review of the evidence base. *Drugs: Education, Prevention and Policy, 11*(2), 149–156.

Kehne, J. H. (2007). The CRF1 receptor, a novel target for the treatment of depression, anxiety and stress-related disorders. *CNS & Neurological Disorders, 6,* 163–182.

Keller, K. B., & Lemberg, L. (2001). Herbal or complementary medicine: Fact or fiction? *American Journal of Critical Care, 10,* 438–443.

Keller, M. B., Ryan, N. D., Strober, M., Klein, R. G., Kutcher, S. P., Birmaher, B., et al. (2001). Efficacy of paroxetine in the treatment of adolescent major depression: A randomized, controlled trial. *Journal of the American Academy of Child and Adolescent Psychiatry, 40,* 762–772.

Kelly, B. D. (2001). St John's wort for depression: What's the evidence? *Hospital Medicine, 62,* 274–276.

Kemp, D. E., Zhao, J., Cazorla, P., Landbloom, R. P., Mackle, M., Snow-Adami, L., et al. (2014). Weight change and metabolic effects of asenapine in patients with schizophrenia and bipolar disorder. *The Journal of Clinical Psychiatry, 75,* 238–245.

Keough, M. T., & O'Conner, R. M. (2014). Clarifying the measurement and the role of the behavioral inhibition system in alcohol misuse. *Alcoholism, Clinical and Experimental Research, 38,* 1470–1479.

Keshavan, M. S. (2013). Renaming schizophrenia: Keeping up with the facts. *Schizophrenia Research, 148,* 1–2.

Keshavan, M. S., Tandon, R., & Nasrallah, H. A. (2013). Renaming schizophrenia: Keeping up with the facts. *Schizophrenia Research, 148,* 1–2.

Kessler, R. C., Chiu, W. T., Demler, O., & Walters, E. E. (2005). Prevalence, severity, and comorbidity of 12-month DSM-IV disorders in the National Comorbidity Survey Replication. *Archives of General Psychiatry, 62*(6), 617.

Kessler, R. C., McGonagle, K. A., Zhao, S., Nelson, C. B., Hughes, M., Eshleman, S., et al. (1994). Lifetime and 12-month prevalence of DSM-II-R psychiatric disorders in the United States. *Archives of General Psychiatry, 51,* 8–19.

Kessler, R. C., Petukhova, M., Sampson, N. A., Zaslovsky, A. M., & Wittchen, H. U. (2012). Twelve month and lifetime prevalence and lifetime morbid risk of anxiety and mood disorders in the United States. *International Journal of Methods in Psychiatric Research, 21,* 169–184.

Khan, A., Leventhal, R. M., Khan, S. R., & Brown, W. A. (2002). Severity of depression and response to antidepressants and placebo: An analysis of the food and drug administration database. *Journal of Clinical Psychopharmacology, 22,* 40–45.

Kiani, J., & Imam, S. Z. (2007). Medicinal importance of grapefruit juice and its interaction with various drugs. *Nutrition Journal, 6,* 6–33.

Kiefer, F., Jahn, H., Tarnaske, T., Helwig, H., Briken, P., Holzbach, R., et al. (2003). Comparing and combining naltrexone and acamprosate in relapse prevention of alcoholism: A double-blind, placebo-controlled study. *Archives of General Psychiatry, 60* (1), 92–99.

Killin, L. O. J., Russ, T. C., Starr, J. M., Abrahams, S., & Della Sala, S. (2014). The effect of funding sources on donepezil randomized controlled trial outcome: A meta-analysis. *British Medical Journal Open, 4,* 1136.

Kim, B., Cho, S. J., Lee, K. S., Lee, J. Y., Choe, A. Y., Lee, J. E., et al. (2013). Factors associated with treatment outcomes in

mindfulness-based cognitive therapy for panic disorder. *Yonsei Medicine, 54,* 1454–1462.

Kim, H. L., Streltzer, J., & Goebert, D. (1999). St. John's wort for depression. *Journal of Nervous and Mental Diseases, 187,* 532–539.

Kim, J. E., Yoon, S. J., Kim, J., Jung, J. Y., Cho, H. B., Shin, E., et al. (2011). Efficacy and tolerability of mirtazapine in treating major depressive disorder with anxiety symptoms: An 8-week open-label, randomized, paroxetine controlled trial. *The International Journal of Clinical Practice, 65,* 323–329.

King, R. A. (1997). Practice parameters for the psychiatric assessment of children and adolescents. *Journal of the American Academy of Child & Adolescent Psychiatry, 36*(Suppl. 10), 1386–1402.

Kinzler, E., Kroner, J., & Helman, E. (1991). Effect of a special kava extract in patients with anxiety, tension, and excitation states of non-psychotic genesis: Double blind study with placebos over 4 weeks. *Arzneimittelforschung, 41,* 584–588.

Kiosses, D. N., Arean, P. A., Teri, L., & Alexopoulos, G. S. (2009). Home-delivered problem adaptation therapy (PATH) for depressed cognitively impaired disabled elders: A preliminary study. *American Journal of Geriatric Psychiatry, 18,* 988–998.

Kiosses, D. N., Arean, A., Teri, L., & Alexopoulos, G. S. (2010). A Home-Delivered Intervention for Depressed, Cognitively Impaired, Disabled Elders. *International Journal of Geriatric Psychiatry, 26,* 256–262.

Kirby, T. (2012). Alcohol as a gateway drug: A study of U.S. 12th graders. *The Journal of School Health, 82,* 371–379.

Kirchmayer, U., Davoli, M., Verster, A. D., Amato, L., Ferri, M., & Perucci, C. A. (2002). A systematic review on the efficacy of naltrexone maintenance treatment in opioid dependence. *Addiction, 97,* 1241–1249.

Kirmayer, L. J., & Ban, L. (2013). Cultural psychiatry: Research strategies and future directions. *Advances in Psychosomatic Medicine, 33,* 97–114.

Kirsch, I., & Low, C. B. (2013). Suggestion in the treatment of depression. *The American Journal of Clinical Hypnosis, 55,* 221–229.

Kishimoto, A., Ogura, C., Hazama, H., & Inoue, K. (1983). Long-term prophylactic effects of carbamazepine in affective disorder. *British Journal of Psychiatry, 143,* 327–331.

Kistorp, T. K., & Laursen, S. B. (2002). Herbal medicines: Evidence and drug interactions in clinical practice. *Ugeskrift for Laeger, 164,* 4161–4165.

Klaus, L., Mechart, D., Mulrow, C. D., & Berner, M. (2002). Effect of Hypericum perforatum (St. John's wort) in major depressive disorder: A randomized controlled trial: Comment. *Journal of the American Medical Association, 288,* 447–448.

Kleijnen, J., & Knipschild, P. (1992). Ginkgo biloba. *Lancet, 340,* 1136–1139.

Klein, D. F. (1967). Importance of psychiatric diagnosis in prediction of clinical drug effects. *Archives of General Psychiatry, 16,* 118–126.

Klein, N. S. (1970). Monoamine oxidase inhibitors: An unfinished, picaresque tale. In F. J. Ayd & B. Blackwell (Eds.), *Discoveries in biological psychiatry* (pp. 209–221). Philadelphia: Lippincott.

Kleindienst, N., & Greil, W. (2002). Inter-episodic morbidity and drop-out under carbamazepine and lithium in the maintenance treatment of bipolar disorder. *Psychological Medicine, 32,* 493–501.

Klesper, T. B., Doucette, W. R., Horton, M. R., Buys, L. M., Ernst, M. E., Ford, J. K., et al. (2000). Assessment of patients' perceptions and beliefs regarding herbal therapies. *Pharmacotherapy, 20,* 83–87.

Kluger, J. (2003). Medicating young minds. *Time, 162,* 48–58.

Knekt, P., Kumpulainen, J., Jarvinen, R., Rissanen, H., Heliovaara, M., Reunanen, A., et al. (2002). Flavonoid intake and risk of chronic disease. *American Journal of Nutrition, 76,* 560–568.

Knickerbocker, B. (2002). Military looks to drugs for battle readiness. *Christian Science Monitor, 8,* 11.

Knudsen, P., Hansen, E. H., Traulsen, J. M., & Eskildsen, K. (2002). Changes in self-concept while using SSRI antidepressants. *Qualitative Health Research, 12,* 932–944.

Koch, C. (2012). *Consciousness: Confessions of a romantic reductionist.* Cambridge, MA: MIT Press.

Kohno, T., Kimura, M., Sasaki, M., Obata, H., Amaya, F., & Saito, S. (2012). Milnacipram inhibits glutamatergic n-methyl-D-Aspartate receptor activity in the spinal dorsal horn neurons. *Molecular Pain, 8,* 45.

Koller, E. A., Cross, J. T., & Schneider, B. (2004). Risperidone associated diabetes mellitus in children. *Pediatrics, 113,* 421–422.

Konstantakopoulos, G., Ploumpidis, D., Oulis, P., Patrikelis, P., Nikitopoulou, S., Papadimitriou, G. N., et al. (2014). The relationship between insight and theory of mind in schizophrenia. *Schizophrenia Research, 152,* 217–222.

Koob, A. (2009). The root of thought: What do glial cells do? *Scientific American, 4,* 12–19.

Korf, D. J. (2002). Dutch coffee shops and trends in cannabis use. *Addictive Behaviors, 27,* 851–866.

Korn, D., & Carlat, D. (2013). Conflicts of interest in medical education: Recommendations from the Pew Task Force on medical conflicts of interest. *Journal of the American Medical Association, 310,* 2397–2398.

Kottler, L., & Devlin, M. J. (2001). Weight gain with antipsychotic medications in children and adolescents. *Child and Adolescent Psychopharmacology News, 6,* 5–9.

Kourmouli, M., Samakouri, M., Mamatsiou, A., Trypsianis, G., Lavaditis, M., & Veletza, S. (2013). Effect of BDNF Val66-Met and serotonin transporter 5-HTTLPR polymorphisms on psychopathological characteristics in a sample of university students. *Psychiatric Genetics, 23,* 188–197.

Kowatch, R. A., Fristad, M., Birmaher, B., Wagner, K. D., Findling, R. L., Hellander, M., et al. (2005). Treatment guidelines for children and adolescents with bipolar disorder. *Journal of the American Academy of Child & Adolescent Psychiatry, 44,* 213–235.

Kraft, I. A. (1968). The use of psychoactive drugs in the outpatient treatment of psychiatric disorders of children. *American Journal of Psychiatry, 124,* 1401–1407.

Kramer, P. D. (1993). *Listening to Prozac: A psychiatrist explores antidepressant drugs and the remaking of the self.* New York: Viking.

Krebs, T. S., & Johansen, P.-O. (2012). Lysergic acid diethylamide (LSD) for alcoholism: meta-analysis of randomized controlled trials. *Journal of Psychopharmacology, 26*(7), 994–1002. doi:10.1177/0269881112439253

Kreshak, A. A., Cantrell, F. L., Clark, R. F., & Tomaszewski, C. A. (2012). A poison center's ten-year experience with flumazenil administration to acutely poisoned adults. *The Journal of Emergency Medicine, 43,* 677–682.

Kronbrot, D. E., Msetfi, R. M., & Grimwood, M. J. (2013). Time perception and depressive realism: Judgment, psychosocial functions and bias. *PLoS One, 8,* 10–19.

Kubik, J. (2002). *S.C.O.P.E.: Student centered outcome plan evaluation.* Avon Lake, OH: Bridge to Success Skill Training.

Kuhlmann, J., Berger, W., Podzuweit, H., & Schmidt, U. (1999). The influence of valerian treatment on reaction time, alertness, and concentration in volunteers. *Pharmacopsychiatry, 32,* 235–241.

Kuhn, R. (1958). The treatment of depressive states with G 22355 (imipramine hydrochloride). *American Journal of Psychiatry, 115,* 459–464.

Kulkarni, S. K., & Naidu, P. S. (2003). Pathophysiology and drug therapy of tardive dyskinesia: Current concepts and future perspectives. *Drugs of Today, 39,* 19–49.

Kupfer, D. J., & Frank, E. (2002). Effect of Hypericum perforatum (St. John's wort) in major depressive disorder: A randomized controlled trial: A reply. *Journal of the American Medical Association, 288,* 449.

Kurtzweil, P. (1996). Medications can aid recovery from alcoholism. *FDA Consumer Magazine, 30,* 22–25.

Kushner, S. F., Khan, A., Lane, R., & Olson, W. H. (2006). Topiramate monotherapy in the management of acute mania: results of four double blind placebo-controlled trials. *Bipolar Disorders, 8,* 15–27.

Kuslak, V. (2003). *Letter to physicians.* Wyeth Pharmmaceuticals, Retrieved August 22, from www.rphlink.com/wyethpharm maceuticals.html. (Cited in Healy, D. Reply to Casey. *Psychotherapy and Psychosomatics, 73,* 261–262)

Kusumaker, V., Lazier, L., MacMaster, F. P., & Santor, D. (2002). Bipolar mood disorder: Diagnosis, etiology, and treatment. In S. Kutcher (Ed.), *Practical child and adolescent psychopharmacology* (pp. 106–133). Cambridge, UK: Cambridge University Press.

Kutcher, S., Boulos, C., Ward, B., Marton, P., Simeon, J., Ferguson, H. B., et al. (1994). Response to desipramine treatment in adolescent depression: A fixed dose, placebo-controlled trial. *Journal of the American Academy of Child and Adolescent Psychiatry, 33,* 686–694.

Kuypers, K. P. C., & Ramaekers, J. G. (2007). Acute dose of MDMA (75 mg) impairs spatial memory for location but leaves contextual processing of visuospatial information unaffected. *Psychopharmacology, 189*(4), 557–563. doi:10.1007/s00213-006-0321-7

Kyaga, S., Lichtenstein, P., Boman, M., Hultman, C., Langstrom, N., & Landen, M. (2011). Creativity and mental disorder: Family study of 300,000 people with severe mental disorder. *The British Journal of Psychiatry, 199,* 373–379.

Kye, C. H., Waterman, G. S., Ryan, N. D., Birmaher, B., Williamson, D. E., Iyengar, S., et al. (1996). A randomized, controlled trial of amitriptyline in acute treatment of adolescent major depression. *Journal of the American Academy of Child and Adolescent Psychiatry, 35,* 1139–1144.

Laakmann, G., Jahn, G., & Schuele, C. (2002). Hypericum perforatum extracts in the treatment of mild to moderate depression: Clinical and pharmacological aspects. *Nervenarzt, 73,* 600–612.

Laaksonen, E., Koski-Jannes, A., Salaspuro, M., Ahtinen, H., & Alho, H. (2008). A randomized, multicentre, open-label, comparative trial of disulfiram, naltrexone and acamprosate in the treatment of alcohol dependence. *Alcohol Alcohol, 43*(1), 53–61.

Labruzza, A. L. (1997). *Using DSM-IV: A clinician's guide to psychiatric diagnosis.* Washington, DC: American Psychiatric Association.

Lachs, M. S., & Pillemer, K. (2004). Elder abuse. *Lancet, 364,* 1263–1272.

Lader, M. (1988). Beta-adrenergic antagonists in neuropsychiatry: An update. *Journal of Clinical Psychiatry, 49,* 213–223.

LaFrance, W. C., Lauterbach, E. C., Coffey, C. E., Salloway, S. P., Kaufer, D. I., Reeve, A., et al. (2000). The use of herbal alternative medicines in neuropsychiatry. *Journal of Neuropsychiatry and Clinical Neurosciences, 12,* 177–192.

Lam, Y. W., Ereshefsky, L., Toney, G. B., & Gonzales, C. (2001). Branded versus generic clozapine: Bioavailability comparison and interchangeability issues. *The Journal of Clinical Psychiatry, 62,* 23–24.

Lambert, M. J. (Ed.). (2004). *Bergin and Garfield's handbook of psychotherapy and behavior change* (5th ed., Michael J. Lambert, Eds.). New York: Wiley.

Lambert, P. A., & Venaud, G. (1992). Use of valpromide in psychiatric therapeutics. *Encephale, 13,* 367–373.

Lapin, I. P., & Oxenkrug, G. F. (1969). Intensification of the central serotonergic processes as a possible determinal of the thymoleptic effect. *Lancet, 1,* 132–136.

Laroche, M. L., Charmes, J. P., Nouaille, Y., Picard, N., & Merle, L. (2006). Is inappropriate medication use a major cause of adverse drug reactions in the elderly? *British Journal of Clinical Pharmacology, 63,* 177–186.

Lauriello, J., Lenroot, R., & Bustillo, J. R. (2003). Maximizing the synergy between pharmacotherapy and psychosocial therapies for schizophrenia. *Psychiatric Clinics of North America, 26,* 191–211.

Lavin, M. R., & Rifkin, A. (1992). Neuroleptic-induced parkinsonism. In J. M. Kane & J. A. Lieberman (Eds.), *Adverse effects of psychotropic medications* (pp. 175–188). New York: Guilford Press.

Law, F. D., Myles, J. S., Daglish, M. R. C., & Nutt, D. J. (2004). The clinical use of buprenorphine in opiate addiction: Evidence and practice. *Acta Neuropsychiatrica, 16,* 246–274.

Lawson, W. B. (1999). The art and science of ethnopharmacotherapy. In J. M. Herrera, W. B. Lawson, & J. J. Sramek (Eds.), *Cross cultural psychiatry* (pp. 67–73). New York: Wiley.

Lawson, W. B., Hepler, N., Holladay, J., & Cuffel, B. (1994). Race as a factor in inpatient and outpatient admissions and diagnosis. *Hospital Community Psychiatry, 45,* 72–74.

Leak, J. A. (1999). Herbal medicine: Is it an alternative or an unknown? A brief review of popular herbals used by patients in a pain and symptom management practice setting. *Current Review of Pain, 3,* 226–236.

Leary, T., Litwin, G. H., & Metzner, R. (1963). Reactions to psilocybin administered in a supportive environment. *The Journal of Nervous and Mental Disease, 137,* 561–573.

Leathwood, P. D., & Chauffard, F. (1982). Quantifying the effects of mild sedatives. *Journal of Psychiatric Research, 17,* 115–122.

Leathwood, P. D., Chauffard, F., Heck, E., & Munoz Box, R. (1982). Aqueous extract of valerian root (Valeriana officinalis L.) improves sleep quality in man. *Pharmacology and Biochemical Behavior, 17,* 65–71.

LeBars, P. L., & Kastelan, J. (2000). Efficacy and safety of Ginkgo biloba extract. *Public Health Nutrition, 3,* 495–499.

LeBars, P. L., Katz, M. M., Berman, N., Itil, T. M., Freedman, A. M., & Schatzberg, A. F. (1997). A placebo-controlled, double-blind randomized trial of an extract of *Ginkgo biloba* for dementia. *JAMA, 278,* 1327–1332.

Lebovitz, H. E. (2003). Metabolic consequences of atypical antipsychotic drugs. *Psychiatric Quarterly, 74,* 277–290.

Lecrubier, Y., Clerc, G., Didi, R., & Keiser, M. (2002). Efficacy of St. John's wort extract WS 5570 in major depression: A double-blind, placebo-controlled trial. *American Journal of Psychiatry, 159,* 1361–1366.

Lee, H. J., Lee, M. S., Kang, R. H., Kim, S. D., Kee, B. S., Kim, Y. H., et al. (2005). Influence of the serotonin transporter promoter gene poly morphism on susceptibility to post traumatic stress disorder. *Depression and Anxiety, 21,* 135–139.

Leichsenring, F., & Salver, S. (2013). A unified protocol for the transdiagnostic psychodynamic treatment of anxiety disorders: An evidence-based approach. *Psychotherapy, 12,* 193–199.

Lemonick, M. D. (2004, June 21). Kids and depression. *Time, 163,* 22–29.

Lencz, T., Smith, C. W., Auther, A. M., Correll, C. U., & Cornblatt, B. A. (2003). The assessment of "prodromal schizophrenia": Unresolved issues and future directions. *Schizophrenia Bulletin, 29,* 717–728.

Leng, Y., Liang, M. H., Ren, M., Marinova, Z., Leeds, P., & Chuang, D. M. (2008). Synergistic neuroprotective effects of lithium and valproic acid or other histone deacetylace inhibitors in neurons: Role of glycogen synthase kinase-3 inhibition. *Journal of Neuroscience, 28,* 2576–2588.

Lenox, R. H., & Manji, H. K. (1998). Lithium. In A. F. Schatzberg & C. B. Nemeroff (Eds.), *Textbook of psychopharmacology* (2nd ed., pp. 379–430). Washington, DC: American Psychiatric Press.

Leo, J. (2002). American preschoolers on Ritalin. *Society, 1,* 52–60.

Leppamaki, S. J., Partonen, T. T., Hurme, J., Haukka, J. K., & Lonnqvist, J. K. (2002). Randomized trial of the efficacy of bright light exposure and aerobic exercise on depressive symptoms and serum lipids. *Journal of Clinical Psychiatry, 63,* 316–321.

Letmaier, M., Schreinzer, D., Wolf, R., & Kasper, S. (2001). Topiramate as a mood stabilizer. *International Clinical Psychopharmacology, 16,* 295–298.

Levy, F., & Hay, D. (2001). *Attention, genes, and ADHD*. Philadelphia: Brunner/Routledge.

Lewin, L. (1998). *Phantastica: a classic survey on the use and abuse of mind-altering plants*. Rochester, VT: Park Street Press.

Lewinsohn, P. M., Klein, D. N., & Seeley, J. (1995). Bipolar disorders in a community sample of older adolescents: Prevalence, phenomenology, comorbidity, and course. *Journal of the American Academy of Child and Adolescent Psychiatry, 34,* 454–464.

Lewis, B. (1973). *The sexual powers of marijuana*. New York: Wyden.

Lewis, R. (1998). Typical and atypical antipsychotics in adolescent schizophrenia: Efficacy, tolerability, and differential sensitivity to extrapyramidal symptoms. *Canadian Journal of Psychiatry, 43,* 596–604.

Libby, A. M., Brent, D. A., Morrato, E. H., Orton, H. D., Allen, R., & Valuck, R. J. (2007). Decline in treatment of pediatric depression after FDA advisory on risk of suicidality with SSRIs. *American Journal of Psychiatry, 164,* 884–888.

Liberty, I. F., Todder, D., Umansky, R., & HarmanBoehm, I. (2004). Atypical antipsychotics and diabetes mellitus: An association. *Israel Medical Association Journal, 6,* 276–279.

Lickey, M. E., & Gordon, B. (1991). *Medicine and mental illness: The use of drugs in psychiatry*. New York: Freeman.

Lieb, R., Schuetz, C. G., Pfister, H., von Sydow, K., & Wittchen, H.-U. (2002). Mental disorders in ecstasy users: a prospective-longitudinal investigation. *Drug and Alcohol Dependence, 68*(2), 195–207.

Lieberman, J. A. (1997). Atypical antipsychotic drugs: The next generation of therapy. *Decade of the Brain, 3,* 3–10.

Lieberman, J. A., Stroup, T. S., McEvoy, J. P., Swartz, M. S., Rosenheck, R. A., Perkins, D. O., et al. (2005). Effectiveness of antipsychotic drugs in patients with chronic schizophrenia. *The New England Journal of Medicine, 353,* 1209–1223.

Liebowitz, M. R., Tourian, K. A., Huang, E., Mele, L., & for the Study 3362 Investigators. (2013). A double-blind, randomized, placebo-controlled study assessing the efficacy and tolerability of desvenlafaxine 10 and 50 mg/day in adult outpatients with major depressive disorder. *BMC Psychiatry, 13,* 3–9.

Liechti, M. E., Gamma, A., & Vollenweider, F. X. (2001). Gender differences in the subjective effects of MDMA. *Psychopharmacology, 154*(2), 161–168.

Liester, M. B., Grob, C. S., Bravo, G. L., & Walsh, R. N. (1992). Phenomenology and sequelae of 3, 4-methylenedioxymethamphetamine use. *The Journal of Nervous and Mental Disease, 180*(6), 345–352; discussion 353–354.

Lillenfeld, S. O., Lynn, S. J., Ruscio, J., & Beyerstein, B. L. (2010). *50 great myths of popular psychology: Shattering widespread misconceptions about human behavior*. New York: Norton.

Lilly, J. (1977). *The deep self: Profound relaxation and the tank isolation technique*. New York: Warner.

Lilly, J. (1996/2006). *The deep self: Consciousness exploration in the isolation tank*. Berkley, CA: Gateway.

Lilly, J. (1997). *The scientist: A metaphysical autobiography*. Berkley, CA: Ronin.

Lim, H. K., & Aizenstein, H. J. (2014). Recent findings and newer paradigms of neuroimaging research in geriatric psychiatry. *Journal of Geriatric Psychiatry, 27,* 3–4.

Lin, K. M. (1996). Psychopharmacology in cross-cultural psychiatry. *Mt. Sinai Journal of Medicine, 63,* 283–284.

Lin, K. M., & Poland, R. E. (1995). Ethnicity, culture, and psychopharmacology. In F. E. Bloom & D. I. Kupfer (Eds.), *Psychopharmacology: The fourth generation of progress* (pp. 1037–1068). New York: Raven Press.

Lin, K. M., Poland, R. E., & Anderson, D. (1995). Psychopharmacology, ethnicity, and culture. *Transcultural Psychiatric Residents Review, 32,* 3–40.

Lin, K. M., Poland, R. E., & Nakasaki, G. (Eds.). (1993). *Psychopharmacology and psychobiology of ethnicity*. Washington, DC: American Psychiatric Association.

Linde, K., & Mulrow, C. D. (2000). St. John's wort for depression. *Cochrane Database System Review, 2,* CD000448.

Linde, K., Ramirez, G., Mulrow, C. D., Pauls, A., Weidenhammer, W., & Melchart, D. (1996). St. John's wort for depression. *British Medical Journal, 313,* 253–258.

Lindenmayer, J. P., & Patel, R. (1999). Olanzapine induced ketoacidosis with diabetes mellitus. *American Journal of Psychiatry, 156,* 1471.

Lindsey, P. L. (2009, September). Psychotropic medication use among older adults; what all nurses need to know. *Journal of Gerontological Nursing, 35,* 28.

Link, B., & Phelan, J. (2001). Conceptualizing stigma. *Annual Review of Sociology, 27,* 363–385.

Litten, R. Z., & Allen, J. P. (1999). Medications for alcohol, illicit drug, and tobacco dependence: An update of research findings. *Journal of Substance Abuse Treatment, 16*(2), 105–112.

Litten, R. Z., & Fertig, J. (1996). International update: New findings on promising medications. *Alcoholism: Clinical and Experimental Research, 20*(Suppl.), 216A–218A.

Livingston, R. (1995). Anxiety and anxiety disorders. In G. O. Gabbard (Ed.), *Treatment of psychiatric disorders* (2nd ed., pp. 229–253). Washington, DC: American Psychiatric Association.

Locke, S. F. (2008). A novel chemical target: A drug for schizophrenia tweaks the brain's levels of glutamate. *Scientific American Mind, 19,* 6.

Loebel, A., Cucchiaro, J., Silva, R., Kroger, H., Sarma, K., Xu, J., et al. (2014). Lurasidone as adjunctive therapy with lithium or valproate for the treatment of bipolar I depression: A randomized, double-blind placebo controlled study. *The American Journal of Psychiatry, 171,* 169–177.

Loera, J. A., Black, S. A., Markides, K. S., Espino, D. C., & Goodwin, J. S. (2001). The use of herbal medicine by older Mexican Americans. *Journals of Gerontology: Series A: Biological Sciences and Medical Sciences, 56A,* M714–M718.

Loimer, N., & Schmid, R. (1992). The use of plasma levels to optimize methadone maintenance treatment. *Drug Alcohol Dependence, 30*(3), 241–246.

Loomer, H. P., Saudners, I. C., & Kline, N. S. (1953). A clinical and pharmacodynamics evaluation of iproniazid as a psychic energizer. *Psychiatric research reports American Psychiatric Association, 8,* 129–141.

Lopez-Munoz, F., & Alamo, C. (2009). Monoaminergic neurotransmission: The history of the discovery of antidepressants from the 1950s until today. *Current Pharaceutical Design, 15,* 1563–1586.

Lopez-Munoz, F., Alamo, C., Rubio, G., & Cuenca, E. (2004). Half a century since the clinical introduction of chlorpromazine and the birth of modern psychopharmacology. *Progress in Neuro-Psychopharmacology & Biological Psychiatry, 28,* 205–208.

Loscher, W., & Rogawski, M. A. (2012). How theories evolved concerning the mechanism of action of barbiturates. *Epilepsia, 53*(Suppl. 8), 12–25.

Lueken, U., Straube, B., Konrad, C., Wittchen, H. U., Strohle, A., Wittman, A., et al. (2013). Neural substrates of treatment response to cognitive behavioral therapy in panic disorder with agoraphobia. *The American Journal of Psychiatry, 170,* 1345–1355.

Lukoff, D., Lu, F. G., & Turner, R. (1996). Diagnosis: A transpersonal clinical approach to religious and spiritual problems. In B. W. Scotton, A. B. Chinen, & J. R. Battista (Eds.), *Textbook of transpersonal psychiatry and psychology* (pp. 231–249). New York: Basic Books.

Lurie, P. MD. MPH. (2005, September 29). *Testimony on the impact of dtc drug advertising on seniors.* Deputy Director, Public Citizens Health Research Group Testimony before the Senate Special Committee on Aging.

Lykouras, L., Agelopoulos, E., & Tzavellas, E. (2002). Improvement of tardive dyskinesia following switch from neuroleptics to olanzapine. *Progress in Neuropsychopharmacology and Biological Psychiatry, 26,* 815–817.

Lynne-Landsman, S. D., Livingston, M. D., & Wagenaar, A. C. (2013). Effects of state medical marijuana laws on adolescent marijuana use. *American Journal of Public Helath, 103,* 1500–1506.

Maack, D. J., Tull, M. T., & Gratz, K. L. (2012). Examining the incremental contribution of behavioral inhibition to generalized anxiety disorder relative to other Axis I disorders and cognitive-emotional vulnerabilities. *Journal of Anxiety Disorders, 26,* 689–695.

MacDonald, J. A. (2001, August 8). Drug ads attract scrutiny of critics. *Akron Beacon Journal,* B1–B4.

Macdonald, K. J., & Young, L. T. (2002). Newer antiepileptic drugs in bipolar disorder: Rationale for use and role in therapy. *Central Nervous System Drugs, 16,* 549–562.

McKeith, I. G., O'Brien, J. T., & Ballard, C. (1999). Diagnosing dementia with Lewy bodies. *Lancet, 354,* 1227–1228.

Mackesy-Amiti, M. E., Fendrich, M., & Goldstein, P. J. (1997). Sequence of drug use among serious drug users: Typical vs. atypical progression. *Drug and Alcohol Dependence, 45,* 185–196.

MacLean, K. A., Johnson, M. W., & Griffiths, R. R. (2011). Mystical experiences occasioned by the hallucinogen psilocybin lead to increases in the personality domain of openness. *Journal of Psychopharmacology (Oxford, England), 25*(11), 1453–1461. doi:10.1177/0269881111420188

Madaan, V., Dvir, Y., & Wilson, D. R. (2008). Child and adolescent schizophrenia: Pharmacological approaches. *Expert Opinion on Pharmacotherapy, 9,* 2053–2068.

Maidment, I. D. (2001). Gabapentin treatment for bipolar disorders. *Annals of Pharmacotherapy, 35,* 1264–1269.

Makhinova, T., & Rascati, K. (2013). Pharmacoeconomics education in US colleges and schools of pharmacy. *American Journal of Pharmaceutical Education, 77,* 145.

Malhi, G. S., Tanious, M., Das, P., Coulston, C. M., & Berk, M. (2013). Potential mechanisms of action of lithium in bipolar disorder. *CNS Drugs, 27,* 135–153.

Malhotra, A. K., Litman, R. E., & Pickar, D. (1993). Adverse effects of antipsychotics. *Drug Safety, 9,* 429–436.

Malik, M., Lake, J., Lawson, W. B., & Joshi, S. V. (2010). Culturally adapted pharmacotherapy and the integrative formulation. *Child and Adolescent Clinics of North America, 19,* 791–814.

Malone, R. P., Luebbert, J., Pena-Ariet, M., Biesecker, K., & Delaney, M. A. (1994). The overt aggression scale in a study of lithium in aggressive conduct disorder. *Psychopharmacology Bulletin, 30,* 215–218.

Maneeton, N., Maneeton, B., Eurviryanukul, K., & Srisurapanant, M. (2013). Efficacy, tolerability and acceptability of bupropion for major depressive disorder: A meta-analysis of randomized, controlled trials comparison with venlafaxine. *Drug Design, Development and Therapy, 7,* 1053–1062.

Manisses Corporation. (2002). Aripriprazole emerging as next great hope for schizophrenia. *Psychopharmacology Update, 13,* 4–5.

Manji, H. L., Bowden, C. L., & Belmaker, R. H. (Eds.). (2000). *Bipolar medications: Mechanisms of action.* Washington, DC: American Psychiatric Press.

Manji, H. L., Moore, G. H., Rajkowska, G., & Chen, S. (2000). Neuroplasticity and cellular resilience in mood disorders. *Molecular Psychiatry, 5,* 578–593.

Mann, J. J., McBride, P. A., Malone, K. M., DeMeo, M., & Keilp, J. (1995). Blunted serotonergic responsivity in depressed inpatients. *Neuropsychopharmacology, 13,* 53–64.

Mann, K., Lehert, P., & Morgan, M. Y. (2004). The efficacy of acamprosate in the maintenance of abstinence in alcohol-dependent individuals: Results of a meta-analysis. *CNS Drugs, 255,* 123–134.

Manos, M. J., Short, E. J., & Findling, R. L. (1999). Differential effectiveness of methylphenidate and Adderall in school-age youths with attention-deficit hyperactivity disorder. *Journal of the American Academy of Child and Adolescent Psychiatry, 38,* 813–819.

MAPS. (2006). *Phase II clinical trial testing the safety and efficacy of 3,4-methylenedioxymethamphetamine (MDMA)-assisted psychotherapy in subjects with chronic posttraumatic stress disorder.*

MAPS. (2009). *MDMA administration in a therapeutic setting in people who have completed the MAPS training program for therapists learning to conduct MDMA-assisted psychotherapy research in subject with PTSD.* Retrieved from http://www.maps.org/mdma/mt1_docs/final_mt1_june_19_09.pdf

MAPS. (2013a). *A manual for MDMA-assisted psychotherapy in the treatment of posttraumatic stress disorder.* Retrieved from http://www.maps.org/research/mdma/MDMA-Assisted_Psychotherapy_Treatment_Manual_Version_6_FINAL.pdf

MAPS. (2013b). *A Placebo-controlled, randomized, blinded, dose finding phase 2 pilot safety study of MDMA-assisted therapy for social anxiety in autistic adults.* Retrieved from http://www.maps.org/research/mdma/MAA1_FINAL_Protocol_22Feb13_redact.pdf

MAPS. (2014). *Exploring mechanisms of action in MDMA-assisted psychotherapy for PTSD.* Retrieved from http://www.maps.org/research/mdma/MP8-S1-substudy_Protocol_FINAL_22-Nov13web.pdf

Maradino, C. (1997). Ephedra falls under FDA jurisdiction. *Vegetarian Times, 241,* 1.

Marazziti, D., Baroni, S., Picchetti, M., Piccinni, A., Carlini, M., Vatteroni, E., et al. (2013). Pharmacokinetics and pharmacodynamics of psychotropic drugs: Effects on sex. *CNS Spectrum, 18,* 118–127.

Marchalant, Y., Baranger, K., Wenk, G. L., Khrestchatisky, M., & Rivera, S. (2012). Can the benefits of cannabinoid receptor stimulation on neuroinflammation, neurogenesis and memory during normal aging be useful in AD prevention? *Journal of Neuroinflammation, 9,* 10.

Marchalant, Y., Brothers, H. M., Norman, G. J., Karelina, K., DeVries, A. C., & Wenk, G. L. (2009). Cannabinoids attenuate the effects of aging upon neuroinflammation and neurogenesis. *Neurobiology of Disease, 34,* 300–307.

Marchalant, Y., Cerbai, F., Brothers, H. M., & Wenk, G. L. (2008). Cannabinoid receptor stimulation is anti-inflammatory and improves memory in old rats. *Neurobiology of Aging, 29,* 1894–1901.

Marchalant, Y., Rosi, S., & Wenk. G. (2006). Anti-inflammatory property of the cannabinoid agonist WIN-55212-2 in a rodent model of chronic brain inflammation. *Neuroscience, 144,* 1516–1522.

Marchetti, S., & Schellens, J. H. (2007). Concise review: Clinical relevance or drug-drug and herb-drug interactions mediated by the ABC transporter ABCB1 (MDR1, P-glycoprotein). *The Oncologist, 12,* 927–941.

Marcotte, D. (1998). Use of topiramate, a new antiepileptic as a mood stabilizer. *Journal of Affective Disorders, 50,* 245–251.

Margulies, D. M., Weintraub, S., Basile, J., Grover, P. J., & Carlson, G. A. (2012). Will disruptive mood dysregulation disorder reduce false diagnosis of bipolar disorder in children? *Bipolar Disorder, 14,* 488–496.

Mark, T. L. (2010). For what diagnoses are psychotropic medications being prescribed? *CNS Drugs, 24,* 319–326.

Mark, T. L., Coffey, R. M., Vandivort-Warren, R., Harwood, H. J., & King, E. C. (2005). U.S. spending for mental health and substance abuse treatment: 1991–2001. *Health Affairs,* 133–142.

Markarian, S. A., Pickett, S. M., Deveson, D. F., & Kanona, B. B. (2013). A model of BIS/BAS sensitivity, emotion regulation difficulties, and depression, anxiety and stress symptoms in relation to sleep quality. *Psychitry Research, 210,* 281–286.

Markowitz, S., & Crullar, A. (2007). Antidepressants and youth? Healing or harmful? *Social Science & Medicine, 64,* 2138–2151.

Marriage, K. (2002). Schizophrenia and related psychosis. In S. Kitchner (Ed.), *Practical child and adolescent psychopharmacology* (pp. 134–158). Cambridge, UK: Cambridge University Press.

Martin, J. L. R., Sainz-Pardo, M., Furukawa, T. A., Martin-Sanchez, E., Seoane, T., & Galan, C. (2007). Benzodiazepines in generalized anxiety disorder: Heterogeneity of outcomes based on a systematic review and meta-analysis of clinical trials. *Journal of Psychopharmacology, 23,* 774–782.

Martin, S. D., Martin, E., Rai, S. S., Richardson, M. A., & Royall, R. (2001). Brain blood flow changes in depressed patients treated with interpersonal psychotherapy or venlafaxine hydrochloride: Preliminary findings. *Archives of General Psychiatry, 58,* 641–648.

Martino, G., Butti, E., & Bacigaluppi, M. (2014). Neurogenesis or non-neurogenesis: That is the question. *The Journal of Clinical Investigation, 124,* 970–973.

Mash, D. (2010). Ibogaine therapy for substance abuse disorders. In D. A. Brizer & R. Castaneda (Eds.), *Clinical addiction psychiatry* (pp. 50–60). Cambridge: Cambridge University Press.

Mason, B. J., Goodman, A. M., Chabac, S., & Lehert, P. (2006). Effect of oral acamprosate on abstinence in patients with alcohol dependence in a double-bind, placebo-controlled trial: The role of patient motivation. *Journal of Psychiatry Research, 40*(5), 383–393.

Mash, D. C., Kovera, C. A., Pablo, J., Tyndale, R. F., Ervin, F. D., Williams, I. C., et al. (2000). Ibogaine: complex pharmacokinetics, concerns for safety, and preliminary efficacy measures. *Annals of the New York Academy of Sciences, 914,* 394–401.

Massachusetts files lawsuit for 'deceptive' marketing of Risperdal. (2011). *Mental Health Weekly.* Retrieved December 4, 2012, from http://www.accessmylibrary.com/article-1G1-266751238/massachusetts-files-lawsuit-deceptive.html

Massoud, F., & Gauthier, S. (2010). Update on the pharmacological treatment of Alzheimer's disease. *Current Neuropharmacology, 8,* 69–80.

Matheson, C. (1998). Privacy and stigma in the pharmacy: Illicit drug users' perspectives and implications for pharmaceutical practice. *Pharmaceutical Journal, 260*(6992), 639–641.

Mathew, S. J., Keegan, J., & Smith, L. (2005). Glutamate modulators as novel interventions for mood disorders. *Revista Brasileira De Psiquiatria, 27,* 243–248.

Mathre, M. L. (Ed.). (1997). *Cannabis in medical practice: A legal, historical, and pharmacological overview of the therapeutic uses of marijuana.* Jefferson, NC: McFarland.

Matsuda, L., Lolait, S. J., Brownstein, J. J., Young, A. C., & Bonner, T. I. (1990). Structure of a cannabinoid receptor and functional expression of the cloned cDNA. *Nature, 365,* 61–65.

Mattick, R. P., Breen, C., & Kimber, J. (2003). Methadone maintenance therapy versus no opioid replacement therapy for opioid dependence. *Cochrane Database System Review,* issue 2, 2209.

McCance-Katz, E. F., Moody, D. E., Morse, G. D., Friedland, G., Pade, P., Baker, J., et al. (2006). Interactions between buprenorphine and antivirals. The nonnucleoside reverse-transcriptase inhibitors efavirnez and delavirdine. *Clinical Infectious Disease, 43,* 224–234.

McCarthy, M. J., Wei, H., Marnoy, Z., Darvish, R. M., McPhie, D. L., Cohen, B. M., et al. (2013). Genetic and clinical factors predict lithium's effects on PER2 gene expression rhythms in cells from bipolar disorder patients. *Tranlational Psychiatry, 3,* 318.

McCarty, C. A., Russo, J., & Rossman, D. C. (2011). Adolescents with suicidal ideation: Health care use and functioning. *Academy of Pediatrics, 11,* 422–426.

McClure, E. B., Kubiszyn, T., & Kaslow, N. J. (2002a). Advances in the diagnosis and treatment of childhood mood disorders. *Professional Psychology: Research and Practice, 33,* 125–134.

McClure, E. B., Kubiszyn, T., & Kaslow, N. J. (2002b). Evidence-based assessment of childhood mood disorders: Reply to Lee and Hunsley. *Professional Psychology: Research, Theory, and Practice, 34,* 113–114.

McDowell, D. M., Levin, F. R., Seracini, A. M., & Nunes, E. V. (2000). Venlafaxine treatment of cocaine abusers with depressive disorders. *The American Journal of Drug and Alcohol Abuse, 26*(1), 25–31.

McGlothlin, W. H., & West, L. J. (1968). The marihuana problem: An overview. *American Journal of Psychiatry, 125,* 126–134.

McGraw, J. (2012). Cytochrome P450 variations in different ethnic populations. *Expert Opinion on Drug Metabolism & Toxicology, 8,* 371–382.

McIntosh, A. M., Job, D. E., Moorhead, W. J., Harrison, L. K., Whalley, H. C., Johnstone, E. C., et al. (2006). Genetic liability to schizophrenia or bipolar disorder and its relationship to brain structure. *American Journal of Medical Genetics Part B (Neuropsychiatric Genetics), 141B,* 76–83.

McIntyre, R. S. (2002). Psychotropic drugs and adverse events in the treatment of bipolar disorders revisited. *Journal of Clinical Psychiatry, 63*(Suppl. 3), 15–20.

McKeage, K., & Plosker, G. L. (2003). Amisulpride: A review of its use in the management of schizophrenia. *CNS Drugs, 18,* 933–956.

McKeganey, N., Russell, C., & Cockayne, L. (2013). Medically assisted recovery from opiate-dependence within the context of the UK drug strategy: Methadone and Suboxone (buprenorphine-naloxone) patients compared. *Journal of Substance Abuse Treatment, 44,* 97–102.

McKeith, I. G., & Obrien, J. (1999). Dementia with lewy bodies. *Australian/New Zealand Journal of Psychiatry, 33,* 800–808.

McKenzie, M. S., & McFarland, B. H. (2007). Trends in antidepressant overdoses. *Pharmacoepidemiology and Drug Safety, 16,* 513–523.

McMahon, F., & DePaulo, J. (1996). Genetics and age at onset. In K. Schulman, M. Tohen, & S. Kutcher (Eds.), *Mood disorders across the life span* (pp. 35–48). New York: Wiley.

McNaughton, N., & Gray, J. H. (2000). Anxiolytic action on the behavioral inhibition system implies multiple types of arousal contribute to anxiety. *Journal of Affective Disorders, 61,* 161–176.

McWilliams, P. (1993). *Ain't nobody's business if you do: The absurdity of consensual crimes in a free society.* Los Angeles: Prelude Press.

Meehl, P. (1962). Schizotaxia, schizotypy, schizophrenia. *American Psychologist, 17,* 827–838.

Megna, J. L., Devitt, P. J., Sauro, M. D., & Mantosh, J. (2001). Gabapentin's effect on agitation in severely and persistently mentally ill patients. *Annals of Pharmcotherapy, 36,* 12–16.

Melzer, H. Y. (1993). New drugs for the treatment of schizophrenia. *Psychiatric Clinics of North America, 16,* 365–385.

Mercola, D. (2012). GlaxoSmithKline: GUILTY in Largest Health Fraud Settlement in US History. Retrieved September 7, 2014, from http://articles.mercola.com/sites/articles/archive/2012/07/16/glaxosmithkline-plead-guilty.aspx

Merrill, R. M., Lyon, J. L., & Matiaco, P. M. (2013). Tardive and spontaneous dyskinesia incidence in the general population. *BMC Psychiatry, 13,* 147–152.

Merton, T. (1968). The Matthew effect in science. *Science, 159,* 59–63.

Messer, T., Schmauss, M., & Lambert-Baumer, J. (2005). Efficacy and tolerability of reboxetine in depressed patients treated in routine clinical practice. *CNS Drugs, 19,* 43–54.

Meyer, H. J. (1967). Pharmacology of kava. *Psychopharmacology Bulletin, 4,* 10–11.

Meyers, H. F. (1993). Biopsychosocial perspective on depression in African-Americans. In K. M. Lin, R. E. Poland, & G. Nakasaki (Eds.), *Psychopharmacology and psychobiology of ethnicity* (pp. 201–222). Washington, DC: American Psychiatric Association.

Michael, N., Erfurth, A., & Ohrmann, P. (2003). Acute mania is accompanied by elevated glutamate/glutamine levels within the left dorsolateral prefrontal cortex. *Psychopharmacology, 168,* 344–346.

Michalak, E. E., Guiraud-Diawara, A., & Sapin, C. (2014). Asenapine treatment and health-related quality of life in patients experiencing bipolar I disorder with mixed episodes: Post-hoc analyses of pivotal trials. *Current Medical Research and Opinion, 30*(4), 711–718.

Miklowitz, D. J., Schneck, C. D., George, E. L., Taylor, D. O., Sugar, C. A., Birmaher, B., et al. (2014). Pharmacotherapy and family-focused treatment for adolescents with Bipolar I and II disorders: A 2-year randomized trial. *The American Journal of Psychiatry, 3,* 213–229.

Milia, A., Pilia, G., Mascia, M. G., Moller, J., Cocco, E., & Marrosu, M. G. (2008). Oxcarbazepine-induced leukopenia. *The Journalof Neuropsychitary, 20,* 502–503.

Miller, L., & Barnnett, S. (2008). Mood lability and bipolar disorder in children and adolescents. *International Review of Psychiatry, 20,* 171–176.

Miller, S. M., Piasecki, C. C., Peabody, M. F., & Lonstein, J. S. (2010). GABA (a) receptor antagonism in the ventrocaudal periaqueductal gray increases anxiety in the anxiety-resistant postpartum rat. *Pharmacology, Biochemistry, and Behavior, 95,* 457–465.

Miron, J. A. (2004). *Drug war crimes: The consequences of prohibition.* Oakland, CA: Independent Institute.

Mischoulon, D. (2002). The herbal anxiolytics kava and valerian for anxiety and insomnia. *Psychiatric Annals, 32,* 55–60.

Mitchell, A. J. (2007). Adherence behavior with psychotropic medication is a form of self medication. *Medical Hypotheses, 68,* 12–21.

Mitchell, P. B., & Malhi, G. S. (2002). The expanding pharmaco-poeia for bipolar disorder. *Annual Review of Medicine, 53,* 173–188.

Mithoefer, M. C. (2013). MDMA-assisted psychotherapy: How different is it from other psychotherapy? *MAPS Bulletin, xxiii*(1), 10–14.

Mithoefer, M. C., Wagner, M. T., Mithoefer, A. T., Jerome, L., & Doblin, R. (2011). The safety and efficacy of 3,4-methylene-dioxymethamphetamine-assisted psychotherapy in subjects with chronic, treatment-resistant posttraumatic stress disorder: the first randomized controlled pilot study. *Journal of Psychopharmacology, 25*(4), 439–452. doi:10.1177/0269881110378371

Mithoefer, M. C., Wagner, M. T., Mithoefer, A. T., Jerome, L., Martin, S. F., Yazar-Klosinski, B., et al. (2013). Durability of improvement in post-traumatic stress disorder symptoms and absence of harmful effects or drug dependency after 3,4-methylenedioxymethamphetamine-assisted psychother-apy: a prospective long-term follow-up study. *Journal of Psychopharmacology (Oxford, England), 27*(1), 28–39. doi:10.1177/0269881112456611

Mitkov, M. V., Trowbridge, R. M., Lockshin, B. N., & Caplan, J. P. (2014). Dermatologic side effects of psychotropic medica-tions. *Psychosomatics, 55,* 1–20.

Miotto, K., McCann, M., Basch, J., Rawson, R., & Ling, W. (2002). Naltrexone and dysphoria: Fact or myth? *American Journal of Addictions, 11,* 151–160.

Model, K. E. (1993). The effect of marijuana decriminalization on hospital emergency room episodes. *Journal of the American Sta-tistical Association, 88,* 11.

Modell, J. G. (1995). The high cost of buspirone. (Letter). *Journal of Clinical Psychiatry, 56,* 375.

Mokhber, N., Azarpazhooh, M. R., Khajehdalueee, M., Velayati, A., & Hopwood, M. (2010). Randomized, single-blind, trial of sertraline and buspirone for treatment of elderly patients with generalized anxiety disorder. *Psychiatry and Clinical Neu-rosciences, 64,* 128–133.

Molino, I., Colucci, L., Fasanaro, A. M., Traini, E., & Amenta, F. (2013). Efficacy of memantine, donepezil, or their association in moderate-severe Alzheimer's disease: A review of clinical trials. *The Scientific World Journal, 2013,* 1–8.

Moody, D. E., Alburges, M. E., Parker, R. J., Collins, J. M., & Strong, J. M. (1997). The involvement of cytochrome P450 3A4 in the N-demethylation of L-a-acetylmethadol (LAAM), norLAAM, and methadone. *Drug Metabolism and Disposition, 25*(12), 1347–1353.

Moore, M. T., & Fresco, D. M. (2012). Depressive realism: A meta-analytic review. *Clinical Psychology Review, 32,* 496–509.

Moreno, F. A., Wiegand, C. B., Taitano, E. K., & Delgado, P. L. (2006). Safety, tolerability, and efficacy of psilocybin in 9 patients with obsessive-compulsive disorder. *The Journal of Clinical Psychiatry, 67*(11), 1735–1740.

Morgenstern, H., & Glazer, W. M. (1993). Identifying risk factors for tardive dyskinesia among chronic outpatients maintained on neuroleptic medications: Results of Yale tardive dyskinesia study. *Archives of General Psychiatry, 50,* 723–733.

Morley, K. I., & Hall, W. D. (2004). Using pharmacogenetics and pharmacogenomics in the treatment of psychiatric disorders: Some ethical and economic considerations. *Journal of Molecular Medicine, 82,* 21–30.

Morral, A. R., McCaffrey, D. F., & Paddock, S. M. (2002). Reas-sessing the marijuana gateway effect. *Addiction, 97,* 1493–1504.

Morris, R. G., TenEyck, M., Barnes, J. C., & Kovandzic, T. V. (2014). The effect of medical marijuana laws on crime: Evi-dence from state panel data, 1990–2006. *PLoS One, 9,* 34–40.

Mosihuzzaman, M. (2012). Herbal medicine in healthcare—an overview. *Natural Product Communications, 7,* 807–812.

Moskowitz, A. S., & Altshuler, L. (1991). Increased sensitivity to lithium-induced neurotoxicity after stroke: A case report. *Journal of Clinical Psychopharmacology, 11,* 272–273.

Mota-Castillo, M., Torruella, A., Engels, B., Perez, J., Dedrick, C., & Gluckman, M. (2001). Valproate in very young children: An open case serves with a brief follow-up. *Journal of Affective Disorders, 67,* 193–197.

MTA Cooperative Group. (1999). A 14 month randomized clinical trial of treatment strategies for attentiondeficit/hyperactivity disorder. *Archives of General Psychiatry, 56,* 1073–1086.

MTA Cooperative Group. (2004). National institute of mental health multimodal treatment study of ADHD follow-up: Changes in effectiveness and growth after the end of treat-ment. *Pediatrics, 113,* 762–769.

Murphy, S. M., & Tyrer, P. (1991). A double-blind comparison of the effects of gradual withdrawal of lorazepam, diazepam and bromazepam in benzodiazepine dependence. *British Journal of Psychiatry, 158,* 511–516.

Murray, N. (2003). *Aldous Huxley: a biography* (1st U.S. Ed.). New York: Thomas Dunne Books/St. Martin's Press.

Murrough, J. W., Perez, A. M., & Stern, J. (2013). Rapid and longer term antidepressant effects of repeated ketamine infusions in treatment-resistant depression. *Biological Psychiatry, 74,* 250–256.

Muthukumaraswamy, S. D., Carhart-Harris, R. L., Moran, R. J., Brookes, M. J., Williams, T. M., Errtizoe, D., et al. (2013). Broadband Cortical Desynchronization Underlies the Human Psychedelic State. *Journal of Neuroscience, 33*(38), 15171–15183. doi:10.1523/JNEUROSCI.2063-13.2013

Mutsatsa, S., & Currid, T. J. (2013). Pharmacogenetics: A reality or a misplaced optimism? *Journal of Psychiatric and Mental Health Nursing, 20,* 315–320.

Nagayama, T., Sinor, A. D., Simon, R. P., Chen, J., Graham, S. H., Jin, K., et al. (1999). Cannabinoids and neuroprotection in global and focal cerebral ischemia and in neuronal cultures. *Journal of Neuroscience, 19,* 2987–2995.

National Institute for Health Care Management. (2002). *Changing patterns of pharmaceutical innovation: A research report by the National Institute for Health Care Management Research and Edu-cation Foundation.* Washington, DC: Author.

National Institute of Mental Health. (1996). *Attention deficit hyperac-tivity disorder* (No. 96-3572). Washington, DC: Author.

National Institute of Mental Health. (2000, September). *Treatment of children with mental disorders.* (No. 00–4702). Retrieved April

22, 2002, from http://www.nimh.nih.gov.publicat/childqa. cfm

National Institutes of Health. (1998). *National Institutes of Health Consensus Development conference statement: Diagnosis and treatment of attention deficit hyperactivity disorder (ADHD). Effectiveness of methylphenidate and adderall in school-age youths with ADHD.* Washington, DC: Author.

Naudet, F., Bruno, M., Philippe, C., Teymann, J. M., Solene, M. A., & Bruno, F. (2013). Which placebo to cure depression? A thought-provoking network meta-analysis. *BMC Medicine, 11,* 1–24.

Naughton, M., Clarke, G., O'Leary, O. F., Cryan, J. F., & Dinan, T. G. (2014). A review of ketamine in affective disorders: current evidence of clinical efficacy, limitations of use and pre-clinical evidence on proposed mechanisms of action. *Journal of Affective Disorders, 156,* 24–35.

Neal, D. L., & Calarco, M. M. (1999). Mental health providers: Role definitions and collaborative practice issues. In R. Balon & M. B. Riba (Eds.), *Psychopharmacology and psychotherapy: A collaborative approach* (pp. 65–110). Washington, DC: American Psychiatric Association.

Neergaard, L. (2004, September 15). U.S. urged to redflag depressed kids' pills. *Cleveland Plain Dealer,* pp. 1, 14.

Neiderdeppe, J., Byrne, S., Avery, R. J., & Cantor, J. (2013). Direct-to-consumer television advertising exposure, diagnosis with high cholesterol, and statin use. *Journal of General Internal Medicine, 10,* 273–279.

Nelson, J. C., & Devenand, D. P. (2011). A systematic review and meta-analysis of placebo-controlled antidepressant trials in people with depression and dementia. *Journal of the American Geriatric Society, 59,* 577–585.

Nelson, J. C., Mankoski, R., Baker, R. A., Carlson, B. X., Eudicone, J. M., Pikalov, A., et al. (2010). Effects of aripiprazole adjunctive to standard antidepressant treatment on the core symptoms of depression: A post-hoc analysis of two large, placebo-controlled studies. *Journal of Affective Disorders, 120,* 133–140.

Nesbitt, A. D., & Goadsby, P. J. (2012). Cluster headache. *BMJ (Clinical Research Ed.), 344,* e2407.

Netjek, V. A. (2012). Race and gender related differences in clinical characteristics and quality of life among outpatients with psychotic disorders. *Journal of Psychiatric Practice, 18,* 329–337.

Newcombe, J. P., & Kerridge, I. H. (2007). Assessment by human research ethics committees of potential conflicts of interest arising from pharmaceutical sponsorship of clinical research. *Internal Medince Journal, 37,* 12–17.

Newcomer, J. W. (2005). Second generation (atypical) antipsychotics and metabolic effects: A comprehensive literature review. *CNS Drugs, 19*(Suppl.), 1–93.

Ng, C. H., & Castle, D. (2010). Pharmacogenetics from ethno-cultural perspectives. *Lanka Journal of Psychiatry, 1,* 29–31.

Ng, C. H., Lin, K. M., Singh, B. S., & Chiu, E. (Eds.). (2008). *Ethno-psychopharmacology: Advances in current practice.* Cambridge: Cambridge University Press.

Nichols, D. E. (2004). Hallucinogens. *Pharmacology & Therapeutics, 101*(2), 131–181. doi:10.1016/j.pharmthera.2003.11.002

Nieoullon, A. (2002). Dopamine and the regulation of cognition and attention. *Progress in Neurobiology, 67,* 53–83.

Niv, N., Shatkin, J. P., Hamilton, A. B., Unutzer, J., Klap, R., & Young, A. S. (2010). The use of herbal medications and dietary supplements by people with mental illness. *Community Mental Health Journal, 46,* 563–569.

Nordfjaern, T. (2013). Prospective associations between benzodiazepine use and later life satisfaction, somatic pain and psychological health among the elderly. *Human Psychopharmacology, 28,* 248–257.

Northridge, M. E., & Mack, R. (2002). Integrating ethnomedicine into public health. *American Journal of Public Health, 92,* 1561.

Notebook numbers. (2004). *Time, 163,* 23.

Nothdurfter, C., Rammes, G., Baghai, T. C., Schule, C., Schumachers, M., Papdopoulos, V., et al. (2011). Translocator protein (18kDa) as a target for novel anxiolytics with a favourable side effect profile. *Journal of Neuroendocrinology, 24,* 82–92.

Novartis Pharmaceuticals (producer). (1998). *Brian's story* [Video]. Hanover, NJ: Novartis Pharmaceuticals Corporation.

Nyer, M., Doorly, J., Durham, K., Yeung, E. S., Freeman, M. P., & Mischoulon, D. (2013). What is the role of alternative treatments in late-life depression? *Psychiatric Clinics of North American, 36,* 577–596.

Ochoa-Sanchez, R., Rainer, Q., Comai, S., Spadoni, G., Bedini, A., Rivara, S., et al. (2012). Anxiolytic effects of the melatonin MT2 receptor partial agonist UCM765: Comparison with melatonin and diazepam. *Progress in Neuro-Psychopharmacology & Biological Psychiatry, 29,* 318–325.

O'Connor, P. G., & Fiellin, D. A. (2000). Pharmacological treatment of heroin dependent patients. *Annals of Internal Medicine, 133,* 40–54.

Office of Diversion Control. (2012). *Title 21 United States Code (USC) Controlled Substances Act.* Retrieved from http://www.deadiversion.usdoj.gov/21cfr/21usc/812.htm

Oguchi-Katayama, A., Monma, A., Sekino, Y., Moriguichi, T., & Sato, K. (2013). Comparative gene expression analysis of the amygdala in autistic rat models produced by pre- and postnatal exposures tovalproic acid. *The Journal of Toxicological Sciences, 38,* 391–402.

Olds, J., & Milner, P. (1954). Positive reinforcement produced by electrical stimulation of septal area and other regions of the rat brain. *Journal of Comparative and Physiological Psychology, 47,* 419–427.

Olfson, M., Gameroff, M. J., Marcus, S. C., & Jensen, P. S. (2003). National trends in the treatment of attention deficit hyperactive disorder. *American Journal of Psychiatry, 160,* 1071–1077.

Olfson, M., Kroenke, K., Wang, S., & Blanco, C. (2014). Trends in office-based mental health care provided by psychiatrists and primary care physicians. *The Journal of Clinical Psychiatry, 75,* 247–253.

Olfson, M., Marcus, S. C., Corey-Lisle, P., Tuomari, A. V., Hines, P., & L'Italien, G. J. (2006). Hyperlipidemia following treatment with antipsychotic medications. *The American Journal of Psychiatry, 163,* 1821–1825.

Olfson, M., Marcus, S. C., Druss, B., Elinson, L., Tanielian, T., & Pincus, H. A. (2002). National trends in the treatment of outpatient depression. *Journal of the American Medical Association, 287,* 203–209.

Olver, J. S., Burrows, G. D., & Norman, T. R. (2001). Third-generation antidepressants: Do they offer advantages over the SSRIs? *Central Nervous System Drugs, 15,* 941–954.

O'Malley, S. S., Jaffe, A. J., Chang, G., Schottenfeld, R. S., Meyer, R. E., & Rounsaville, B. (1992). Naltrexone and coping skills therapy for alcohol dependence: A controlled study. *Archive of General Psychiatry, 49,* 881–887.

Omnibus Budget Reconciliation Act of 1987, Pub. L No. 100-203, Subtitle C: Nursing Home Reform, (1987).

Organon. (2003). *Life without depression.* Retrieved October 10, 2004, from www.remeronsoltab.com

Ostacher, M. J., Perlis, R. H., Nierenberg, A. A., Calabrese, J., Stange, J. P., Salloum, I., et al. (2010). Impact of substance use disorders on recovery from episodes of depression in bipolar disorder patients: Prospective data from the systematic treatment enhancement program for bipolar disorder (STEP-BD). *The American Journal of Psychiatry, 167,* 289–297.

Ostad, H. E., Heimke, C., & Pfuhlmann, B. (2012). Therapeutic drug monitoring for antidepressant drug treatment. *Current Pharmaceutical Design, 18,* 5818–5827.

Ott, J. (1993). *Pharmacotheon.* Occidental, CA: Natural Products.

Ouzir, M., Azorin, J. M., Adida, M., Boussaoud, D., & Battas, O. (2012). Insight in schizophrenia: From conceptualization to neuroscience. *Psychiatry and Clinical Neurosciences, 66,* 167–179.

Owens, E. B., Hinshaw, S. P., Arnold, L. F., Cantwell, D. P., Elliott, G., Hechtman, L., et al. (2003). Which treatment for whom for ADHD? *Moderators of Treatment Response in the MTA, 71,* 540–550.

Pacchiarotti, I., Bond, D. J., Baldessarini, R. J., Nolen, W. A., Grunze, H., Licht, R. W., et al. (2013). The International Society for Bipolar Disorders (ISBD) task force report on antidepressant use in bipolar disorders. *The American Journal of Psychiatry, 170,* 1249–1262.

Pacifici, R., Zuccaro, P., Farré, M., Pichini, S., Di Carlo, S., Roset, P. N., et al. (2000). Immunomodulating activity of MDMA. *Annals of the New York Academy of Sciences, 914,* 215–224.

Padala, P. R., Burke, W. J., Bhatia, S. C., & Petty, F. (2007). Treatment of apathy with methylphenidate. *The Journal of Neuropsychiatry and Clinical Neurosciences, 19,* 81–83.

Padala, P. R., Burke, W. J., Shostrom, V. K., Bhatia, S. C., Wengel, S. P., Potter, J. F., et al. (2010). Methylphenidate for apathy and functional status in dementia of the Alzheimer type. *American Journal of Geriatric Psychiatry, 18,* 371–374.

Padhy, R., Saxena, K., Remsing, L., Huemer, J., Plattner, B., & Steiner, H. (2011). Symptomatic response to divalproex in subtypes of conduct disorder. *Child Psychiatry and Human Development, 42,* 584–593.

Pae, C. U. (2013). Sertindole: Dilemmas for its use in clinical practice. *Expert Opinion Druug Safety, 12,* 321–326.

Pai, N., Deng, C., Vella, S. L., Castle, D., & Huang, F. (2012). Are there different neural mechanisms responsible for three stages of weight gain development in antipsychotic therapy: Temporally based hypothesis. *Asian Journal of Psychiatry, 5,* 315–318.

Paille, F. M., Guelfi, J. D., Perkins, A. C., Royer, R. J., Steru, L., & Parot, P. (1995). Double-blind randomized multicenter trial of acamprosate in maintaining abstinence from alcohol. *Alcohol Alcohol, 30*(2), 239–247.

Pande, A. C., Crockatt, G. J., Janney, C. A., Werth, J. L., & Tsaroucha, G. (2000). Gabapentin in bipolar disorder: A placebo-controlled trial of adjunctive therapy. *Bipolar Disorders, 2,* 249–255.

Paparrigopoulos, T., Tzavellas, E., Karaiskos, D., & Llappas, I. (2008). Intranasal zaleplon abuse. *American Journal of Psychiatry, 165,* 1488–1489.

Pappadopulos, E., Jensen, P. S., Schur, S. B., MacIntyre , J. C., Ketner, S., Van Oreden, K., et al. (2002). "Real world" atypical antipsychotic prescribing practices in public child and adolescent inpatient settings. *Schizophrenia Bulletin, 28,* 111–121.

Paragas, M. G. (1984). Lithium adverse reactions in psychiatric patients. *Pharmacology, Biochemistry, and Behavior, 21*(Suppl. 21), 65–69.

Paris, J. (2009). The bipolar spectrum: A critical perspective. *Harvard Review of Psychiatry, 17,* 206–213.

Park, J. S. (2013). Direct to consumer (DTC) antidepressant advertising and consumer misperceptions about the chemical imbalance theory of depression: The moderating role of skepticism. *Health Marketing Quarterly, 30,* 362–378.

Parker, G., & Brotchie, H. (2011). Mood effects of the amino acids tryptophan and tyrosine. *Acta Psychiatrica Scandinavica, 124,* 417–426.

Parker, V., Wong, A. H., Boon, H. S., & Seeman, M. V. (2001). Adverse reactions to St. John's wort. *Canadian Journal of Psychiatry/Revue Canadienne De Psychiatre, 46,* 77–79.

Parry, W. (2004, April 13). Ban on ephedra upheld; appeals of makers denied. *Cleveland Plain Dealer,* p. A6.

Patterson, L. E. (1996). Strategies for improving medication compliance. *Essential Psychopharmacology, 1,* 70–79.

Paul, G. L. (1967). Strategy of outcome research in psychotherapy. *Journal of Consulting Psychology, 31,* 109–118.

Paulose-Ram, R., Safran, M. A., Jonas, B. S., Gu, Q., & Orwig, D. (2007). Trends in psychotropic medication use among U.S. adults. *Pharmacoepidemiology and Drug Safety, 16,* 560–570.

Payte, J. T. (1991). A brief history of methadone in the treatment of opioid dependence: A personal perspective. *Journal of Psychoactive Drugs, 23*(2), 103–107.

Payte, J. T. (2002). Opioid agonist treatment of addiction. *ASAM Review Course in Addiction Medicine.* Retrieved April 2, 2014, from http:www/jtpayte.com

Payte, J. T., Zweben, J. E., & Martin, J. (2003). Opioid maintenance treatment. In A. W. Graham, T. K. Schultz, M. F. Mayo-Smith, R. K. Ries, & B. B. Wilford (Eds.), *Principles of addiction medicine* (pp.751–766). Maryland: American Society of Addiction Medicine.

Pearce, E. F., & Murphy, J. A. (2014). Vortioxetine for the treatment of depression. *The Annals of Pharmacotherapy, 9,* 1542–1546.

Penn, D., & Corrigan, P. (2002). The effects of stereotype suppression on stereotype stigma. *Schizophrenia Research, 55,* 269–276.

Perlis, R. H. (2007). Genetic predictors of antidepressant treatment response: Progress toward clinical pharmacogenetics. *Primary Psychiatry, 14,* 54–59.

Peroutka, S. J., Newman, H., & Harris, H. (1988). Subjective effects of 3, 4-methylenedioxymethamphetamine in recreational users. *Neuropsychopharmacology: Official Publication of the American College of Neuropsychopharmacology, 1*(4), 273–277.

Perry, E. K. (2002). Plants of the gods: Ethnic routes to altered consciousness. In E. K. Perry & H. Ashton (Eds.), *Neurochemistry of consciousness: Neurotransmitters in mind* (pp. 205–225). Philadelphia: J. Benjamins.

Perry, P. J., Alexander, B., & Liskow, B. I. (2006). *Psychotropic drug handbook* (8th ed.). Washington, DC: American Psychiatric Association.

Peselow, E. D., Dunner, D. L., Fieve, R. R., & Lautin, A. (1980). Lithium carbonate and weight gain. *Journal of Affective Disorders, 2,* 303–310.

Peters, R., Beckett, N., Forette, F., Tuomilehto, J., Clarke, R., Burch, M., et al. (2008). Incident dementia and blood pressure lowering in the hypertension in the very elderly trial cognitive function assessment (HYVET-COG): A double-blind, placebo controlled, trial. *Lancet Neurology, 7,* 683–689.

Petersen, M. (2009). *Our daily meds: How pharmaceutical companies transformed themselves into slick marketing machines and hooked the nation on prescription drugs.* New York: Crichton.

Petkova, E., Tarpey, T., Huang, L., & Deng, L. (2013). Interpreting meta-regression: Application to recent controversy in antidepressant efficacy. *Statistics in Medicine, 32,* 2875–2892.

The Pfizer settlement. (2004). *Journal News.com.* Retrieved May 20, 2004, from www.thejournalnews. com.newsroom/051604/edpfizer.html

Phelps, L., Brown, R. T., & Power, T. J. (2002). *Pediatric psychopharmacology: Combining medical and psychosocial interventions.* Washington, DC: American Psychological Association.

Pi, E. H., Gutierrez, M. A., & Gray, G. E. (1993). Tardive dyskinesia: Cross-cultural perspectives. In K. M. Lin, R. E. Poland, & R. E. Nakasaki (Eds.), *Psychopharmacology and psychobiology of ethnicity* (pp. 153–167). Washington, DC: American Psychiatric Association.

Pies, R. W. (2000). Adverse neuropsychiatric reactions to herbal and over-the-counter "antidepressants." *Journal of Clinical Psychiatry, 61,* 815–820.

Pies, R. W. (2005). *Handbook of essential psychopharmacology* (2nd ed.). Washington, DC: American Psychiatric Association.

Pies, R. W., & Rogers, D. P., (2005). *Handbook of essential psychopharmacology* (2nd ed.). Washington, DC: American Psychiatric Association

Pilar-Cuellar, F., Vidal, R., Diaz, A., Castro, E., dos Anjos, S., Pascual-Brazo, J., et al. (2013). Neural plasticity and proliferation in the generation of antidepressant effects: Hippocampal implication. *Neural Plasticity, 2013,* 21–42.

Pinna, G. (2014). Targeting neurosteroidogenesis as therapy for PTSD. *Frontiers in Pharmacology, 10,* 389.

Pirastu, R., Fais, R., Messina, M., Bini, V., Spiga, S., Falconieri, D., & Diana, M. (2005). Impaired decision-making in opiate-dependent subjects: Effect of pharmacological therapies. *Drug and Alcohol Dependence, 83,* 163–168.

Pisciotta, A. V. (1992). Hematologic reactions associated with psychotropic drugs. In J. M. Kane & J. A. Lieberman (Eds.), *Adverse effects of psychotropic medications* (pp. 376–394). New York: Guilford.

Pitchot, W., Scantamburlo, G., & Asseau, M. (2011). Tricyclic antidepressants and monoamine oxidaseinhibitors-do they still have a role in the treatment of depression? *Revue Medicalae De Liege, 66,* 144–152.

Placidi, G. P., Oquendo, M. A., Malone, K. M., Huang, Y. Y., Ellis, S. P., & Mann, J. J. (2001). Aggressivity, suicide attempts, and depression: Relationship to cerebrospinal fluid monoamine metabolite levels. *Biological Psychiatry, 50,* 783–791.

Polanyi, M. (1958). *Personal knowledge: Towards a postcritical philosophy.* Chicago: University of Chicago Press.

Polinski, J. M., Maclure, M., Marshall, B., Agnew-Blais, J., Patrick, A. R., & Schneeweiss, S. (2008). Does knowledge of medication prices predict physicians' support for cost effective prescribing policies? *The Canadian Journal of Clinical Pharmacology, 15,* 286–294.

Polyakova, M., Sonnabend, N., Sander, C., Mergl, R., Schroeter, M. L., & Schonknecht, P. (2014). Prevalance of minor depression in elderly persons with and without mild cognitive impairment: A systematic review. *Journal of Affective Disorders, 152,* 23–28.

Pomerantz, J. M. (2003). Antidepressants used as placebos: Is that good practice? *Drug Benefit Trends, 15,* 32–33.

Post, R. M. (2010). Letter to the editor regarding "A critical appraisal of lithium's efficacy and effectiveness: The last 60 years. *Bipolar Disorders, 12,* 455–456.

Post, R. M., Weiss, S. R., & Chuang, D. M. (1992). Mechanisms of action of anticonvulsants in affective disorders: Comparison with lithium. *Journal of Clinical Psychopharmacology, 12*(Suppl. 1), 23–25.

Pradel, V., Delga, C., Rouby, F., Micallef, J., & Lapeyre-Mestre, M. (2010). Assessment of abuse potential of benzodiazepines from a prescription database using doctor shopping as an indicator. *CNS Drugs, 24,* 611–620.

Prakash, S. (2002). Actions by drug company Parke-Davis to promote the drug neurotin for uses that had not yet been approved by the government. Transcript of story run December 19, 2002. *All Things Considered, National Public Radio.* Retrieved from http://www.npr.org/templates/story/story.php?storyId=885153

Prakash, S. (2003). Drug companies marketing promotion in the name of education. Transcript of story run January 16, 2003. *All Things Considered, National Public Radio.* Retrieved from http://www.npr.org/templates/story/story.php?storyId=885153

Prescrier International. (2011). Quetiapine: A me-too neuroleptic; no panacea. *Prescriber International, 20,* 257–261.

Presti, D. E., & Nichols, D. E. (2006). Biochemistry and neuropharmacology of psilocybin mushrooms. In R. Metzner & D. Darling (Eds.), *Sacred mushroom of visions: teonanácatl:: A sourcebook on the psilocybin mushroom.* Rochester, VT: Park Street Press.

Preston, J. D., O'Neal, J. H., & Talaga, M. C. (2002). *Handbook of clinical psychopharmacology for therapists* (3rd ed.). Oakland, CA: New Harbinger.

Price, L. H., & Heninger, G. R. (1994). Lithium in the treatment of mood disorders. *New England Journal of Medicine, 331,* 591–598.

Priest, R., Vize, C., Roberts, M., & Tylee, A. (1996). Lay people's attitudes to treatment of depression: Results of opinion poll for defeat depression campaign just before its launch. *British Medical Journal, 313,* 858–859.

Procyshyn, R. M., Barr, A. M., Brickell, T., & Honer, W. G. (2010). Medication errors in psychiatry: A comprehensive review. *CNS Drugs, 24,* 595–609.

Psychlink. (1998, September 9). *Access to atypical antipsychotics: A public debate* [Video]. New York: Interactive Medical Network.

Puig-Antich, J., Perel, J., Lupatkin, W., Chambers, W. J., Tabrizi, M. A., King, J., et al. (1987). Imipramine in prepubertal major depressive disorders. *Archives of General Psychiatry, 44,* 81–89.

Puyat, J. H., Daw, J. R., Cunningham, C. M., Law, M. R., Wong, S. T., Greyson, D. L., et al. (2013). Racial and ethnic disparities in the use of antipsychotic medication: A systematic review and meta-analysis. *Social Psychiatry and Psychiatric Epidemiology, 48,* 1861–1873.

Quigley, P., Barnett, S., Bulat, Y., & Friedman, R. (2014). Reducing falls and fall-related injuries in mental health: A 1-year multihospital falls collaborative. *Journal of Nursing Care and Quality, 29,* 51–59.

Quinones, A. R., Thielke, S. M., Beaver, K. A., Trivedi, R. B., Williams, C., & Fan, V. S. (2014). Racial and ethnic differences in receipt of antidepressants and psychotherapy by veterans with chronic depression. *Psychiatric Services, 65,* 193–200.

Rabins, P. V., & Black, B. S. (2010). Ethical issues in geriatric psychiatry. *International Review of Psychiatry, 22,* 267–273.

Radin, D. (1997). *The conscious universe: The scientific truth of psychic phenomena.* San Francisco: Harper.

Rado, J. T., & Janicak, P. G. (2014). Long-term efficacy and safety of iloperidone: An update. *Neuropsychiatric Disease and Treatment, 10,* 409–415.

Raghavan, R., Brown, D. S., Allaire, B. T., Garfield, L. D., Ross, R. E., & Snowden, L. R. (2014). Racial/ethnic differences in Medicaid expenditures on psychotropic medications among maltreated children. *Child Abuse & Neglect, 16,* 720–731.

Rahman, S., Robbins, T. W., Hodges, J. R., Mehta, M. A., Nestor, P. J., Clark, L., et al. (2006). Methylphenidate ('Ritalin') can ameliorate abnormal risk-taking behavior in the frontal variant of frontotemporal dementia. *Neuropsychopharmacology, 31,* 651–658.

Rambos, S., Oosting, R., Amara, D. A., Kung, H. F., Blier, P., Mendelsohn, M., et al. (1998). Serotonin receptor 1A knockout: An animal model of anxiety-related disorder. *Proceedings of the National Academy of Sciences United States of America, 95,* 14476–14481.

Rapelli, P., Fabritius, C., Alho, H., Salaspuro, M., Wahlbeck, K., & Kalska, H. (2007). Methadone vs. buprenorphine/naloxone during opioid substitution treatment: A naturalistic comparison of cognitive performance relative to healthy controls. *BMC Clinical Pharmacology, 7,* 1–10.

Rapoport, J. (2013). Pediatric psychopharmacology: Too much or too little? *World Psychiatry, 12,* 118–122.

Rapp, A., Dodds, A., Walkup, J. T., & Rynn, M. (2013). Treatment of pediatric anxiety disorders. *Annals of the New York Academy of Sciences, 13,* 52–61.

Rasmussen, N. (2008). *On speed: The many lives of amphetamine.* New York: New York University Press.

Ravindran, L. N., & Stein, M. B. (2009). Pharmacotherapy of PTSD: premises, principles, and priorities. *Brain Research, 1293,* 24–39. doi:10.1016/j.brainres.2009.03.037

Ray, U. S., Mukhopadhyaya, S., Purkayastha, S. S., Asnani, V., Tomer, O. S., Prashad, R., et al. (2001). Effect of yogic exercises on physical and mental health of young fellowship course trainees. *Indian Journal of Physiology and Pharmacology, 45,* 37–53.

Recheneberg, K., & Humphries, D. (2013). Nutritional interventions in depression and perinatal depression. *Yale Journal of Biology and Medicine, 86,* 127–137.

Redvers, A., Laugharne, R., Kanagaratnam, G., & Srinivasan, G. (2001). How many patients self-medicate with St. John's wort? *Psychiatric Bulletin, 25,* 254–256.

Reidboard, S. (2009). *Abilify for depression?.* Retrieved April 13, 2014, from http://blog.stevenreidbordmd.com/?p=8

Remschmidt, H. (2002). Early-onset schizophrenia as a progressive-deteriorating developmental disorder: Evidence from child psychiatry. *Journal of Neural Transmission, 109,* 101–117.

Reneman, L., Schilt, T., de Win, M. M., Booij, J., Schmand, B., van den Brink, W., et al. (2006). Memory function and serotonin transporter promoter gene polymorphism in ecstasy (MDMA) users. *Journal of Psychopharmacology (Oxford, England), 20*(3), 389–399. doi:10.1177/0269881106063266

Resnick, R. B. (1998). *A practitioner's experience with naltrexone.* American Society of Addiction Medicine, 29th Annual Scientific Conference, New Orleans, LA.

Reuters Medical News. (2001, September 5). *Cannabis spray helps ease chronic pain.* Retrieved October 14, 2004, from News in Science, www.abc.net.au/science/news/pring/ print_358716. htm

Rex, A., Morgenstern, E., & Fink, H. (2002). Anxiolyticlike effects of Kava-Kava in the elevated plus maze test: A comparison with diazepam. *Progress in Neuropsychopharmacology & Biological Psychiatry, 26,* 855–860.

Reynolds, C. F., Butters, M. A., Lopez, O., Pollock, B. G., Dew, M. A., Mulsant, B. H., et al. (2011). Maintenance treatment of depression in old age: A randomized, double-blind, placebo-controlled evaluation of the efficacy and safety of donepezil combined with antidepressant pharmacotherapy. *Archives of General Psychiatry, 68,* 51–60.

Ricaurte, G. A. (2003). Retraction. *Science, 301,* 1479.

Ricaurte, G. A., Yuan, J., Hatzidimitriou, G., Cord, B. J., & McCann, U. D. (2002). Severe dopaminergic neurotoxicity in primates after a common recreational dose regimen of MDMA ("ecstasy"). *Science, 297,* 2260–2263.

Ricciardiello, L., & Jornaro, P. (2013). Beyond the cliff of creativity: A novel key to bipolar disorder and creativity. *Medical Hypothese, 80,* 534–543.

Rickels, K., & Rynn, M. (2002). Pharmacotherapy of generalized anxiety disorder. *Journal of Clinical Psychiatry, 63,* 9–16.

Rickels, K., Schweizer, E., Case, W. G., & Greenblatt, D. J. (1991). Long term therapeutic use of benzodiazepines. I. Effects of abrupt discontinuation. *Archives of General Psychiatry, 47,* 899–907.

Rico-Villademoros, F., Rodriguez-Lopez, C. M., Morillas-Arques, P., Vilchez, J. S., Hidalgo, J., & Calandre, E. P. (2012). Amisulpride in the treatment of fibromyalgia: An uncontrolled study. *Clinical Rheumatology, 31,* 1371–1375.

Riddle, M. A., Geller, B., & Ryan, N. (1993). Another sudden death in a child treated with desipramine. *Journal of the American Academy of Child and Adolescent Psychiatry, 32,* 792–797.

Riddle, M. A., Kastelic, E., & Frosch, E. (2001). Pediatric psychopharmacology. *Journal of the Child Psychological Psychiatrist, 42,* 73–90.

Riddle, M. A., King, R. A., Hardin, M. T., Scahill, L., Ort, S. I., Chappell, P., et al. (1991). Behavioral side effects of fluoxetine in children and adolescents. *Journal of Child and Adolescent Psychopharmacology, 1,* 193–198.

Riddler, M. A., Walkup, J. T., & Vitiello, B. (2008). Introduction: Issues and viewpoints in pediatric psychopharmacology. *International Review of Psychiatry, 20,* 119–120.

Rivara, F. P., & Cummings, P. (2002). Publication bias: The problem and some suggestions. *Archives of Pediatric and Adolescent Medicine, 156,* 424–425.

Rivas-Vasquez, R. (2001). Ziprasidone: Pharmacological and clinical profile of the newest atypical antipsychotic. *Professional Psychology: Research and Practice, 32,* 662–665.

Roberts, T. B., & Winkleman, M. (Eds.). (2007). *Psychedelic medicine: New evidence for hallucinogenic substances as treatments.* New York: Praeger.

Robinson, G. E. (2002). Women and psychopharmacology. *Medscape Women's Health E-Journal, 7,* 1–8. Retrieved October 14, 2004, from www.medscape.com/viewarticle/423938

Roccaforte, W. H., & Burke, W. J. (1990). Use of psychostimulants for the elderly. *Hospital & Community Psychiatry, 41,* 1330–1333.

Rodriguez, T. (2013). Gut bacteria may exacerbate depression. *Scientific American Mind, 24,* 8.

Rogers, C. R. (1957). The necessary and sufficient conditions of therapeutic personality change. *Journal of Consulting Psychology, 21,* 95–103.

Rogers, G., Elston, J., Garside, R., Roome, C., Taylor, R., Younger, P., et al. (2009). The harmful health effects of recreational ecstasy: a systematic review of observational evidence. *Health Technology Assessment (Winchester, England), 13*(6), iii–iv, ix–xii, 1–315. doi:10.3310/hta13050

Rojansky, N., Wang, K. E., & Halbreich, U. (1992). Reproductive and adverse effects of psychotropic drugs. In J. M. Kane & J. A. Lieberman (Eds.), *Adverse effects of psychotropic drugs* (pp. 356–375). New York: Guilford Press.

Rosen, D. M. (2007). *FDA approves ABILIFY(R) (aripiprazole) as the first medication for add-on treatment of MDD.* Retrieved May 20, 2014, from http://www.eurekalert.org/pub_releases/2007-11/bs-faa112007.php

Rosenberg, D. R., Holttum, J., & Gershon, S. (1994). *Textbook of pharmacotherapy for child and adolescent disorders.* New York: Brunner/Mazel.

Rosenheck, R., Chang, S., Choe, Y., Cramer, J., Xu, W., Henderson, W., et al. (2000). Medication continuation and compliance: A comparison of patients treated with clozapine and haloperidol. *Journal of Clinical Psychiatry, 61,* 382–386.

Rosenson, J., Smollin, C., Sporer, K. A., Blanc, P., & Olson, K. R. (2007). Patterns of ecstasy-associated hyponatremia in California. *Annals of Emergency Medicine, 49*(2), 164–171, 171.e1. doi:10.1016/j.annemergmed.2006.09.018

Rosenthal, J. Z., Boyer, P., Vialet, C., Hwang, E., & Tourian, K. A. (2013). Efficacy and safety of desvenlafaxine 50 mg/d for prevention of relapse in major depressive disorder: A randomized controlled trial. *Journal of Clinical Psychiatry, 74,* 158–166.

Ross, C. A. (1995). Errors of logic in biological psychiatry. In C. A. Ross & A. Pam (Eds.), *Pseudoscience in biological psychiatry: Blaming the body* (pp. 85–128). New York: Wiley.

Ross, C. A., & Pam, A. (1995). *Pseudoscience in biological psychiatry: Blaming the body.* New York: Wiley.

Ross, C. C. (2012). Do antidepressants really work? *Psychology Today.* Retrieved March 15, 2014, from http://www.psychologytoday.com/blog/real-healing/201202/do-anti-depressants-really-work

Ross, J. S., & Kravitz, R. L. (2013). Direct-to-consumer television advertising: Time to turn off the tube? *Journal of General Internal Medicine, 28,* 862–864.

Roth, M. D., Arora, A., Barsky, S. H., Kleerup, E. C., Simmons, M. S., & Tashkin, D. P. (1998). Airway inflammation in young marijuana and tobacco smokers. *American Journal of Respiratory and Critical Care Medicine, 157,* 1–9.

Ruck, C. A., Bigwood, J., Staples, D., Ott, J., & Wasson, R. G. (1979). Entheogens. *Journal of Psychedelic Drugs, 11*(1–2), 145–146.

Ruiz, P., Strain, E. C., & Langrod, J. (2007). *The substance abuse handbook.* New York: LWW.

Russell, A. T. (2001). Childhood-onset schizophrenia. In G. O. Gabbard (Ed.), *Treatments of psychiatric disorders* (pp. 339–358). Washington, DC: American Psychiatric Association.

Russo-Neustadt, A., Beard, R. C., & Cotman, C. W. (1999). Exercise, antidepressant medications, and enhanced brain derived neurotrophic factor expression. *Neuropsychopharmacology, 21,* 679–682.

Ryan, J. B., Katsiyannis, A., Losinski, M., Reid, R., & Ellis, C. (2014). Review of state medication policies/guidelines regarding psychotropic medications in public schools. *Journal of Child and Family Studies, 23,* 704–715.

Ryan, N. D. (2002). Depression. In S. Kutcher (Ed.), *Practical child and adolescent psychopharmacology* (pp. 91-105). Cambridge, UK: Cambridge University Press.

Ryan, N. D., Bhatara, V. S., & Perel, J. M. (1999). Mood stabilizers in children and adolescents. *Journal of the American Academy of Child and Adolescent Psychiatry, 38,* 529–536.

Rybakowski, J. K., Abramowicz, M., Dragowski, J., Chlopocka-Wozniak, M., Mihalak, M., & Czekalski, S. (2012). Screening for the markers of kidney damage in men and women on long-term lithium treatment. *Medical Science Monitor: Medical Journal of Experimental and Clinical Research, 18,* 656–660.

Sabanovic, S., Bennett, C. C., Chang, W. L., & Huber, L. (2013). PARO robot affects diverse interaction modalities in group sensory therapy for older adults with dementia. *International Conference on Robotics,* 665–669.

Sabzwari, S. R., Qidwai, W., & Bhanji, S. (2013). Polypharmacy in the elderly: A cautious trail to tread. *The Journal of the Pakistan Medical Association, 63,* 624–627.

Sachs, G. S., Nierenberg, A. A., Calabrese, J. R., Marrgell, L. B., Wisniewski, S. R., Gyulai, L., et al. (2007). Effectiveness of adjunctive antidepressant treatment for bipolar depression. *New England Journal of Medicine, 356,* 1711–1722.

Safer, D. S., Zito, J. M., & Fine, E. M. (1996). Increased methylphenidate usage for attention deficit disorders in the 1990s. *Pediatrics, 98,* 1084–1088.

Sahling, D. L. (2009). Pediatric bipolar disorder: Underdiagnosed or fiction? *Ethical Human Psychology and Psychiatry, 11,* 215–228.

Saitz, R., & O'Malley, S. S. (1997). Pharmacotherapies for alcohol abuse: Withdrawal and treatment. *Medicine Clinical North America, 81*(4), 881–907.

Salmon, P. (2001). Effects of physical exercise on anxiety, depression, and sensitivity to stress: A unifying theory. *Clinical Psychology Review, 21,* 33–61.

Santos, C., Costa, J., Santos, J., Vaz-Carneiro, A., & Lunet, N. (2010). Caffiene intake and dementia: a systematic review and meta-analysis. *Journal of Alzheimers Disease, 20,* 187–207.

Sapolsky, R. (2005). *Biology and human behavior* (2nd cd.). Chantilly, VA: The Teaching Company.

Sarris, J. (2013). St John's wort for the treatment of psychiatric disorders. *Psychiatric Clinics of North America, 36,* 65–72.

Sarris, J., Fava, M., Schweitzer, I., & Mischoulon, D. (2012). St John's wort (Hypericum perforatum) versus sertraline and placebo in major depressive disorder: Continuation data from a 26-week RCT. *Pharmacopsychiatry, 5,* 275–278.

Sarris, J., & Kavanaugh, D. J. (2009). Kava and St. John's wort: Current evidence for use in mood and axiety disorders. *The Journal of Alternative and Complementary Medicine, 15,* 827–836.

Sarris, J., Stough, C., Bousman, C. A., Wahid, Z. T., Murray, G., Teschke, R., et al. (2013). Kava in the treatment of generalized anxiety disorder: A double-blind, randomized, placebo-controlled study. *Journal of Clinical Psychopharmacology,* 643–648.

Sasagawa, M., Martzen, M. R., Kelleher, W. J., & Wenner, C. A. (2008). Positive correlation between the use of complementary and alternative medicine and internal health locus of control. *Explore, 4,* 38–41.

Sasaki, T., Matsuki, N., & Ikegaya, Y. (2011). Action-potential modulation during axonal conduction. *Science, 331,* 599–601.

Satcher, D. (2001). Report of the Surgeon Generals Conference on Children's Mental Health: A National Action Agenda. *American Journal of Health Education, 32,* 179–182.

Satlin, A., & Wasserman, C. (1997). Overview of geriatric psychopharmacology. In S. L. McElroy (Ed.), *Psychopharmacology across the lifespan* (pp. 143–172). Washington, DC: American Psychiatric Association.

Saunders, S. K., Morzorati, A., & Shekhar, S. (1995). Priming of experimental anxiety by repeated subthreshold GABA blockade in the rat amygdala. *Brain Research, 699,* 250–259.

Sayre, J. (2000). The patient's diagnosis: Explanatory models of mental illness. *Qualitative Health Research, 10,* 71–83.

Schaefer, E. J., Bongard, V., Beiser, A. S., Lamon-Fava, S., Robins, S. J., Au, R., et al. (2006). Plasma phosphatidylcholine decosahaxaenoic acid content and risk of dementia and Alzheimer disease: The framingham heart study. *Archives of Neurology, 63,* 1545–1550.

Schaller, J. L., & Behar, D. (1999). Quetiapine for refractory mania in a child. *Journal of the American Academy of Child and Adolescent Psychiatry, 38,* 498–499.

Schatzberg, A. F. (1997). Serotonin reuptake inhibitor discontinuation syndrome: A hypothetical definition. *Journal of Clinical Psychiatry, 58*(Suppl. 7), 5–10.

Schatzberg, A. F., Cole, J. O., & DeBattista, C. (1997). *Manual of clinical psychopharmacology* (3rd ed.). Washington, DC: American Psychiatric Press.

Schatzberg, A. F., Cole, J. O., & DeBattista, C. (2010). *Manual of clinical pharmacology* (7th ed.). Washington, DC: American Psychiatric Association.

Schatzberg, A. F., & Nemeroff, C. B. (Eds.). (1998). *The American Psychiatric Association textbook of psychopharmacology* (2nd ed.). Washington, DC: American Psychiatric Association.

Scheffler, R. M., Brown, T. T., Fulton, B. D., Hinshaw, S. P., Levine, P., & Stone, S. (2009). Positive association between attention-deficit/hyperactivity disorder medication use and academic achievement during elementary school. *Pediatrics, 123,* 1273–1279.

Schilt, T., de Win, M. M. L., Koeter, M., Jager, G., Korf, D. J., van den Brink, W., et al. (2007). Cognition in novice ecstasy users with minimal exposure to other drugs: a prospective cohort study. *Archives of General Psychiatry, 64*(6), 728–736. doi:10.1001/archpsyc.64.6.728

Schlosser, E. (1997). More reefer madness. *Atlantic Monthly, 279,* 90–102.

Schorr, M. (2004). Neurotrophic factor improves motor function in Parkinson's patients. *Medscape Medical News*. Retrieved June 11, 2004, from www.medscape.com/viewarticle/474873_print

Schou, M. (1978). The range of clinical uses of lithium. In F. N. Johnson & S. Johnson (Eds.), *Lithium in medical practice* (pp. 34–57). Baltimore, MD: University Park Press.

Schou, M. (1997). Forty years of lithium treatment. *Archives of General Psychiatry, 54*, 9–13.

Schowalter, J. E. (2008). How to manage conflicts of interest with industry? *International Review of Psychiatry, 20*, 127–133.

Schreiber, F., Heimlich, C., Schweitzer, C., & Stangier, R. (2013). Cognitive therapy for social anxiety disorder: The impact of the 'self focused attention and safety behaviours experiement' on the course of treatment. *Behavioural and Cognitive Psychotherapy, 9*, 1–9.

Schreiber, R., & Hartrick, G. (2002). Keeping it together: How women use the biomedical explanatory model to manage the stigma of depression. *Mental Health Nursing, 23*, 91–105.

Schulman, K. A., & Linas, B. P. (1997). Pharacoeconomics: State of the art in 1997. *Americna Review of Public Health, 18*, 529–548.

Schultes, R., Hoffman, A., & Rätsch, C. (2001). *Plants of the gods: Their sacred, healing and hallucinogenic powers*. New York: Healing Arts.

Schwartz, J. M., & Begley, S. (2002). *The mind and the brain: Neuroplasticity and the power of mental force*. New York: Regan.

Schwartz, R. (1987). Marijuana: An overview. *Pediatric Clinics of North America, 34*, 305–317.

Schwieler, L., Engberg, G., & Erhardt, S. (2004). Clozapine modulates midbrain dopamine neuron firing via interaction with the NMDA receptor complex. *Synapse, 52*, 114–122.

Scott, J., & Pope, M. (2002). Nonadherence with mood stabilizers: Prevalence and predictors. *Journal of Clinical Psychiatry, 63*, 384–390.

Seabury, S. A., Goldman, D. P., Kalsekar, I., Sheehan, J. J., Labmeier, K., & Lakdawalla, D. N. (2014). Formulary restrictions on atypical antipsychotics: Impact on costs for patients with schizophrenia and bipolar disorder in medicaid. *AJMC.com*. Retrieved April 11, 2014, from http://www.ajmc.com/publications/issue/2014/2014-vol20-n2/Formulary-Restrictions-on-Atypical-Antipsychotics-Impact-on-Costs-for-Patients-With-Schizophrenia-and-Bipolar-Disorder-in-Medicaid

Sechter, D., Peuskens, J., Fleurot, O., Rein, W., Lecrubier, Y., & the Amisulpride Study Group. (2002). Amisulpride vs. Risperidone in chronic schizophrenia. *Neuropsychopharmacology, 27*, 1071–1081.

Sedky, K., & Lippmann, S. (2006). Psychotropic medications and leukopenia. *Current Drug Targets, 7*, 1191–1194.

Seeman, M. V., & Seeman, N. (2012). The meaning of antipsychotic medication to patients with schizophrenia. *Journal of Psychiatric Practice, 18*, 338–348.

Seeman, P. (2014). Clozapine, a fast-off D2 antipsychotic. *ACD Chemical Neuroscience, 5*, 24–29.

Segraves, R. T., & Balon, R. (2013). Antidepressant induced sexual dysfunction in men. *Pharmacology, Biochemistry, and Behavior, 11*, 183–192.

Selikoff, I. J., Robitzek, E. H., & Ornstein, G. G. (1952). Treatment of pulmonary tuberculosis with hydrazine derivatives of isonicotinic acid. *Journal of the American Medical Association, 150*, 973–980.

Senate Special Committee on Illegal Drugs. (2002). *Discussion paper on cannabis*. Canada: Author. Retrieved October 14, 2004, from http://www.parl.gc.ca/37/1/parlbus/ commbus/senate/com-e/ille-e/library-e/summarye.pdf

Sernyak, M. J., Desai, R., Stolar, M., & Rosenheck, R. (2001). Impact of clozapine on completed suicide. *American Journal of Psychiatry, 158*, 931–937.

Sewell, R. A., Halpern, J. H., & Pope, H. G. (2006). Response of cluster headache to psilocybin and LSD. *Neurology, 66*(12), 1920–1922. doi:10.1212/01.wnl.0000219761.05466.43

Shaw, E. (1986). Lithium noncompliance. *Psychiatric Annals, 16*, 583–587.

Sheard, M. H. (1971). Effect of lithium on human aggression. *Nature, 230*, 113–114.

Sheard, M. H. (1975). Lithium in the treatment of aggression. *Journal of Nervous and Mental Disease, 160*, 108–118.

Sheard, M. H., & Marini, J. L. (1978). Treatment of human aggressive behavior: Four case studies of the effect of lithium. *Comprehensive Psychiatry, 19*, 37–45.

Sheard, M. H., Marini, J. L., Bridges, C. I., & Wagner, E. (1976). The effect of lithium on impulsive aggressive behavior in man. *American Journal of Psychiatry, 133*, 1409–1413.

Sheean, G. L. (1991). Lithium neurotoxicity. *Clinical and Experimental Neurology, 28*, 112–127.

Shelton, R. C., Keller, M. B., Gelenbert, A., Dunner, D. L., Hirschfeld, R., Thase, M. E., et al. (2001). Effectiveness of St. John's wort in major depression: A randomized, controlled trial. *Journal of the American Medical Association, 285*, 1978–1986.

Shifrin, D. (1998). Three-year study documents nature of television violence. *American Academy of Pediatrics News, 8*, 1.

Shors, T. J., Miesegaes, G., Beylin, A., Zhao, M., Rydel, T., & Gould, E. (2001). Neurogenesis in the adult is involved in the formation of trace memories. *Nature, 410*, 372–376.

Shrank, W. H., Liberman, J. N., Fischer, M. A., Girdish, C., Brennan, T. A., & Choudhry, N. K. (2011). Physician perceptions about generic drugs. *The Annals of Pharmacotherapy, 45*, 31–38.

Shufman, E., & Witztum, E. (2000). Cannabis—a drug with dangerous implications for mental health. *Harefuah, 138*, 410–413.

Shulgin, A., & Nichols, D. E. (1978). Characterization of three new psychotomimetics. In *The psychopharmacology of hallucinogens* (pp. 74–83). New York: Pergamon Press.

Shuman, M. D., Trgoboff, E., Demler, T. L., & Opler, L. A. (2014). Exploring the potential effect of polypharmacy on the hematologic profiles of clozapine patients. *Journal of Psychiatric Practice, 20*, 50–58.

Shumilov, M., & Touitou, E. (2010). Buspirone transdermal administration for menopausal syndromes, in vitro and in animal model studies. *International Journal of Pharmaceutics, 387*, 26–33.

Siegel, R. K. (1989). *Intoxication: Life in pursuit of artificial paradise.* New York: Dutton.

Sifaneck, S. J. (1995). Keeping off, stepping on and stepping off: The steppingstone theory reevaluated in the context of the Dutch cannabis experience. *Contemporary Drug Problems, 22,* 483–512.

Silberg, J., Pickles, A., Rutter, M., Hewitt, J., Simonoff, E., Maes, H., et al. (1999). The influences of genetic factors and life stressors on depression among adolescent girls. *Archives of General Psychiatry, 56,* 225–232.

Silverstein, D. D., & Spiegel, A. D. (2001). Are physicians aware of the risks of alternative medicine? *Journal of Community Health: The Publication for Health Promotion & Disease Prevention, 26,* 159–174.

Silverstein, F. S., Boxer, L., & Johnson, M. F. (1983). Hematological monitoring during therapy with carbamazepine in children. *Annals of Neurology, 13,* 685–686.

Silverstone, T., & Romans, S. (1996). Long-term treatment of bipolar disorder. *Drugs, 51,* 367–382.

Sinclair, J. D. (2001). Evidence about the use of naltrexone and for different ways of using it in the treatment of alcoholism. *Alcohol & Alcoholism, 36*(1), 2–10.

Singh, J., Chen, G., & Canuso, C. M. (2012). Antipsychotics in the treatment of bipolar disorder. *Handbook of Experimental Pharmacology, 212,* 187–212.

Sipkoff, M. (2003). *Glaxo-Apotex ruling could impact future patent cases.* Retrieved May 14, 2014, from http://drugtopics.modernmedicine.com/drug-topics/news/glaxo-apotex-ruling-could-impact-future-patent-cases?page=full

Skolnick, P., Layer, R. T., Popik, P., Nowak, G., Pauli, A., & Trullas, R. (1996). Adaptation of N-methyl-D-aspartate (NMDA) receptors following antidepressant treatment: Impliations for the pharmacotherapy of depression. *Pharmacopsychiatry, 29,* 23–26.

Slejko, J. F., Libby, A. M., Nair, K. V., Valuck, R. J., & Campbell, J. D. (2013). Pharmacoeconomics and outcomes research degree-granting PhD programs in the United States. *Research in Social and Administrative Pharmacy: RSAP, 9,* 108–113.

Slifman, N. R., Obermeyer, W. R., Musser, S. M., Correll, W. A., Chichowicz, S. M., & Love, L. A. (1998). Contamination of botanical dietary supplements by digitalis lanata. *New England Journal of Medicine, 339,* 806–811.

Smeets, C. H., Smallbrugge, M., Gerritsen, D. L., Nelissen-Vrancken, M. H., Wetzels, R. B., van der Spek, K., et al. (2013). Improving psychotropic drug prescription in nursing home patients with dementia: Design of a cluster randomized controlled trial. *BMC Psychiatry, 13,* 280–282.

Smith, H. (2000). *Cleansing the doors of perception: The religious significance of entheogenic plants and chemicals.* New York: Tarcher.

Smith, J. A. (1953). The use of the isopropyl derivative of isonicotinylhydrazine (Marsilid) in the treatment of mental disease. *American Practice, 4,* 519–520.

Smith, N. T. (2002). A review of published literature into cannabis withdrawal symptoms in human users. *Addiction, 97,* 621–632.

Snyder, S. H., Banerjee, S. P., Yamanura, H. I., & Greenberg, A. (1974). Drugs, neurotoxins, and schizophrenia. *Science, 188,* 1243–1245.

Snyder, S. H. (1996). *Drugs and the brain.* New York: Scientific American Library.

Sobo, S. (1999, October 1). Mood stabilizers and mood swings: In search of a definition. *Psychiatric Times.* Retrieved April 13, 2014, from http://www.psychiatrictimes.com/mood-disorders/mood-stabilizers-and-mood-swings-search-definition

Sochting, I., O'Neal, E., Third, B., Rogers, J., & Ogrodniczuk, J. S. (2013). An integrative group therapy model for depression and anxiety later in life. *International Journal of Group Psychotherapy, 63,* 502–523.

Soeffing, J. M., Martin, L. D., Fingerhood, M. I., Jasinski, D. R., & Rastegar, D. A. (2009). Buprenorphine maintenance treatment in a primary care setting: Outcomes at 1 year. *Journal of Substance Abuse Treatment, 37,* 426–430.

Solanto, M. C., Arnsten, A. T. F., & Castellanos, F. X. (2001). *Stimulant drugs and ADHD: Basic and clinical neuroscience.* New York: Oxford University Press.

Soloman, P. R., Adams, F., Silver, A., Zimmer, J., & DeVeaux, R. (2002). Ginkgo for memory enhancement: A randomized control trial. *Journal of the American Medical Association, 288,* 835–840.

Sommer, B. R., & Schatzberg, A. F. (2002). Ginkgo biloba and related compounds in Alzheimer's disease. *Psychiatric Annals, 32,* 13–18.

Sommers-Flanagan, J., & Sommers-Flanagan, R. (1996). Efficacy of antidepressant medication with depressed youth: What psychologists should know. *Professional Psychology: Research and Practice, 27,* 145–153.

Sonovion Pharmaceuticals. (2012). *Package insert for lunestra/eszopiclone.* Retrieved April 6, 2014, from http://www.lunesta.com/pdf/PostedApprovedLabelingText.pdf

Sopko, M. A., Ehret, M. J., & Grgas, M. (2008). Desvenlafaxine: Another "me too" drug? *The Annals of Pharmacotherapy, 42,* 1439–1446.

Sopolsky, R. (2005). *Biology and human behavior. The neurological origins of individuality* (2nd ed.). Chantilly, VA: The Teaching Company.

Soutullo, C. A., Chang, K. D., Diez-Suarez, A., Figueroa-Quintana, A., Escamilla-Canales, I., Rapado-Castro, M., et al. (2005). Bipolar disorder in children and adolescents: International perspective on epidemiology and phenomenology. *Bipolar Disorders, 7,* 497–506.

Sowell, T. (2002). *Controversial essays.* Stanford, CA: Hoover Institution.

Spanemberg, L., Nogueira, E. L., da Silva, C. T., Dargel, A. A., Menezes, F. S., & Cataldo Neto, A. (2011). High prevalence and prescription of benzodiazepines for elderly: Data from psychiatric consultation to patients from an emergency room of a general hospital. *General Hospital Psychiatry, 33,* 45–50.

Spector, N., & Doherty, M. (2007). Development of a standardized medication assistant curriculum. *JONA's Healthcare Law, Ethics, and Regulation, 9,* 119–124.

Speigel, D. A., Wiegel, M., Baker, S. L., & Greene, K. A. (2000). Pharmacological management of anxiety disorders. In D. I. Mostofsky & D. H. Barlow (Eds.), *The management of anxiety disorders* (pp. 36–65). Boston: Allyn and Bacon.

Spencer, T., Biederman, J., & Wilens, T. (2002). Attention deficit/hyperactivity disorder. In S. Kutcher (Ed.), *Practical child and adolescent psychopharmacology* (pp. 230–264). Cambridge, UK: Cambridge University Press.

Spielmans, G. I. (2002). Effect of Hypericum perforatum (St. John's wort) in major depressive disorder: A randomized controlled trial: A reply. *Journal of the American Medical Association, 288,* 446–447.

Stafford, N. (2012, September–October). Possible implications of recent research into the gut-brain axis on people with mental health problems. *Mental Health Today,* 22.

Stafford, P. G. (1992). *Psychedelics encyclopedia* (3rd expanded ed.). Berkeley, CA: Ronin Pub.

Stafford, P. G., & Golightly, B. H. (1967). *LSD The Problem-Solving Psychedelic.* Award Books.

Stahl, S. M. (2000). *Essential psychopharmacology: Neuroscientific basis and practical applications.* Cambridge, UK: Cambridge University Press.

Stahl, S. M. (2002). Don't ask, don't tell, but benzodiazepines are still the leading treatments for anxiety disorder. *Journal of Clinical Psychiatry, 63,* 756–757.

Stahl, S. M. (2013). *Essential psychopharmacology: Neuroscientific basis and practical applications* (4th ed.). Cambridge, UK: Cambridge University Press.

Stahl, S. M., Hauger, R. L., Rausch, J. L., Fleischaker, H. C., & Hubbell-Alberts, H. C. (1995). Downregulation of serotonin receptor subtypes by nortriptyline and adinozalam in major depressive disorder: Neuroendocrine and platelet markers. *Clinical Neuropharmacology, 16*(Suppl. 3), S19–S31.

Stanilla, J. K., & Simpson, G. M. (1995). Drugs to treat extrapyramidal side effects. In A. F. Schatzberg & C. B. Nemeroff (Eds.), *American Psychiatric Association textbook of psychopharmacology* (pp. 289–299). Washington, DC: American Psychiatric Association.

Stanton, S. P., Keck, P. E., & McElroy, S. L. (1997). Treatment of acute mania with gabapentin. *The American Journal of Psychiatry, 154,* 287.

Stein, D. J., Ipser, J. C., Baldwin, D. S., & Bandelow, B. (2007). Treatment of obsessive-compulsive disorder. *CNS Spectrums, 12*(2 Suppl. 3), 28–35.

Stein, M. C. (2002). Are herbal products dietary supplements or drugs? An important question for public safety. *Clinical Pharmacology and Therapeutics, 71,* 411–413.

Sterke, C. S., Ziere, G., van Beeck, E. F., Looman, C. W., & van der Cammen, T. J. (2012). Dose-reponse relationship between selective serotonin reuptake inhibitors and injurious falls: A study in nursing home residents with dementia. *British Journal of Clinical Pharmacology, 18,* 210–221.

Stevens, P. (2009). *Substance abuse counseling: Theory and practice* (4th ed.). Upper Saddle River, NJ: Merrill/Pearson.

Stivers, R. (2001). *Technology as magic: The triumph of the irrational* New York: Continuum.

Stober, G., Ben-Shachar, D., Cardon, M., Falkai, P., Fonteh, A. N., Gawlik, M., et al. (2009). Schizophrenia: From the brain to peripheral markers. A consensus paper of the WFSBP task force on biological markers. *The World Journal of Biological Psychiatry, 10,* 127–155.

Stolaroff, M. J., & Multidisciplinary Association for Psychedelic Studies. (2004). *The secret chief revealed.* Sarasota, FL: Multidisciplinary Association for Psychedelic Studies.

Stone, K. J., Viera, A. J., & Parman, C. L. (2003). Off-label applications for SSRIs. *American Family Physician, 68,* 498–504.

Strain, E. C., Walsh, S. L., Preston, K. L., Liebson, I. A., & Bigelow, G. E. (1997). The effects of buprenorphine in buprenorphine-maintained volunteers. *Psychopharmacology (Berlin), 129*(4), 329–338.

Strassman, R. J. (1984). Adverse reactions to psychedelic drugs. A review of the literature. The *Journal of Nervous and Mental Disease, 172*(10), 577–595.

Stratkowski, S. M., McElroy, S. L., Keck, P. E., & West, S. A. (1996). Racial influences on diagnosis in psychotic mania. *Journal of Affective Disorders, 39,* 157–162.

Streator, S. E., & Moss, J. T. (1997). Identification of offlabel antidepressant use and costs in a network model HMO. *Drug Benefit Trends, 9,* 48–56.

Strickland, T. L., Lin, K.-M., Fu, P., Anderson, D., & Zheng, Y. (1995). *Comparison of lithium ratio between African-American and Caucasian bipolar patients. Biological Psychiatry, 37,* 325–330.

Studerus, E., Gamma, A., Kometer, M., & Vollenweider, F. X. (2012). Prediction of Psilocybin Response in Healthy Volunteers. *PLoS ONE, 7*(2), e30800. doi:10.1371/journal.pone.0030800

Substance Abuse and Mental Health Services Administration (SAMHSA). (2007). *The DASIS Report: Heroin-Changes in how it is used: 1995–2005.* Rockville, MD: Author.

Substance Abuse and Mental Health Services Administration (SAMHSA). (2009). *The TEDS Report: Heroin and other opiate admissions to substance abuse treatment.* Rockville, MD: Author.

Substance Abuse and Mental Health Services Administration (SAMSA). (2013). *National survey on drug use and health.* Retrieved May 22, 2014, from http://www.samhsa.gov/data/NSDUH/2k12MH_FindingsandDetTables/Index.aspx

Sucher, N. J., Awobuluyi, M., Choi, Y. B., & Lipton, S. A. (1996). NMDA receptors: From genes to channels. *Trends in Psychopharmacological Science, 17,* 348–355.

Sue, D. W., Arredondo, P., & McDavis, R. J. (1992). Multicultural counseling competencies and standards: A call to the profession. *Journal of Counseling and Development, 70,* 477–486.

Sugrue, M., Seger, M., Dredge, G., Davies, D. J., Ieraci, S., Bauman, A., et al. (1995). Evaluation of the prevalence of drug and alcohol abuse in motor vehicle trauma in Southwestern Sydney. *Australian and New Zealand Journal of Surgery, 65,* 853–856.

Sullivan, G., & Lukoff, D. (1990). Sexual side effects of antipsychotic medication: Evaluation and interventions. *Hospital and Community Psychiatry, 41,* 1238–1241.

Sullivan, R. J., & Hagen, E. H. (2002). Psychotropic substance-seeking: Evolutionary path or adaptation? *Addiction, 97,* 389–400.

Suurkula, J. (1996). *Junk DNA: Over 95 percent of DNA has largely unknown function.* Retrieved May 2, 2004, from http://www.psrast.org/junkdna.htm

Swanson, J., Wigal, S., Greenhill, L., Browne, R., Walik, B., Lerner, M., et al. (1998). Analog classroom assessment of adderall in children with ADHD. *Journal of the American Academy of Child and Adolescent Psychiatry, 37,* 519–526.

Swazy, J. P. (1974). *Chlorpromazine in psychiatry.* Cambridge, MA: MIT Press.

The system: A weekly check-up on health care costs and coverage section. (2002). *Washington Post,* p. F3. Retrieved July 2002, from http://www.washingtonpost.com

Szalavitz, M. (2010). How a study of a failed antidepressant shows that antidepressants really work. *Time, 10,* 32–34.

Szasz, T. (1992). *Our right to drugs: The case for a free market.* Syracuse, NY: Syracuse University Press.

Szymanksi, S., Cannon, T. D., Gallagher, F., Erwin, R. J., & Gur, R. E. (1996). Course of treatment response to first-episode and chronic schizophrenia. *American Journal of Psychiatry, 153,* 519–525.

Taira, M., Hashimoto, T., Takamatsu, T., & Maeda, K. (2006). Subjective response to neuroleptics: The effect of a questionnaire about neuroleptic side effects. *Progress in Neuro-Psychopharmacology & Biological Psychiatry, 30,* 1139–1142.

Tait, R. C., & Chibnall, J. T. (2014). Racial/ethnic disparities in the assessment and treatment of pain: Psychosocial perspectives. *The American Psychologist, 69,* 131–141.

Takeda Pharmaceuticals. (2013). *Introducing Brintellix (vortioxetine).* Chicago, IL: Author.

Talib, H. J., & Alderman, E. M. (2013). Gynocologica and reproductive health concerns of adolescents using selected psychotropic medications. *Pediatric and Adolescent Gynecology, 26,* 7–15.

Tan, C. C., Yu, J. T., Wang, H. F., Meng, Z. F., Wang, C., Jiang, T., et al. (2014). Efficacy and safety of donepezil, galantamine, rivastigmine and memantine for the treatment of Alzheimer's disease: A systematic review and meta-analysis. *Journal of Alzheimer's Disease, 3,* 223–231.

Tan, C. C., Yu, J. T., Wang, H. F., Tan, M. S., Meng, X. F., Wang, C., et al. (2014). Efficacy and safety of donepezil, galantamine, rivastigmine and memantine for the treatment of Alzheimer's disease: A systematic review and meta-analysis. *Journal of Alzheimer's Disease, 3,* 450–459.

Tangamornsuksan, W., Chaiyakunapruk, N., Somkrua, R., Lohitnavy, M., & Tassaneeyakul, W. (2013). Relationship between the HLA-B★1502 allel and carbamazcpine-induced Stevens-Johnson syndrome and toxic epidermal necrolysis: A systematic review and meta-analysis. *JAMA Dermatololgy, 149,* 1025–1032.

Tanner, L. (2004, September 9). Medical journals' policy aims to help enlighten public. *Cleveland Plain Dealer,* p. A16.

Tart, C. T. (Ed.). (1997). *Body, mind, spirit: Exploring the parapsychology of spirituality.* Charlottesville, VA: Hampton Roads.

Tart, C. T. (2000). *On being stoned: A psychological study of marijuana intoxication.* Lincoln, NE: Authors Guild. Originally published 1971.

Tashkin, E. (1999). Effects of marijuana on the lung and its defenses against infection and cancer. *School Psychology International, 20,* 23–37.

Task Force on Financial Conflicts of Interest in Clinical Research. (2001). *Protecting subjects, preserving trust, promoting progress: Policy and guidelines for the oversight of individual financial interests in human subjects research.* Washington, DC: Association of American Medical Colleges.

Taylor, M. J., Rudkin, L., Bullemor-Day, P., Lubin, J., Chukwujetwu, C., & Hawton, K. (2013). Strategies for managing sexual dysfunction induced by antidepressant medication. *The Cochrane Database of Systematic Reviews,* issue 5, 1469–1493.

Teasdale, J. D., Segal, Z. V., Williams, J. M., Ridgeway, V. A., Soulsby, J. M., & Lau, M. A. (2000). Prevention of relapse/recurrence in major depression by mindfulness-based cognitive therapy. *Journal of Consulting and Clinical Psychology, 68,* 615–623.

Teasdale, J. D., Segal, Z., & Williams, J. M. (1999). How does cognitive therapy prevent depressive relapse and why should attentional control (mindfulness) training help? *Behavior Research and Therapy, 33,* 25–39.

Teicher, M. H., Glod, C., & Cole, J. O. (1990). Emergence of intense suicidal preoccupation during fluoxetine treatment. *American Journal of Psychiatry, 147,* 207–211.

Temin, P. (1980). *Taking your medicine: Drug regulation in the United States.* Cambridge, MA: Harvard University Press.

Thaker, G. K., & Tamminga, C. A. (2001). Schizophrenia and other psychotic disorders. In G. O. Gabbard (Ed.), *Treatment of psychiatric disorders* (3rd ed., pp. 1005–1025). Washington, DC: American Psychiatric Press.

Thase, M. E., Entsuah, A. R., & Rudolph, R. L. (2001). Remission rates during treatment with venlafaxine or selective serotonin reuptake inhibitors. *British Journal of Psychiatry, 178,* 234–241.

Thomas, C. R., & Holzer, C. E. (2006). The continuing shortage of child and adolescent psychiatrists. *Journal of the Academy of Child & Adolescent Psychiatry, 49,* 1023–1031.

Thomas, E. A., & Petrou, S. (2013). Network-specific mechanisms may explain the paradoxical effects of carbamazepine and phenytoin. *Epilipsia, 54,* 1195–1202.

Thompson, R. F. (2000). *The brain: A neuroscience primer* (3rd ed.). New York: Worth Publishers.

Thorgrimsen, L., Spector, A., Wiles, A., & Orrell, M. (2003). Aroma therapy for dementia. *The Cochrane Database of Systematic Reviews, 3,* 315–319.

Thurber, S., Ensign, J., Punnett, A. F., & Welter, K. (1995). A meta-analysis of antidepressant outcome studies that involved children and adolescents. *Journal of Clinical Psychology, 51,* 340–345.

Tilkian, A. G., Schroeder, J. S., Kao, J., & Hultgren, H. (1976). The cardiovascular effects of lithium in man. *American Journal of Medicine, 61,* 665–670.

Toftegard, A. L., Voigt, H. M., Rosenberg, J., & Gogenur, I. (2013). Pharmacological treatment of depression in women with breast cancer: A systematic review. *Breast Cancer Research and Treatment, 141,* 325–330.

Tohen, M., Baker, R. W., Altshuler, L. L., Zarate, C. A., Suppes, T., Ketter, T. A., et al. (2002). Olanzapine versus divalproex in the treatment of acute mania. *American Journal of Psychiatry, 159,* 1011–1017.

Tomlin, S. L., Jenkins, A., Lieb, W. R., & Franks, N. P. (1999). Preparation of barbiturate optical isomers and their effects on GABA (A) receptors. *Anesthesiology, 90,* 1714–1722.

Tone, A. (2009). *The age of anxiety: A history of America's turbulent affair with tranquilizers.* New York: Basic.

Toren, P., Ratner, S., Laor, N., & Weizman, A. (2004). Benefit-risk assessment of atypical antipsychotics in the treatment of schizophrenia and comorbid disorders in children and adolescents. *Drug Safety: An International Journal of Medical Toxicology and Drug Experience, 27,* 1135–1136.

Trincavelli, M. L., Da Pozzo, E., Daniele, S., & Martini, C. (2012). The GABAA-BZR complex as target for the development of anxiolytic drugs. *Current Topics in Medicinal Chemistry, 12,* 254–269.

Tseng, W. S., (2001). *Handbook of cultural psychiatry.* San Diego: Academic Press.

Tseng, W. S. (2003). *Clinician's guide to cultural psychiatry.* San Diego, CA: Academic Press.

Tsuang, M. T., Stone, W. S., & Faraone, S. V. (2000). Toward prevention of schizophrenia. *Biological Psychiatry, 48,* 349–356.

Turk, C. L., Heimberg, R. G., & Hope, D. A. (2001). Social phobia and social anxiety. In D. H. Barlow (Ed.), *Clinical handbook of psychological disorders: A stepby-step treatment manual* (3rd ed., pp. 99–136). New York: Guilford Press.

Turner, W. J. (1964). SCHIZOPHRENIA AND ONEIRO-PHRENIA*: A clinical and biological note. *Transactions of the New York Academy of Sciences, 26*(3 Series II), 361–368. doi:10.1111/j.2164-0947.1964.tb01257.x.

Twemlow, S. W., Fonagy, P., Sacco, F. C., & Brethour, J. R. (2006). Teachers who bully students: A hidden trauma. *The International Journal of Social Psychiatry, 52,* 187–198.

Tyler, V. E. (1994). *Herbs of choice: The therapeutic use of phytomedicinals.* New York: Pharmaceutical Products Press.

Tzourio, C., Anderson, C., Chapman, N., Woodward, M., Neal, B., MacMahon, S., et al. (2003). Effects of blood pressure lowering with perindopril a dindapamide therapy on dementia and cognitive decline in patients with cerebrovascular disease. *Archives of Internal Medicine, 163,* 1069–1075.

U.S. Department of Health and Human Services. (2001). *Report of the surgeon general's conference on children's mental health: A national action agenda.* Rockville, MD: U.S. Department of Health and Human Services, Substance Abuse and Mental Health Administration, Center for Mental Health Services, National Institute of Mental Health.

U.S. Department of Health and Human Services. (2009). Emerging issues in the use of methadone. *Substance Abuse Treatment Advisory, 9,* 1–8.

U.S. Department of Health and Human Services, Substance Abuse and Mental Health Services Administration, Center for Behavioral Health Statistics and Quality, (2009). *National survey on drug use and health*

U.S. Department of Justice. (2012). *Abbott Labs to pay $1.5 billion to resolve criminal and civil investigations of off-label promotion of Depakote.* Retrieved April 13, 2014, from http://www.justice.gov/opa/pr/2012/May/12-civ-585.html

Udenfriend, S., Weissback, H., & Bogdanski, D. F. (1957). Effect of iproniazid on serotonin metabolism in vivo. *Journal of Pharmacologic Therapeutics, 120,* 255–260.

Van Apeldoorn, F. J., Stant, A. D., van Hout, W. J. P. J., Mersch, P. P. A., & den Boer, J. A. (2014). Cost effectiveness of CBT, SSRI and CBT + SSRI in the treatment for panic disorder. *Acta Psychiatrica, Scandinavica, 129,* 286–295.

Van der Hooft, C. S., & Stricher, B. H. (2002). Ephedrine and ephedra in weight loss products and other preparations. *Nederlands Tijdschrift Coor Geneeskunde, 146,* 1335–1336.

Van Gundy, K. (2010). A life-course perspective on the "gateway hypothesis." *Journal of Health and Social Behavior, 51,* 244–259.

Van Luijn, J. C. F. (2012). Is there a role for pharmacoeconomics in decision making? *Pharacoeconomics, 30,* 979–980.

Van Praag, H., Christie, B. R., Sejnowski, T. J., & Gage, F. H. (1999). Running enhances neurogenesis, learning and long-term potentiation in mice. *Proceedings of the National Academy of Sciences of the United States of America, 96,* 13427–13431.

Vasanthaku, B. N. (2001). *Medical malpractice: A comprehensive analysis.* New York: Auburn House.

Veilleux, J. C., Covin, P. J., Anderson, J., York, C. & Heinz, A. J. (2010). A review of opioid dependence treatment: Pharmacological and psychosocial interventions to treat opioid addiction. *Clinical Psychology Review, 30,* 155–166.

Ventola, C. L. (2011). Direct-to-consumer pharmaceutical advertising. *Pharmacy and Therapeutics, 36,* 681–684.

Vermani, M., Milosevic, I., Smith, F., & Katzman, M. A. (2005). Herbs for mental illness: Effectiveness and interaction with conventional medicine. *The Journal for Family Practice, 54,* 789–800.

Viesselman, J. O. (1999). Antidepressant and antimanic drugs. In J. S. Werry & M. G. Aman (Eds.), *Practitioner's guide to psychoactive drugs for children and adolescents* (2nd ed., pp. 249–296). New York: Plenum.

Vinarova, E., Uhlir, V., Stika, J., & Vinar, O. (1972). Side effects of lithium administration. *Activas Nervosa Superior, 14,* 105–107.

Vinkers, C. A., Cryan, J. F., Olivier, B., & Groenink, L. (2010). Elucidating GABAa and GABAb receptor funtions in anxiety using the stress-induced hyperthermia paradigm: A review. *The Open Pharmacology Journal, 4,* 1–14.

Vitiello, B., & Jensen, P. S. (1995). Developmental perspectives in pediatric psychopharmacology. *Psychopharmacology Bulletin, 31,* 75–81.

Vitiello, B., & Jensen, P. S., (1997). Medication development and testing of children and adolescents. *Archives of General Psychiatry, 54,* 871–876.

Vitry, A., Hoile, A. P., Gilbert, A. L., Esterman, A., & Luszcz, M. A. (2010). The risk of falls and fractures associated with persistent use of psychotropic medications in elderly people. *Archives of Gerontology and Geriatrics, 50,* 1–4.

Volavka, J., Czobor, P., Sheitman, B., Lindenmayer, J. P., Citrome, L., McEvoy, J. P., et al. (2002). Clozapine, olanzapine, risperidone, and haloperidol in the treatment of patients with chronic schizophrenia and schizoaffective disorder. *American Journal of Psychiatry, 159,* 255–262.

Volkow, N. D., Ding, Y., Fowler, J. S., Wang, G., Logan, J., Gatley, J. S., et al. (1995). Is methylphenidate like cocaine? *Archives of General Psychiatry, 52,* 456–463.

Vollenweider, F. X., & Kometer, M. (2010). The neurobiology of psychedelic drugs: implications for the treatment of mood disorders. *Nature Reviews Neuroscience, 11*(9), 642–651. doi:10.1038/nrn2884

Volp, A. (2002). Effect of Hypericum perforatum (St. John's wort) in major depressive disorder: A randomized controlled trial: Comment. *Journal of the American Medical Association, 288,* 447.

Volpicelli, J. R., Alterman, A. I., Hayashida, M., & O'Brien, C. P. (1992a). Naltrexone in the treatment of alcohol dependence. *Archives of General Psychiatry, 49,* 876–880.

Volz, H. P. (1997). Controlled clinical trials of hypericum extracts in depressed patients: An overview. *Pharmacopsychiatry, 30*(Suppl. 2), 72–76.

Volz, H. P., & Laux, P. (2000). Potential treatment for subthreshold and mild depression: A comparison of St. John's wort extracts and fluoxetine. *Comprehensive Psychiatry, 41,* 133–137.

Volz, H. P., Murck, H., Kasper, S., & Moeller, H. J. (2002). St. John's wort extract (LI 160) in somatoform disorders: Results of a placebo-controlled trial. *Psychopharmacology, 164,* 294–300.

Vonnegut, K. (1991). *Fates worse than death: An autobiographical collage.* New York: Berkley.

Von Sydow, K., Lieb, R., Pfister, H., Höfler, M., & Wittchen, H.-U. (2002). Use, abuse and dependence of ecstasy and related drugs in adolescents and young adults—a transient phenomenon? Results from a longitudinal community study. *Drug and Alcohol Dependence, 66*(2), 147–159.

Voruganti, L. N., Slomka, P., Zabel, P., Mattar, A., & Awad, A. G. (2001). Cannabis induced dopamine release: An in-vivo SPECT study. *Psychiatry Research, 107,* 173–177.

Wafford, K. A., & Ebert, B. (2006). Gaboxadol— a new awakening in sleep. *Current Opinion in Pharmacology, 6,* 30–36.

Wagner, K. D., & Fershtman, M. (1993). Potential mechanism of desipramine-related sudden death in children. *Psychosomatics, 34,* 80–83.

Wagner, K. D., Kowatch, R. A., Emslie, G. J., Findling, R. L., Wilens, T. E., McCague, K., et al. (2006). A double-blind randomized, placebo controlled trial of oxcarbazepine in the treatment of bipolar disorder in children and adolescents. *The American Journal of Psychiatry, 163,* 1179–1186.

Wagner, K. D., Weller, E. B., Carlson, G. A., Sachs, G., Biederman, J., Frazier, J. A., et al. (2002). An open-label trial of divalproex in children and adolescents with bipolar disorder. *Journal of the American Academy of Child and Adolescent Psychiatry, 41,* 1224–1230.

Wahlbeck, K., Cheine, M., Essali, A., & Adams, C. (1999). Evidence of clozapine's effectiveness in schizophrenia: A systematic review and meta-analysis of randomized trials. *American Journal of Psychiatry, 156,* 990–999.

Wallace, B. A. (1999). A Buddhist response. In Z. Houshmand, R. B. Livingston, & B. A. Wallace (Eds.), *Consciousness at the crossroads: Conversations with the Dalai Lama on brain science and Buddhism* (pp. 33–36). Ithaca, NY: Snow Lion, 1999.

Walsh, M. A., Royal, A., Bronw, L. H., Barrantes-Vidal, N., & Kwapil, T. R. (2012). Looking for bipolar spectrum psychopathology: Identification and expression in daily life. *Comprehensive Psychiatry, 53,* 409–421.

Walsh, R. N., & Vaughan, F. (1980). *Beyond ego: Transpersonal dimensions in psychology.* Los Angeles: Tarcher.

Walter, G., & Rey, J. M. (1999). Use of St. John's wort by adolescents with a psychiatric disorder. *Journal of Child and Adolescent Psychopharmacology, 9,* 307–311.

Walter, G., Rey, J. M., & Harding, A. (2000). Psychiatrists' experience and views regarding St. John's wort and alternative treatments. *Australian and New Zealand Journal of Psychiatry, 34,* 992–996.

Wang, Z., & Woolverton, W. L. (2006). Estimating the relative reinforcing strength of (±)-3,4-methylenedioxymethamphetamine (MDMA) and its isomers in rhesus monkeys: comparison to (+)-methamphetamine. *Psychopharmacology, 189*(4), 483–488. doi:10.1007/s00213-006-0599-5

Warden, D., Rush, A. J., Trivedi, M. H., Fava, M., & Wisniewski, S. R. (2007). The STAR*D project results: A comprehensive review of findings. *Current Psychiatry Reports, 9,* 449–459.

Warnecke, G. (1991). Psychosomatic dysfunctions in the female climacteric: Clinical effectiveness and tolerance of kava extract KS 1490. *Fortschritte der Medizin, 109,* 119–122.

Warner, C., & Shoaib, M. (2005). How does bupropion work as a smoking cessation aid? *Addiction Biology, 10,* 219–231.

Warner, L. A., Kessler, R. C., Hughes, M., Anthony, J. C., & Nelson, C. B. (1995). Prevalence and correlates of drug use and dependence in the United States: Results from the National Comorbidity Survey. *Archives of General Psychiatry, 52,* 219–229.

Washton, A. M., Gold, M. S., & Pottash, A. C. (1984). Successful use of naltrexone in addicted physicians and business executives. *Advanced Alcohol Substance Abuse, 4*(2), 89–96.

Watson, S. J., Benson, J. A., & Joy, J. E. (2000). Marijuana and medicine: Assessing the science base. *Archives of General Psychiatry, 57,* 547–552.

Watts, A. W. (1973). *What is reality? Sound recording from philosophy and society.* San Anselmo, CA: Electronic University.

Weathers, F. W., Keane, T. M., & Davidson, J. R. (2001). Clinician-administered PTSD scale: a review of the first ten years of research. *Depression and Anxiety, 13*(3), 132–156.

Weber, S. S., Saklad, S. R., & Kastenholz, K. V. (1992). Bipolar affective disorders. In M. A. Koda-Kimble, L. Y. Young, W. A. Kradjan, & B. J. Guglielmo (Eds.), *The clinical use of drugs* (pp. 62–90). Vancouver, WA: Applied Therapeutics.

Webster's new universal unabridged dictionary. (1989). New York: Barnes & Noble.

Wegman, J. (2009). *Prestiq: New antidepressant or merely patent extender?* Retrieved May 13, 2014, from http://www.psycho-logytoday.com/blog/pharmatherapy/200909/pristiq-new-antidepressant-or-merely-patent-extender

Weiden, P., Aquila, R., & Standard, J. (1996). Atypical antipsychotic drugs and long-term outcome of schizophrenia. *Journal of Clinical Psychiatry, 57*(Suppl. 11), 53–60.

Weiden, P. J. (2012). Iloperidone for the treatment of schizophrenia: An updated clinical review. *Clinical Schizophrenia and Related Psychoses, 6,* 34–44.

Weiden, P. J., Citrome, L., Alva, G., Brams, M., Glick, I. D., Jackson, R., et al. (2014). A trial evaluating gradual- or immediate – switch strategies from risperidone, olanzapine or aripiprazole to iloperidone in patients with schizophrenia. *Schizophrenia Research, 153,* 160–168.

Weil, A., & Rosen, W. (1993). *From chocolate to morphine: Everything you need to know about mind altering drugs* (rev. Ed.). Boston: Houghton Mifflin.

Weissman, M. M., Bruce, M. L., Leaf, P. J., Florio, L. P., & Holzer, C. (1991). Affective disorders. In L. N. Robins & D. A. Regier (Eds.), *Psychiatric disorders of America: The epidemiologic catchment area study* (pp. 53–80). New York: Free Press.

Weizman, R., & Weizman, A. (2001). Use of atypical antipsychotics in mood disorders. *Current Opinion in Investigational Drugs, 2,* 940–950.

Weller, E. B., Weller, R. A., & Fristad, M. A. (1995). Bipolar disorder in children: Misdiagnosis, underdiagnosis, and future directions. *Journal of the American Academy of Child and Adolescent Psychiatry, 34,* 709–714.

Wenk, G. (2014). *Marijuana may help prevent Alzheimer's but research hits a dead end.* Retrieved April 21, 2014, from http://blog.seattlepi.com/marijuana/2014/03/02/marijuana-may-prevent-alzheimers-but-research-hits-dead-end/#13130103=0&19612101=0

Werler, M. M., Ahrens, J. A., Bosco, J. L., Mitchell, A. A., Anderka, M. T., Gilboa, S. M., et al. (2011). Use of antiepileptic medications in pregnancy in relation to risks of birth defects. *Annals of Epidemiology, 21,* 842–850.

Werry, J. S. (1999). Introduction: A guide for practitioners, professionals, and public. In J. S. Werry & M. G. Aman (Eds.), *Practitioner's guide to psychoactive drugs for children and adolescents* (pp. 3–22). New York: Plenum.

West, A. P. (1996). Excitotoxic aspects of lithium neurotoxicity. *Psycholoquy, 7,* 14–32.

West, A. P., & Melzer, H. Y. (1979). Paradoxical lithium neurotoxicity: Five case reports and an hypothesis about risk for neurotoxicity. *American Journal of Psychiatry, 136,* 963–966.

West, S. A. (1997). Child and adolescent psychopharmacology. In S. L. McElroy (Ed.), *Psychopharmacology across the lifespan* (pp. 129–142). Washington, DC: American Psychiatric Association.

Westermeyer, J. (1989). *Psychiatric care of migrants: A clinical guide.* Washington, DC: American Psychiatric Association.

Wheatley, D. (1997). LI 160, an extract of St. John's wort, versus amitriptyline in mildly to moderately depressed outpatients: A controlled 6-week clinical trial. *Pharmacopsychiatry, 30*(Suppl. 2), 77–80.

Wheatley, D. (1999). Hypericum in seasonal affective disorder (SAD). *Current Medical Research and Opinion, 15,* 33–37.

Wheatley, D. (2001). Kava-kava in the treatment of generalized anxiety disorder. *Primary Care Psychiatry, 7,* 97–100.

Wheatley, D. (2002). Effect of Hypericum perforatum (St. John's wort) in major depressive disorder: A randomized controlled trial: Comment. *Journal of the American Medical Association, 288,* 446.

Whiskey, E., Werneke, U., & Taylor, D. (2001). A systematic review and meta-analysis of hypericum perforatum in depression: A comprehensive review. *International Clinical Psychopharmacology, 16,* 239–252.

White, W. (2013). *A life in addiction psychiatry: An interview with Dr. Herb Kleber.* Retrieved from http://www.williamwhitepapers.com/pr/2013%20Dr.%20%20Herb%20Kleber.pdf

Wikler, A. (1948). Recent progress in research on the neurophysiologic basis of morphine addiction. *American Journal of Psychiatry, 105,* 329–338.

Wilber, K. (1995). *Sex, ecology, spirituality: The spirit of evolution.* Boston: Shambhala.

Wilber, K. (1997). *The eye of spirit: An integral vision for a world gone slightly mad.* Boston: Shambhala.

Wilber, K. (1999). *The collected works of Ken Wilber* (Vol. 3). Boston: Shambhala.

Wilber, K. (2000). *A theory of everything: An integral vision for business, politics, science, and spirituality.* Boston: Shambhala.

Wilber, K. (2003). *Kosmic consciousness* [Audio interview with Tami Simon]. Boulder, CO: Sounds True Productions.

Williams, J. T., Christie, M. J., & Manzoni, O. (2001). Cellular and synaptic adapations mediating opioid dependence. *Psychological Review, 81*(299), 299–343.

Williams, S. H. (2005). Medications for treating alcohol dependence. *American Family Physician, 72*(9), 1775–1780.

Williamson, E. M., & Evans, F. J. (2000). Cannabinoids in clinical practice. *Drugs, 60,* 1303–1314.

Williamson, R. S. (1983). International illicit drug traffic: The United States response. *United Nations Bulletin on Narcotics, 35,* 33–45.

Willutzki, U., Teismann, T., & Schulte, D. (2012). Psychotherapy for social anxiety disorder: Long term effectiveness of resource-oriented cognitive behavioral therapy and cognitive therapy in social anxiety disorder. *Journal of Clinical Psychology, 68,* 581–591.

Wilson, D. (2010). *For $520 million, Astrazeneca settles case over marketing of drug.* Retrieved May 4, 2014, from http://www.nbcnews.com/id/28677805/ns/health-health_care/t/eli-lilly-settles-zyprexa-lawsuit-billion/#.U2aoEvldU3k

Wilson, R. A. (1992). *Right where you are sitting now: Further tales of the illuminati.* Berkeley, CA: Ronin.

Wilson, R. A. (1993). *Sex and drugs: A journey beyond limits* (4th ed.). Phoenix, AZ: New Falcon.

Wilson, R. A. (2002). *TSOG: The thing that ate the constitution and other everyday monsters.* Tempe, AZ: New Falcon Publications.

Winblad, B., Grossberg, G., Frolich, L., Farlow, M., Zechner, S., Nagel, J., et al. (2007). IDEAL: A 6-month, double-blind, placebo-controlled study of the first skin patch for Alzheimer disease. *Neurology, 69*, S14–22.

Winkler, P., & Csémy, L. (2014). Self-Experimentations with Psychedelics among Mental Health Professionals: LSD in the Former Czechoslovakia. *Journal of Psychoactive Drugs, 46*(1), 11–19. doi:10.1080/02791072.2013.873158

Wirshing, D. A., Wirshing, W. C., Kysar, L., Berisford, M. A., Goldstein, D., Pashdag, J., et al. (1999). Novel antipsychotics: Comparison of weight gain liabilities. *Journal of Clinical Psychiatry, 60*, 358–363.

Witte, S., Loew, D., & Gaus, W. (2005). Meta-analysis of the efficacy of the acetonic kava-kava extract WS 1490 in patients with non-psychotic anxiety disorders. *Phytotherapy Research, 19*, 183–188.

Wolfe, F. (1989). Fibromyalgia: The clinical syndrome. *Rheumatic Disorders Clinics of North America, 2*, 1–18.

Wolitsky-Taylor, K., Operskalski, J. T., Ries, R., Craske, M. G., & Roy-Byrne, P. (2011). Understanding and treating comorbid anxiety disorders in substance users: Review and future directions. *Journal of Addiction Medicine, 5*, 233–247.

Wolraich, M. L., Hannah, J. N., Pinnock, T. Y., Baumgaertel, A., & Brown, J. (1996). Comparison of diagnostic criteria for attention deficit hyperactivity disorder in a county-wide sample. *Journal of the American Academy of Child and Adolescent Psychiatry, 35*, 319–324.

Womack, C. A. (2013). Ethical and epistemic issues in direct-to-consumer drug advertising: Where is patient agency? *Medical Health Care and Philosophy, 16*, 275–280.

Wong, A. H., Smith, M., & Boon, H. S. (1998). Herbal remedies in psychiatric practice. *Archives of General Psychiatry, 55*, 1033–1044.

Wood, A. J. J. (2001). Racial differences in the response to drugs–pointers to genetic differences. *New England Journal of Medicine, 344*, 1394–1396.

Wooltorton, E., & Sibbald, B. (2002). Ephedra/ephedrine: Cardiovascular and CNS effects. *Canadian Medical Association Journal, 166*, 633.

World Health Organization (WHO). (1992). *The ICD-10 classification of mental and behavioural disorders: Clinical descriptions and diagnostic guidelines*. Geneva: Author.

World Health Organization (WHO). (2004). *The use of stems in the selection of International Nonproprietary Names (INN) for pharmaceutical substances*. Geneva, Switzerland: Author.

World Health Organization (WHO). (2009). *Guidelines for the psychosocially assisted pharmacological treatment of opioid dependence*. Switzerland: WHO Press.

Worley, J., & McGuinness, T. M. (2010). Promoting adherence to psychotropic medication for youth – part 1. *Journal of Psychosocial Nursing, 48*, 19–25.

Wozniak, J., Biederman, J., Spencer, T., & Wilens, T. (1997). Pediatric psychopharmacology. In A. J. Gelenberg & E. L. Bassuk (Eds.), *The practitioner's guide to psychoactive drugs* (4th ed., pp. 385–415). New York: Plenum.

Wright, R. (1994). *The moral animal: Why we are the way we are: The new science of evolutionary psychology*. New York: Vintage.

Wurtzel, E. (1994). *Prozac nation: A memoir*. New York: Houghton Mifflin.

Wyatt, R. J., Henter, I. D., & Jamison, J. C. (2001). Lithium revisited: Savings brought about by the use of lithium, 1970–1991. *Psychiatric Quarterly, 72*, 149–166.

Yager, J., Siegfried, S. L., & DiMatteo, T. L. (1999). Use of alternative remedies by psychiatric patients: Illustrative vignettes and a discussion of the issues. *American Journal of Psychiatry, 156*, 1432–1438.

Yalom, I. (1995). *The theory and practice of group psychotherapy* (4th ed.). New York: Basic Books.

Yatham, L. N. (2002). The role of novel antipsychotics in bipolar disorders. *Journal of Clinical Psychiatry, 63*(Suppl. 3), 10–40.

Yatham, L. N., Kusumakar, V., Calabrese, J. R., Rao, R., Scarrow, G., & Kroeker, G. (2002). Third generation anticonvulsants in bipolar disorder: A review of efficacy and summary of clinical recommendations. *Journal of Clinical Psychiatry, 63*, 275–283.

Yen, C. F., Cheng, C. P., Huang, C. F., Yen, J. Y., Ko, C. H., & Chen, C. S. (2008). Quality of life and its association with insight, adverse effects of medication and use of atypical antipsychotics in patients with bipolar disorder and schizophrenia in remission. *Bipolar Disorders, 10*, 617–624.

Yeo, B. K. (1997). What you need to know: Addiction–prescribing naltrexone. *Singapore Medical Journal, 38*(2), 92–93.

Yerkes, R. M., & Dodson, J. D. (1908). The relation of strength of stimulus to rapidity of habit formation. *Journal of Comprehensive Neurologic and Psychology, 18*, 459–482.

Zajicek, A. (2009). The National Institutes of Health and the best pharmaceuticals for children act. *Pediatric Drugs, 11*, 45–47.

Zammit, G. (2009). Comparative tolerability of newer agents for insomnia. *Drug Safety, 32*, 735–748.

Zarate, C. A., Machado-Viera, R., Henter, I., Ibrahim, L., Diazgranados, N., & Salvadore, G. (2010). Glutamatergic modulators: The future for treatmeing mood disorders? *Harvard Review of Psychiatry, 18*, 293–303.

Zarate, C. A., Singh, J., & Carlson, P. J. (2006). A randomized trial of an N-methyl-D-aspartate antagonist in treatment resistant major depression. *Archives of General Psychiatry, 63*, 856–864.

Zarate, C. A., & Tohen, M. (1996). Epidemiology of mood disorders throughout the life cycle. In K. Schuman, M. Tohen, & S. Kutcher (Eds.), *Mood disorders across the life span* (pp. 17–34). New York: Wiley.

Zeiner, P. (1995). Body growth and cardiovascular function after extended treatment (1.75 years) with methylphenidate in boys with attention deficit hyperactivity disorder. *Journal of Child and Adolescent Psychopharmacology, 5*, 129–138.

Zeller, E. A., Barsky, J., Fouts, J. R., Kirchheimer, W. F., & Van Orden, L. S.(1952). Influence of isonicotinic acid hydrazide (INH) and 1-isonicotinic-2-isopropyl-hydrazide (IIH) on bacterial and mammalian enzymes. *Experientia, 8*, 349.

Zhu, H., Cottrell, J. E., & Kass, I. S. (1997). The effect of thiopental and propofol on NMDA- and AMPA-mediated glutamate excitotoxicity. *Anesthesiology, 87*, 944–951.

Zillman, E. A., Spiers, M. V. & Culbertson, W. (2007). *Principles of neuropsychology* (2nd ed.). Belmont, CA: Wadsworth.

Zito, J. M., Safer, D. L., de Jong-van den Berg, L. T. W., Janhsen, K., Fegert, J. M., Gardner, J. F., et al. (2008). A three-country comparison of psychotropic medication prevalence in youth. *Child and Adolescent Psychiatry and Mental Health, 2,* 1–8.

Zito, J. M., Safer, D. J, dosReis, S., Gardner, J. F., Boles, M., & Lynch, F. (2000). Trends in prescribing psychotropic medications to preschoolers. *JAMA, 283,* 1025–1030.

Zito, J. M., Safer, D. J., dosReis, S., Gardner, J. F., Boles, M., Lynch, F., et al. (2003). Psychotropic practice patterns for youth: A 10-year perspective. *Archives of Pediatric and Adolescent Medicine, 157,* 17–25.

Zito, J. M., Tobi, H., de Jong-van den Bert, L. T. W., Fegert, J. M., Safer, D. J., Janhsen, K., et al. (2006). Antidepressant prevalence for youths: A multi-national study. *Pharmacoepidemiology and Drug Safety, 15,* 793–798.

Zuckerman, B., Frank, D., Hingson, R., Amaro, H., Levenson, S. M., Kayne, H., et al. (1989). Effects of maternal marijuana and cocaine use on fetal growth. *New England Journal of Medicine, 320,* 762–768.

Zuidema, S. U., dr Jonghe, J. F., Verhey, F. R., & Koopmans, R. T. (2011). Psychotropic drug prescription in nursing home patients with dementia: Influence of environmental correlates and staff distress on physicians' prescription behavior. *International Psychogeriatrics, 23,* 1623–1639.

Zweben, J. E., & Payte, J. T. (1990). Methadone maintenance in the treatment of opioid dependence: A current perspective. *West Journal of Medicine, 152,* 588–599.

Name Index

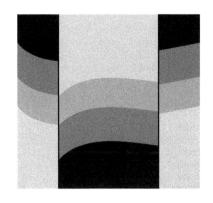

Subject Index

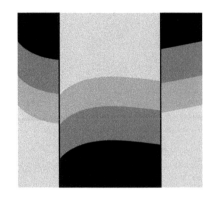